Hematopathology

Editor

ALIYAH R. SOHANI

SURGICAL PATHOLOGY CLINICS

www.surgpath.theclinics.com

Consulting Editor
JASON L. HORNICK

June 2023 • Volume 16 • Number 2

ELSEVIER

1600 John F. Kennedy Boulevard • Suite 1800 • Philadelphia, Pennsylvania, 19103-2899

http://www.theclinics.com

SURGICAL PATHOLOGY CLINICS Volume 16, Number 2
June 2023 ISSN 1875-9181, ISBN-13: 978-0-323-96075-5

Editor: Taylor Hayes
Developmental Editor: Diana Grace Ang

Surgical Pathology Clinics (ISSN 1875-9181) is published quarterly by Elsevier Inc., 360 Park Avenue South, New York, NY 10010. Months of issue are March, June, September, and December. Business and Editorial Office: Elsevier Inc., 1600 John F. Kennedy Blvd., Ste. 1800, Philadelphia, PA 19103-2899. Accounting and Circulation Offices: Elsevier Inc., 3251 Riverport Lane, Maryland Heights, MO 63043. Periodicals postage paid at New York, NY and at additional mailing offices. Subscription prices are $246.00 per year (US individuals), $354.00 per year (US institutions), $100.00 per year (US students/residents), $294.00 per year (Canadian individuals), $402.00 per year (Canadian Institutions), $295.00 per year (foreign individuals), $402.00 per year (foreign institutions), and $120.00 per year (international students/residents), $100.00 per year (Canadian students/residents). Foreign air speed delivery is included in all *Clinics*' subscription prices. All prices are subject to change without notice. **POSTMASTER:** Send address changes to *Surgical Pathology Clinics*, Elsevier, 3251 Riverport Lane, Maryland Heights, MO 63043. **Customer Service: 1-800-654-2452 (US). From outside the United States, call 1-314-447-8871. Fax: 1-314-447-8029. E-mail: JournalsCustomerServiceusa@elsevier.com (for print support)** and **JournalsOnlineSupport-usa@elsevier.com (for online support)**.

Reprints. For copies of 100 or more, of articles in this publication, please contact the Commercial Reprints Department, Elsevier Inc., 360 Park Avenue South, New York, NY 10010-1710. Tel. 212-633-3874; Fax: 212-633-3820; E-mail: reprints@elsevier.com.

Surgical Pathology Clinics of North America is covered in *MEDLINE/PubMed (Index Medicus)*.

Contributors

CONSULTING EDITOR

JASON L. HORNICK, MD, PhD
Director of Surgical Pathology and Immunohistochemistry, Brigham and Women's Hospital, Professor of Pathology, Harvard Medical School, Boston, Massachusetts, USA

EDITOR

ALIYAH R. SOHANI, MD
Professor of Pathology, Department of Pathology, Massachusetts General Hospital and Harvard Medical School, Boston, Massachusetts, USA

AUTHORS

NADINE AGUILERA, MD
University of Virginia Health System, Charlottesville, Virginia, USA

AARON AUERBACH, MD, MPH
Joint Pathology Center, Silver Spring, Maryland, USA

JACOB R. BLEDSOE, MD
Director of Hematopathology, Department of Pathology, Boston Children's Hospital, Harvard Medical School, Boston, Massachusetts, USA

JENNIFER CHAPMAN, MD
Professor of Clinical Pathology, Director, Division of Hematopathology, Department of Pathology and Laboratory Medicine, University of Miami Hospital/Sylvester Comprehensive Cancer Center, Miami, Florida, USA

ELIZABETH L. COURVILLE, MD
Associate Professor, Department of Pathology, University of Virginia Health, Charlottesville, Virginia, USA

ANDREW L. FELDMAN, MD
Department of Laboratory Medicine and Pathology, Mayo Clinic, Rochester, Minnesota, USA

MEGAN J. FITZPATRICK, MD
Hospital Pathology Associates, Minneapolis, Minnesota, USA

JULIA T. GEYER, MD
Department of Pathology and Laboratory Medicine, Weill Cornell Medicine, NewYork-Presbyterian Hospital, Immunopathology, New York, New York, USA

MARK GIRTON, MD
University of Virginia Health System, Charlottesville, Virginia, USA

MICHAEL J. KLUK, MD, PhD
Department of Pathology and Laboratory Medicine, Weill Cornell Medicine, Molecular Hematopathology Laboratory, New York, New York, USA

ALEXANDRA E. KOVACH, MD
Director of Hematopathology, Division of Laboratory Medicine, Department of Pathology

and Laboratory Medicine, Children's Hospital Los Angeles, Associate Professor, Clinical Pathology, Keck School of Medicine of USC, University of Southern California, Los Angeles, California, USA

ABNER LOUISSAINT, Jr, MD, PhD
Associate Professor of Pathology, Aziz and Nur Hamzaogullari Endowed Scholar in Hematologic Malignancies, Harvard Medical School, Medical Director, Core Labatory, Hematology Section, Department of Pathology,Massachusetts General Hospital, Boston, Massachusetts, USA

FABIENNE LUCAS, MD, PhD
Clinical Pathology Resident, Department of Pathology, Brigham and Women's Hospital, Boston, Massachusetts, USA

MARIO L. MARQUES-PIUBELLI, MD
Department of Translational Molecular Pathology, The University of Texas MD Anderson Cancer Center, Houston, Texas, USA

L. JEFFREY MEDEIROS, MD
Department of Hematopathology, The University of Texas MD Anderson Cancer Center, Houston, Texas, USA

ROBERTO N. MIRANDA, MD
Department of Hematopathology, The University of Texas MD Anderson Cancer Center, Houston, Texas, USA

ANDREA P. MOY, MD
Assistant Attending Pathologist, Department of Pathology and Laboratory Medicine, Memorial Sloan Kettering Cancer Center, New York, New York, USA

MANDAKOLATHUR R. MURALI, MD
Medical Director of Clinical Immunology Laboratory, Division of Rheumatology, Allergy and Immunology, Departments of Pathology and Medicine, Massachusetts General Hospital, Harvard Medical School, Boston, Massachusetts, USA

VALENTINA NARDI, MD
Department of Pathology, Massachusetts General Hospital, Harvard Medical School, Boston, Massachusetts, USA

IFEYINWA OBIORAH, MD, PhD
Assistant Professor, Department of Pathology, University of Virginia Health, Charlottesville, Virginia, USA

NAOKI OISHI, MD, PhD
Department of Pathology, University of Yamanashi, Chuo, Yamanashi, Japan

MELISSA P. PULITZER, MD
Attending Pathologist, Department of Pathology and Laboratory Medicine, Memorial Sloan Kettering Cancer Center, New York, New York, USA

GORDANA RACA, MD, PhD
Director of Clinical Cytogenomics Laboratory, Division of Genomic Medicine, Department of Pathology and Laboratory Medicine, Center for Personalized Medicine, Children's Hospital Los Angeles, Professor, Clinical Pathology, Keck School of Medicine, University of Southern California, Los Angeles, California, USA

SAM SADIGH, MD
Associate Pathologist, Department of Pathology, Brigham and Women's Hospital, Boston, Massachusetts, USA

GRAHAM W. SLACK, MD
Department of Pathology and Laboratory Medicine, BC Cancer, Vancouver, British Columbia, Canada

ALIYAH R. SOHANI, MD
Professor of Pathology, Department of Pathology, Massachusetts General Hospital and Harvard Medical School, Boston, Massachusetts, USA

JOHN STEWART, MD
Department of Pathology, The University of Texas MD Anderson Cancer Center, Houston, Texas, USA

Contents

Preface: Evolving Concepts in Diagnostic Hematopathology xi

Aliyah R. Sohani

Immunoglobulin G4-Related Disease, Lymphadenopathy, and Lymphoma: Histopathologic Features and Diagnostic Approach 177

Jacob R. Bledsoe

Lymphadenopathy occurring in patients with immunoglobulin G4 (IgG4)-related disease, termed IgG4-related lymphadenopathy, shows morphologic heterogeneity and overlap with other nonspecific causes of lymphadenopathy including infections, immune-related disorders, and neoplasms. This review describes the characteristic histopathologic features and diagnostic approach to IgG4-related disease and IgG4-related lymphadenopathy, with comparison to nonspecific causes of increased IgG4-positive plasma cells in lymph nodes, and with emphasis on distinction from IgG4-expressing lymphoproliferative disorders.

Hematopathology of Severe Acute Respiratory Syndrome Coronavirus 2 Infection and Coronavirus Disease-19 197

Fabienne Lucas and Sam Sadigh

Coronavirus disease 2019 is caused by severe acute respiratory syndrome coronavirus 2 and is associated with pronounced hematopathologic findings. Peripheral blood features are heterogeneous and very often include neutrophilia, lymphopenia, myeloid left shift, abnormally segmented neutrophils, atypical lymphocytes/plasmacytoid lymphocytes, and atypical monocytes. Bone marrow biopsies and aspirates are often notable for histiocytosis and hemophagocytosis, whereas secondary lymphoid organs may exhibit lymphocyte depletion, pronounced plasmacytoid infiltrates, and hemophagocytosis. These changes are reflective of profound innate and adaptive immune dysregulation, and ongoing research efforts continue to identify clinically applicable biomarkers of disease severity and outcome.

Immunodeficiency-Associated Epstein-Barr Virus-Positive B-cell Lymphoproliferative Disorders: A Review and New Paradigm 213

Jennifer Chapman

Sources of immune deficiency and dysregulation (IDD) are being increasingly recognized and defined, as are IDD-related B-cell lymphoproliferative lesions and lymphomas occurring in these patients. In this review, basic biology of Epstein-Barr virus (EBV) as it relates to classification of EBV-positive B-cell lymphoproliferative disorders (LPDs) is reviewed. Also discussed is the new paradigm of classification of IDD-related LPDs adopted by the fifth edition World Health Organization classification. IDD-related EBV-positive B-cell hyperplasias, LPDs, and lymphomas are discussed with particular attention to unifying and unique features that assist with recognition of these IDD-related lesions and their classification scheme.

Navigating the Heterogeneity of Follicular Lymphoma and its Many Variants: An Updated Approach to Diagnosis and Classification 233

Abner Louissaint Jr.

Follicular lymphoma (FL) is a lymphoid neoplasm composed of follicle center (germinal center) B cells, with varying proportions of centrocytes and centroblasts, that usually has a predominantly follicular architectural pattern. Over the past decade, our understanding of FL has evolved significantly, with new recognition of several recently defined FL variants characterized by distinct clinical presentations, behaviors, genetic alterations, and biology. This manuscript aims to review the heterogeneity of FL and its variants, to provide an updated guide on their diagnosis and classification, and to describe how approaches to the histologic subclassification of classic FL have evolved in current classification schemes.

Modern Classification and Management of Pediatric B-cell Leukemia and Lymphoma 249

Alexandra E. Kovach and Gordana Raca

Although pediatric hematopathology overlaps with that of adults, certain forms of leukemia and lymphoma, and many types of reactive conditions affecting the bone marrow and lymph nodes, are unique to children. As part of this series focused on lymphomas, this article (1) details the novel subtypes of lymphoblastic leukemia seen primarily in children and described since the 2017 World Health Organization classification and (2) discusses unique concepts in pediatric hematopathology, including nomenclature changes and evaluation of surgical margins in selected lymphomas.

Current Concepts in Nodal Peripheral T-Cell Lymphomas 267

Naoki Oishi and Andrew L. Feldman

This review summarizes the current understanding of mature T-cell neoplasms predominantly involving lymph nodes, including ALK-positive and ALK-negative anaplastic large cell lymphomas, nodal T-follicular helper cell lymphoma, Epstein-Barr virus–positive nodal T/NK-cell lymphoma, and peripheral T-cell lymphoma (PTCL), not otherwise specified. These PTCLs are clinically, pathologically, and genetically heterogeneous, and the diagnosis is made by a combination of clinical information, morphology, immunophenotype, viral positivity, and genetic abnormalities. This review summarizes the pathologic features of common nodal PTCLs, highlighting updates in the fifth edition of the World Health Organization classification and the 2022 International Consensus Classification.

Hodgkin Lymphoma and Its Differential Diagnosis: New Twists on an Old Challenge 287

Aliyah R. Sohani

Hodgkin lymphoma is a B-cell neoplasm that typically presents with localized, nodal disease. Tissues are characterized by few large neoplastic cells, usually comprising less than 10% of tissue cellularity, present in a background of abundant nonneoplastic inflammatory cells. This inflammatory microenvironment, although key to the pathogenesis, can make diagnosis a challenge because reactive conditions, lymphoproliferative diseases, and other lymphoid neoplasms may mimic Hodgkin lymphoma and vice versa. This review provides an overview of the classification of Hodgkin lymphoma, its differential diagnosis, including emerging and recently recognized entities, and strategies to resolve challenging dilemmas and avoid diagnostic pitfalls.

Breast Implant-Associated Anaplastic Large Cell Lymphoma: Updates in Diagnosis and Specimen Handling 347

Mario L. Marques-Piubelli, L. Jeffrey Medeiros, John Stewart, and Roberto N. Miranda

Pathologic staging including assessment of margins is essential for the proper management of patients with breast implant-associated anaplastic large-cell lymphoma (BIA-ALCL). As most patients present with effusion, cytologic examination with immunohistochemistry and/or flow cytometry immunophenotyping are essential for diagnosis. Upon a diagnosis of BIA-ALCL, en bloc resection is recommended. When a tumor mass is not identified, a systematic approach to fixation and sampling of the capsule, followed by pathologic staging and assessment of margins, is essential. Cure is likely when lymphoma is contained within the en bloc resection and margins are negative. Incomplete resection or positive margins require a multidisciplinary team assessment for adjuvant therapy.

Aggressive Cutaneous Lymphomas and Their Mimics 361

Andrea P. Moy and Melissa P. Pulitzer

Cutaneous lymphomas encompass a heterogeneous group of neoplasms with a wide spectrum of clinical presentations, histopathologic features, and prognosis. Because there are overlapping pathologic features among indolent and aggressive forms and with systemic lymphomas that involve the skin, clinicopathologic correlation is essential. Herein, the clinical and histopathologic features of aggressive cutaneous B- and T-cell lymphomas are reviewed. Indolent cutaneous lymphomas/lymphoproliferative disorders, systemic lymphomas, and reactive processes that may mimic these entities are also discussed. This article highlights distinctive clinical and histopathologic features, increases awareness of rare entities, and presents new and evolving developments in the field.

Controversies in the Spleen: Histiocytic, Dendritic, and Stromal Cell Lesions 385

Aaron Auerbach, Mark Girton, and Nadine Aguilera

Histiocytic, dendritic, and stromal cell lesions that occur in the spleen are challenging diagnostically, not well studied due to their rarity, and therefore somewhat controversial. New techniques for obtaining tissue samples also create challenges as splenectomy is no longer common and needle biopsy does not afford the same opportunity for examination of tissue. Characteristic primary splenic histiocytic, dendritic, and stromal cell lesions are presented in this paper with new molecular genetic findings in some entities that help differentiate these lesions from those occurring in non-splenic sites, such as soft tissue, and identify possible molecular markers for diagnosis.

Molecular Diagnostics of Plasma Cell Neoplasms 401

Megan J. Fitzpatrick, Mandakolathur R. Murali, and Valentina Nardi

Genetic characterization of myeloma at diagnosis by interphase fluorescence in situ hybridization and next-generation sequencing (NGS) can assist with risk stratification and treatment planning. Measurable residual disease (MRD) status after treatment, as evaluated by next-generation flow cytometry or NGS on bone marrow aspirate material, is one of the most important predictors of prognosis. Less-invasive tools for MRD assessment such as liquid biopsy approaches have also recently emerged as potential alternatives.

Current Landscape of Ancillary Diagnostic Testing in Chronic Lymphocytic Leukemia 411

Julia T. Geyer and Michael J. Kluk

Chronic lymphocytic leukemia (CLL) is the most common adult leukemia and is a heterogeneous disease with variable patient outcomes. A multidisciplinary technical evaluation, including flow cytometry, immunohistochemistry, molecular and cytogenetic analyses, can comprehensively characterize a patient's leukemia at diagnosis, identify important prognostic biomarkers, and track measurable residual disease; all of which can impact patient management. This review highlights the key concepts, clinical significance, and main biomarkers detectable with each of these technical approaches; the contents are a helpful resource for medical practitioners involved in the workup and management of patients with CLL.

Diagnostic Flow Cytometry in the Era of Targeted Therapies: Lessons from Therapeutic Monoclonal Antibodies and Chimeric Antigen Receptor T-cell Adoptive Immunotherapy 423

Ifeyinwa Obiorah and Elizabeth L. Courville

Therapeutic monoclonal antibodies (therapeutic mAb) and adoptive immunotherapy have become increasingly more common in the treatment of hematolymphoid neoplasms, with practical implications for diagnostic flow cytometry. Their use can reduce the sensitivity of flow cytometry for populations of interest owing to downregulation/loss of the target antigen, competition for the target antigen, or lineage switch. Expanded flow panels, marker redundancy, and exhaustive gating strategies can overcome this limitation. Therapeutic mAb have been reported to cause pseudo-light chain restriction, and awareness of this potential artifact is key. Established guidelines do not yet exist for antigen expression by flow cytometry for therapeutic purposes.

Diagnostic, Prognostic, and Predictive Role of Next-Generation Sequencing in Mature Lymphoid Neoplasms 433

Graham W. Slack

Lymphoma is a clinically and biologically heterogeneous disease. Next-generation sequencing (NGS) has expanded our understanding of this heterogeneity at the genetic level, refining disease classification, defining new entities, and providing additional information that can be used in diagnosis and management. This review highlights some of the NGS findings in lymphoma and how they can be used as genetic biomarkers to aid diagnosis and prognosis and guide therapy.

SURGICAL PATHOLOGY CLINICS

FORTHCOMING ISSUES

September 2023
Liver Pathology: Diagnostic Challenges, Practical Considerations and Emerging Concepts
Lei Zhao, *Editor*

December 2023
Gastrointestinal Pathology
Rondell Graham, *Editor*

March 2024
Soft Tissue Pathology
Gregory W. Charville, *Editor*

RECENT ISSUES

March 2023
Endocrine Pathology
Nicole A. Cipriani, *Editor*

December 2022
Genitourinary Pathology
Ming Zhou, *Editor*

September 2022
Pancreatobiliary Pathology
Aartur D. Singhi, *Editor*

SERIES OF RELATED INTEREST
Clinics in Laboratory Medicine
http://www.labmed.theclinics.com/
Hematology/Oncology Clinics
https://www.hemonc.theclinics.com

Preface
Evolving Concepts in Diagnostic Hematopathology

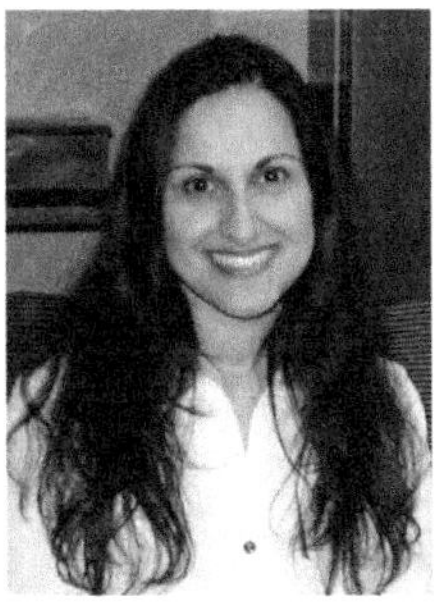

Aliyah R. Sohani, MD
Editor

This collection of articles in *Surgical Pathology Clinics* explores new diagnostic entities and concepts, areas of controversy or evolving understanding, and emerging techniques that aid in diagnosis, prognosis, or predictive response to targeted therapies, with a focus on lymphoid neoplasms. The publication of this issue follows the development of two updated paradigms of disease classification in our field: the 5th edition of the WHO Classification of Haematolymphoid Tumours and the 2022 International Consensus Classification. The entities of focus span the gamut from nonneoplastic to indolent to aggressive neoplastic conditions, beginning with complications of inflammatory diseases affecting the hematopoietic system and lymphoid tissues, including a novel coronavirus that has given rise to a once-in-a-generation global pandemic. The next area of focus includes categories of lymphoproliferative diseases and lymphomas for which novel subtypes and variants are newly or recently recognized and approaches to their diagnostic workup or specimen handling. Some of these newer variants arise more commonly in pediatric populations and require different approaches to management and therapy that are more conservative or localized in nature, thereby emphasizing the pathologist's role in calling attention to this possibility and guiding appropriate management. Certain sites of disease, such as the skin, breast, and spleen, may be inherently challenging and require nuances in their diagnostic approach. Finally, various techniques have led to a paradigm shift, perhaps none more than the routine availability of next-generation sequencing, which has spawned unique considerations in terms of disease (re)classification, prognostication, and prediction to targeted therapies. Specific attention is given to the broader role of molecular diagnostic techniques in the evaluation of pediatric lymphoid neoplasms, chronic lymphocytic leukemia, and plasma cell neoplasms. Flow cytometry continues to hold an important and growing role in hematopathology diagnostics, and issues that arise following novel and targeted therapies are explored and emphasized. I am so grateful to all the contributors to this issue for their time and for sharing their valuable insights and diagnostic expertise. It is our collective hope that the articles in this issue will serve as an important and contemporary resource in our ever-evolving field.

Aliyah R. Sohani, MD
Department of Pathology
Massachusetts General Hospital
55 Fruit Street, WRN 219
Boston, MA 02114, USA

E-mail address:
arsohani@mgh.harvard.edu

Surgical Pathology 16 (2023) xi
https://doi.org/10.1016/j.path.2023.02.003

Immunoglobulin G4-Related Disease, Lymphadenopathy, and Lymphoma

Histopathologic Features and Diagnostic Approach

Jacob R. Bledsoe, MD

KEYWORDS

• IgG4 • IgG4-related disease • Lymphadenopathy • IgG4-related lymphadenopathy • Lymphoma

Key points

- Lymphadenopathy is common in patients with established extranodal immunoglobulin G4-related disease (IgG4-RD) and is referred to as "IgG4-related lymphadenopathy."
- The finding of increased IgG4-positive plasma cells in lymph nodes is nonspecific and may be seen in heterogeneous immune-related, infectious, and neoplastic processes.
- Increased IgG4-positive plasma cells (>100 per high-power field) and IgG4/IgG ratio (>40%) within interfollicular and/or fibrotic regions of a lymph node is the most specific feature for true IgG4-RD.
- An initial diagnosis of IgG4-RD should not be rendered on a lymph node specimen. When IgG4-RD is suspected, correlation with clinical and laboratory findings, and investigation for extranodal lesions is required.
- IgG4-expressing lymphoproliferative disorders should be routinely excluded as part of the diagnostic workup for IgG4-RD and lymphadenopathy.

ABSTRACT

Lymphadenopathy occurring in patients with immunoglobulin G4 (IgG4)-related disease, termed IgG4-related lymphadenopathy, shows morphologic heterogeneity and overlap with other nonspecific causes of lymphadenopathy including infections, immune-related disorders, and neoplasms. This review describes the characteristic histopathologic features and diagnostic approach to IgG4-related disease and IgG4-related lymphadenopathy, with comparison to nonspecific causes of increased IgG4-positive plasma cells in lymph nodes, and with emphasis on distinction from IgG4-expressing lymphoproliferative disorders.

OVERVIEW

Immunoglobulin G4-related disease (IgG4-RD) is a chronic immune-mediated disorder characterized by the development of mass-forming fibrosing lesions at one or more bodily sites. IgG4-RD is characterized by distinct clinicopathologic features including elevated serum IgG4 levels, increased IgG4-positive plasma cells in tissue sections, and characteristically a good response to immunosuppressive therapy.[1] IgG4-RD may involve nearly any organ, and most patients will develop lymphadenopathy at some point in their clinical course.[2–4]

Histopathologically the plasma cell-rich infiltrate of IgG4-RD may lead to consideration of alternative plasmacytic and lymphoplasmacytic pathologies including infections, other immune-related

Department of Pathology, Boston Children's Hospital, Harvard Medical School, 300 Longwood Avenue, Boston, MA 02115, USA
E-mail address: jacob.bledsoe@childrens.harvard.edu

Surgical Pathology 16 (2023) 177–195
https://doi.org/10.1016/j.path.2023.01.002
1875-9181/23/

disorders, and neoplasms, and these cases often cross the desks of hematopathologists. Therefore, pathologists in general and hematopathologists in particular need to be familiar with key histopathologic features that prompt recognition of IgG4-RD and should be aware of diagnostic criteria and differential diagnosis. The histopathology of IgG4-RD involving lymph nodes, termed IgG4-related lymphadenopathy, is heterogeneous and may be nonspecific and subtle. Significant morphologic overlap exists between IgG4-related lymphadenopathy, other reactive patterns of lymphadenopathy, and IgG4-expressing lymphoproliferative disorders. The aim of this review is to provide a diagnostically useful summary of the clinicopathologic features of IgG4-RD with an emphasis on simplifying the diagnostic approach to IgG4-related lymphadenopathy and its differential diagnosis.

PATHOPHYSIOLOGY

The etiology of IgG4-RD is unknown. Recent advances in our understanding of the immunologic mechanisms of the disease have implicated CD4-positive cytotoxic T lymphocytes, M2 macrophages, and activated B cells as likely contributors to the development of fibrosis through cytokine production resulting in the activation of fibroblasts.[5–7] The dramatic therapeutic response to glucocorticoids and B-cell depletion confirm that B cells play an important role in contributing to disease activity. The role of the IgG4 molecule and IgG4-positive plasma cells is uncertain and may be a secondary phenomenon or, given the potential anti-inflammatory properties of IgG4, may be an attempt to dampen the immune response.[7] BATF-positive T-follicular helper (Tfh) lymphocytes appear to play a key role in promoting class-switch of B cells to IgG4 through secretion of IL-4 and possibly IL-10.[8,9]

EPIDEMIOLOGY

IgG4-RD is predominantly a disease of older men, with an average age of approximately 50 to 60 years at initial diagnosis, and a male:female ratio of 2 to 4:1 in most studies.[4,10,11] Most cases occur after 40 years of age.[11] However, IgG4-RD does occur in younger adults and bona fide cases of pediatric IgG4-RD exist, though are extraordinarily uncommon.[12] Based on the limited number of reported cases, pediatric IgG4-RD tends to occur most commonly in children over age 10 and does not demonstrate the male predominance seen in adult IgG4-RD.[12,13] The estimated incidence of IgG4-RD is difficult to accurately ascertain given the rarity of the disease and reporting bias, but is likely at minimum 1 in 100,000 people given under-recognition of the disease.[14]

CLINICAL FEATURES

The initial presentation of IgG4-RD most commonly involves tumor-like enlargement of one or more, often exocrine, organs. The most common visceral sites involved by IgG4-RD are the submandibular glands, orbit/lacrimal glands, and pancreaticobiliary tract, each being involved in approximately one-quarter of cases.[2,4] Systemic IgG4-RD or involvement of three or more organs is present in approximately 30% to 40% of cases.[2,4] The disease may occur almost anywhere, and other sites of non-nodal involvement include (in approximately decreasing order of occurrence) the retroperitoneum, lung, kidney, aorta, meninges, mediastinum, and others.[4] Orbital IgG4-RD is reportedly the most common site of involvement in the pediatric population, making up at least 40% to 50% of cases.[12,13]

In superficial sites such as the submandibular gland or orbit, a visible mass-like enlargement of involved structures is commonly the presenting symptom. In deep sites, the tumefactive lesion of IgG4-RD typically becomes apparent due to organ dysfunction caused by mass effect on adjacent structures. The classic example is IgG4-related pancreatitis presenting with jaundice and pancreatic mass lesion, which is often concerning for a pancreatic malignancy. In such cases, imaging modalities showing mass-like enlargement or fibrosis at one or more sites play a key role in the diagnosis of IgG4-RD.[15]

LYMPHADENOPATHY

Lymphadenopathy is frequent in IgG4-RD, occurring in an estimated 40% to 60% of cases,[2,3] and may precede visceral involvement. In most cases, lymphadenopathy is present at the time of initial IgG4-RD diagnosis.[16] Lymphadenopathy is most often limited to the anatomic region or compartment of the site of visceral involvement, but may be multicentric or generalized. In one study on biopsy-proven IgG4-related lymphadenopathy, lymphadenopathy outside of the region of visceral involvement was present in 40% of cases.[16] Recognition of characteristic histopathologic features in a lymph node specimen may prompt initial consideration of IgG4-RD diagnosis, particularly if IgG4-RD is not suspected clinically, or if the diagnosis is not already established based on documented visceral involvement. However, given the relative nonspecificity of increased IgG4-positive plasma cells in lymph nodes, in the absence of previously established extranodal IgG4-RD it is not prudent to make a definitive initial diagnosis of IgG4-RD solely based on lymph node morphology.[17] In a minor subset of cases (<5%), lymph nodes may be the predominant or only site of involvement without extranodal disease, and the finding of a pseudotumor-like pattern akin to extranodal IgG4-RD (as described below), along with compelling clinical and laboratory findings, may help facilitate IgG4-RD diagnosis in this uncommon situation.[16]

LABORATORY FEATURES

Correlation of morphologic findings with laboratory testing is essential for the diagnosis of IgG4-RD. An elevated serum IgG4 level is the most well-known laboratory finding in IgG4-RD, though it is neither sensitive nor specific for the diagnosis.[18] One study on a Western cohort showed that increased serum IgG4 was present in only about half of patients with active IgG4-RD diagnosis.[4] Overall a serum IgG4 elevated above the normal range has been shown to be relatively sensitive (approximately 80–90%) but with a lower specificity of approximately 60% to 80%, with higher values being more specific for IgG4-RD.[18–20] It is important to recognize that elevated serum IgG4 levels can be found in other heterogeneous inflammatory, immune-related, and neoplastic disorders, and without clinical and morphologic context should be interpreted with caution.[20–22] Given that IgG4-expressing plasma cell neoplasms and B-cell lymphomas with plasmacytic differentiation may also be associated with an elevated serum IgG4, serum protein electrophoresis should be performed in patients being evaluated for IgG4-RD, along with immunofixation if a monoclonal protein is identified.[23–25] Additional characteristically abnormal laboratory values in IgG4-RD include decreased complement levels, elevated serum IgE, peripheral eosinophilia, and elevated C-reactive protein (CRP).[4,26]

HISTOPATHOLOGY

IMMUNOGLOBULIN G4-RELATED DISEASE

Morphology

The classic triad of IgG4-RD histopathology is a plasma cell-rich inflammatory infiltrate with (1) an increase in the absolute number of IgG4-positive plasma cells and an increased ratio of IgG4-positive plasma cells to IgG-positive plasma cells (IgG4/IgG ratio) >40%; with (2) associated storiform fibrosis, that is, a cartwheel-like pattern of fibrosis; and (3) obliterative phlebitis, with partial or complete occlusion of veins by the fibroinflammatory infiltrate (Figs. 1–3).[1] Depending on the age of the lesion, varying degrees of fibrosis and inflammatory infiltrate may be present. For example, active or relatively new lesions typically have a prominent inflammatory infiltrate, whereas in older lesions the inflammatory component is reduced and the fibrosis may be more extensive, including some cases with an extensively sclerotic appearance (see Fig. 1). In addition to plasma cells, a less prominent infiltrate of eosinophils is almost always present as part of the fibroinflammatory infiltrate of IgG4-RD, and is a useful diagnostic clue.

Obliterative phlebitis is often the most subtle of the classic histopathologic features of IgG4-RD, though it is arguably the most specific for the disease (see Fig. 2). Completely obliterated veins may be indistinct and the addition of an elastic stain is valuable for their detection. Understanding of the normal distribution of veins in a particular tissue type will often facilitate recognition of obliterative phlebitis when a vein is absent from its expected location. For example, veins are typically present adjacent to arteries of similar caliber, and when a vein is not easily identified in an inflammatory background suggestive of IgG4-RD then closer examination of H&E and elastic stains may demonstrate obliterative phlebitis.

Immunohistochemistry

Immunohistochemical staining for IgG and IgG4 is necessary for evaluation of IgG4-RD. Recommendations for quantification of IgG4-positive plasma cells include counting and averaging the three high-power fields (HPF) with the highest number of IgG4-positive plasma cells, counting and averaging the number of IgG-positive plasma cells in the corresponding fields on IgG immunohistochemical stain, and calculating a ratio of IgG4/IgG-positive plasma cells using the averages.[1] Using this technique, an average absolute value of IgG4-positive plasma cells and average IgG4/IgG ratio can be determined. In some cases, IgG immunohistochemical staining is obscured by high background staining, and a CD138 stain may be used as a rough surrogate for IgG under the assumption that most plasma cells will be IgG-positive. The recommended cutoffs for absolute numbers of IgG4-positive plasma cells varies by tissue type and by method of tissue sampling (Table 1).[1] At all sites an IgG4/IgG ratio of >40% is required for diagnosis of IgG4-RD (see Fig. 3). In general, larger amounts of evaluable tissue allow for more optimal assessment of the number of IgG4-positive plasma cells and a more secure diagnosis. Therefore, in limited biopsies, a lower cutoff number of IgG4-positive plasma cells is used to arrive at a diagnosis of 'suspicious for IgG4-RD' than in larger excision specimens.

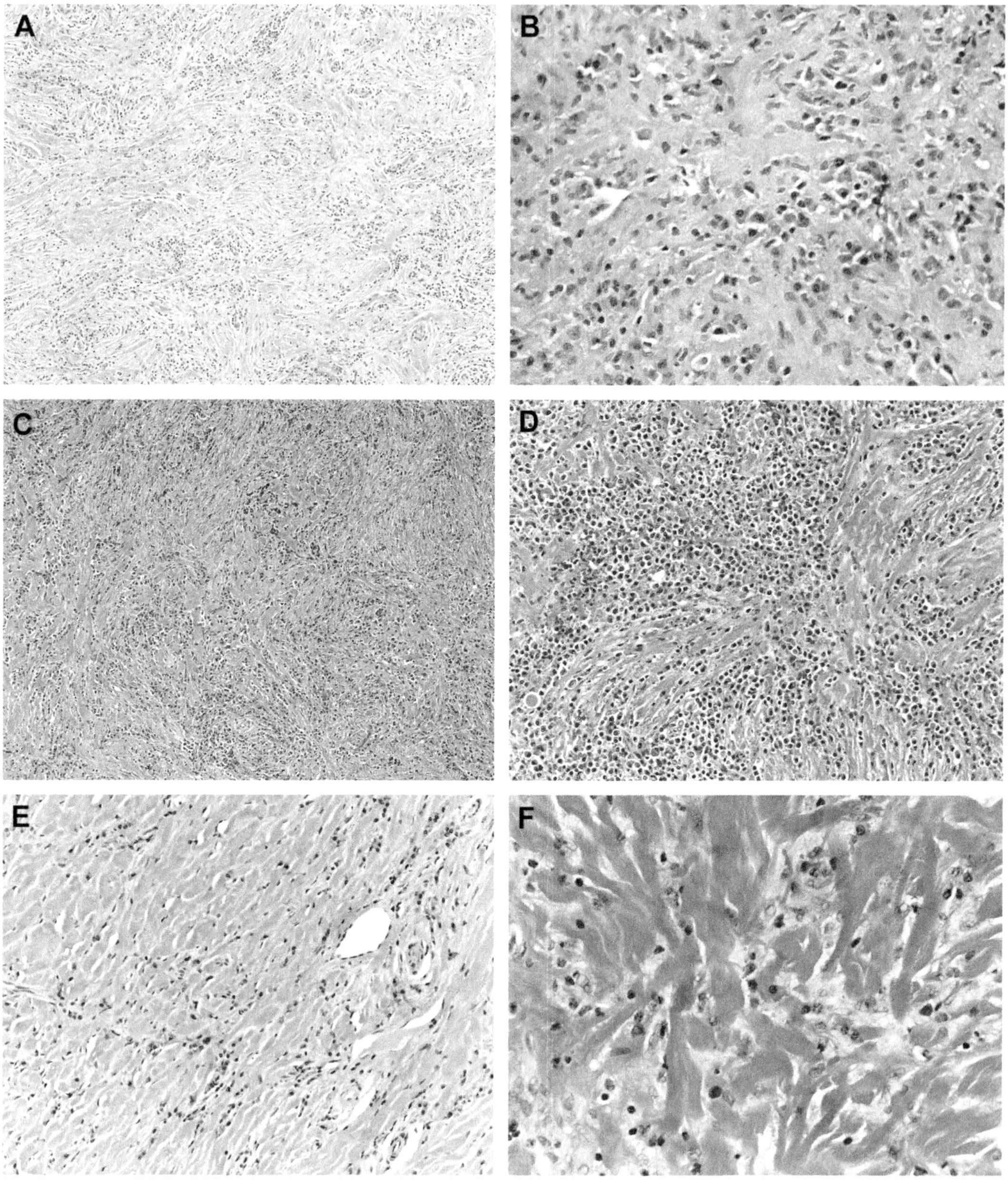

Fig. 1. Morphologic features of the fibroinflammatory infiltrate of IgG4-RD. IgG4-RD is characterized by a plasmacytic infiltrate associated with fibrosis with a storiform pattern and admixed eosinophils (*A*, *B*). Lesions may vary from markedly cellular (*C*, *D*) to markedly fibrotic with less prominent inflammatory infiltrate (*E*, *F*). (Image F courtesy of Dr Vikram Deshpande.)

When considering a diagnosis of IgG4-RD, it is also recommended to routinely evaluate plasma cell clonality by immunohistochemistry or in situ hybridization for kappa and lambda light chains.[17] In IgG4-RD, plasma cells should be polytypic, whereas in an IgG4-expressing lymphoid or plasma cell neoplasm, the IgG4-positive plasma cells demonstrate monoclonal light chain expression.[24] IgG4-positive extranodal marginal zone lymphoma (EMZL) with plasmacytic differentiation is the classic example of such a neoplasm, and its sites of involvement have significant overlap with IgG4-RD, resulting in a potential diagnostic pitfall.[24,25,27]

Diagnostic Terminology

Recommended terminology for the histopathologic diagnosis of cases with features of IgG4-RD

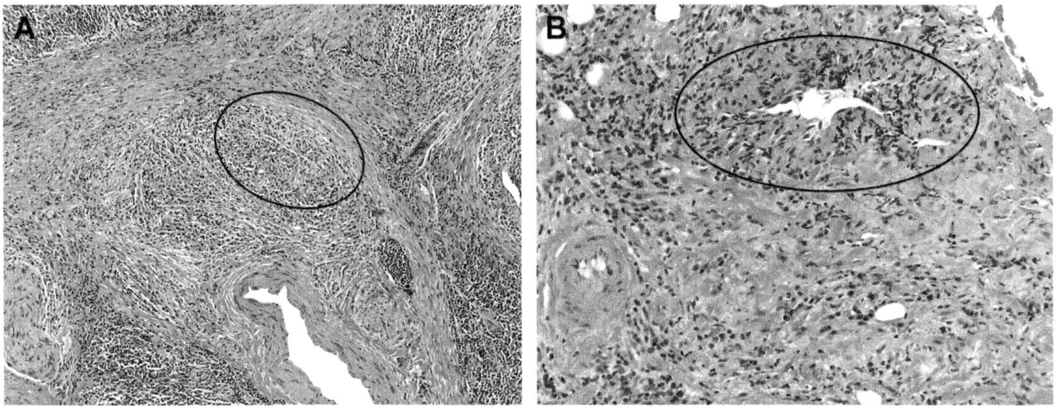

Fig. 2. Obliterative phlebitis. Obliterated veins are often best appreciated by identification of an artery without a patent adjacent vein but with a nodule of mixed inflammation (*A*, oval). Closer examination may reveal a vein partially obliterated by fibrosis and admixed inflammatory cells (*A, B, ovals*).

integrates (1) the tissue type, (2) the number and proportion of IgG4-positive plasma cells, and (3) the presence or absence of a dense lymphoplasmacytic infiltrate, storiform fibrosis, and/or obliterative phlebitis. Using these features, cases can be placed into three categories: "histologically highly suggestive of IgG4-RD," "suspicious for IgG4-RD," or "unlikely to be IgG4-RD."[1] Referring to the consensus criteria for the diagnosis of IgG4-RD is useful when considering how to report a

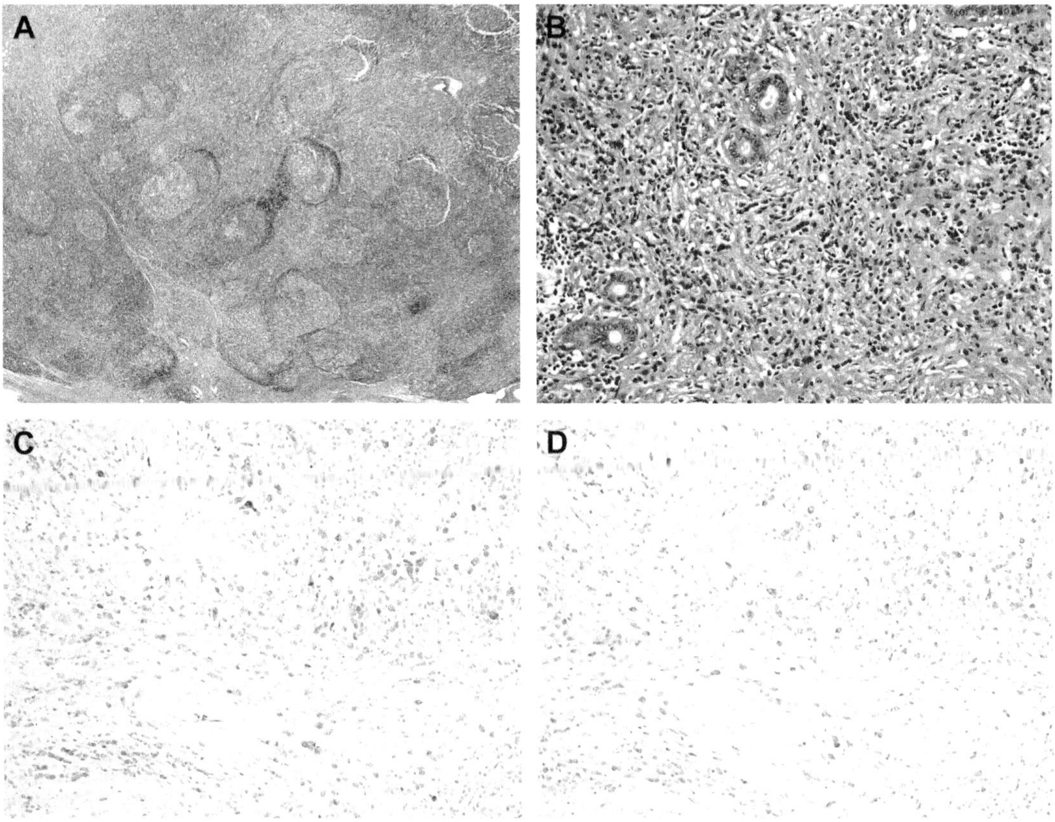

Fig. 3. IgG4-related sialadenitis. Low power (*A*) shows fibrous accentuation of the submandibular lobules/acini with frequent reactive follicles. The fibroinflammatory infiltrate is composed of frequent plasma cells and admixed eosinophils in a background of fibrosis (*B*). Immunohistochemistry for IgG (*C*) and IgG4 (*D*) shows a marked increase in IgG4-positive plasma cells and IgG4/IgG plasma cell ratio of >40%.

Table 1
Recommended cutoff values of immunoglobulin G4-positive cells per high-power field by site[a]

Site	IgG4+ per HPF
Orbit	>100
Salivary gland	>100
Lung	>50 (excision)
Pancreas	>50 (excision), >10 (biopsy)
Bile duct	>50 (excision)
Liver	>50 (excision)
Kidney	>30 (excision), >10 (biopsy)
Aorta	>50
Retroperitoneum	>30

[a] The above values are recommended cutoffs for "highly suspicious for IgG4-RD" provided that two of the three following features are also present: dense lymphoplasmacytic infiltrate, storiform fibrosis, obliterative phlebitis. IgG4/IgG ratio >40% is required.

specific case.[1] Cases that meet criteria for "histologically highly suggestive of IgG4-RD" have been shown to more commonly truly represent IgG4-RD than the other diagnostic categories.[28] Use of this terminology is recommended in all cases due to the fact that it is difficult to definitively establish the diagnosis of IgG4-RD based on histopathology in isolation. Rather, the histopathologic findings must be correlated with other clinical and laboratory findings, including serum IgG4, before a definitive diagnosis of IgG4-RD can be established.

IMMUNOGLOBULIN G4-RELATED LYMPHADENOPATHY

IgG4-related lymphadenopathy is a term used to describe lymphadenopathy occurring in a patient with an established diagnosis of IgG4-RD, based on known extranodal IgG4-RD. Many studies have shown that increased IgG4-positive plasma cells occur in lymph nodes in various disease states other than IgG4-RD, including other autoimmune disorders, infections, and neoplasia.[24,29–35] Based on this fact, it is recommended that the term 'IgG4-related lymphadenopathy' be used to denote only cases of bona fide IgG4-RD involving lymph nodes, rather than as a general term for a lymph node with increased IgG4-positive plasma cells. Given that the interpretation of the significance of increased IgG4-positive plasma cells in lymph nodes is complex, it is also recommended that an initial diagnosis of IgG4-RD not be made on a lymph node specimen.[17] Further complicating this issue, many described morphologic patterns of IgG4-related lymphadenopathy are nonspecific, though knowledge of these patterns is useful to prompt further diagnostic work-up.[16]

Morphology

The morphologic spectrum of IgG4-related lymphadenopathy is broad. In some patients with known IgG4-RD, lymph nodes will have no abnormal morphologic features and no increase in IgG4-positive plasma cells.[16] This is likely related to activity of disease and distance of the lymph node from the site of extranodal/visceral involvement. However, abnormal morphologic changes are present in most IgG4-RD patients with enlarged lymph nodes. Initial descriptions of lymph node morphology in patients with IgG4-RD with enlarged lymph nodes identified five characteristic patterns. These include (1) Castleman disease (CD)-like pattern, (2) follicular hyperplasia-like pattern, (3) interfollicular expansion pattern, (4) progressive transformation of germinal centers (PTGC)-type pattern, and (5) inflammatory pseudotumor-like pattern.[36–38] Although in isolation these H&E morphologic patterns are nonspecific, in the setting of increased IgG4-positive plasma cells (>100 per HPF) and increased IgG4/IgG plasma cell ratio (>40%), the above patterns raise the possibility of IgG4-RD. The PTGC-like pattern is classically characterized by increased IgG4-positive plasma cells and IgG4/IgG ratio within reactive follicles, whereas the other patterns contain increased IgG4 parameters in an interfollicular distribution.[38] Subsequent studies have suggested that an isolated increase in IgG4 parameters within follicles is nonspecific and seen commonly in reactive lymphadenopathy unrelated to IgG4-RD.[16] Other uncommon morphologic patterns of lymphadenopathy that may occur in patients with IgG4-RD, including infectious mononucleosis-like changes,[39] and rarely Rosai-Dorfman disease-like changes.

Castleman disease-like pattern

Lymph nodes with the CD-like pattern demonstrate increased interfollicular (ie, outside of follicles) IgG4-positive plasma cells with admixed eosinophils, along with morphologic features typical of CD including follicles with penetration by a hyalinized vessel ("lollipop follicle"), an "onion-skin" arrangement of mantle zone B cells, and increased interfollicular vascularity (**Fig. 4**). Regions of parenchymal or capsular fibrosis may be present and if fibrotic regions contain increased IgG4-positive plasma cells this suggests IgG4-RD.[16] In contrast to the atrophic follicles of CD, the CD-like pattern of IgG4-related

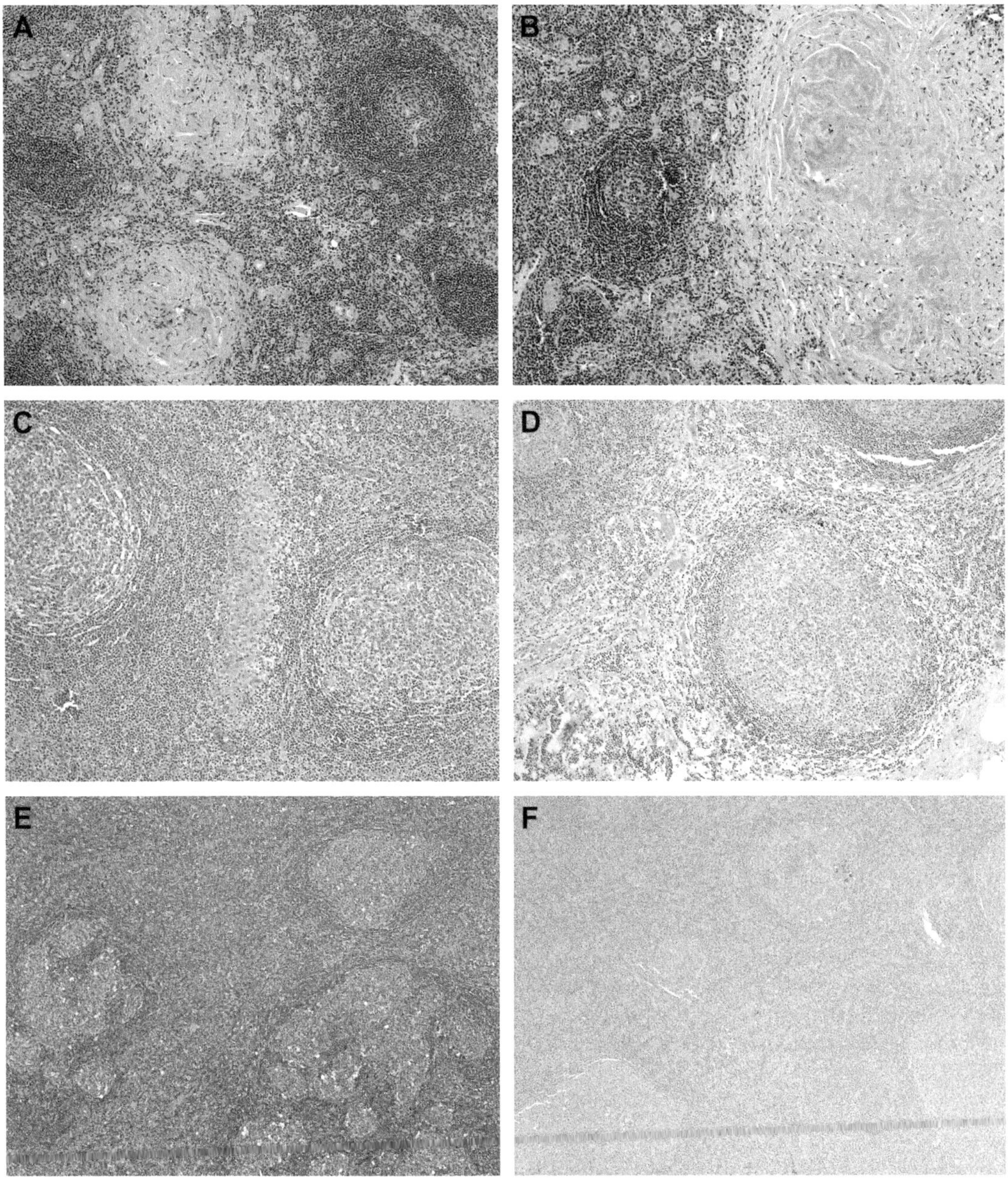

Fig. 4. Relatively nonspecific patterns of IgG4-related lymphadenopathy. The CD-like (*A, B*) pattern is characterized by follicles with an onion skin-like arrangement of mantle zone B cells with prominent interfollicular vascularity. Parenchymal or capsular fibrosis may be present. The follicular hyperplasia-like pattern (*C, D*), with a perifollicular granuloma (*C*). The PTGC-like pattern has characteristics of follicular hyperplasia with foci of PTGC (*E, F*).

lymphadenopathy more often has follicles of normal size or hyperplastic follicles.[32,38]

Follicular hyperplasia and progressive transformation of germinal center-like patterns

The follicular hyperplasia pattern of IgG4-related lymphadenopathy is characterized by enlarged follicles with reactive germinal centers and increased IgG4-positive plasma cells, classically in an interfollicular distribution (see Fig. 4).[40] The PTGC-like pattern has features of follicular hyperplasia with enlarged follicles showing PTGC changes including the extension of mantle zone B cells into follicles with follicle fragmentation (see Fig. 4). The PTGC-like pattern is classically described with increased IgG4-positive plasma cells within follicles.[41] Studies have shown that the PTGC-like pattern of IgG4-related lymphadenopathy occurs most commonly in cervical lymph nodes and may be associated with the subsequent development of submandibular IgG4-related sialadenitis.[41] Outside of this particular scenario the finding of an isolated increase of intrafollicular IgG4-positive plasma cells is largely nonspecific.[16]

Interfollicular expansion pattern

The interfollicular expansion pattern is characterized by prominent interfollicular zones containing many IgG4-positive plasma cells admixed with small lymphocytes, eosinophils, histiocytes, and scattered immunoblasts. Follicles are infrequent or absent (Fig. 5). When identified with increased interfollicular IgG4-positive plasma cells and IgG4/IgG ratio, this pattern has been found to be highly specific for IgG4-RD.[16]

Inflammatory pseudotumor-like pattern

The inflammatory pseudotumor-like pattern of IgG4-related lymphadenopathy has many morphologic features that are similar to extranodal IgG4-RD, including broad areas of nodal fibrosis containing increased IgG4-positive plasma cells and IgG4/IgG ratio and usually admixed eosinophils (Fig. 6). The capsule is fibrotic and subcapsular fibrosis is typically prominent. Fibrosis frequently extends into perinodal soft tissue and may be storiform in a pattern. Occasionally fibrous bands surround reactive follicles imparting a "nodular sclerosis" pattern akin to nodular sclerosis classic Hodgkin lymphoma. On H&E morphology, this pattern may closely mimic syphilitic lymphadenitis. The inflammatory pseudotumor-like pattern is highly specific for IgG4-RD.[16]

Diagnostic approach to immunoglobulin G4-related lymphadenopathy

A diagnostic approach to categorize lymph nodes with increased IgG4-positive plasma cells has been proposed (Fig. 7)[16,17] In the absence of increased IgG4-positive plasma cells (>100 per HPF) and increased IgG4/IgG plasma cell ratio (>40%), a diagnosis of IgG4-related lymphadenopathy cannot be rendered and the above morphologic patterns are nonspecific. The presence of increased IgG4 parameters within follicles is also largely nonspecific, perhaps with the exception of the PTGC-like pattern occurring in cervical lymph nodes.[16,41] Indeed, one study showed that an isolated increase in intrafollicular IgG4-positive plasma cells and IgG4/IgG ratio (even at levels >100 per HPF and >40% IgG4/IgG ratio) was seen more commonly in nonspecific causes of lymphadenopathy than in true IgG4-RD.[16] In contrast, the presence of increased IgG4 parameters in extrafollicular regions (between follicles, in interfollicular regions, or in regions of parenchymal or capsular fibrosis) had higher specificity for bona fide IgG4-RD.[16] In particular, the interfollicular expansion and inflammatory pseudotumor-like patterns were highly specific for true IgG4-related lymphadenopathy.[16]

Other diagnostically useful features of IgG4-related lymphadenopathy include the finding of capsular fibrosis containing a mixed cellularity infiltrate including frequent IgG4-positive plasma cells and admixed eosinophils (Fig. 8). Perifollicular granulomas partially or completely encircling follicles are also characteristic (see Fig. 8),[42] though not specific, particularly if IgG4 parameters are not increased, as similar granulomas may be seen in nodular lymphocyte predominant Hodgkin lymphoma and some infections, including toxoplasma lymphadenitis. Phlebitis is occasionally seen in IgG4-related lymphadenopathy and may suggest the diagnosis, though obliterative phlebitis is uncommon (see Fig. 8).

DIFFERENTIAL DIAGNOSIS

The differential diagnosis of both extranodal IgG4-RD and IgG4-related lymphadenopathy is broad and includes other inflammatory and immune-mediated disorders, infections, and neoplasms.

IMMUNOGLOBULIN G4-EXPRESSING LYMPHOPROLIFERATIVE DISORDERS

IgG4-expressing lymphoproliferative disorders are a significant diagnostic pitfall in the differential diagnosis of IgG4-RD and IgG4-related lymphadenopathy and show an overlap of both pathologic and laboratory features. IgG4-expressing lymphoproliferative disorders may be associated with elevated serum IgG4 levels; however, serum protein electrophoresis with immunofixation may demonstrate that the elevated serum IgG4 is monoclonal.[43] In contrast, IgG4-RD is a nonneoplastic process with polyclonal IgG4-positive plasma cells and without a serum monoclonal protein. Morphologically, both IgG4-RD and IgG4-expressing lymphoproliferative disorders have an extensive plasmacytic infiltrate with increased IgG4-positive plasma cells and increased IgG4/IgG ratio. Given these considerations, evaluation of plasma cell clonality by immunohistochemistry or in situ hybridization for kappa and lambda light chains is recommended to confirm polyclonality in

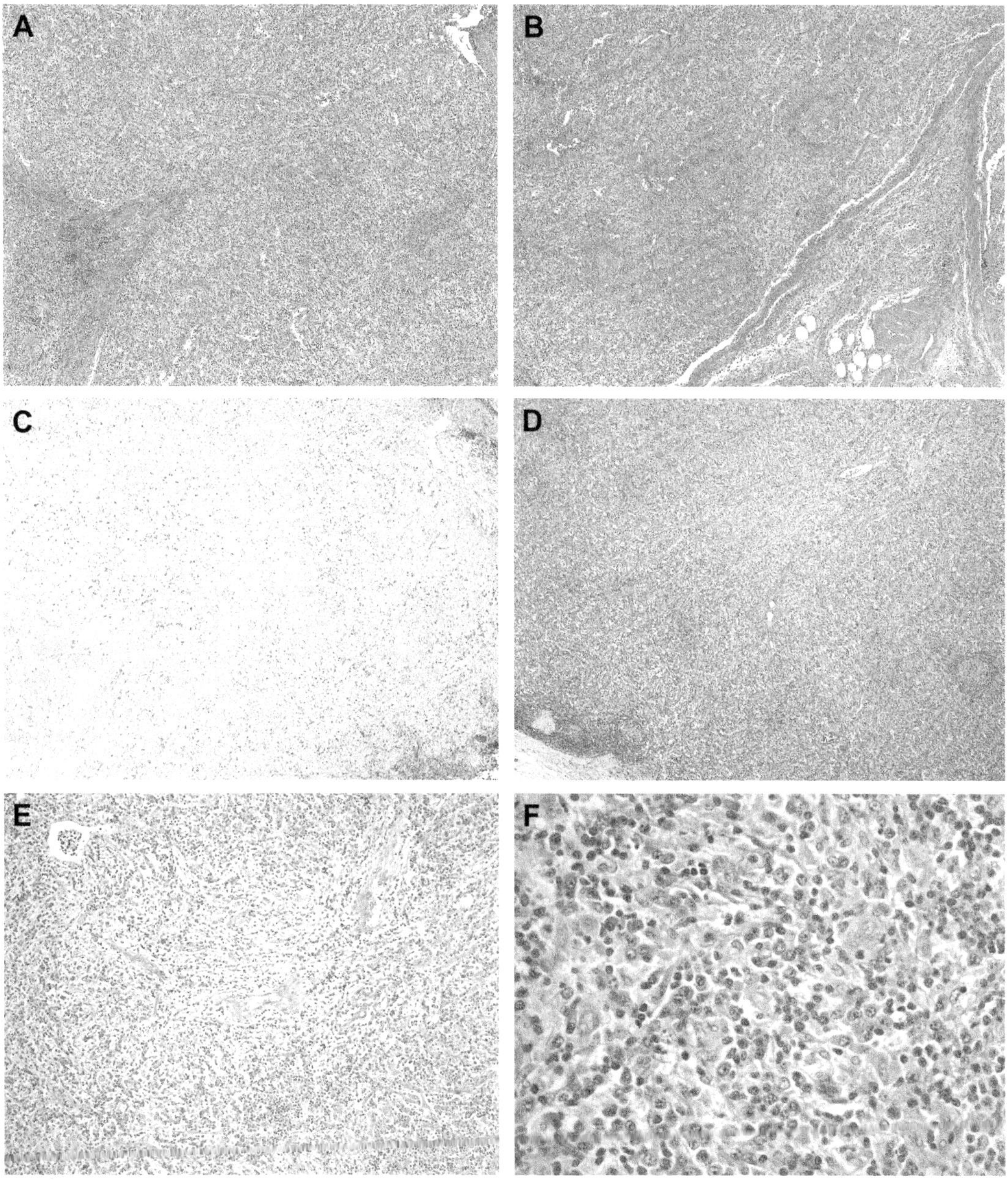

Fig. 5. Interfollicular expansion pattern of IgG4-related lymphadenopathy. Lymph node (*A–C*) with marked expansion of interfollicular zones (*A*) with few small residual follicles (*B*) and increased IgG4-positive plasma cells in interfollicular regions (*C*). Another case (*D–F*) with similar morphology along with associated fine strands of interfollicular fibrosis (*E*); the inflammatory infiltrate includes frequent plasma cells admixed with small lymphocytes, occasional immunoblasts, and eosinophils (*F*).

all cases in which a diagnosis of IgG4-RD is suspected.[17]

IgG4-expressing lymphoproliferative disorders occur in two groups: B-cell lymphomas with plasmacytic differentiation (**Fig. 9**) and plasma cell neoplasms. The former group is predominantly made up of IgG4-positive marginal zone lymphomas (MZL) with plasmacytic differentiation, including nodal MZL and extranodal MZL of mucosa-associated lymphoid tissue (EMZL).[16,44] Although IgG4 is uncommonly expressed in EMZL in general, it is expressed more frequently, in approximately 30% to 40% of cases, in cutaneous and meningeal EMZL.[25,27] Involvement of the salivary glands or orbit is also well-described.[24,45] The morphologic and

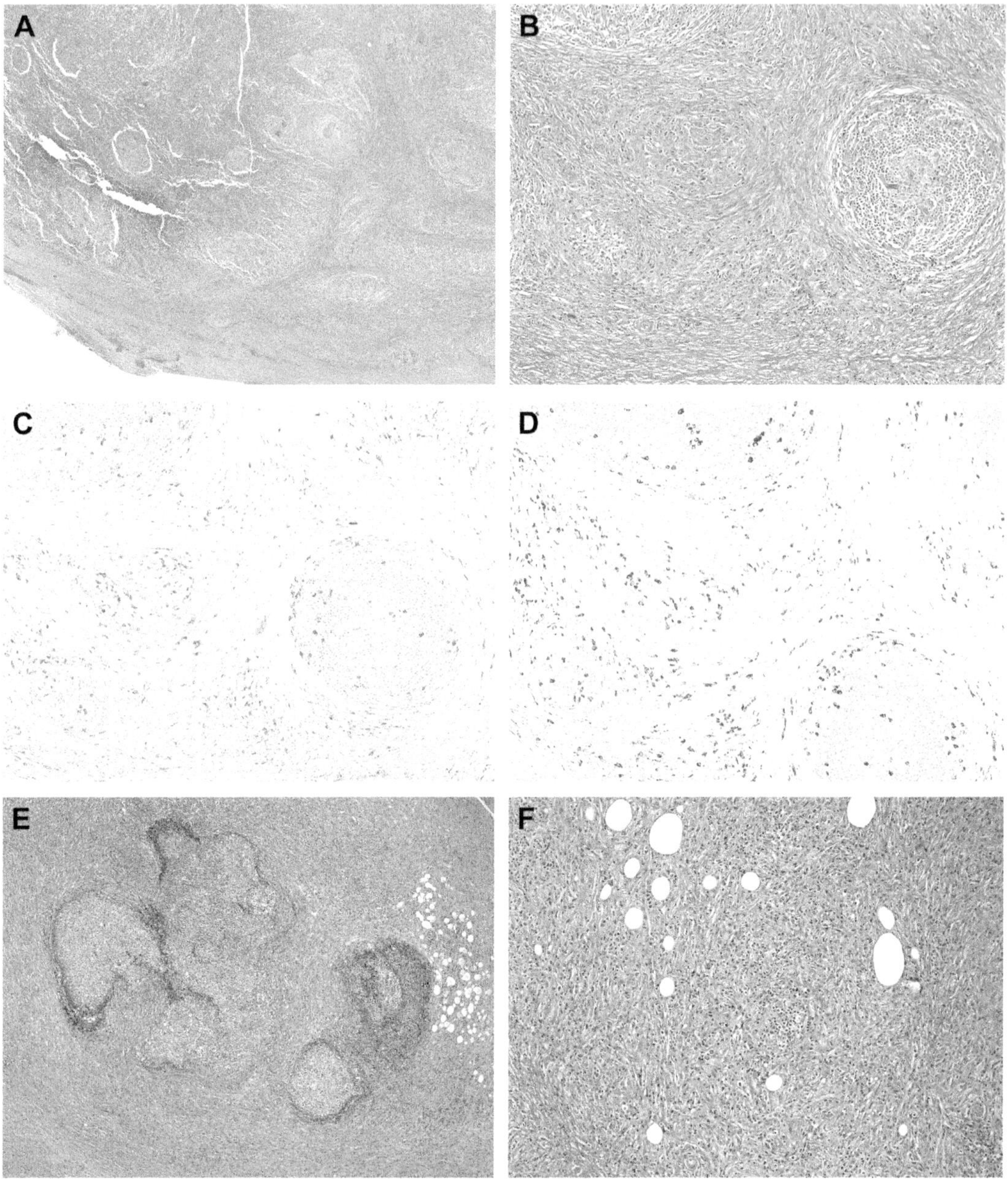

Fig. 6. Inflammatory pseudotumor-like pattern of IgG4-related lymphadenopathy. One case (*A–D*) with marked capsular, subcapsular, and parenchymal fibrosis (*A*), with a storiform pattern (*B*), and with increased IgG4-positive plasma cells and IgG4/IgG ratio (*C*: IgG, *D*: IgG4). Another case (*E, F*) with marked fibrosis imparting a "nodular sclerosis"-like pattern around islands of inflammatory cells (*E*), and with an extension of the fibroinflammatory infiltrate into surrounding perinodal adipose tissue (*F*).

immunophenotypic features are similar to non-IgG4-expressing MZL. Interestingly, frequent clonal IgG4-positive plasma cells with abundant cytoplasmic immunoglobulin inclusions (Mott cells) were described in 5 of 6 cases in one series (see **Fig. 9**).[24] IgG4-expressing plasma cell neoplasms occur infrequently, comprising 4% of IgG-positive multiple myeloma cases in one series, and may show an association with plasmablastic morphology.[23]

A diagnosis of an IgG4-expressing lymphoma or plasma cell neoplasm does not imply that the patient had a preceding or concurrent diagnosis of IgG4-RD, or that the lymphoproliferative process evolved from underlying IgG4-RD.[24] In fact, to date there has been no reported instance in which

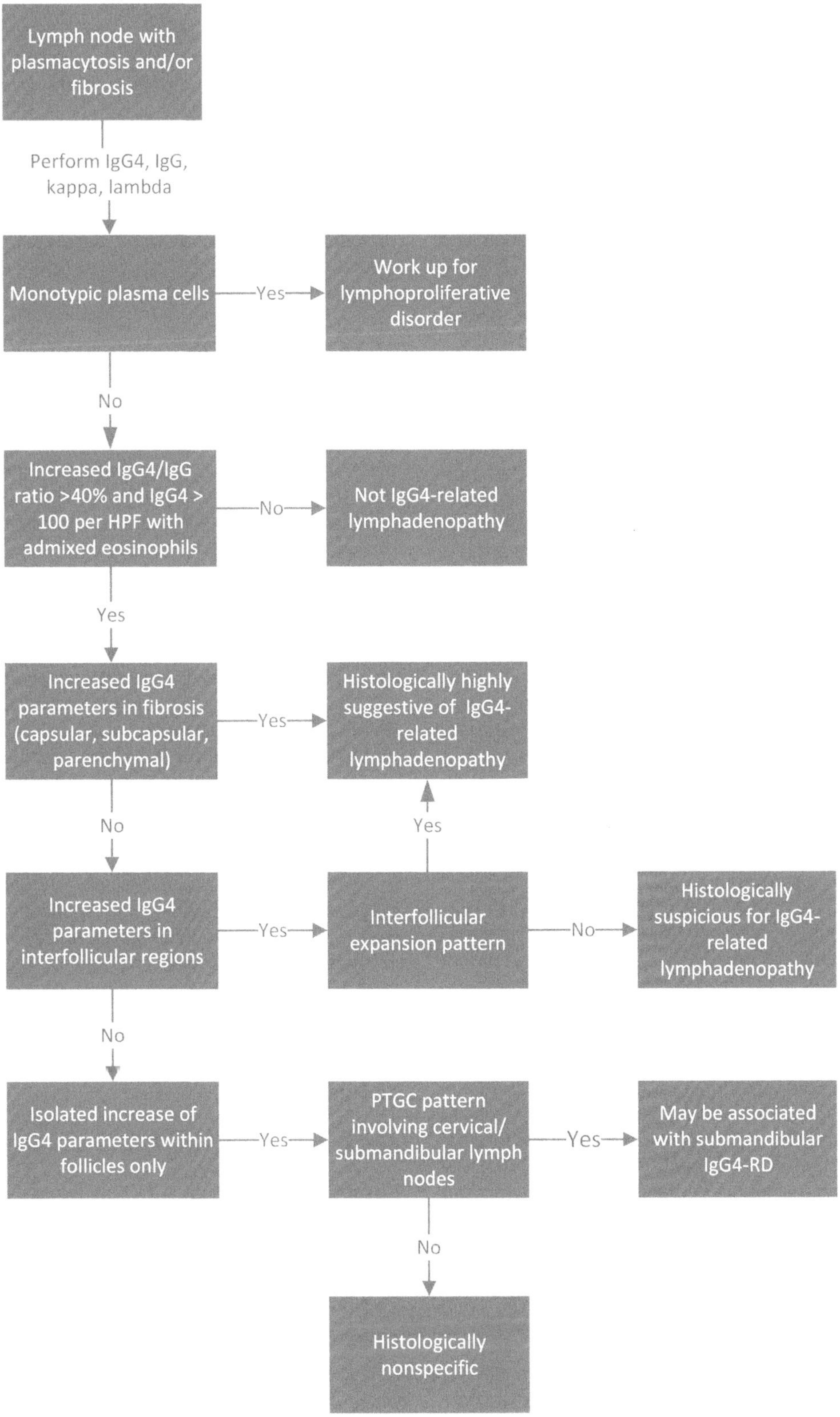

Fig. 7. An approach for workup and reporting of lymph nodes with features of IgG4-related lymphadenopathy such as plasmacytosis, fibrosis, and/or increased IgG4-positive plasma cells. In patients without previously

IgG4-RD has been shown to be definitively clonally related to a subsequent lymphoid or plasma cell neoplasm. Supporting this conjecture, in most described cases of IgG4-expressing lymphoproliferative disorders, the patients had no reported history of IgG4-RD. However, several cases of lymphoma occurring in sites with prior or concurrent involvement by IgG4-RD have been described, suggesting that the lymphoma may arise in the setting of chronic inflammation and antigenic stimulation related to IgG4-RD.[46] Only rare cases have been described in which an IgG4-expressing lymphoma occurs in a patient with established IgG4-RD.[46]

Some studies have suggested that patients with IgG4-RD may have an increased risk of developing of neoplasia, including lymphoma.[47–49] Most reported cases of lymphomas occurring in patients with IgG4-RD are from Asia and are B-cell lymphomas, particularly EMZL.[44–46,48,50] Data from the Western world are more limited, but in addition to MALT lymphomas, DLBCL has been reported in a larger proportion of cases.[46,48] Lymphoma may occur concurrently with the diagnosis of IgG4-RD or may develop subsequently, and in the latter scenario, IgG4-related lymphadenopathy is commonly present between the times of IgG4-RD and lymphoma diagnoses.[46] Notably, most lymphomas that occur in patients with IgG4-RD do not express IgG4.[46]

ATYPICAL IMMUNOGLOBULIN G4-POSITIVE PLASMACYTIC PROLIFERATIONS

Further complicating the distinction between IgG4-RD and IgG4-expressing lymphomas are descriptions of atypical IgG4-expressing plasmacytic proliferations that demonstrate apparent oligoclonality or monotypia but do not meet criteria for malignancy (**Fig. 10**).[24] Such processes can occur in nodal or extranodal locations and are characterized by collections of IgG4-positive plasma cells with monotypic light chain expression within discrete microanatomic compartments rather than as a diffuse infiltrate with architectural destruction or effacement. This most commonly occurs in the setting of reactive follicular lymphoid hyperplasia with increased intrafollicular IgG4-positive plasma cells that appear to be light-chain restricted.[24] Similar proliferations may occur outside of follicles.

Atypical IgG4-positive plasmacytic proliferations have been described both in patients with and without known IgG4-RD. In most such cases, given the restricted localization of the apparently monotypic IgG4-positive plasma cells, the finding is of uncertain significance but raises concern for lymphoma or for the development of a clonal plasma cell population in a background of IgG4-RD. In some cases, atypical IgG4-positive plasmacytic proliferations may represent partial involvement of a specimen by an IgG4-positive lymphoma.[24]

CASTLEMAN DISEASE

Hyper-IL-6 syndromes, including Castleman disease, rheumatoid arthritis, and systemic lupus erythematosus, are immune-mediated disorders that commonly have lymphadenopathy characterized by follicular hyperplasia with interfollicular plasmacytosis, and may contain increased IgG4-positive plasma cells.[32,51] The plasma cell type of CD, in particular, may show overlapping features with the CD-like pattern of IgG4-related lymphadenopathy.[32] In the CD-like pattern of IgG4-related lymphadenopathy, follicles are more often normal in size or hyperplastic, whereas in CD, follicles are typically regressive and atrophic (**Fig. 11**).[52] The plasma cell type of CD classically contains regions with a sheet-like distribution of plasma cells with hemosiderin deposition and without admixed eosinophils, a pattern that would be uncommon in IgG4-related lymphadenopathy.[32] The presence of HHV8-positive plasmablastic cells within CD-type follicles supports the diagnosis of HHV8-associated multicentric CD (see **Fig. 11**). Neutrophil infiltration may be seen in hyper-IL-6 syndromes but is not typical of IgG4-RD.[32] Clinical and laboratory studies, including elevated serum IL-6, persistently elevated CRP, and elevated IgA and IgM, may be useful to distinguish CD and rheumatoid arthritis from IgG4-RD.[51]

ROSAI–DORFMAN DISEASE

Rosai-Dorfman disease (RDD, or "sinus histiocytosis with massive lymphadenopathy") may be accompanied by increased IgG4-positive plasma cells in an interfollicular pattern resulting in misdiagnosis as IgG4-RD.[30] The classic RDD

established extranodal IgG4-RD a definitive initial diagnosis of IgG4-RD should not be rendered on a lymph node specimen. In cases where a diagnosis of IgG4-related lymphadenopathy is suspected, a statement recommending correlation with clinical and laboratory features, including serum IgG4 level, investigation for extranodal fibrosing lesions, and exclusion of other disorders that can have increased nodal IgG4-positive plasma cells, is prudent.

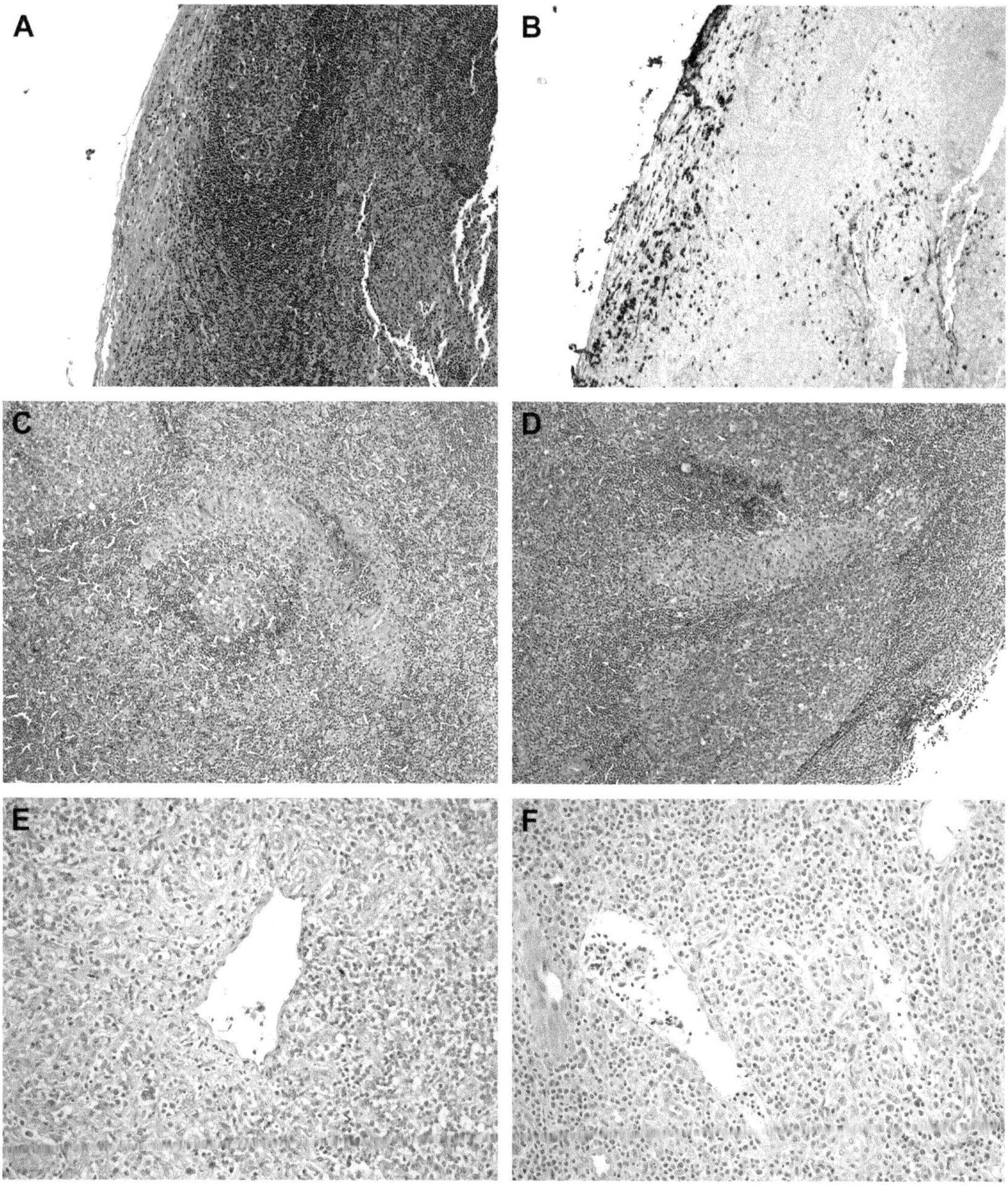

Fig. 8. Other features of IgG4-related lymphadenopathy. Lymph node capsular fibrosis (*A*) containing increased IgG4-positive plasma cells (*B*) is a finding suggestive of IgG4-related lymphadenopathy. Perifollicular granulomas partly or completely encircling reactive lymphoid follicles (*C, D*), or phlebitis (*E, F*) may be seen occasionally in IgG4-related lymphadenopathy.

morphologic feature is emperipolesis, the finding of S100-positive histiocytes with enlarged atypical nuclei and intact intracytoplasmic inflammatory cells, typically present in a sinusoidal pattern (see **Fig. 11**). Emperipolesis is not typically present in IgG4-related lymphadenopathy and strongly suggests RDD. Rarely, a small number of histiocytes with emperipolesis may be identified in IgG4-related lymphadenopathy (see **Fig. 11**), or atypical IgG4-positive plasmacytic proliferations.[24] Recent studies have shown that RDD histiocytes frequently have strong expression of cyclin D1 and OCT2 by immunohistochemistry.[53,54] The finding of an MAPK pathway mutation would also support the diagnosis of RDD.

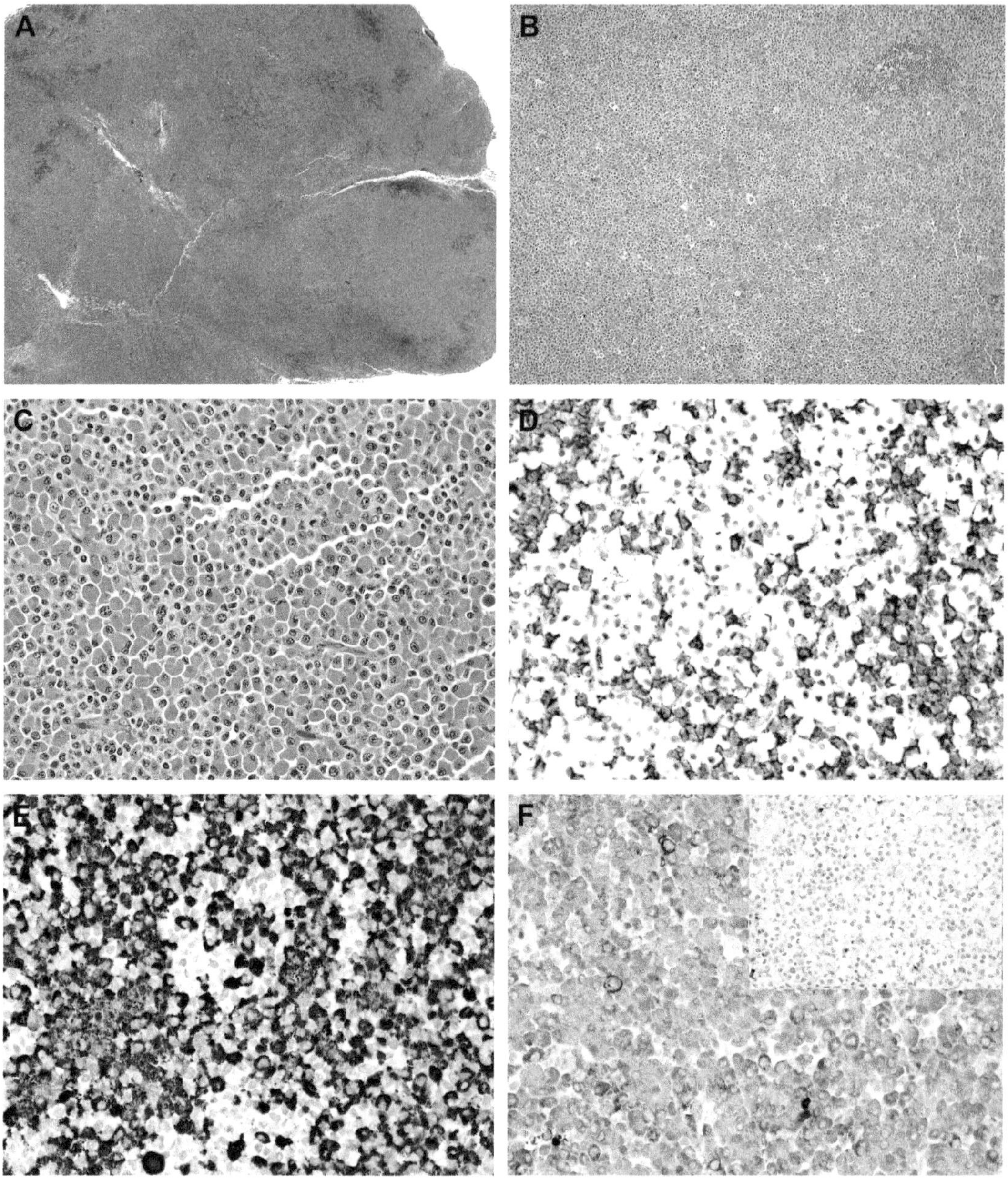

Fig. 9. IgG4-expressing lymphoma. An IgG4-expressing orbital MALT lymphoma with extensive plasmacytic differentiation. Orbital tissue shows a marked plasmacytic infiltrate including abundant Mott cells, admixed with fewer small lymphocytes (*A–C*). Immunohistochemistry for CD20 (*D*) shows that most lymphocytes are B cells. The plasma cells express IgG4 (*E*) and lambda light chain (*F*), and do not express kappa light chain (*F inset*).

SYPHILITIC LYMPHADENITIS

Syphilitic lymphadenitis is a close mimic of the inflammatory pseudotumor-like pattern of IgG4-related disease, and commonly shows storiform fibrosis with marked plasmacytic infiltrate, as well as phlebitis (see **Fig. 11**). In most cases of syphilis, IgG4-positive plasma cells are not increased or only mildly increased. However, studies have shown that increased IgG4-positive plasma cells can occur in the setting of syphilis, as well as other chronic infections such as mastoiditis and aortitis.[55] Use of a silver stain or Treponema immunohistochemistry is useful to verify the diagnosis of syphilis.

NEOPLASIA

IgG4-positive plasma cells may be increased within the inflammatory background of solid

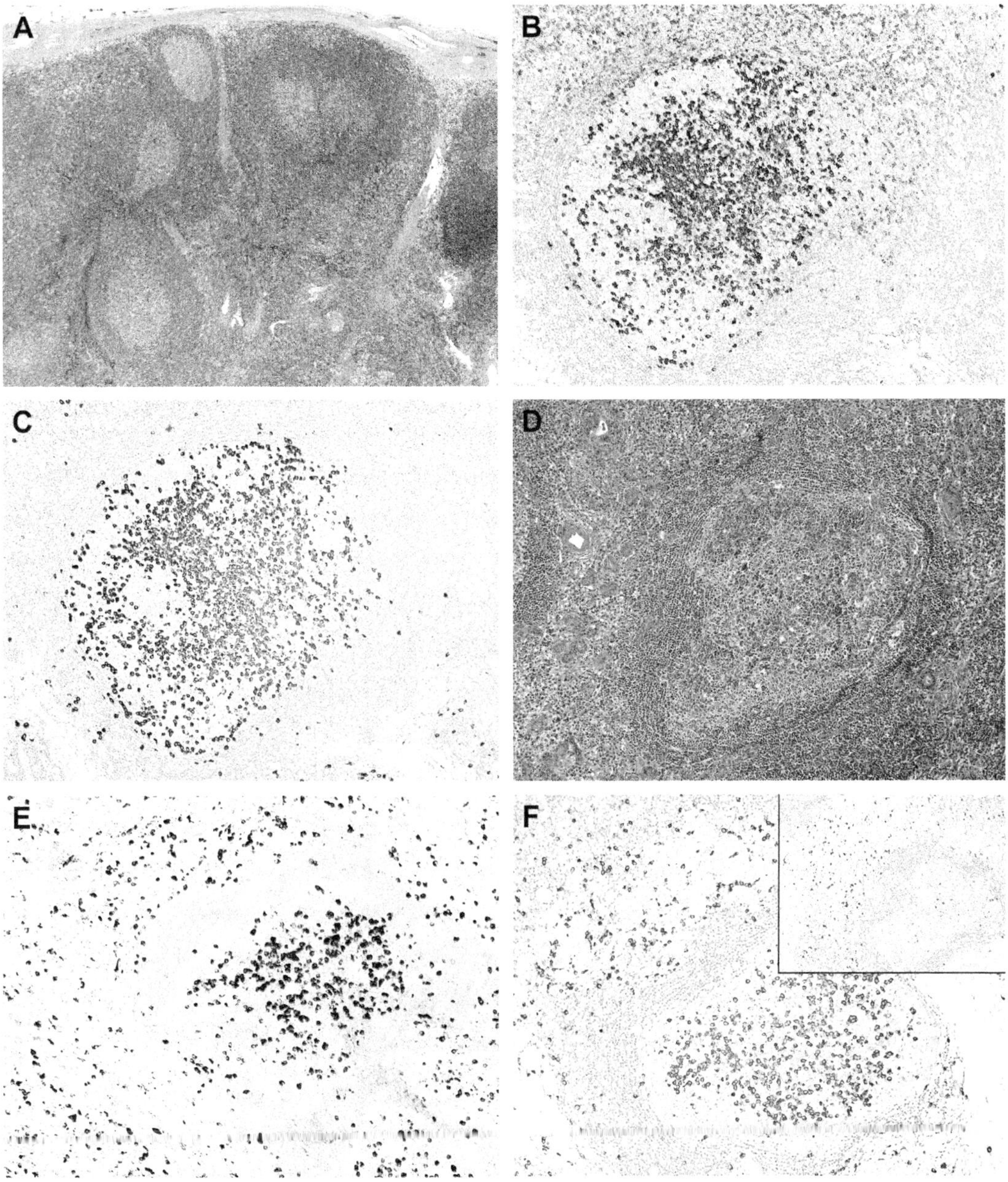

Fig. 10. Atypical IgG4-positive plasmacytic proliferations. An enlarged lymph node (*A, C*) with follicular hyperplasia (*A*). Several reactive follicles contained a marked increase in plasma cells expressing IgG4 (*B*) and kappa light chain (*C*; kappa immunohistochemistry [IHC]). A submandibular mass (*D, F*) with features of IgG4-related sclerosing sialadenitis including many reactive follicles. IgG4-positive plasma cells were increased in number and proportion in both extrafollicular and intrafollicular regions (*E*; IgG4). Within follicles the IgG4-positive plasma cells appear kappa-restricted (*F*; kappa IHC), whereas extrafollicular plasma cells appear polytypic (*F inset*; lambda IHC). (Images D–F courtesy of Dr Judith Ferry.)

tumors[1,29,34] and lymphomas.[24,56] As discussed above, IgG4-expressing lymphomas are a significant diagnostic pitfall.

The interfollicular expansion pattern of IgG4-related lymphadenopathy may morphologically resemble angioimmunoblastic T-cell lymphoma (AITL) by exhibiting a mixed inflammatory infiltrate of small lymphocytes, plasma cells, scattered large immunoblasts, and eosinophils.[36,37,57] However, the neoplastic T cells of AITL demonstrate cytologic atypia, a Tfh immunophenotype including reactivity for CD10, BCL6, PD1, ICOS, and/or CXCL13, are

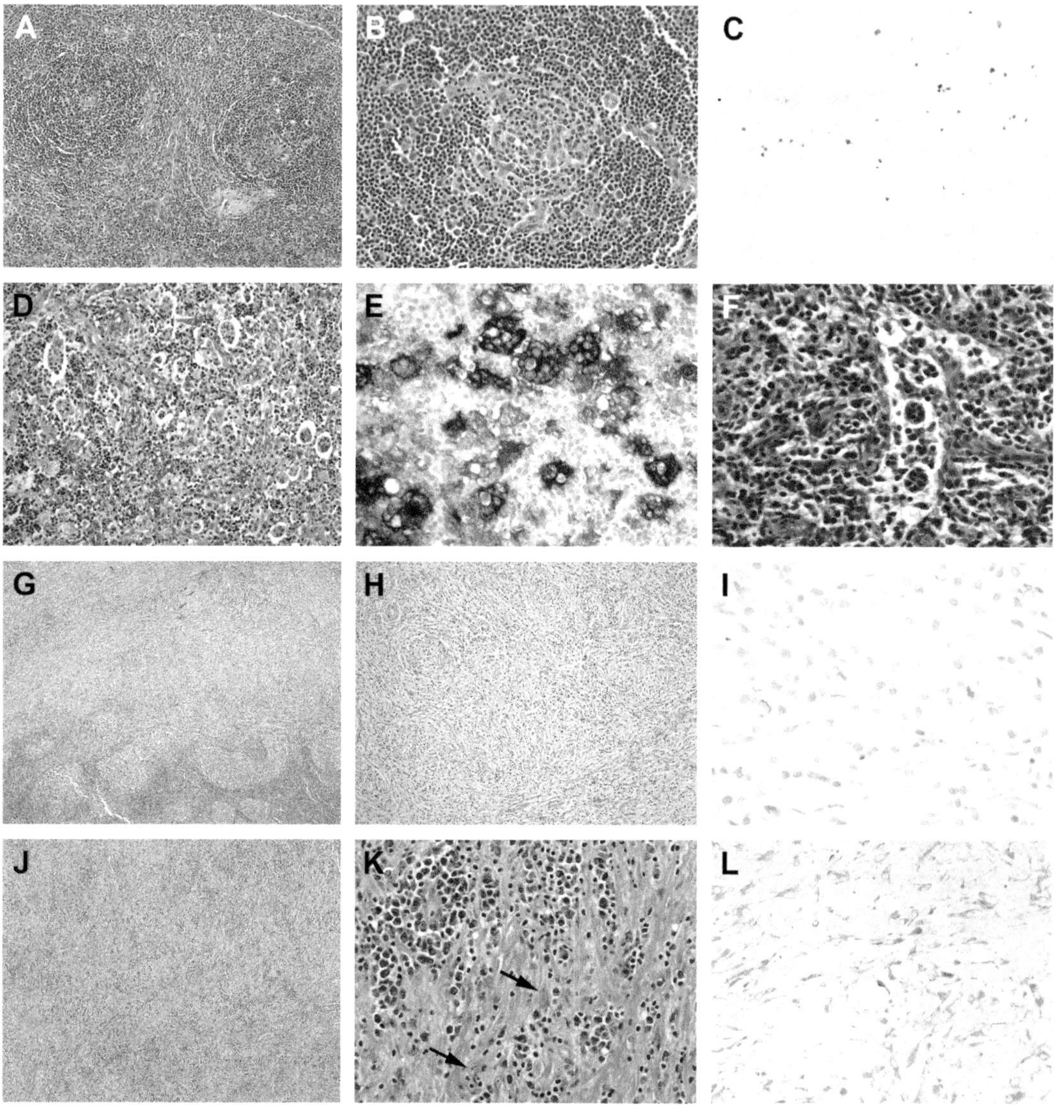

Fig. 11. Differential diagnosis of IgG4-related lymphadenopathy and IgG4-RD. HHV8-associated multicentric Castleman disease (*A–C*) showing atrophic/regressive follicles with interfollicular plasmacytosis (*A*). Large plasmablastic cells are seen around the atrophic follicles (*B*) that express HHV8 (*C*). Rosai–Dorfman disease (*D, E*) with enlarged histiocytes with conspicuous emperipolesis surrounding mixed inflammation including many plasma cells (*D*). The atypical histiocytes express S100 (*E*). Very rarely, a few histiocytes with features of emperipolesis may be seen in lymph nodes from patients with established IgG4-related disease (*F*). Syphilitic lymphadenitis (*G–I*) with marked capsular and parenchymal fibrosis (*G*) with abundant plasmacytic infiltrate and regions of storiform fibrosis (*H*). Treponema immunohistochemistry (*I*) highlights spirochetes confirming the diagnosis of syphilis. IMT (*J–L*) mimicking IgG4-related disease with marked fibrosis and plasmacytosis including foci of storiform fibrosis (*J, K*). Stromal cells demonstrate cytologic atypia (*K, arrows*), a finding not seen in IgG4-RD that should prompt consideration of IMT. Immunohistochemistry for ALK1 (*L*) highlights the atypical stromal cells. (Images J–K courtesy of Dr Vikram Deshpande.)

associated with expanded follicular dendritic cell meshworks, and have clonally rearranged T-cell receptor genes, *TRG* and/or *TRB*.[58] IgG4-positive plasma cells are not typically increased in AITL.[57] Interestingly, EBV-positive cells may be increased in IgG4-related lymphadenopathy, similar to AITL.[57]

Inflammatory myofibroblastic tumor (IMT) may demonstrate marked fibrosis that is storiform in pattern, obliterative phlebitis, and markedly increased IgG4-positive plasma cells, resulting in misdiagnosis as IgG4-RD.[34] The presence of cytologically atypical myofibroblastic cells is not a feature of IgG4-RD and should prompt consideration of IMT (see **Fig. 11**). Immunohistochemistry for ALK1 and ROS1 and/or FISH or molecular fusion analysis may help to identify the genetic abnormality of IMT and confirm that diagnosis.[34]

OTHER ENTITIES

Increased IgG4-positive plasma cells may be present in nodal and extranodal sites in a wide number of disorders other than IgG4-RD. These include chronic smoldering infections such as aortitis, sialadenitis, and mastoiditis,[59,60] Kimura disease,[61] angiolymphoid hyperplasia with eosinophilia,[62] and vasculitis including granulomatosis with polyangiitis and eosinophilic granulomatosis with polyangiitis,[63] among others.

SUMMARY

The finding of increased IgG4-positive plasma cells within lymph nodes is not specific for IgG4-RD and may be seen in a range of reactive and neoplastic conditions including IgG4-expressing lymphoproliferative disorders. The term "IgG4-related lymphadenopathy" should therefore be used to indicate lymphadenopathy occurring in a person with established IgG4-RD rather than as a general term for increased IgG4-positive plasma cells in lymph nodes from patients without known IgG4-RD. Although recognition of the described morphologic patterns of IgG4-related lymphadenopathy, including CD-like, follicular hyperplasia, PTGC-like, interfollicular expansion, and inflammatory pseudotumor-like patterns, is useful to prompt consideration of IgG4-related lymphadenopathy, many of these patterns overlap with nonspecific causes of reactive lymphadenopathy. The finding of increased IgG4-positive plasma cells (>100 per HPF) and IgG4/IgG ratio >40% within expanded interfollicular or fibrotic regions of a lymph node appears to be the most specific feature for IgG4-RD. In general, an initial diagnosis of IgG4-RD should not be made based solely on lymph node morphology. Correlation with laboratory and clinical features, including serum IgG4 levels and investigation for extranodal fibroinflammatory lesions, is indicated when morphologic features suggestive of IgG4-related lymphadenopathy are identified in a patient without previously established IgG4-RD. When considering a diagnosis of IgG4-related lymphadenopathy, knowledge of the differential diagnosis, including other inflammatory, immune-related, and IgG4-expressing lymphoproliferative disorders, is essential to avoid misdiagnosis.

DISCLOSURES

There are no conflicts of interest.

ACKNOWLEDGMENTS

The author would like to acknowledge Drs Vikram Deshpande and Judith Ferry for contribution of images for this review article, and general guidance in the subject of IgG4-related disease and lymphadenopathy.

REFERENCES

1. Deshpande V, Zen Y, Chan JK, et al. Consensus statement on the pathology of IgG4-related disease. Mod Pathol 2012;25:1181–92.
2. Zen Y, Nakanuma Y. IgG4-related disease: a cross-sectional study of 114 cases. Am J Surg Pathol 2010;34:1812–9.
3. Lin W, Lu S, Chen H, et al. Clinical characteristics of immunoglobulin G4–related disease: a prospective study of 118 Chinese patients. Rheumatology 2015;54:1982–90.
4. Wallace ZS, Deshpande V, Mattoo H, et al. IgG4-related disease: clinical and laboratory features in one hundred twenty-five patients. Arthritis Rheumatol 2015;67:2466–75.
5. Mattoo H, Mahajan VS, Maehara T, et al. Clonal expansion of CD4(+) cytotoxic T lymphocytes in patients with IgG4-related disease. J Allergy Clin Immunol 2016;138:825–38.
6. Mattoo H, Stone JH, Pillai S. Clonally expanded cytotoxic CD4+ T cells and the pathogenesis of IgG4-related disease. Autoimmunity 2017;50:19–24.
7. Perugino CA, Stone JH. IgG4-related disease: an update on pathophysiology and implications for clinical care. Nat Rev Rheumatol 2020;16:702–14.
8. Akiyama M, Suzuki K, Yamaoka K, et al. Number of circulating follicular helper 2 T cells correlates with IgG4 and interleukin 4 levels and plasmablast numbers in IgG4-related disease. Arthritis Rheumatol 2015;67:2476–81.
9. Akiyama M, Suzuki K, Yasuoka H, et al. Follicular helper T cells in the pathogenesis of IgG4-related disease. Rheumatology 2018;57:236–45.
10. Martínez-Valle F, Fernández-Codina A, Pinal-Fernández I, et al. IgG4-related disease: evidence from six recent cohorts. Autoimmu Rev 2017;16:168–72.
11. Uchida K, Masamune A, Shimosegawa T, et al. Prevalence of IgG4-related disease in Japan based on nationwide survey in 2009. Int J Rheumatol 2012;2012:358371.
12. Karim F, Loeffen J, Bramer W, et al. IgG4-related disease: a systematic review of this unrecognized disease in pediatrics. Pediatr Rheumatol Online J 2016;14:1460.

13. Akca ÜK, Atalay E, Cüceoğlu MK, et al. IgG4-related disease in pediatric patients: a single-center experience. Rheumatol Int 2022;42:1177–85.
14. Umehara H, Okazaki K, Masaki Y, et al. Comprehensive diagnostic criteria for IgG4-related disease (IgG4-RD), 2011. Mod Rheumatol 2012;22: 21–30.
15. Kurowecki D, Patlas MN, Haider EA, et al. Cross-sectional pictorial review of IgG4-related disease. Br J Radiology 2019;92:20190448.
16. Bledsoe JR, Ferry JA, Neyaz A, et al. IgG4-related Lymphadenopathy. Am J Surg Pathol 2021;45: 178–92.
17. Cheuk W., Zen Y., Ferry J.A., et al., IgG4-related disease. In: WHO Classification of Tumours Editorial Board. Haematolymphoid tumours [Internet; beta version ahead of print.] Lyon (France): International Agency for Research on Cancer; 2022. (WHO classification of tumours series, 5th ed.; vol. 11). Available at: https://tumourclassification.iarc.who.int/chapters/63.
18. Carruthers MN, Khosroshahi A, Augustin T, et al. The diagnostic utility of serum IgG4 concentrations in IgG4-related disease. Ann Rheum Dis 2015;74:14–8.
19. Chen LYC, Mattman A, Seidman MA, et al. IgG4-related disease: what a hematologist needs to know. Haematologica 2019;104:444–55.
20. Culver EL, Sadler R, Simpson D, et al. Elevated serum IgG4 levels in diagnosis, treatment response, organ involvement, and relapse in a prospective IgG4-related disease UK cohort. Am J Gastroenterol 2016;111:733–43.
21. Ebbo M, Grados A, Bernit E, et al. Pathologies associated with serum IgG4 elevation. Int J Rheumatol 2012;2012(8):602809.
22. Terasaki Y, Ikushima S, Matsui S, et al. Comparison of clinical and pathological features of lung lesions of systemic IgG4-related disease and idiopathic multicentric Castleman's disease. Histopathology 2017;70:1114–24.
23. Geyer JT, Niesvizky R, Jayabalan DS, et al. IgG4 plasma cell myeloma: new insights into the pathogenesis of IgG4-related disease. Mod Pathol 2014; 27:375–81.
24. Bledsoe JR, Wallace ZS, Deshpande V, et al. Atypical IgG4+ plasmacytic proliferations and lymphomas: characterization of 11 cases. Am J Clin Pathol 2017;148:215–35.
25. Venkataraman G, Rizzo KA, Chavez JJ, et al. Marginal zone lymphomas involving meningeal dura: possible link to IgG4-related diseases. Mod Pathol 2011;24:355–66.
26. Della-Torre E, Mattoo H, Mahajan VS, et al. Prevalence of atopy, eosinophilia, and IgE elevation in IgG4-related disease. Allergy 2014;69:269–72.
27. Brenner I, Roth S, Puppe B, et al. Primary cutaneous marginal zone lymphomas with plasmacytic differentiation show frequent IgG4 expression. Mod Pathol 2013;26:1568–76.
28. Bateman AC, Culver EL. IgG4-related disease-experience of 100 consecutive cases from a specialist centre. Histopathology 2017;70:798–813.
29. Strehl JD, Hartmann A, Agaimy A. Numerous IgG4-positive plasma cells are ubiquitous in diverse localised nonspecific chronic inflammatory conditions and need to be distinguished from IgG4-related systemic disorders. J Clin Pathol 2011;64: 237–43.
30. Menon MP, Evbuomwan MO, Rosai J, et al. A subset of Rosai-Dorfman disease cases show increased IgG4-positive plasma cells: another red herring or a true association with IgG4-related disease? Histopathology 2014;64:455–9.
31. Rollins-Raval MA, Felgar RE, Krasinskas AM, et al. Increased numbers of IgG4-positive plasma cells may rarely be seen in lymph nodes of patients without IgG4-related sclerosing disease. Int J Surg Pathol 2011;20:47–53.
32. Sato Y, Kojima M, Takata K, et al. Multicentric Castleman's disease with abundant IgG4-positive cells: a clinical and pathological analysis of six cases. J Clin Pathol 2010;63:1084–9.
33. Asano N, Sato Y. Rheumatoid lymphadenopathy with abundant IgG4(+) plasma cells : a case mimicking IgG4-related disease. J Clin Exp Hematop 2012;52:57–61.
34. Taylor MS, Chougule A, MacLeay AR, et al. Morphologic overlap between inflammatory myofibroblastic tumor and IgG4-related disease: lessons from next-generation sequencing. Am J Surg Pathol 2019;43:314–24.
35. Martinez LL, Friedländer E, van der Laak JAWM, et al. Abundance of IgG4+ plasma cells in isolated reactive lymphadenopathy is no indication of IgG4-related disease. Am J Clin Pathol 2014;142:459–66.
36. Cheuk W, Chan JKC. Lymphadenopathy of IgG4-related disease: an underdiagnosed and overdiagnosed entity. Semin Diagn Pathol 2012;29:226–34.
37. Cheuk W, Yuen HKL, Chu SYY, et al. Lymphadenopathy of IgG4-related sclerosing disease. Am J Surg Pathol 2008;32:671–81.
38. Sato Y, Yoshino T. IgG4-Related Lymphadenopathy. Int J Rheumatol 2012;2012:572539.
39. Chen Y-R, Chen Y-J, Wang M-C, et al. A newly recognized histologic pattern of IgG4-related lymphadenopathy: expanding the morphologic spectrum. Am J Surg Pathol 2018;42:977–82.
40. Sato Y, Notohara K, Kojima M, et al. IgG4-related disease: historical overview and pathology of hematological disorders. Pathol Int 2010;60:247–58.
41. Sato Y, Inoue D, Asano N, et al. Association between IgG4-related disease and progressively transformed germinal centers of lymph nodes. Mod Pathol 2012; 25:956–67.

42. Bateman AC, Ashton-Key MR, Jogai S. Lymph node granulomas in immunoglobulin G4-related disease. Histopathology 2015;67:557–61.
43. Geyer JT, Deshpande V. IgG4-associated sialadenitis. Curr Opin Rheumatol 2011;23:95–101.
44. Ferry JA. IgG4-related lymphadenopathy and IgG4-related lymphoma: moving targets. Diagn Histopathol 2013;19:128–39.
45. Cheuk W, Yuen HKL, Chan ACL, et al. Ocular adnexal lymphoma associated with IgG4+ chronic sclerosing dacryoadenitis: a previously undescribed complication of IgG4-related sclerosing disease. Am J Surg Pathol 2008;32:1159–67.
46. Bledsoe JR, Wallace ZS, Stone JH, et al. Lymphomas in IgG4-related disease: clinicopathologic features in a Western population. Virchows Arch 2018;472:839–52.
47. Yu T, Wu Y, Liu J, et al. The risk of malignancy in patients with IgG4-related disease: a systematic review and meta-analysis. Arthritis Res Ther 2022;24:14.
48. Takahashi N, Ghazale AH, Smyrk TC, et al. Possible association between IgG4-associated systemic disease with or without autoimmune pancreatitis and non-Hodgkin lymphoma. Pancreas 2009;38:523–6.
49. Yamamoto M, Takahashi H, Tabeya T, et al. Risk of malignancies in IgG4-related disease. Mod Rheumatol 2014;22:414–8.
50. Kubota T, Moritani S, Yoshino T, et al. Ocular adnexal marginal zone B cell lymphoma infiltrated by IgG4-positive plasma cells. J Clin Pathol 2010;63:1059–65.
51. Satou A, Notohara K, Zen Y, et al. Clinicopathological differential diagnosis of IgG4-related disease: A historical overview and a proposal of the criteria for excluding mimickers of IgG4-related disease. Pathol Int 2020;70:391–402.
52. Zoshima T, Yamada K, Hara S, et al. Multicentric Castleman disease with tubulointerstitial nephritis mimicking IgG4-related disease: two case reports. Am J Surg Pathol 2016;40:495–501.
53. Ravindran A, Goyal G, Go RS, et al. Rosai-Dorfman disease displays a unique monocyte-macrophage phenotype characterized by expression of OCT2. Am J Surg Pathology 2021;45:35–44.
54. Baraban E, Sadigh S, Rosenbaum J, et al. Cyclin D1 expression and novel mutational findings in Rosai-Dorfman disease. Brit J Haematol 2019;186:837–44.
55. Tse JY, Chan MP, Ferry JA, et al. Syphilis of the aerodigestive tract. Am J Surg Pathol 2018;42:472–8.
56. Nowak V, Agaimy A, Kristiansen G, et al. Increased IgG4-positive plasma cells in nodular-sclerosing Hodgkin lymphoma: a diagnostic pitfall. Histopathology 2019;76:244–50.
57. Takeuchi M, Sato Y, Yasui H, et al. Epstein-Barr virus–infected cells in IgG4-related lymphadenopathy with comparison with extranodal IgG4-related disease. Am J Surg Pathol 2014;38:946–55.
58. Xie Y, Jaffe ES. How I diagnose angioimmunoblastic T-cell lymphoma. Am J Clin Pathol 2021;156:1–14.
59. Siddiquee Z, Zane NA, Smith RN, et al. Dense IgG4 plasma cell infiltrates associated with chronic infectious aortitis: implications for the diagnosis of IgG4-related disease. Cardiovasc Pathol 2012;21(6):470–5.
60. Deshpande V, Zane NA, Kraft S, et al. Recurrent mastoiditis mimics IgG4 related disease: a potential diagnostic pitfall. Head Neck Pathol 2016;10:314–20.
61. Wang X, Ng C, Yin W. A comparative study of Kimura's disease and IgG4-related disease: similarities, differences and overlapping features. Histopathology 2021;79:801–9.
62. Hamaguchi Y, Fujimoto M, Matsushita Y, et al. IgG4-related skin disease, a mimic of angiolymphoid hyperplasia with eosinophilia. Dermatology 2012;223:301–5.
63. Ferry JA, Klepeis V, Sohani AR, et al. IgG4-related orbital disease and its mimics in a Western population. Am J Surg Pathol 2015;39:1688–700.

Hematopathology of Severe Acute Respiratory Syndrome Coronavirus 2 Infection and Coronavirus Disease-19

Fabienne Lucas, MD, PhD, Sam Sadigh, MD*

KEYWORDS

• COVID-19 • SARS-CoV-2 • Neutrophilia • Lymphopenia • Dysgranulopoiesis
• Atypical lymphocytes • Lymphadenopathy • Hemophagocytic lymphohistiocytosis

- Coronavirus disease 2019 (COVID-19) disease is accompanied by an array of hematologic alterations.
- Peripheral blood abnormalities are present in most COVID-19 patients but are heterogeneous. They very often include neutrophilia, lymphopenia, myeloid left shift, abnormally segmented neutrophils, atypical lymphocytes/plasmacytoid lymphocytes, and atypical monocytes.
- Bone marrow biopsies and aspirates may show left-shifted maturation, occasional erythroid dysplasia, and evidence of hemophagocytic lymphohistiocytosis.
- Secondary lymphoid organs often show lost/hypoplastic germinal centers, altered lymphocyte compositions, sinus histiocytosis/hemophagocytosis, and plasmacytoid proliferations.

ABSTRACT

Coronavirus disease 2019 is caused by severe acute respiratory syndrome coronavirus 2 and is associated with pronounced hematopathologic findings. Peripheral blood features are heterogeneous and very often include neutrophilia, lymphopenia, myeloid left shift, abnormally segmented neutrophils, atypical lymphocytes/plasmacytoid lymphocytes, and atypical monocytes. Bone marrow biopsies and aspirates are often notable for histiocytosis and hemophagocytosis, whereas secondary lymphoid organs may exhibit lymphocyte depletion, pronounced plasmacytoid infiltrates, and hemophagocytosis. These changes are reflective of profound innate and adaptive immune dysregulation, and ongoing research efforts continue to identify clinically applicable biomarkers of disease severity and outcome.

OVERVIEW

Individuals with coronavirus disease 2019 (COVID-19), the disease caused by severe acute respiratory syndrome coronavirus 2 (SARS-CoV-2), exhibit a range of pulmonary, cerebral, myocardial, hepatic, and renal dysfunctions. Large-scale autopsy studies have documented multi-organ pathology findings[1,2] with substantial remodeling in lung epithelial, immune, and stromal compartments and evidence of multiple paths of failed tissue regeneration.[3] SARS-CoV-2 infection is also associated with pronounced hematologic alterations. During acute infection, peripheral blood abnormalities are present that occur in a complex network of innate and adaptive immune dysregulation,[4] some of which can serve as clinical biomarkers of disease severity and outcome.[5,6] Secondary lymphoid organs often show lymphocyte depletion and

Department of Pathology, Brigham and Women's Hospital, 75 Francis Street, Boston, MA 02115, USA
* Corresponding author:
E-mail address: ssadigh@bwh.harvard.edu

Surgical Pathology 16 (2023) 197–211
https://doi.org/10.1016/j.path.2023.01.007

occasionally hemophagocytosis.[7,8] Hemophagocytic lymphohistiocytosis (HLH) is also common in bone marrow biopsies and aspirates.[9–11] We herein review currently well-established and clinically relevant hematopathologic findings in patients with COVID-19 and discuss their diagnostic and prognostic relevance. Although COVID-19 is also associated with pronounced hemostasis-/thrombosis-related changes, a review of this comprehensive topic is beyond the scope of this article and can be found elsewhere.[12]

PERIPHERAL BLOOD FEATURES

QUANTITATIVE CHANGES

Peripheral blood key features are summarized in **Box 1**. Initial studies reported that complete blood counts (CBCs) and white blood cell differential counts from patients admitted with COVID-19 were notable for leukocytosis, absolute neutrophilia, and lymphopenia, especially in the intensive care unit (ICU) compared with non-ICU patients.[13–15] Early meta-analyses confirmed that lymphopenia is frequent in acute COVID-19,[16,17] and that patients with severe and fatal disease had significantly increased white blood counts (WBCs) and absolute neutrophil counts (ANCs), decreased absolute lymphocyte counts (ALCs), platelet and eosinophil counts, and decreased hemoglobin compared with those with non-severe disease and survivors.[17] In subsequent single-institution studies, lymphopenia, neutrophilia, and thrombocytopenia remained prominent features,[18–21] while eosinopenia and monocytosis occurred at highly varying frequencies.[19–21]

When directly compared with SARS-CoV-2 negative patients, WBCs in SARS-CoV-2-positive patients varied widely but were generally lower.[22–25] Similarly, lymphopenia was frequent, and ALCs tended to be lower when compared with SARS-CoV-2-negative patients, but often failed to reach statistical significance.[22–26] Neutrophilia was frequent, and ANCs were not significantly different from negative patients in some,[22–24] but significantly lower in other studies.[25] In some studies, significantly lower absolute eosinophil,[24–26] basophil,[25] and monocyte counts[23,25] were present in positive patients. Hemoglobin values appeared to be highly variable, and findings included anemia in a proportion of SARS-CoV-2-positive patients,[22,24,26,27] but also increased hemoglobin in other populations.[23,25]

QUALITATIVE CHANGES

Qualitative (morphologic) changes affecting all cell lineages are found in blood smears from up to 100% of patients with COVID-19 (see **Box 1**), including circulating apoptotic cells.[6] One of the most striking findings is dysgranulopoiesis (**Fig. 1**). Neutrophils demonstrate a range of abnormal nuclear shapes, such as pseudo-Pelger–Huët morphology, nuclear hyposegmentation or hypersegmentation, and ring-shaped nuclei.[18–20,23,24,26–28] Abnormal granulation patterns are frequent.[18–20,22–24,26,27,29] Several studies reported apoptotic, pyknotic, disintegrating, or smudged neutrophils,[18,21,22,24,26] potentially reflecting neutrophil extracellular traps (NET), enzymatic webs released by activated neutrophils.[30] In addition, left-shifted myeloid cells can be found, occasionally with leukoerythroblastosis (**Fig. 2**).[18,22–24,26,27,31] Pronounced morphologic changes are also present within the lymphoid lineage (see **Fig. 2**), and several types of atypical and/or enlarged lymphocytes have been observed.[6,20,23,24,26,27] These include plasmacytoid lymphocytes, occasionally with bizarre-shaped nuclei and pseudopods,[20,23,24,26,27] large granular lymphocytes (LGLs),[20,23] atypical lymphocytes,[23] and lymphocytes with pronounced cytoplasmic vacuoles.[23,26] Some studies reported a small proportion of circulating plasma cells or Mott cells.[22,26] Vacuolization, including numerous large coalescing vacuoles, has been seen in monocytes (see **Fig. 2**),[23,24,26] along with blue-green cytoplasmic inclusions.[29] Vacuolated eosinophils have been noted,[19,23] as well as increased large or giant platelets,[18,19,21,22] occasionally with pseudopodia formations.[18]

When directly compared with patients without COVID-19, the most significant morphologic findings included left-shifted myeloid cells, smudged neutrophils, neutrophil vacuolation, pseudo-Pelger–Huët anomaly, non-segmented and ring neutrophils, atypical lymphocytes, plasma cells/plasmacytic cells, pyknotic cells, and large/ giant platelets (see **Box 1**).[22,24]

MORPHOLOGY SCORES

Several morphology scores have been developed. Using abnormalities in granulocytes, lymphocytes, monocytes, maturational left shift, and pyknotic cells, with a scoring scale of zero to five, no patient with COVID-19 had score zero, whereas 27%, 42%, and 26% had score one, two, and three, respectively, with a score range of zero to two in non-COVID-19 blood smears.[26] Another study scored WBC morphology using a four-point scale

Box 1
Peripheral blood key features

Frequent quantitative changes	WBC ↕ Neutrophils ↑ Lymphocytes ↓ Eosinophils may be ↓ Basophils may be ↓ Monocytes may be ↓ Hemoglobin ↕ Platelets ↕

Frequent qualitative changes	• Atypical lymphocytes:
	  ○ Plasmacytoid[a]
	  ○ Circulating plasma cells[a]
	  ○ Large granular lymphocytes (LGLs)
	  ○ Cytoplasmic vacuoles
	• Myeloid left shift ± leukoerythroblastosis[a]
	• Smudged neutrophils[a]
	• Neutrophil vacuolation[a]
	• Abnormal neutrophil segmentation:
	  ○ Hyposegmentation or hypersegmentation[a]
	  ○ Pseudo-Pelger–Huët[a]
	  ○ Ring-shaped nuclei[a]
	• Abnormal neutrophil granulation, cytoplasmic inclusions:
	  ○ Varying toxic granulation
	  ○ Hypogranularity
	  ○ Blue-green inclusions
	  ○ Howell-Jolly body-like inclusions
	  ○ Döhle bodies
	• Large or giant platelets[a]
	• Pyknotic cells[a]
	• Eosinophils with multiple vacuoles
	• Monocyte vacuolization

Association with severe disease including death	• High WBC count
	• Increasing neutrophilia
	  ○ Higher number of left-shifted/immature granulocytes
	  ○ Ring-shaped neutrophils
	  ○ Significant toxic granulation
	• Continuing decline in ALC
	  ○ LGLs and reactive lymphocytes
	• Decline in absolute monocyte and eosinophil counts
	  ○ Monocyte vacuolization
	• Low platelet count
	• Neutrophil to lymphocyte ratio (NLR) ↑
	• Platelet to neutrophil ratio (PNR) ↑

[a] Most significant morphologic findings in COVID-19 patients when compared with patients without COVID-19.

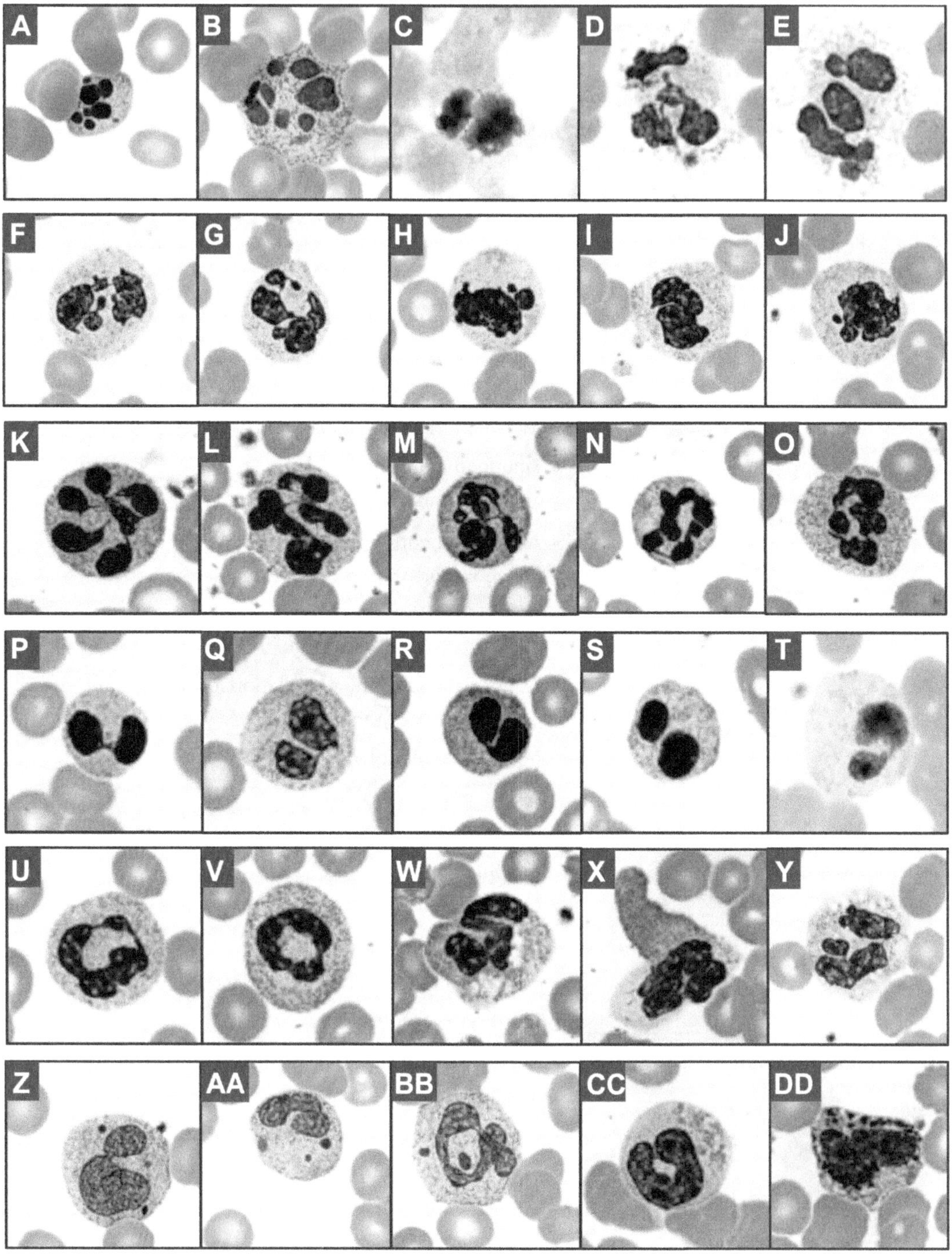

Fig. 1. Abnormal granulopoiesis in peripheral blood smears: (*A–E*) apoptotic/pyknotic, disintegrating, and smudged neutrophils; (*F–J*) abnormally segmented nuclei, including (*K–O*) hypersegmentation, (*P–T*) pseudo-Pelger–Huët morphology, and (*U, V*) ring forms. Abnormal granulation can feature (*W–Y*) toxic granules, cytoplasmic vacuolization, patchy hypogranularity, and (*Z–BB*) Döhle body-like inclusions or apparent nuclear fragments. Abnormally granulated eosinophils (*CC*) and basophils (*DD*) can be seen.

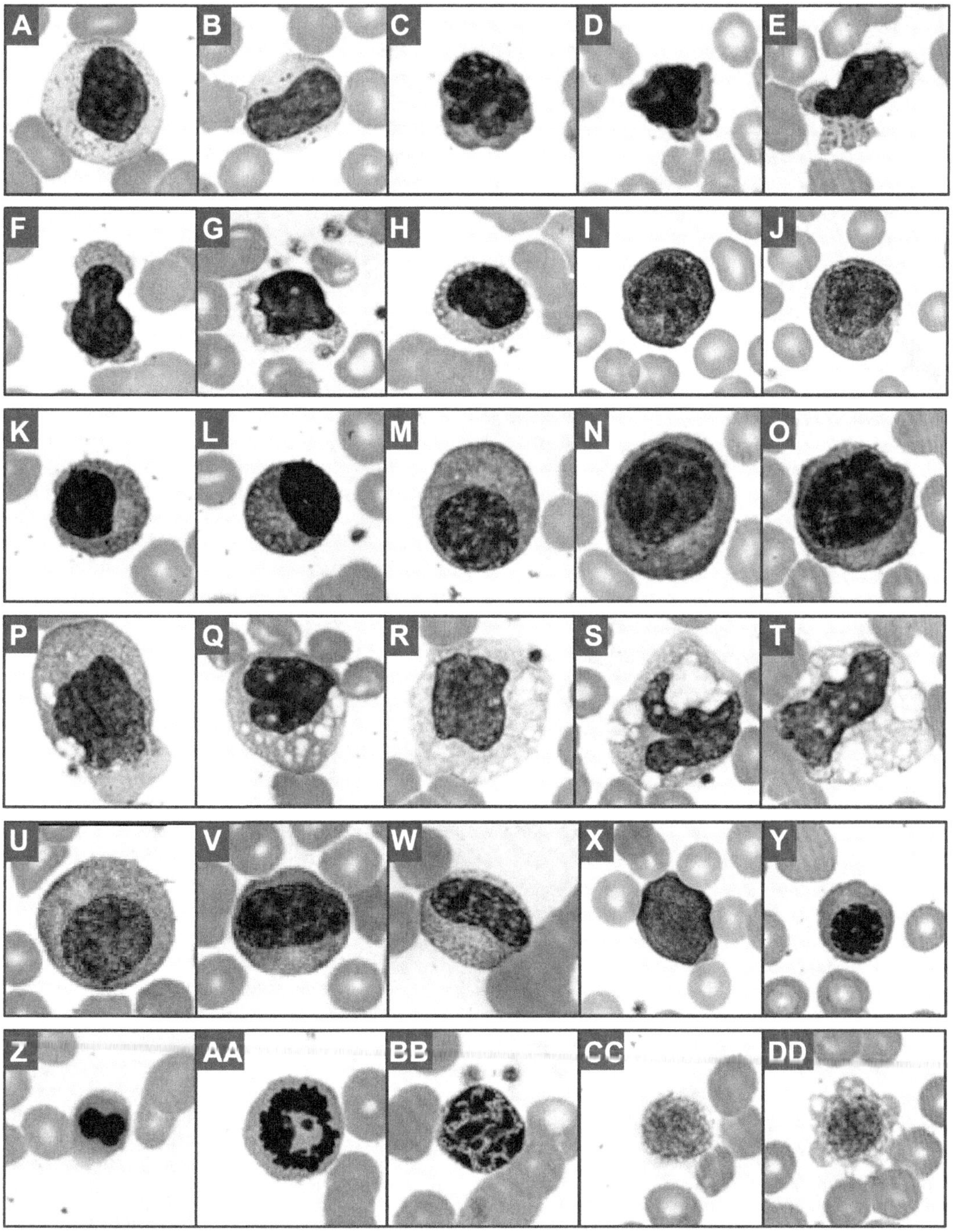

Fig. 2. Atypical lymphocytes and other COVID-19-related blood findings: (*A*, *B*) large granular lymphocytes; (*C–O*) atypical lymphocytes can show a spectrum of features, with nuclear irregularities, variably coarse chromatin, deeply basophilic cytoplasm, occasionally with cytoplasmic blebs, granules or vacuolization; (*K–O*) plasma cells or plasmacytoid forms can include irregular enlarged forms. (*P–T*) Monocytes can show coarser granules or varying degrees of prominent coalescing vacuolization. (*U–Y*) Left-shifted myeloid cells and leukoerythroblastosis; (*Z–AA*) budding erythroid nucleus and mitotic figure, (*BB*) pyknotic cell, and (*CC–DD*) giant platelets.

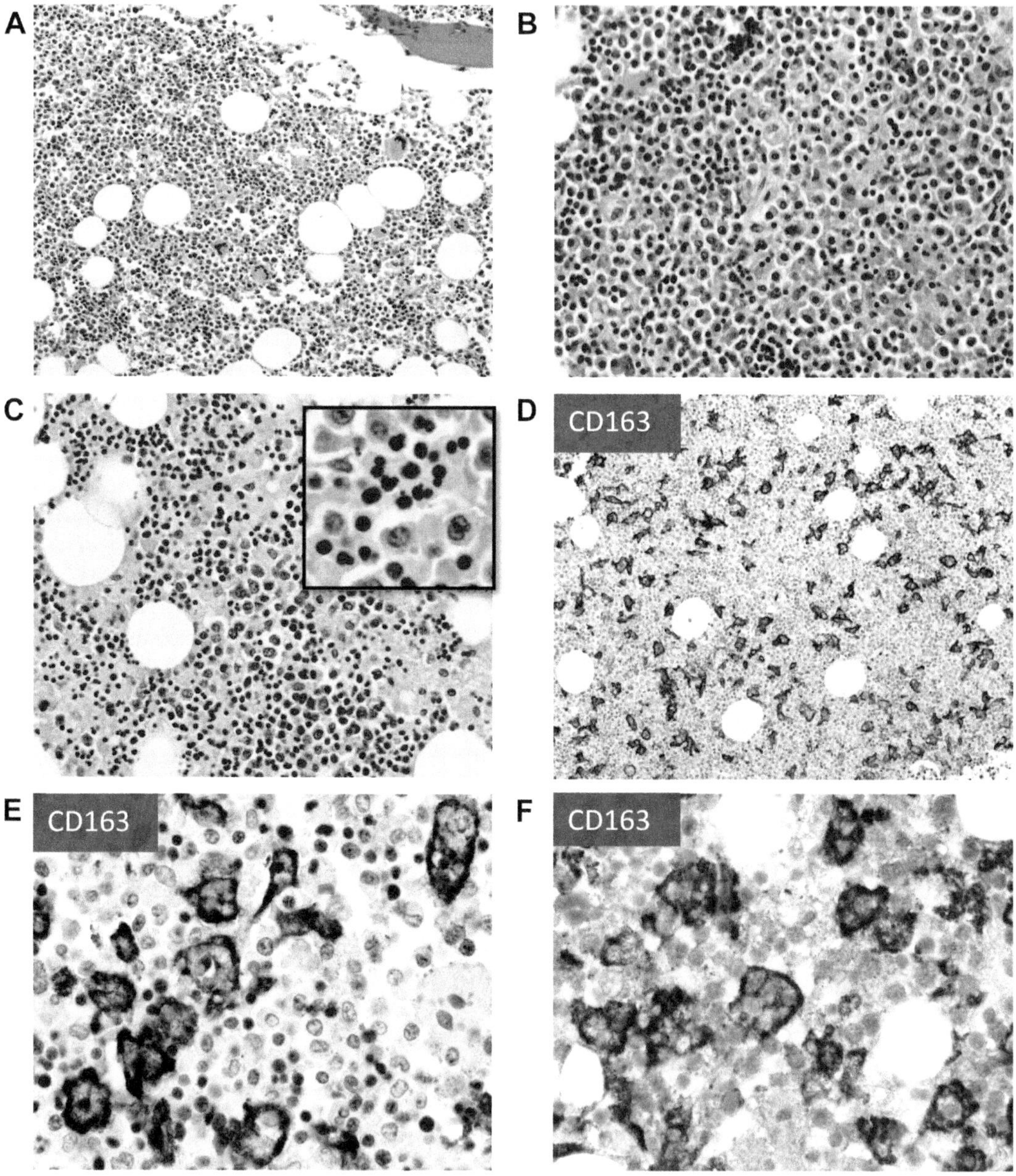

Fig. 3. Bone marrow biopsy findings: H&E sections (A–C, from four different decedents) show varying cellularity with frequent hypercellularity, maturing trilineage hematopoiesis with frequent myeloid left shift (*A*, *B*), and occasional decreased M:E ratio (*C*). There may be pronounced dyserythropoiesis (*C-inlay*) and varying degrees of histiocytosis and hemophagocytosis that may not be readily appreciated on H&E sections but are unearthed with immunohistochemistry for histiocytic markers (eg, CD163) (*D*, *E*). Autopsy cases kindly provided by Dr Olga Pozdnyakova.

(0: absent; 1: present in ≤10% of cell lineage; 2: present in 11% to 25%; 3: present in >25%).[23] When directly compared with negative ICU patients, positive patients showed significantly fewer monocytes with abnormal vacuolization, whereas the presence of atypical lymphocytes, especially plasmacytoid forms, was more predictive of COVID-19 infection.

ASSOCIATION WITH DISEASE SEVERITY AND OUTCOME

Several parameters and ratios between blood cells have been associated with disease severity and outcome, including death[23–26,32–34] (see **Box 1**). When applying the score by Gabr and colleagues, patients with higher scores had

Box 2
Key features in spleen and lymph nodes

Spleen	• White pulp atrophy or depletion • Absence of marginal zones • Increased ratio of red: white pulp • Lymphoplasmacytic infiltrates • Immunoblast infiltrates • Red pulp necrosis • Red pulp congestion • Hemorrhage	• Defective germinal centers • Absence of TFH cells • Altered lymphocyte subsets • Hemophagocytosis • Extramedullary megakaryocytes
Lymph nodes	• Lymphocyte depletion • Absent or hypoplastic germinal centers • Sinus histiocytosis • Increased immunoblasts and plasmablasts • Vascular congestion with vascular transformation of sinuses • Hemorrhage	

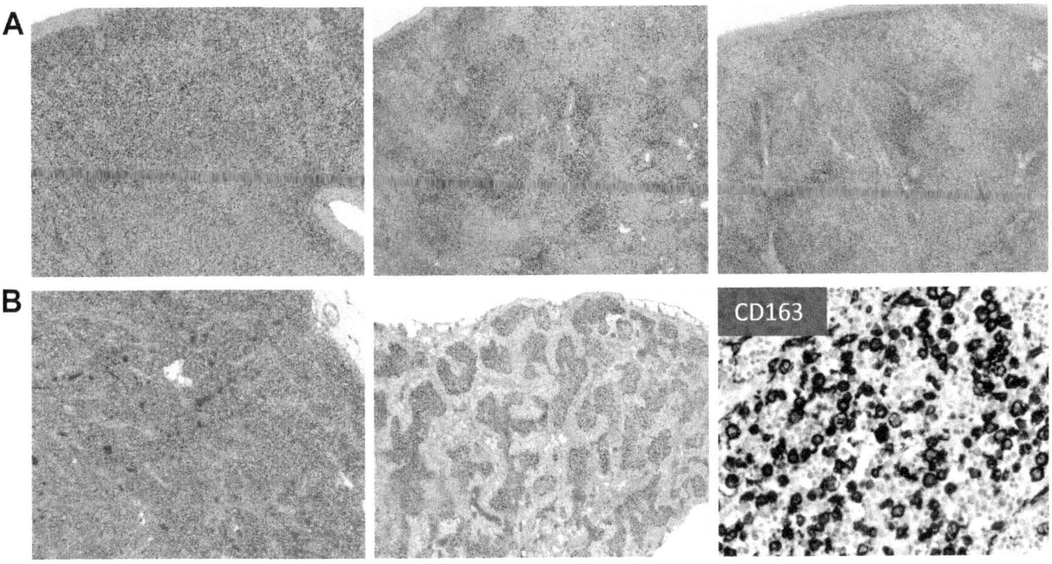

Fig. 4. Common findings in spleen (*A*) and lymph node (*B*): Spleens show diminished white pulp and increased red-to-white pulp ratio, with areas of hemorrhage (*A*). On low magnification, lymph nodes show attenuation of follicular architecture (*B*, *left*) and varying degrees of sinus histiocytosis (*B*, *middle*), with some cases also showing prominent hemophagocytosis (*B*, *right*, highlighted by CD163).

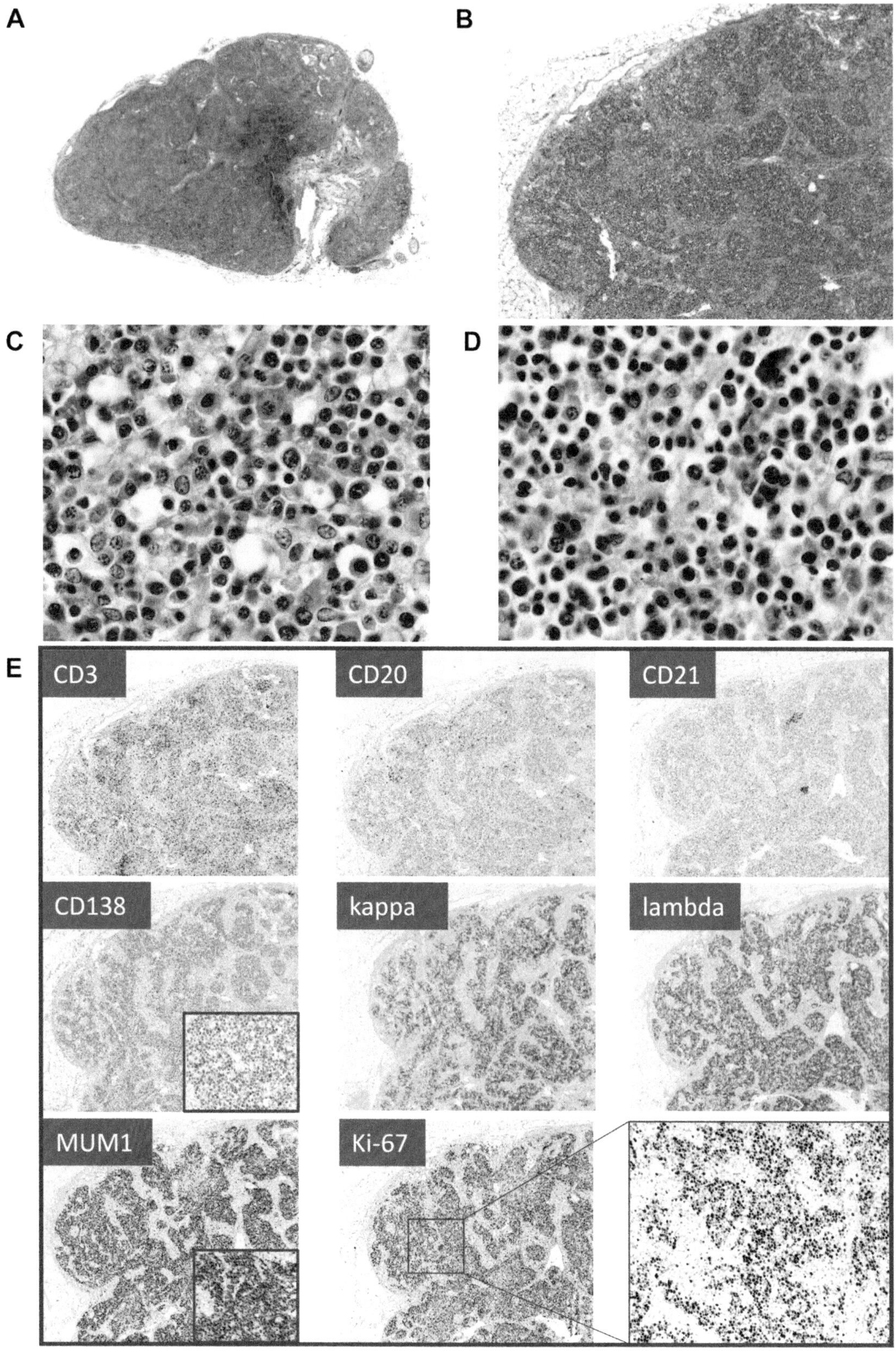

Fig. 5. Lymph node showing lymphocyte depletion and prominent polyclonal plasmacytosis with increased proliferation in acute infection: (*A*, *B*) show an architecturally intact lymph node with patent subcapsular and

generally unfavorable outcomes.[26] Myeloid left shift was associated with requiring ICU admission, whereas atypical lymphocytes and monocytes with large coalescent cytoplasmic vacuoles were associated with non-ICU patients in one study.[23] In contrast, Gabr and colleagues found significantly more atypical monocytes in ICU patients,[26] whereas Pezeshki and colleagues did not identify any statistically significant associations between blood findings and clinical course.[21] Importantly, several non-hematologic factors (eg, age, gender), and other laboratory parameters (including ferritin, C-reactive protein, interleukin-6) are often associated with death, and machine learning-based algorithms have been employed for diagnosis and prediction of care needs and outcome.[35–37]

BONE MARROW FEATURES

Examination of bone marrow aspirations and biopsies from individuals with COVID-19 showed varying cellularity (normocellular to hypercellular), mostly maturing trilineage hematopoiesis with occasional myeloid left shift, occasional dyserythropoiesis, increased pleomorphic megakaryocytes with focal clustering, increased polyclonal plasma cells, lymphocytosis, and varying degrees of histiocytosis and hemophagocytosis[8–11,38,39] (Fig. 3). The latter is an important finding as it provides histopathologic evidence of secondary development of HLH, a life-threatening inflammatory syndrome associated with significant mortality. Based on these findings, it has been suggested to promptly perform bone marrow aspiration and biopsy in COVID-19 patients with suspected HLH to guide appropriate treatment.[11]

SPLEEN AND LYMPH NODE FEATURES

ACUTE INFECTION

The key features are summarized in Box 2 and Fig. 4. Several autopsy studies have described splenic white pulp atrophy or depletion, absence of marginal zones, increased red-to-white pulp ratio, and hemophagocytosis in a subset of COVID-19 decedents.[7,8] In addition, varying degrees of lymphoplasmacytic infiltrates in the red pulp and immunoblasts in the white pulp were noted. Other occasional findings included extensive red pulp necrosis, red pulp congestion, and frank hemorrhage.[40]

Similarly, lymphocyte depletion or absence of germinal centers and hemophagocytosis (see Fig. 4) are frequent in lymph nodes (approximately 20% of patients).[8] When present, germinal centers may be hypoplastic, whereas sinus histiocytosis and increased immunoblasts and plasmablasts are frequently noted in sinuses and within the paracortex.[7,8,40] Other features may include vascular congestion with vascular transformation of sinuses and hemorrhage.[40] Immunohistochemistry (IHC)-based studies further highlighted a defect of germinal center structure, with T-follicular helper (TFH) cells and germinal center formation largely absent in draining hilar lymph nodes, which correlated with reduced Immunoglobulin M (IgM) and Immunoglobulin G (IgG) levels compared with convalescent COVID-19 patients.[41] Another study demonstrated decreased T lymphocytes in most examined lymph nodes, with a disproportionate decrease of CD8+ T cells, and relative preservation of B lymphocytes.[40]

A comprehensive analysis of lymphoid architecture and lymphocyte populations of thoracic lymph nodes and spleens from patients with early and late COVID-19 revealed the absence of lymph node and splenic germinal centers and depletion of Bcl-6-expressing B cells, but the preservation of activation-induced cytidine deaminase-positive B cells.[42] In addition, Bcl-6+ TFH-cell generation and differentiation were defective, whereas abundant T-helper 1 (TH1) cells and aberrant TNF-alpha production were seen. Interestingly, extramedullary megakaryocytes and clusters of erythroid precursors were noted in several studies,[38,40] and their role in COVID-19-related hemostatic and thrombotic alterations is an area of active research.

Fig. 5 highlights a lymph node showing lymphocyte depletion and prominent plasmacytosis with an increased proliferation rate. Despite being polyclonal, plasma cells and plasmacytoid forms can

medullary sinuses, many with reactive histiocytosis. There are almost no apparent follicles and lymphocytes are diminished, with the parenchyma (*C, D*) mostly replaced by a population of small to medium-sized plasma cells and plasmacytoid forms with occasional markedly enlarged, hyperchromatic nuclei or binucleated forms, as well as ones with more dispersed chromatin and prominent nucleoli. (*E*) CD3+ T cells and CD20+ B cells are markedly reduced, with only rare CD21+ follicular dendritic cell meshworks. The plasma cell population shows dim-to-negative CD138, uniform MUM1 expression, and considerably increased Ki-67 proliferation (approximately 50%) but polytypic kappa and lambda light chain expression.

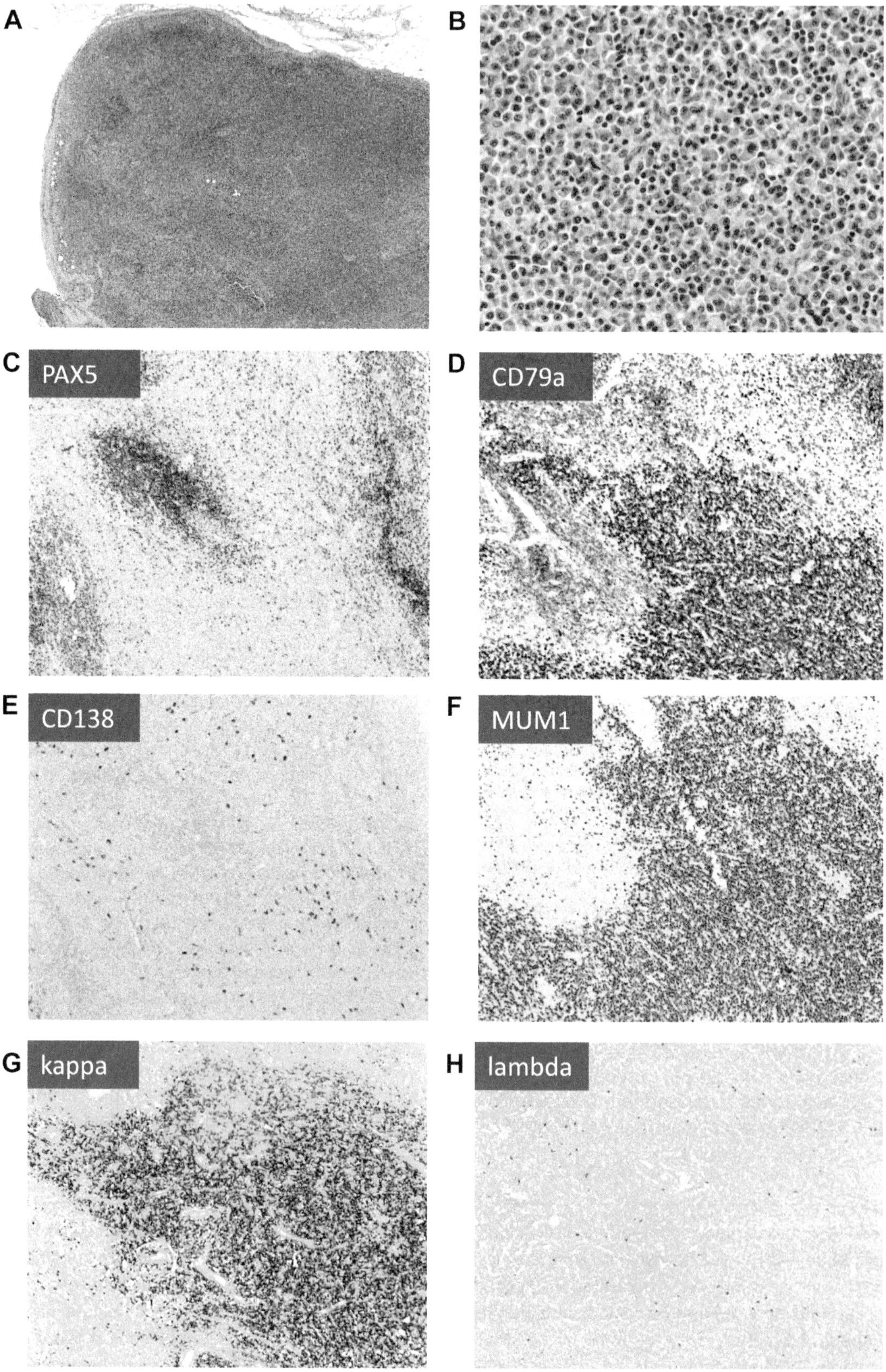

Fig. 6. Kappa-predominant plasmacytoid proliferation in a patient with a history of lymphoma: A patient with stage IV diffuse large B-cell lymphoma developed new FDG-avid lymphadenopathy concerning recurrent lymphoma (note: case has previously been published,[55] new images were taken for this publication with permission).

be markedly enlarged, include hyperchromatic and binucleated forms, and show a plasmablast-like immunophenotype (MUM1+, CD138 variable/negative). These features can pose a diagnostic challenge, especially in patients with pre-existing hematologic conditions, and extensive ancillary studies may be warranted to exclude a neoplastic process (Fig. 6). Similarly, careful exclusion of an underlying malignancy, or autoimmune or infectious disease, is advised in the workup of mediastinal lymphadenopathy, which has been noted in up to 66% of patients with COVID-19 and is frequently associated with inferior outcomes.[43,44]

COVID-19 POST-VACCINATION LYMPHADENOPATHY

There is a growing body of evidence highlighting the diagnostic dilemmas related to COVID-19 post-vaccination lymphadenopathy. This often affects axillary lymph nodes at the ipsilateral injection site and occurs at an overall rate of 14%, but varies widely in published cohort studies and clinical trials.[45] Although ultimately there is spontaneous resolution, the reported duration varies, and lymphadenopathy post-COVID-19 vaccination can persist for weeks[45,46] or even months.[47] To avoid unnecessary workup, especially in women undergoing routine breast cancer screening and patients with a pre-existing malignancy, recommendations for imaging and imaging-based additional workup have been developed.[48] In individuals who underwent a biopsy for further workup, cytologic smears and histologic sections have generally shown reactive features with follicular hyperplasia, prominent germinal centers, and paracortical expansion[49–51] (Fig. 7). However, rare cases of lymphoma have been described, highlighting that malignancy should remain an important differential diagnostic consideration.[52,53]

ANCILLARY TESTING: FLOW CYTOMETRY

A plethora of cytometry-based studies has explored COVID-19-associated immune-subset alterations. Although currently not clinically used, this has provided meaningful insights into disease pathogenesis, severity, and outcome.[54] Flow cytometry testing has been employed in various patient cohorts and settings, and the available knowledge continues to rapidly evolve. A comprehensive and up-to-date review is, therefore, beyond the scope of this article.

DIFFERENTIAL DIAGNOSIS

The differential diagnosis of COVID-19 generally includes infection with another pathogen, co-infection, and other inflammatory conditions. The findings of left-shifted myeloid lineage cells, leukoerythroblastosis, and enlarged platelets point to early release of immature forms from the bone marrow, reflecting a stress response that may be seen in several infectious and inflammatory conditions. Ultimately, microbiology and laboratory studies are required for further workup.

Lymphadenopathy or splenomegaly in the setting of COVID-19 infection, recovery, or vaccination is likely a reactive feature. However, underlying malignancy, autoimmune conditions, or infectious (particularly viral) lymphadenopathies cannot be completely excluded, and clinical correlation and ancillary studies are needed.

SUMMARY

The inflammatory response to COVID-19 infection is reflected in prominent hematopathologic alterations. Peripheral blood findings are heterogeneous, but several alterations have emerged as markers for disease severity and outcome. Bone marrow biopsies and aspirates may show varying degrees of histiocytosis and hemophagocytosis, whereas myeloid left shift is frequent, and erythroid dysplasia might be present. Lymph node and spleen germinal centers are often hypoplastic or absent, and lymphocyte compositions may be altered. In addition, the presence of plasmacytoid proliferations with plasmablast-like immunophenotypes might require extensive workup to exclude malignancy. As knowledge continues to evolve, more specific diagnostic or predictive

H&E sections (*A, B*) show an interfollicular expansion by numerous small lymphocytes, epithelioid histiocytes, and focal sheets of plasmacytoid cells variably positive for PAX5 (*C*), positive for CD79a (*D*), negative for CD138 (*E*), and positive for MUM1 (*F*) with marked excess kappa (*G*) light chain expression compared with lambda (*H*). However, molecular studies showed polyclonal immunoglobulin heavy chain gene (*IGH*) rearrangements, absence of clonal aberrancies by cytogenetics, and lymphadenopathy resolved over time without evidence of lymphoma recurrence.

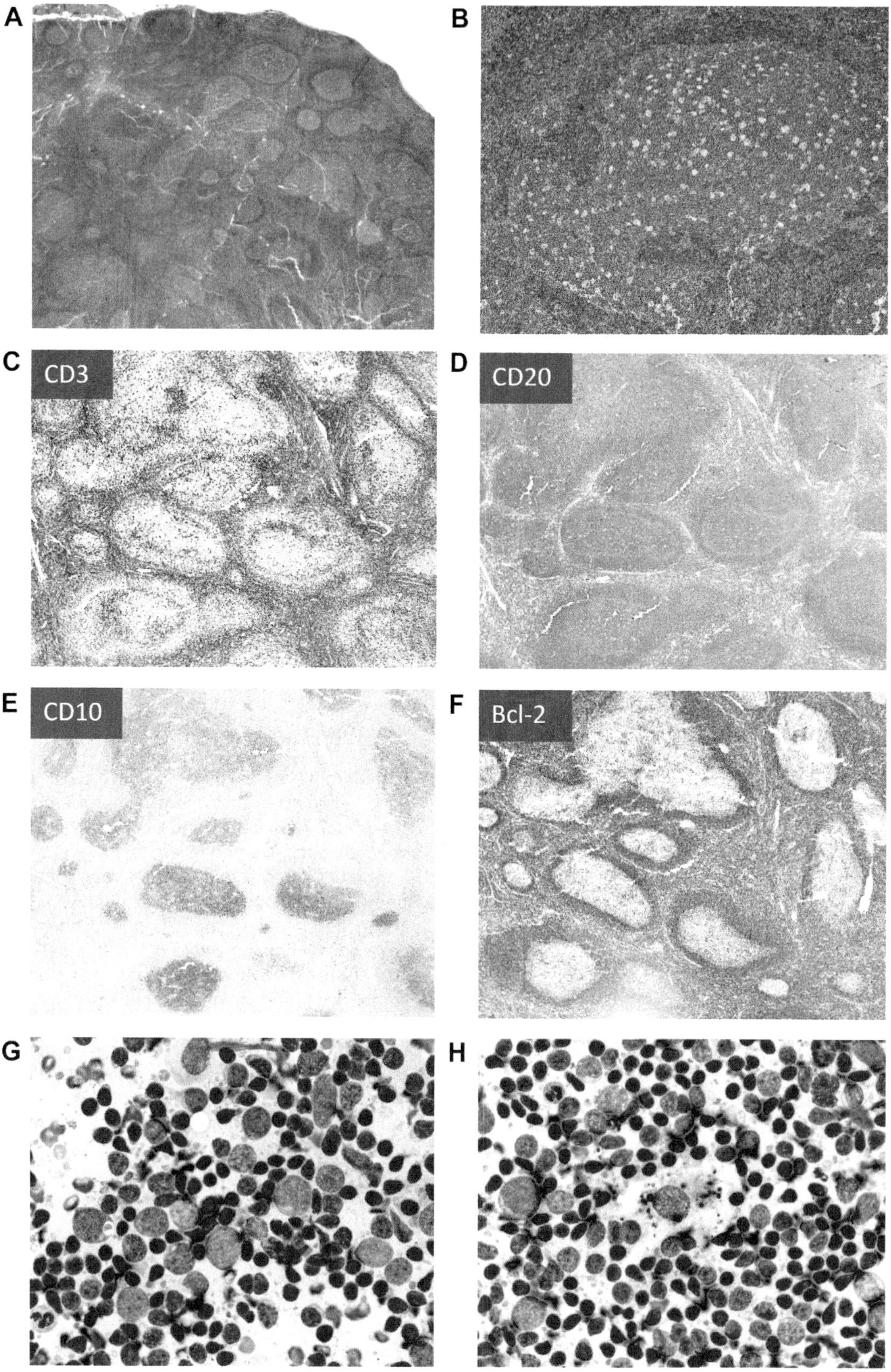

Fig. 7. Histologic and cytologic findings of COVID-19 vaccine-related lymphadenopathy: An individual in their twenties suddenly developed axillary, cervical, and supraclavicular lymphadenopathy (up to 2 cm in greatest dimension) 1 week after receiving the second mRNA COVID-19 vaccine in the deltoid muscle. H&E sections (*A*, *B*) and IHC for CD3 (*C*), CD20 (*D*), CD10 (*E*), and Bcl-2 (*F*) of lymph nodes (ipsilateral to vaccine site) show marked

biomarkers that are amenable for clinical diagnostic testing will likely appear.

CLINICS CARE POINTS

Key points

- Peripheral blood abnormalities can be heterogeneous and dynamic, depending on the disease course and disease severity (see Box 1).
- Serial CBCs with comprehensive morphologic analysis might predict the disease course and clinical severity in newly-diagnosed hospitalized COVID-19 patients.
- A clinical suspicion of HLH may necessitate bone marrow aspiration and biopsy in COVID-19 patients, and IHC for histiocyte markers may be helpful to visualize hemophagocytosis.
- Secondary lymphatic organs may show pronounced atypical features and must be distinguished from other viral lymphadenopathies and malignancies.

DISCLOSURE

The authors have nothing to disclose. Written permission was obtained for select cases.

REFERENCES

1. Hooper JE, Padera RF, Dolhnikoff M, et al. A Postmortem Portrait of the Coronavirus Disease 2019 (COVID-19) Pandemic: A Large Multi-institutional Autopsy Survey Study. Arch Pathol Lab Med 2021;145(5):529–35.
2. von Stillfried S, Bülow RD, Röhrig R, et al, German Registry of COVID-19 Autopsies (DeRegCOVID), DeRegCOVID Collaborators. First report from the German COVID-19 autopsy registry. Lancet Reg Health Eur 2022;15:100330.
3. Delorey TM, Ziegler CGK, Heimberg G, et al. COVID-19 tissue atlases reveal SARS-CoV-2 pathology and cellular targets. Nature 2021;595(7865):107–13.
4. Ahern DJ, Ai Z, Ainsworth M, et al. A blood atlas of COVID-19 defines hallmarks of disease severity and specificity. Cell 2022;185(5):916–38.e58.
5. Terpos E, Ntanasis-Stathopoulos I, Elalamy I, et al. Hematological findings and complications of COVID-19. Am J Hematol 2020;95(7):834–47.
6. Bell R, Zini G, d'Onofrio G, et al. The hematology laboratory's response to the COVID-19 pandemic: A scoping review. Int J Lab Hematol 2021;43(2):148–59.
7. Satturwar S, Fowkes M, Farver C, et al. Postmortem Findings Associated With SARS-CoV-2: Systematic Review and Meta-analysis. Am J Surg Pathol 2021;45(5):587–603.
8. Hammoud H, Bendari A, Bendari T, et al. Histopathological Findings in COVID-19 Cases: A Systematic Review. Cureus 2022;14(6):e25573.
9. Harris CK, Hung YP, Nielsen GP, et al. Bone Marrow and Peripheral Blood Findings in Patients Infected by SARS-CoV-2. Am J Clin Pathol 2021;155(5):627–37.
10. Dandu H, Yadav G, Malhotra HS, et al. Hemophagocytic histiocytosis in severe SARS-CoV-2 infection: A bone marrow study. Int J Lab Hematol 2021;43(6):1291–301.
11. Ioannou M, Zacharouli K, Doukas SG, et al. Hemophagocytic lymphohistiocytosis diagnosed by bone marrow trephine biopsy in living post-COVID-19 patients: case report and mini-review. J Mol Histol 2022;53(4):753–62.
12. Conway EM, Mackman N, Warren RQ, et al. Understanding COVID-19-associated coagulopathy. Nat Rev Immunol 2022;22(10):639–49.
13. Huang C, Wang Y, Li X, et al. Clinical features of patients infected with 2019 novel coronavirus in Wuhan, China. Lancet Lond Engl 2020;395(10223):497–506.
14. Guan W jie, Ni Z, Hu Y, et al. Clinical Characteristics of Coronavirus Disease 2019 in China. N Engl J Med 2020;382(18):1708–20.
15. Fan BE, Chong VCL, Chan SSW, et al. Hematologic parameters in patients with COVID-19 infection. Am J Hematol 2020;95(6):E131–4.
16. Rodriguez-Morales AJ, Cardona-Ospina JA, Gutiérrez-Ocampo E, et al. Clinical, laboratory and imaging features of COVID-19: A systematic review and meta-analysis. Travel Med Infect Dis 2020;34:101623.
17. Henry BM, de Oliveira MHS, Benoit S, et al. Hematologic, biochemical and immune biomarker abnormalities associated with severe illness and

reactive lymphoid hyperplasia. Aspirate smears (*G, H*) show a polymorphous mixture of small and large lymphocytes, occasional admixed inflammatory cells, tingible-body macrophages, and lymphoglandular bodies (cytoplasmic fragments). Case and images kindly provided by Dr Amy Duffield.

mortality in coronavirus disease 2019 (COVID-19): a meta-analysis. Clin Chem Lab Med CCLM 2020; 58(7):1021–8.
18. Zini G, Bellesi S, Ramundo F, et al. Morphological anomalies of circulating blood cells in COVID-19. Am J Hematol 2020;95(7):870–2.
19. Ahnach M, Ousti F, Nejjari S, et al. Peripheral Blood Smear Findings in COVID-19. Turk J Haematol Off J Turk Soc Haematol 2020;37(4):310–2.
20. Schapkaitz E, De Jager T, Levy B. The characteristic peripheral blood morphological features of hospitalized patients infected with COVID-19. Int J Lab Hematol 2021;43(3):e130–4.
21. Pezeshki A, Vaezi A, Nematollahi P. Blood cell morphology and COVID-19 clinical course, severity, and outcome. J Hematop 2021;14(3):221–8.
22. Sadigh S, Massoth LR, Christensen BB, et al. Peripheral blood morphologic findings in patients with COVID-19. Int J Lab Hematol 2020;42(6):e248–51.
23. Pozdnyakova O, Connell NT, Battinelli EM, et al. Clinical Significance of CBC and WBC Morphology in the Diagnosis and Clinical Course of COVID-19 Infection. Am J Clin Pathol 2021;155(3):364–75.
24. Jain S, Meena R, Kumar V, et al. Comparison of hematologic abnormalities between hospitalized coronavirus disease 2019 positive and negative patients with correlation to disease severity and outcome. J Med Virol 2022;94(8):3757–67.
25. Chandler CM, Reid MC, Cherian S, et al. Comparison of Blood Counts and Markers of Inflammation and Coagulation in Patients With and Without COVID-19 Presenting to the Emergency Department in Seattle, WA. Am J Clin Pathol 2021;156(2): 185–97.
26. Gabr H, Bastawy S, Abdel Aal AA, et al. Changes in peripheral blood cellular morphology as diagnostic markers for COVID-19 infection. Int J Lab Hematol 2022;44(3):454–60.
27. Nazarullah A, Liang C, Villarreal A, et al. Peripheral Blood Examination Findings in SARS-CoV-2 Infection. Am J Clin Pathol 2020;154(3):319–29.
28. Singh A, Sood N, Narang V, et al. Morphology of COVID-19–affected cells in peripheral blood film. BMJ Case Rep 2020;13(5):e236117.
29. Cantu MD, Towne WS, Emmons FN, et al. Clinical significance of blue-green neutrophil and monocyte cytoplasmic inclusions in SARS-CoV-2 positive critically ill patients. Br J Haematol 2020;190(2):e89–92.
30. Ackermann M, Anders HJ, Bilyy R, et al. Patients with COVID-19: in the dark-NETs of neutrophils. Cell Death Differ 2021;28(11):3125–39.
31. Mitra A, Dwyre DM, Schivo M, et al. Leukoerythroblastic reaction in a patient with COVID-19 infection. Am J Hematol 2020;95(8):999–1000.
32. Lippi G, Plebani M, Henry BM. Thrombocytopenia is associated with severe coronavirus disease 2019 (COVID-19) infections: A meta-analysis. Clin Chim Acta Int J Clin Chem 2020;506:145–8.
33. Azghar A, Bensalah M, Berhili A, et al. Value of hematological parameters for predicting patients with severe coronavirus disease 2019: a real-world cohort from Morocco. J Int Med Res 2022;50(7), 3000605221109381.
34. Chan AS, Rout A. Use of Neutrophil-to-Lymphocyte and Platelet-to-Lymphocyte Ratios in COVID-19. J Clin Med Res 2020;12(7):448–53.
35. Adamidi ES, Mitsis K, Nikita KS. Artificial intelligence in clinical care amidst COVID-19 pandemic: A systematic review. Comput Struct Biotechnol J 2021; 19:2833–50.
36. Magunia H, Lederer S, Verbuecheln R, et al. Machine learning identifies ICU outcome predictors in a multicenter COVID-19 cohort. Crit Care Lond Engl 2021;25(1):295.
37. Famiglini L, Campagner A, Carobene A, et al. A robust and parsimonious machine learning method to predict ICU admission of COVID-19 patients. Med Biol Eng Comput 2022;1–13.
38. Rapkiewicz AV, Mai X, Carsons SE, et al. Megakaryocytes and platelet-fibrin thrombi characterize multi-organ thrombosis at autopsy in COVID-19: A case series. EClinicalMedicine 2020;24:100434.
39. Prieto-Pérez L, Fortes J, Soto C, et al. Histiocytic hyperplasia with hemophagocytosis and acute alveolar damage in COVID-19 infection. Mod Pat*hol* 2020;33(11):2139–46.
40. Bryce C, Grimes Z, Pujadas E, et al. Pathophysiology of SARS-CoV-2: the Mount Sinai COVID-19 autopsy experience. Mod Pathol 2021;34(8):1456–67.
41. Duan Y, Xia M, Ren L, et al. Deficiency of Tfh Cells and Germinal Center in Deceased COVID-19 Patients. Curr Med Sci 2020;40(4):618–24.
42. Kaneko N, Kuo HH, Boucau J, et al. Loss of Bcl-6-Expressing T Follicular Helper Cells and Germinal Centers in COVID-19. Cell 2020;183(1):143–57.e13.
43. Lee JE, Jeong WG, Nam BD, et al. Impact of Mediastinal Lymphadenopathy on the Severity of COVID-19 Pneumonia: A Nationwide Multicenter Cohort Study. J Korean Med Sci 2022;37(22):e78.
44. Khatri G, Priya null, Saleem MB, et al. Mediastinal lymphadenopathy: A serious complication in COVID-19 patients. Ann Med Surg (Lond) 2022;79: 104039.
45. Bshesh K, Khan W, Vattoth AL, et al. Lymphadenopathy post-COVID-19 vaccination with increased FDG uptake may be falsely attributed to oncological disorders: A systematic review. J Med Virol 2022; 94(5):1833–45.
46. Garreffa E, Hamad A, O'Sullivan CC, et al. Regional lymphadenopathy following COVID-19 vaccination: Literature review and considerations for patient

management in breast cancer care. Eur J Cancer Oxf Engl 2021;159:38–51.
47. Yu Q, Jiang W, Chen N, et al. Misdiagnosis of Reactive Lymphadenopathy Remotely After COVID-19 Vaccination: A Case Report and Literature Review. Front Immunol 2022;13:875637.
48. Schiaffino S, Pinker K, Magni V, et al. Axillary lymphadenopathy at the time of COVID-19 vaccination: ten recommendations from the European Society of Breast Imaging (EUSOBI). Insights Imaging 2021;12(1):119.
49. García-Molina F, Cegarra-Navarro MF, Andrade-Gonzales RJ, et al. Cytologic and histologic features of COVID-19 post-vaccination lymphadenopathy. CytoJournal 2021;18:34.
50. Tan NJH, Tay KXJ, Wong SBJ, et al. COVID-19 post-vaccination lymphadenopathy: Report of cytological findings from fine needle aspiration biopsy. Diagn Cytopathol 2021;49(12):E467–70.
51. Hagen C, Nowack M, Messerli M, et al. Fine needle aspiration in COVID-19 vaccine-associated lymphadenopathy. Swiss Med Wkly 2021;151:w20557.
52. Sekizawa A, Hashimoto K, Kobayashi S, et al. Rapid progression of marginal zone B-cell lymphoma after COVID-19 vaccination (BNT162b2): A case report. Front Med 2022;9:963393.
53. Mizutani M, Mitsui H, Amano T, et al. Two cases of axillary lymphadenopathy diagnosed as diffuse large B-cell lymphoma developed shortly after BNT162b2 COVID-19 vaccination. J Eur Acad Dermatol Venereol JEADV 2022;36(8):e613–5.
54. Chattopadhyay PK, Filby A, Jellison ER, et al. A cytometrist's guide to coordinating and performing COVID-19 research. Cytometry 2021;99(1):11–8.
55. Evans MG, Crymes A, Crombie JL, et al. Monotypic plasmacytoid cells mimicking lymph node malignancy in the setting of COVID-19 recovery. Am J Hematol 2022;97(5):666–7.

Immunodeficiency-Associated Epstein-Barr Virus-Positive B-cell Lymphoproliferative Disorders
A Review and New Paradigm

Jennifer Chapman, MD

KEYWORDS

• EBV • Lymphoproliferative disorder • Immune deficiency–associated lymphoma

Key points

- Epstein-Barr virus is oncogenic, in particular when host immunity is compromised, allowing EBV to express its full genome. Viral-derived antigens exhibit homology to human antiapoptotic molecules, signal transducers, and cytokines, thereby promoting EBV infection, cell immortalization, and transformation. A "second hit" is usually required to cause cancer.
- EBV-positive immune deficiency–related lymphoproliferative disorders (LPDs) are clinically, histopathologically, and biologically heterogeneous as a group but show similar features among different immune deficiency states.
- Classification of EBV-positive LPDs can be difficult and often requires extensive histopathologic evaluation and correlation with clinical features.

ABSTRACT

Sources of immune deficiency and dysregulation (IDD) are being increasingly recognized and defined, as are IDD-related B-cell lymphoproliferative lesions and lymphomas occurring in these patients. In this review, basic biology of Epstein-Barr virus (EBV) as it relates to classification of EBV-positive B-cell lymphoproliferative disorders (LPDs) is reviewed. Also discussed is the new paradigm of classification of IDD-related LPDs adopted by the fifth edition World Health Organization classification. IDD-related EBV-positive B-cell hyperplasias, LPDs, and lymphomas are discussed with particular attention to unifying and unique features that assist with recognition of these IDD-related lesions and their classification scheme.

EPSTEIN-BARR VIRUS: BACKGROUND AND BASIC CONCEPTS

Epstein-Barr virus (EBV) is a member of the Herpesviridae family (human herpes virus type 4 [HHV-4]) and is a lymphotropic double-stranded DNA virus that infects B cells and epithelial cells. The name Herpesviridae is derived from the Greek word "herpein," meaning "to creep," terminology that refers to the latent and recurring infectious cycles that characterize Herpesviridae (Table 1). Humans are the only known definitive host of EBV, and approximately 90% of the world's population is infected.[1] Most infections result in lifelong asymptomatic carrier states. However, there exists variation in outcomes of EBV infection according to geographic distribution, including high prevalence of EBV-positive nasopharyngeal carcinoma in areas of

Division of Hematopathology, Department of Pathology and Laboratory Medicine, University of Miami Hospital/Sylvester Comprehensive Cancer Center, 1400 Northwest 12th Avenue, Miami, FL 33136, USA
E-mail address: Jchapman@med.miami.edu
Twitter: @Nodesallday (J.C.)

Surgical Pathology 16 (2023) 213–231
https://doi.org/10.1016/j.path.2023.01.008
1875-9181/23/

surgpath.theclinics.com

Table 1
Characteristics of Herpesviridae family

Human Herpesvirus (HHV) Name	Alternate Virus Name	Disease Caused	Target Cell During Primary Infection (Lytic Phase)	Reservoir Cell Type During Latency
HHV-1	Herpes simplex virus-1 (HSV-1)	Oral herpes	Mucoepithelial	Neuron
HHV-2	Herpes simplex virus-2 (HSV-2)	Genital herpes	Mucoepithelial	Neuron
HHV-3	Varicella zoster virus (VZV)	Chickenpox, shingles	Mucoepithelial	Neuron
HHV-4	*Epstein-Barr virus (EBV)*	*Many*	*B cell*	*B cell*
HHV-5	Cytomegalovirus (CMV)	Many	Monocyte, lymphocyte, epithelial cells	Monocyte, lymphocyte
HHV-6	HHV-6 variant A or B	Roseola infantum	T cell	T cell
HHV-7	HHV-7			
HHV-8	Kaposi sarcoma herpesvirus (KSHV)/HHV-8	Kaposi sarcoma, primary effusion lymphoma, KSHV/ HHV-8–positive diffuse large B-cell lymphoma, KSHV/ HHV-8-positive germinotropic lymphoproliferative disorder	B cell	B cell

China, EBV-positive endemic Burkitt lymphoma in sub-Saharan Africa, and infectious mononucleosis in teenagers and young adults in the Western world.[1] EBV is also causally associated with hemophagocytic lymphohistiocytosis, numerous lymphomas and lymphoproliferative disorders (LPDs), and other epithelial and sarcomatous neoplasms. The variability of EBV sequalae according to geographic location and human demographic is now known to be related to genetic variability of EBV strains and status of the host immune system.[2]

Despite its ubiquitous nature, EBV-related symptomatic diseases and cancers occur in only a small minority of infected people; this is because following an initial acute EBV infection, the intact human immune system encourages EBV to exist in a latent state where it can avoid host immune response and its own eradication (**Fig. 1**). The latent stages of EBV produce only few viral proteins and are not particularly immunogenic or oncogenic. Upon changes to host immunity, which occur in a minority of people, EBV may shift to more immunogenic and oncogenic latency stages.

EPSTEIN-BARR VIRUS: LATENCY

EBV does not have efficient lytic replication. Therefore, its replication is largely reliant on infection of host B cells, establishment of latency, production of stable EBV episome, and replication of the episome in synchrony with replication of the host genome in proliferating infected cells.[3,4] There are at least 4 latency stages of EBV each characterized by distinct gene expression programs that are associated with stage of B-cell differentiation, host immunity, and type of LPD that may arise (**Fig. 2**, **Table 2**).[4]

EBV initially infects naïve B cells after entrance through the oral mucosa.[5] During initial infection, EBV is in a highly immunogenic gene expression program known as latency III. Latency III is a "growth program" in which EBV's oncogenic antigens are expressed, promoting B-cell proliferation and immortalization and potentially oncogenesis. Hosts with intact immunity mount a vigorous humoral and CD4-positive and CD8-positive T-cell–mediated response to this primary infection and during occasional bouts of EBV reactivation that occur throughout life.[5] In fact, enumerations of EBV-specific T cells show that approximately 1% to 5% of circulating T cells in normal people may be specific for EBV.[5–7] This immune response encourages EBV to alter its gene expression program away from latency III to avoid its own eradication; thus, EBV enters alternate latency stages where it exists as an episome within B cells.

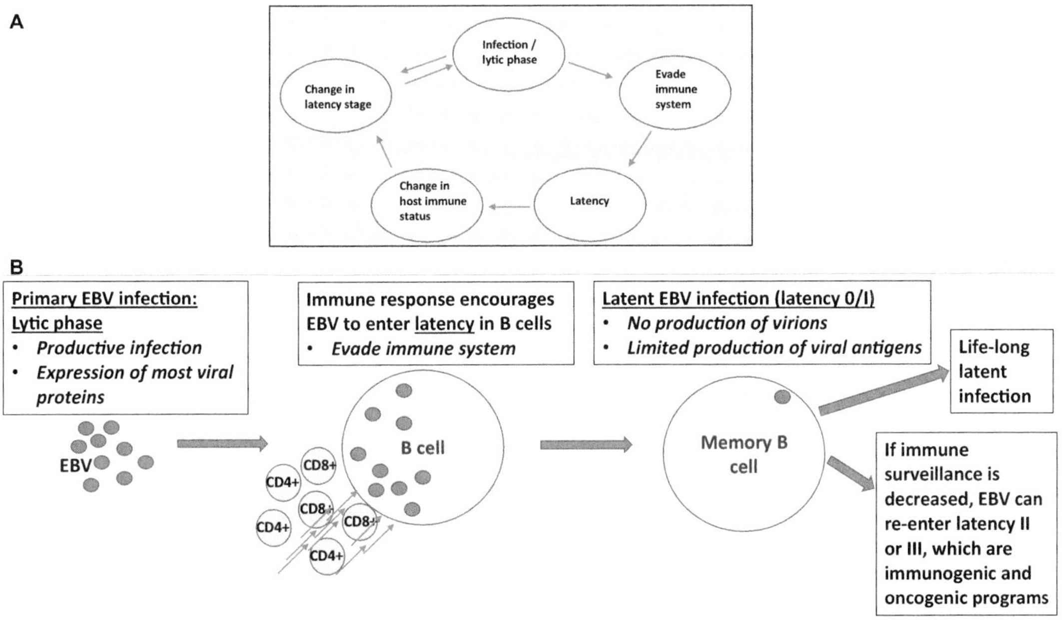

Fig. 1. EBV life cycle. At the time of initial infection, EBV is in lytic phase. Upon infection of B cells, EBV needs to avoid host immune response to preserve itself, and therefore EBV enters latency. EBV can remain latent throughout the life of the host or can enter into more immunogenic latency stages or lytic phase upon changes to host immune system status (*A*). In lytic phase, EBV infection is productive (produces virions), and most of the viral genome is expressed. In latency, there is no production of virions and only limited production of viral antigens (*B*).

As EBV-infected naïve B cells home to lymphoid tissues and into germinal centers, EBV enters latency stage II (see Fig. 2). Latency II is a "rescue program" in which EBV-derived antigens provide signals for infected cells to survive and differentiate into memory B cells. EBV-infected B cells that should otherwise be programmed to undergo apoptosis as part of the normal germinal center

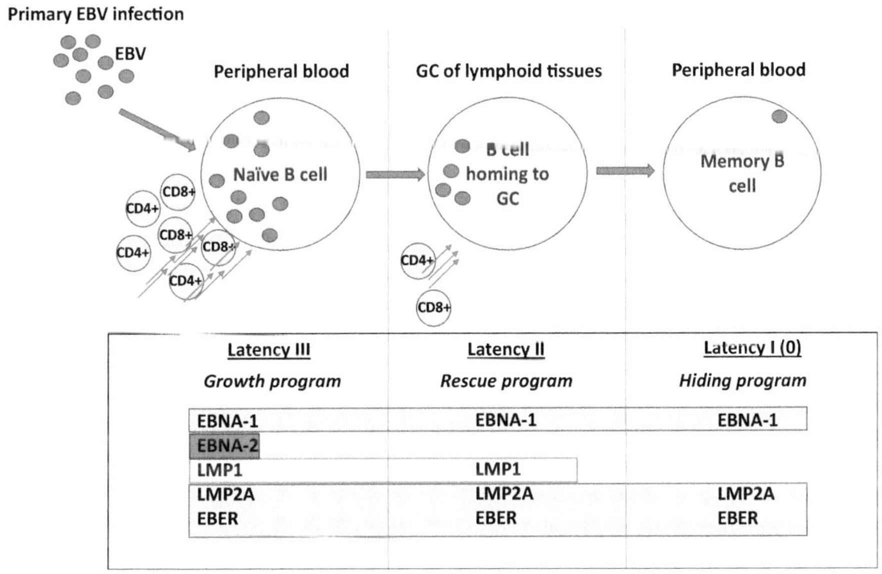

Fig. 2. EBV latency stage and EBV antigens expressed according to B-cell differentiation stage. EBER, Epstein-Barr–encoded RNAs; EBNA, Epstein-Barr nuclear antigen; GC, germinal center; LMP, latent membrane protein.

Table 2
Characteristics of Epstein-Barr virus latency programs

Latency Type	Program	EBV Antigens Expressed	Associated Lymphoproliferative Disorders, Lymphomas, and Other Neoplasms[a]
Latency I	Hiding	EBNA-1, LMP-2A, EBER	Burkitt lymphoma, HIV-associated DLBCL (immunoblastic), PEL, monomorphic PTLD
Latency II	Rescue	EBNA-1, LMP-1, LMP-2A, EBER	CHL, EBV + DLBCL NOS, EBV + MCU, other IDD-associated LPD, NK/T-cell lymphomas, epithelial tumors
Latency III	Growth	EBNA-1, EBNA-2 (all 6 EBNAs), LMP-1, LMP2A, EBER	HIV-associated DLBCL (centroblastic), PTLD, other IDD-associated LPD, CI-DLBCL (PAL), FA-LBCL, some PEL, LyG, infectious mononucleosis

Abbreviations: CHL, classic Hodgkin lymphoma; CI-DLBCL, diffuse large B-cell lymphoma associated with chronic inflammation; DLBCL, diffuse large B-cell lymphoma; EBER, EBV-encoded small RNAs; EBNA, Epstein-Barr nuclear antigen; FA-LBCL, fibrin-associated large B-cell lymphoma; IDD, immune deficiency/dysregulation; LMP, latent membrane protein; LPD, lymphoproliferative diseases; LyG, lymphomatoid granulomatosis; MCU, mucocutaneous ulcer; NOS, not otherwise specified; PAL, pyothorax-associated lymphoma; PEL, primary effusion lymphoma.

[a] Classification nomenclature taken from both WHO revised fourth edition and WHO fifth edition.

reaction can be "rescued" by cell survival signals provided by EBV. For example, B cells that normally undergo apoptosis because they do not have a functional B-cell receptor (BCR) can be "rescued" in latency II by EBV-derived viral proteins that mimic the BCR.[8]

EBV-infected cells surviving the germinal center reaction then transition to latency I or latency 0, EBV's gene expression programs in memory B cells (see Fig. 2, see Table 2). In latency 0, only noncoding RNA is transcribed from the episome.[4] Latency I is an EBV "hiding program." Most viral-derived antigens are not expressed and those expressed are not overtly immunogenic, so the virus effectively "hides" from immune system eradication. Because the EBV gene expression program in latency I is not overtly immunogenic or oncogenic, tumors arising in latency I generally require additional oncogenic "hits" (in addition to EBV) and tend to have minimal immune cell response in the tumor microenvironment.

EBV-derived antigens expressed in latency include nuclear antigens (EBNA 1, 2, 3a, 3b, 3c, 5), latent membrane proteins (LMP1, LMP2A, LMP2B), Epstein-Barr–encoded RNAs (EBER 1, 2), viral capsid antigen, membrane antigen, and early antigen (see Table 2; Table 3). EBNA-1, unlike all other EBNAs, is expressed in latency I, II, and III and is therefore found in all EBV-related malignancies. The ubiquitous nature of EBNA-1 indicates its critical role in ensuring stable persistence of the EBV genome in latently infected cells.[9] EBNA-1 also promotes the expression of other EBV-derived latency genes.[10] In contrast, EBNA-2 is highly immunogenic and recognized by cytotoxic T cells, thus its expression is only tolerated in the context of severely compromised T-cell immunity. EBNA-2 is a key regulator of other viral-encoded genes and host genes and is directly oncogenic by inducing transition of resting B cells through the G0/G1 checkpoint, promoting immortalization of EBV-infected cells.[11] EBNA-2 is expressed in latency III and present in tumors arising in the context of significant immune deficiency. LMP-1 is also oncogenic and expressed in latency II and III. LMP-1 acts as a constitutive CD40-like receptor that induces activation of multiple cellular signaling pathways including NF-κB and JAK/STAT.[12] LMP-1 also activates BCL2, promoting B-cell survival via its antiapoptotic action, and is involved in modulation of the interaction of EBV-infected cells and the microenvironment, including regulating angiogenesis and invasiveness.[13] LMP-2A is expressed in all latency stages and is also oncogenic. This antigen mimics the BCR, thereby rescuing germinal center B cells lacking a functional BCR from apoptosis.[8] EBERs are short, noncoding RNAs that are expressed abundantly in all EBV-infected cells in all latency stages and likely contribute to tumorigenesis by promoting resistance to apoptosis and inducing interleukin-10 expression, which acts as an autocrine growth factor for B lymphocytes.[14] Of note, development of EBV-associated cancers generally requires a second "hit" in addition to the oncogenic mechanisms of EBV.

Table 3
Characteristics and proposed function(s) of EBV-derived antigens

Viral Antigen	Latency State Expressed	Proposed Function
EBNA-1	All	Replication and maintenance of the viral genome (episomal) in latently infected cells; regulation of transcription through positive and negative regulation of viral promoters by phosphorylation; antiapoptosis.
EBNA-2	III	*Directly oncogenic*: regulates both viral and B-cell gene expression; is a key regulator of other viral-encoded genes (LMP1 and LMP2); and induces transition of resting B cell from G0/G1, promoting immortalization of EBV-infected cells.
LMP-1	II, III	*Directly oncogenic*: acts as a constitutive CD40-like receptor inducing expression of NF-κB and downstream signaling; activates BCL2, promoting B-cell survival via its antiapoptotic action; and modulates interaction between EBV-infected cells and microenvironment, including regulating angiogenesis and invasiveness.
LMP-2A	All	*Oncogenic*: mimics the B-cell receptor, thereby rescuing germinal center B cells lacking a functional B-cell receptor from apoptosis; polymerizes without antigen activation.
EBER	All	Short, noncoding RNAs that are *likely oncogenic*: promotes resistance to apoptosis and induces interleukin-10 expression, which acts as an autocrine growth factor for B lymphocytes.

Abbreviations: EBER, EBV-encoded small RNAs; EBNA, Epstein-Barr nuclear antigen; LMP, latent membrane protein.

In clinical practice, EBV is most commonly detected in formalin-fixed, paraffin-embedded tissues by in situ hybridization using commercially available RNA probes against EBER. LMP-1 detection by immunohistochemistry (IHC) is used to support classification of EBV in latency II, and EBNA-2 detection by IHC is used to support classification of EBV in latency III (Fig. 3).

EPSTEIN-BARR VIRUS–ASSOCIATED B-CELL LESIONS: GENERAL CLASSIFICATION

EBV-associated B-cell lymphomas and LPDs include lesions that, by definition, occur in immune competent states and those that occur in the context of immune deficiency or dysregulation (IDD) (Fig. 4). EBV-positive diffuse large B-cell lymphoma (DLBCL) and lymphomatoid granulomatosis occur *without known IDD*. At this time, because age-related immune senescence is poorly defined and has no objective measure, EBV-positive DLBCL and lymphomatoid granulomatosis can occur in patients with possible age-related immune senescence. Recently the existence of EBV-positive large B-cell lymphomas (LBCL) arising in association with breast implants has also been reported and in a series of cases showed morphologic and clinical overlap with breast implant–associated anaplastic large cell lymphoma.[15] Because they are not IDD-associated, these lymphomas are not reviewed herein.

EBV-associated LPDs and lymphomas occurring in the context of *known (localized or systemic) IDD* are more common and include the specifically defined entities of DLBCL associated with chronic inflammation (CI-DLBCL), fibrin-associated LBCL (FA-LBCL), and EBV-positive mucocutaneous ulcer (MCU), as well as the more heterogeneous groups of EBV positive hyperplasias, B-cell LPDs, and lymphomas (see Fig. 4; Fig. 5). Plasmablastic lymphomas (PBL) are specifically defined lymphomas that are usually EBV-positive and frequently arise in IDD, but not always.

EBV may also be present in a subset of other B-cell lymphomas that are more often EBV-negative. These lymphomas include a subset of Burkitt lymphoma, classic Hodgkin lymphoma (CHL), and rare low-grade B-cell lymphomas of follicular, marginal zone or lymphoplasmacytic lymphoma type. Because these lymphomas are only sometimes associated with EBV, their EBV-positive subset is not classified as a separate lymphoma entity by the World Health Organization (WHO) classification scheme. The fifth edition WHO classification intends to capture the EBV-positive subset of

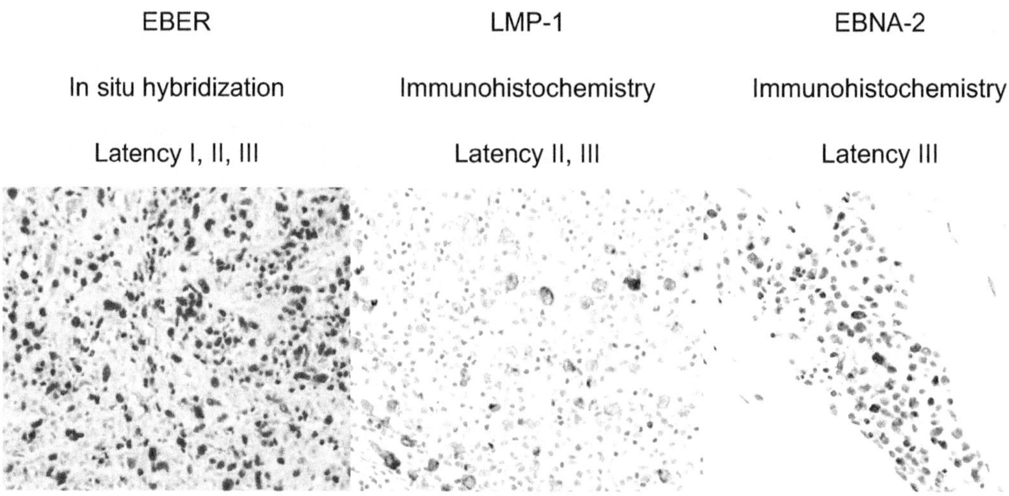

Fig. 3. EBV-derived antigens commonly detected in clinical practice in FFPE tissues.

otherwise EBV-negative lymphomas based on their frequent association with IDD and thus classify them as IDD-associated lymphomas or LPDs, as described later (see **Fig. 5**).[16] The exception to this is Burkitt lymphoma, where EBV-positive and EBV-negative tumors have increasingly recognized biological distinctions, thus classification of Burkitt lymphoma as EBV-

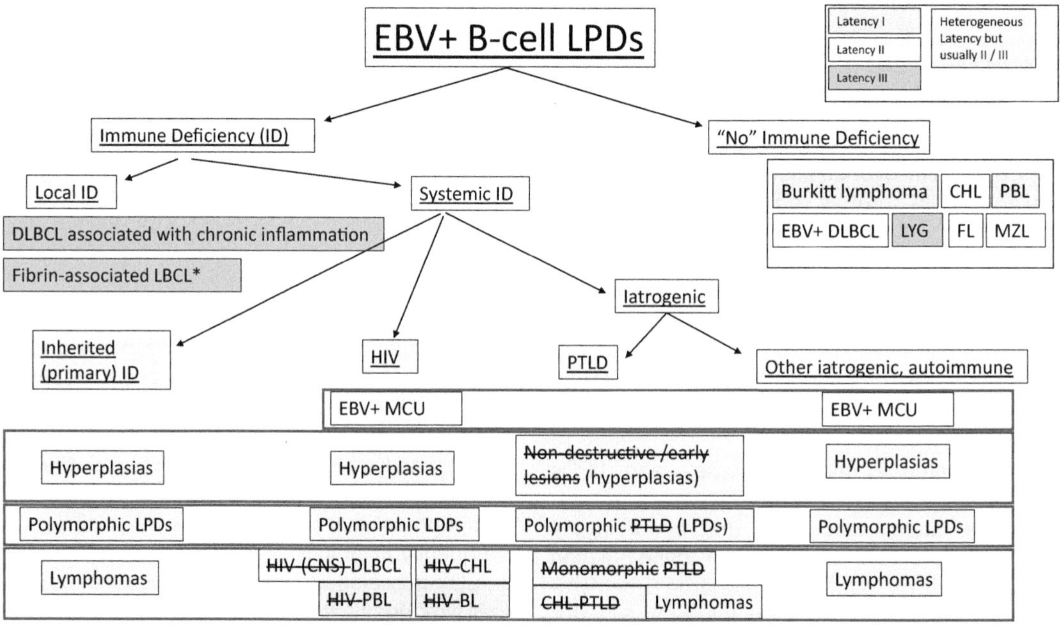

Fig. 4. EBV-associated LPDs and lymphomas according to immune deficiency and dysregulation (IDD) states as organized in the revised fourth edition WHO classification. EBV-associated hyperplasias, polymorphic lesions/lymphoproliferative diseases (LPDs), and lymphomas with similar histopathologic and clinical features are now known to occur across different IDD states (*red boxes*). Therefore, the fifth edition WHO classification has reorganized the naming structure of the IDD-related lesions to include the lesion, viral association, and source of IDD. In the fifth edition WHO classification, LPDs and lymphomas arising posttransplantation are no longer separately classified as posttransplantation LPDs (PTLDs) and those arising in HIV are no longer separately classified as HIV-lymphomas. Strikeouts indicate terminologies no longer recommended in the fifth edition WHO classification scheme. [a]Fibrin-associated large B-cell lymphoma is a new entity in the fifth edition WHO classification that includes lymphomas previously classified as diffuse large B-cell lymphoma arising in chronic inflammation (considered a subtype of DLBCL, NOS in the fourth edition WHO classification). NOS, not otherwise specified.

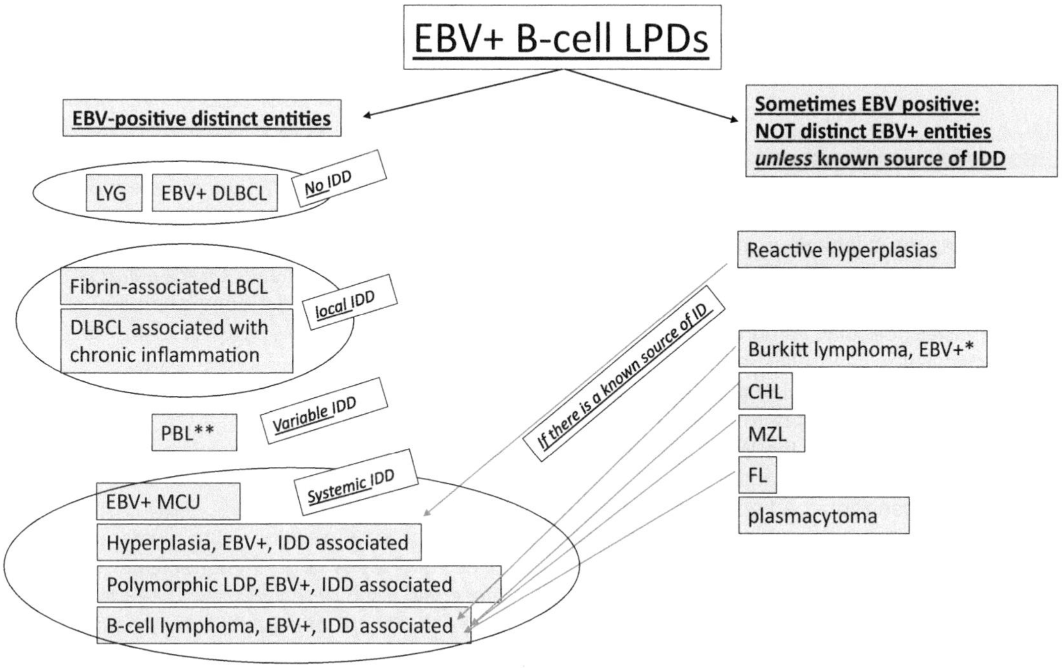

Fig. 5. EBV-associated LPDs and lymphomas include distinct entities and lesions that are not distinct entities when EBV-positive. [a]Burkitt lymphoma (BL) is an exception in that the fifth edition WHO classification now recommends classifying BL as EBV-positive versus EBV-negative. [b]Rare plasmablastic lymphomas (PBL) are EBV-negative.

positive versus EBV-negative is now recommended by the fifth edition WHO classification.[16]

Primary effusion lymphoma and its solid variant are frequently EBV-positive but also Kaposi sarcoma herpes virus (KSHV)/HHV-8–positive, unlike the aforementioned LPDs that are negative for KSHV/HHV-8. When both EBV and KSHV/HHV-8 are positive, the lesion is classified according to KSHV/HHV-8 positivity as primary effusion lymphoma or other KSHV/HHV-8–associated LPD (KSHV/HHV-8–positive DLBCL, KSHV/HHV-8–positive germinotropic LPD). KSHV/HHV-8–associated lesions are not discussed further in this review.

EPSTIEN-BARR VIRUS–ASSOCIATED B-CELL LYMPHOPROLIFERATIVE DISORDERS AND IMMUNE DEFICIENCY/DYSREGULATION STATES

Conceptually, IDD may be localized to an anatomic site or be systemic. Localized IDD usually occurs in body cavities or other confined spaces, arising in the context of prolonged local chronic inflammation. Systemic forms of IDD are many but were historically organized into 4 main categories by the revised fourth edition of the WHO classification: primary inherited immunodeficiencies (now known as inborn errors of immunity), human immunodeficiency virus (HIV) infection, posttransplantation, and other/iatrogenic immunodeficiency. Other iatrogenic immune deficiencies most commonly include IDD associated with autoimmune disorders and their treatments. Other sources of IDD that are increasingly recognized, but that do not yet have objective measures in clinical practice, include immune senescence and immune system dysregulation in the setting of polychemotherapy and immune modulatory agents for previous solid tumors or hematologic malignancies.

The organization of IDD-associated lesions by IDD state allowed for the recognition that although these LPDs include a wide spectrum of lesions ranging from hyperplasias to high-grade lymphomas, this spectrum is overlapping across different IDD states. This concept was reviewed at the 2015 Society for Hematopathology/European Association for Haematopathology (SH/EAHP) workshop.[17,18] As a result, a proposal by Natkunam and colleagues was published, suggesting a 3-part unifying nomenclature that includes the name of the lesion (eg, hyperplasia, polymorphic lesion, lymphoma, and so forth), presence or absence of virus (eg, EBV or HHV-8), and the specific IDD setting (eg, posttransplantation, HIV, methotrexate-associated, and so forth) for all IDD-related LPDs.[19] This naming system has now been adapted by the fifth edition WHO classification scheme that reorganizes the IDD-associated LPDs according to their common histologies.[16]

B-CELL OR PLASMA CELL REACTIVE HYPERPLASIAS

Example diagnosis: infectious mononucleosis-like immunoblastic hyperplasia, EBV-positive, autoimmune disease–related (rheumatoid arthritis)

Hyperplasias (follicular, immunoblastic/infectious mononucleosis-like, and plasma cell) occurring in IDD states may form clinical masses but histologically show maintenance of normal tissue architecture. In the fifth edition of the WHO classification, KSHV/HHV-8–positive multicentric Castleman disease is also organized as a hyperplasia arising in the setting of IDD, but this lesion is not discussed here because it is not EBV-related.[16]

As in the immune competent setting, follicular hyperplasias show prominent, sometimes expansile hyperplastic germinal centers. The follicles may be increased in number and size and have expanded dark zones and attenuated mantle zones, but nodal architecture is maintained, as is the normal germinal center B-cell immunophenotype. In some cases, there may be associated paracortical, plasma cell, and/or immunoblastic hyperplasia. EBV-positive cells must be identified to link the hyperplastic lesion to an IDD state and is currently the method used to resolve the diagnosis of follicular hyperplasia versus follicular hyperplasia, EBV-positive, HIV-associated, for example; this is generally accomplished by in situ hybridization staining for EBER, which is present in all EBV latency phases and is therefore a sensitive detection method.

All people latently infected with EBV, which includes approximately 90% of people on Earth, may have few, scattered EBV-positive cells in normal tissues identifiable by EBER staining. There is general agreement that the finding of rare, scattered EBV-positive small lymphoid cells is normal, does not suggest IDD, and should not cause a hyperplasia to be classified as an IDD-associated lesion. There is also general agreement that increased numbers and/or clusters of EBV-positive cells is atypical and raises the possibility of IDD if acute infectious mononucleosis is excluded. At this time, however, there is no firmly established threshold beyond which the number of EBV-positive cells is considered abnormal. In a study reviewing the distribution of EBER-positive cells in normal tonsils, most contained fewer than 10 EBER-positive cells per tissue section.[20] In a report analyzing EBER staining in negative staging bone marrows in patients without EBV-related cancers, up to 4 EBER-positive cells were seen in the entire staging bone marrow core biopsy in 34% of cases.[21] In hyperplasias arising in IDD, EBER-positive cells typically exceed these thresholds and are present in interfollicular and/or follicular compartments.

Plasmacytic hyperplasias show increased small lymphocytes and lymphoplasmacytic cells in the paracortex and increased plasma cells in the interfollicular and sinusoidal compartments. Although increased in number, plasma cells are overall maintained within their normal expected compartments within the lymph node and are generally polytypic.

Infectious mononucleosis-like immunoblastic hyperplasias are characterized by expanded interfollicular foci of admixed small lymphocytes, plasma cells, and scattered to clustered, variably sized, and often large immunoblasts, but overall preserved tissue architecture. These lesions may show significant overlap with polymorphic LPDs, EBV-positive LBCLs, and CHL, especially in small biopsies where architecture cannot be fully evaluated. Immunoblastic hyperplasias may contain significantly increased EBV-positive cells that can be evenly distributed or present in clusters, similar to those seen in acute infectious mononucleosis. Importantly, EBV-positive cells are of *variable size and appearance* in infectious mononucleosis-like immunoblastic hyperplasias, which helps to distinguish these lesions from EBV-positive lymphomas that have relatively more monomorphic EBV-positive cells. Correlation with clinical features may be necessary to separate these lesions from acute infectious mononucleosis. Reactive hyperplasias are composed of polytypic and polyclonal B cells and plasma cells, and EBV-positive hyperplasias usually regress spontaneously or with immune reconstitution, if possible.

In the revised fourth edition of the WHO classification of posttransplantation lymphoproliferative disorders (PTLDs), the reactive hyperplasias comprised the nondestructive lesions, which had previously been termed "early" lesions. The terms "early lesion" and "nondestructive lesion" are no longer preferred in the fifth edition of the WHO classification.

POLYMORPHIC B-CELL LYMPHOPROLIFERATIVE DISORDERS

Example diagnosis: polymorphic B-cell lymphoproliferative disorder, EBV-positive, iatrogenic/therapy-related (methotrexate).

Polymorphic LPDs are *destructive* hematolymphoid proliferations composed of heterogeneous populations of hematolymphoid cells. Unlike the hyperplastic lesions, polymorphic LPDs disrupt normal tissue architecture; however, they fall short of meeting criteria for a diagnosis of lymphoma. These lesions are usually nodal but may be extranodal and may occur with or without identifiable sources of IDD; EBV-positive cases are usually IDD-associated. Classification of these lesions may be difficult and somewhat subjective because of their relatively nonspecific diagnostic criteria that reflect the nature of these lesions as existing on a biological spectrum between hyperplasias and bona fide lymphomas.

Polymorphic LPDs are composed of variable populations of small lymphoid cells, plasma cells, immunoblasts, and large B cells, the latter in variable amount and with variable Hodgkin-like morphology (Fig. 6). These lesions are recognized and characterized by their B-cell component showing a *range* of differentiation along the B-cell maturation spectrum through the lymphocyte—immunoblast—plasma cell stages. This heterogeneity of B-cell appearance and presence of B cells and plasma cells across the complete maturation spectrum is one of the most useful features for separating this lesion from EBV-positive DLBCL and CHL. Necrosis and an angioinvasive and/or angiodestructive pattern may be present, mimicking that of lymphomatoid granulomatosis. Despite their polymorphic appearance, these lesions often have monoclonal and monotypic B cells and plasma cells. Polymorphic LPDs are usually EBER- and LMP-1–positive, and sometimes EBNA2-positive (latency II or III), supporting the presence of underlying IDD that allows EBV to transition out of latency 0/I. In situations where immunosuppression can be withdrawn, these lesions may respond to immune reconstitution, as EBV in latency II or III is immunogenic. For patients in whom immunosuppression cannot be withdrawn, high-risk, or nonresponder patients, treatment may involve donor T cells, EBV-specific T cells, surgery, radiation, immunotherapy, and/or chemotherapy.[5] In the revised fourth edition of the WHO classification, these lesions comprised the "polymorphic PTLDs," a term no longer recommended in the fifth edition of the WHO classification.[16]

EPSTEIN-BARR VIRUS–POSITIVE MUCOCUTANEOUS ULCER

Example diagnosis: mucocutaneous ulcer, EBV-positive, iatrogenic/therapy-related (methotrexate).

EBV-positive MCU is a distinct EBV-positive LPD that often presents as a solitary ulcerated

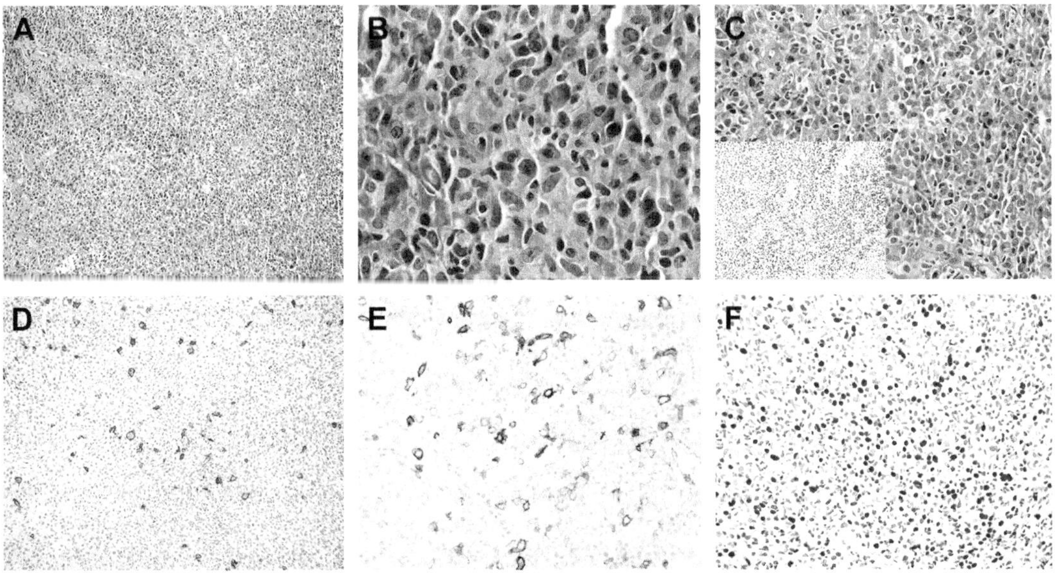

Fig. 6. Polymorphic B-cell lymphoproliferative disorder, EBV-positive, iatrogenic/therapy-related (methotrexate). Hematoxylin and eosin (H&E)-stained tissue sections of retroperitoneal mass show an atypical polymorphic hematolymphoid infiltrate effacing the normal architecture (*A*). The infiltrate consists of small lymphocytes, plasma cells, atypical plasmablasts, immunoblasts, and histiocytes (*B*). In most foci plasma cells predominate (*C*) and are kappa light chain restricted (*C, inset*). CD20 highlights only scattered B cells that are variable in size and include scattered large immunoblasts (*D*). CD30 highlights immunoblasts with variable staining intensity (*E*). In situ hybridization for EBER is positive in frequent cells that vary in size and morphologic appearance (*F*).

lesion in the oropharyngeal mucosa of patients with history of iatrogenic immunosuppression or age-related immune senescence.[22,23] In addition to oropharyngeal mucosa, skin and gastrointestinal tract can be involved. Since its original description, EBV-positive MCU has been expanded to include cases in persons living with HIV (PLWH) and when lesions are multiple, particularly if involving only a single anatomic site.[23] If lesions involve multiple different anatomic sites, including different cutaneous sites, they likely go beyond the intended spectrum of EBV-positive MCU. EBV-positive MCU are usually ulcerated and painful and should have a well-circumscribed border grossly and histologically. There is an absence of systemic involvement and no masses.

Similar to polymorphic LPDs, EBV-positive CHL, and some EBV-positive DLBCL, EBV-positive MCU contains a polymorphic hematolymphoid infiltrate that includes EBV-positive large B cells and variable Hodgkin-like cells in a background rich in T cells (**Fig. 7**). Angioinvasion and necrosis may be present. In addition to a well-defined margin histologically, there is often a bandlike rim of small T lymphoid cells encircling the deep margin of the lesion. EBV-positive cells include small and large lymphocytes, including Hodgkin-like cells that typically express CD30 and variable pan-B-cell markers but usually not CD15. B-cell marker expression may be downregulated. Although individual EBV-positive Hodgkin-like cells may be histologically similar to those seen in CHL, EBV-positive DLBCLs, and polymorphic LPDs, in EBV-positive MCU they show a spectrum of sizes and are present in mucosal lesions with well-defined borders, unlike CHL and DLBCL. This distinction is critical, as EBV-positive MCU usually regresses spontaneously or with reduction of immunosuppression. EBV-positive MCU with plasmacytic/plasmablastic differentiation and with features overlapping with EBV-positive polymorphic B-cell LPD are reported.[24]

LYMPHOMAS ARISING IN IMMUNE DEFICIENCY/DYSREGULATION: GENERAL FEATURES

Lymphomas arising in IDD settings are frequently EBV-positive and may involve nodal or extranodal sites (including allografts), with more frequent extranodal presentations compared with lymphomas in immune competent people. In the era of combination antiretroviral therapy (cART), primary central nervous system (CNS) DLBCL, DLBCL, Burkitt lymphoma, and CHL remain the most common lymphomas in PLWH, although the incidence of primary CNS DLBCL and DLBCL have decreased significantly with cART. Lymphomas arising in autoimmune and iatrogenic IDD are more heterogeneous.

EBV-positive LBCLs arising in IDD share some common characteristics, including the following: (1) lymphoma cells tend to have morphologic and immunophenotypic variability, existing on a spectrum from DLBCL-like to CHL-like across individual cases, as well as in different foci within a single case; (2) they more frequently show plasmacytic, immunoblastic, and/or plasmablastic morphologic and immunophenotypic differentiation; (3) most are of nongerminal center B-cell immunophenotype with expression of MUM1 and BCL6 (variable) and absence of CD10 (except Burkitt lymphoma and some PBL); (4) antigen expression is more variable, including expression of some plasma cell markers by LBCLs, dim BCL2 expression in Burkitt lymphoma, and variable or overlapping expression of CD30 and/or CD15 and pan-B-cell markers in large or Hodgkin-like cells; (5) EBV latency is II or III except in Burkitt lymphoma and some PBL, where it is usually latency I; (6) EBV-positive tumors are characterized by lower tumor mutational burden and some recurrent cytogenetic and molecular abnormalities (described in the following section).

It is important to recognize that among EBV-positive B-cell lymphomas, there may be significant overlap between the polymorphic LPDs, DLBCLs, and CHLs, and well-defined diagnostic borders between these entities that reliably distinguish all cases do not exist; this is likely related to the biological spectrum of these lesions in the context of EBV infection and IDD and our attempts to define borders that are not naturally occurring in all cases. Under these circumstances, discussion with clinical colleagues that integrates clinical, imaging, and histopathologic features is critical for developing best treatment strategies.

DIFFUSE LARGE B-CELL LYMPHOMA, EPSTEIN-BARR VIRUS–POSITIVE, ARISING IN IMMUNE DEFICIENCY/DYSREGULATION

Example diagnosis: DLBCL, EBV-positive, iatrogenic/therapy-related (posttransplantation, solid organ).

DLBCL may be EBV-positive or EBV-negative and may occur in the context of known or no known IDD. Classification of these lesions integrates these features. Therefore, in the diagnosis of all DLBCL, knowledge of EBV and immune system status affects lymphoma classification. In

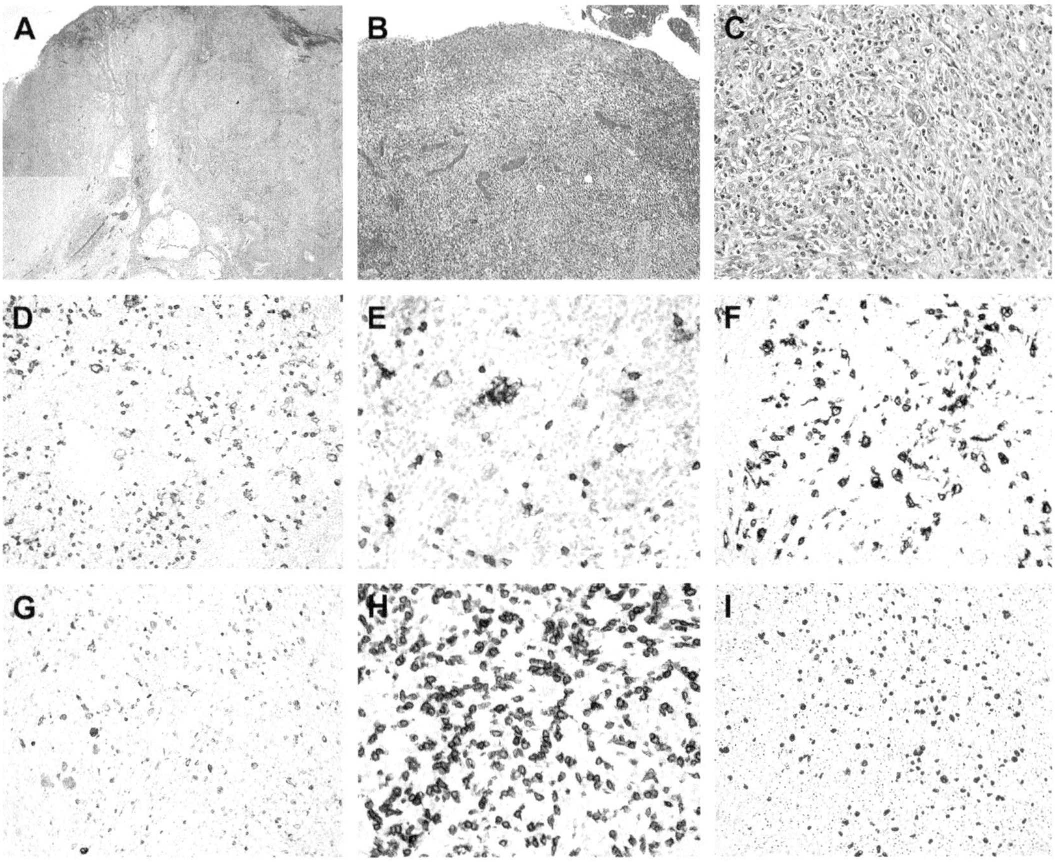

Fig. 7. EBV-positive mucocutaneous ulcer arising in a patient with a history of autoimmune hepatitis and nephritis on immunosuppressive therapy. H&E-stained tissue sections of terminal ileum show ulcerated mucosa with an underlying hematolymphoid infiltrate (*A, B*). The infiltrate has a well-circumscribed border and is focally surrounded by a band of small lymphoid cells (*A, inset*). Beneath the mucosal ulceration is an atypical infiltrate composed mostly of small lymphocytes and histiocytes with scattered large lymphoid cells with variable immunoblastic and Hodgkin-like morphology (*B, C*). CD20 immunohistochemical stain is positive in scattered small lymphocytes and immunoblasts with variable expression in Hodgkin-like cells (*D, E*). CD30 is strongly expressed in immunoblasts and Hodgkin-like cells (*F*), whereas CD79a shows more variable expression (*G*). CD3 highlights frequent small T cells (*H*). EBER is positive in frequent cells with variable morphology, including Hodgkin-like cells (*I*).

EBV-positive cases, history of known IDD separates DLBCL, EBV-positive, and IDD-associated from EBV-positive DLBCL.[16] In EBV-negative cases, those with known IDD are classified as IDD-associated and those without known IDD are classified as DLBCL, not otherwise specified, according to the fifth edition of the WHO classification.[16]

DLBCL is the most common lymphoma reported in IDD states. EBV positivity varies with IDD source, ranging from approximately 40% in posttransplantation settings to approximately 75% in cases of iatrogenic IDD.[18] Histologically, these lymphomas exist as a spectrum ranging from usual DLBCL (sheets of medium to large cells) to CHL-like or T-cell/histiocyte-rich LCBL-like lesions with prominent, mixed polymorphic or T-cell/histiocyte-rich backgrounds.[18] Most IDD-associated DLBCL are activated B-cell type and EBV latency II or III regardless of IDD source.

When sheets of medium or large cells are present and show a preserved B-cell expression program, the diagnosis of DLBCL is usually clear (Fig. 8). These cases may express CD30, but when expression of CD20 and other pan-B-cell markers (CD79a, PAX5, OCT2, BOB1) is diffuse and strong, classification as DLBCL is reproducible. Cases with a polymorphic or T-cell/histiocyte-rich background and those containing more prominent Hodgkin-like cells or showing gray-zone (overlapping DLBCL/CHL) immunophenotypes are diagnostically challenging due to their potentially significant overlap with polymorphic LPDs and CHL[25] (Fig. 9). Extensive immunophenotyping, clonality

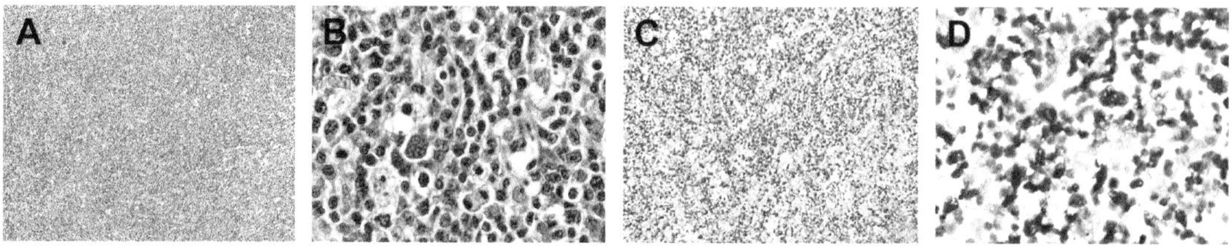

Fig. 8. DLBCL, EBV-positive, iatrogenic/therapy-related (posttransplantation, solid organ). H&E-stained tissue sections of excisional lymph node biopsy show nodal architectural effacement and diffuse involvement by lymphoma (*A*). Lymphoma cells are medium to large and include centroblasts and occasional cells with eccentric nuclei imparting an immunoblastic/plasmablastic appearance; scattered multinucleated cells with Hodgkin-like features are also seen (*B*). In situ hybridization for EBER is diffusely positive (*C*) with EBER-positive cells being medium to large and occasionally Hodgkin-like (*D*).

and mutational analysis, and correlation with clinical details may be required to assist with development of best treatment approach. The frequency and extent of histopathologic overlap between DLBCL and CHL exceeds that seen in non–IDD-related cases, suggesting that IDD-associated EBV-positive LBCLs exist on a morphologic and immunophenotypic spectrum that reflects a common underlying biology.[17,19]

If immune suppression can be withdrawn, these lesions may respond to immune reconstitution and/or treatment with rituximab monotherapy. In patients in whom immune suppression cannot or should not be decreased, or in high-risk or nonresponder patients, treatment usually involves lymphoma-directed combination chemotherapy and may also involve immunotherapy, donor T cells, and/or EBV-specific T cells.[5]

CLASSIC HODGKIN LYMPHOMA, EPSTEIN-BARR VIRUS–POSITIVE, ARISING IN IMMUNE DEFICIENCY/DYSREGULATION

Example diagnosis: CHL, EBV-positive, HIV-associated.

EBV-positive CHL comprises approximately 30% of all CHL and may or may not be IDD-associated.[26] Cases of IDD-associated CHL are classified as such regardless of EBV status, although the vast majority are EBV-positive. However, unlike in DLBCL, cases of EBV-positive CHL arising in the setting of intact immunity are not classified separately but are classified as CHL.

Regardless of immune status, evidence for a causative role for EBV in development of EBV-positive CHL includes the following: anti-EBV serum antibody titer is increased before

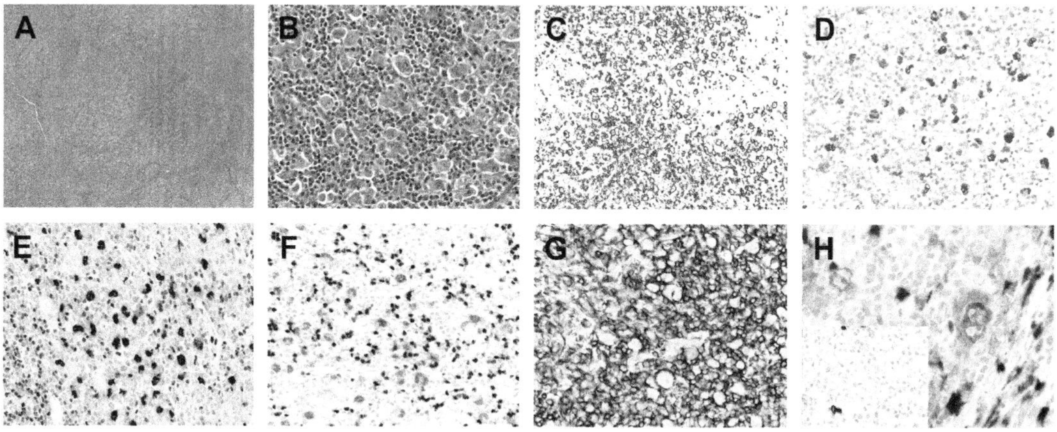

Fig. 9. DLBCL, EBV-positive, iatrogenic/therapy-related (posttransplantation, multivisceral). H&E-stained tissue sections of excisional lymph node biopsy show nodal architectural effacement and extensive involvement by lymphoma (*A*). Lymphoma cells are large with prominent Hodgkin-like features present in a background of small lymphocytes and occasional histiocytes (*B*). Lymphoma cells express strong and diffuse CD20 (*C*) and are positive for EBER (*D*) with strong co-expression of OCT2 (*E*), weak coexpression of PAX5 (*F*), and variable, but mostly positive, expression of CD45 (*G*). Lymphoma cells show variable cytoplasmic (but not membranous) staining for CD30 (*H*) and are negative for CD15 (*H, inset*). Not pictured is that lymphoma cells additionally expressed CD79a.

development of CHL and is restricted to EBV-positive CHL cases; people with history of acute infectious mononucleosis are at increased risk for development of EBV-positive CHL (temporal association of approximately 3 years postinfection); EBV genome is monoclonal and usually persists throughout disease and in all involved sites in an individual person; the frequency of EBV-positive CHL far exceeds the expected statistically random chance of development of EBV-positive CHL based on frequency of bystander EBV-positive cells.[26–31] EBV-encoded EBER and LMP1, as well as LMP2A and EBNA1, may be present in EBV-positive CHL, consistent with latency II or III. In terms of mechanism of oncogenesis, EBV antigens LMP1, LMP2A, and EBNA1 are implicated as contributors via their oncogenic mechanisms discussed previously. EBV positivity in CHL has been associated with significantly worse overall survival, with the negative impact of EBV preferentially seen in patients older than 50 years.[32]

CHL arising in IDD is usually histologically and immunophenotypically similar to CHL in immune competent states, with most IDD-associated cases being EBV-positive and of mixed cellularity or nodular sclerosis types (Figs. 10 and 11). However, as discussed earlier, CHL cells in the IDD setting may show variable morphology and an atypical immunophenotype, including expression of pan-B-cell markers (see Fig. 10). Although these features may initially suggest gray-zone lymphoma, those tumors are usually mediastinal, are not common in the IDD setting, and are EBV-negative, allowing this distinction in most IDD-related cases. More difficult is the overlap of EBV-positive IDD-associated CHL with B-cell LPD, DLBCL, and MCU (see Fig. 10). As described earlier, correlation with clinical features, site of involvement, and careful and extensive immunophenotypic analysis may be required to resolve these diagnostic dilemmas. In the differential diagnosis with EBV-positive MCU, site of involvement and clinical features of the lesion are important and, in general, involvement of a mucosal or cutaneous site is unlikely in CHL. Not all cases of LBCL with overlapping DLBCL/CHL features can be resolved, and some likely exist on an IDD-related LBCL spectrum, as described earlier.

In terms of treatment, clinical approaches may include attempts at reduction of immune suppression when possible, but most cases require lymphoma-directed combination chemotherapy as would be applied in the immune-competent setting. In CHL arising in PLWH, the addition of cART combined with chemotherapy has led to improved long-term survival compared with that of non–HIV-positive people.[33]

BURKITT LYMPHOMA, EPSTEIN-BARR VIRUS–POSITIVE, ARISING IN IMMUNE DEFICIENCY/DYSREGULATION

Example diagnosis: Burkitt lymphoma, EBV-positive, iatrogenic/therapy-related (posttransplantation, solid organ).

Similar to DLBCL and CHL, Burkitt lymphoma may arise in the context of IDD or no known IDD and may be EBV-positive or EBV-negative. In the context of intact immunity, EBV status is of increasing importance, as new insights into Burkitt lymphoma biology support distinct underlying molecular features depending on EBV status; this fascinating discussion is beyond the scope of this review. Burkitt lymphoma arising in IDD states are classified as IDD-associated lymphomas regardless of EBV status (Fig. 12).

IDD-associated Burkitt lymphoma is most frequent in PLWH and may show greater variability in terms of variation of lymphoma cell morphology and immunophenotype compared with classic Burkitt lymphoma. Importantly, a subset of IDD-related Burkitt lymphoma may show immunoblastic or plasmacytoid differentiation and be EBV-positive, features that overlap with PBL. Careful evaluation of complete immunophenotypic, cytogenetic, and molecular features is important in these cases. IDD-associated Burkitt lymphoma is clinically aggressive and requires treatment with high-intensity chemotherapeutic regimens, which have considerably improved patient survival.[34]

PLASMABLASTIC LYMPHOMA ARISING IN IMMUNE DEFICIENCY/DYSREGULATION

Example diagnosis: PBL, EBV-positive, HIV-associated.

PBL were initially described in the context of HIV, and most PBL occur in IDD settings that are now also known to include posttransplantation, immunosuppressive therapy, and rarely, autoimmune diseases. PBL occurring without known IDD are usually seen in elderly people, possibly arising in the context of immune senescence. EBV is positive in most cases, usually in latency I or II, in the context of EBV reactivation.

PBL are large cell lymphomas with predominantly immunoblastic/plasmablastic morphology and occasional plasmacytic morphology that express a mature plasma cell immunophenotype (CD38+, VS38c+, CD138+, MUM1+, light chain+, ± CD79a) and are negative for CD20 with decreased or negative expression of PAX5 (Fig. 13). MYC protein expression is frequently

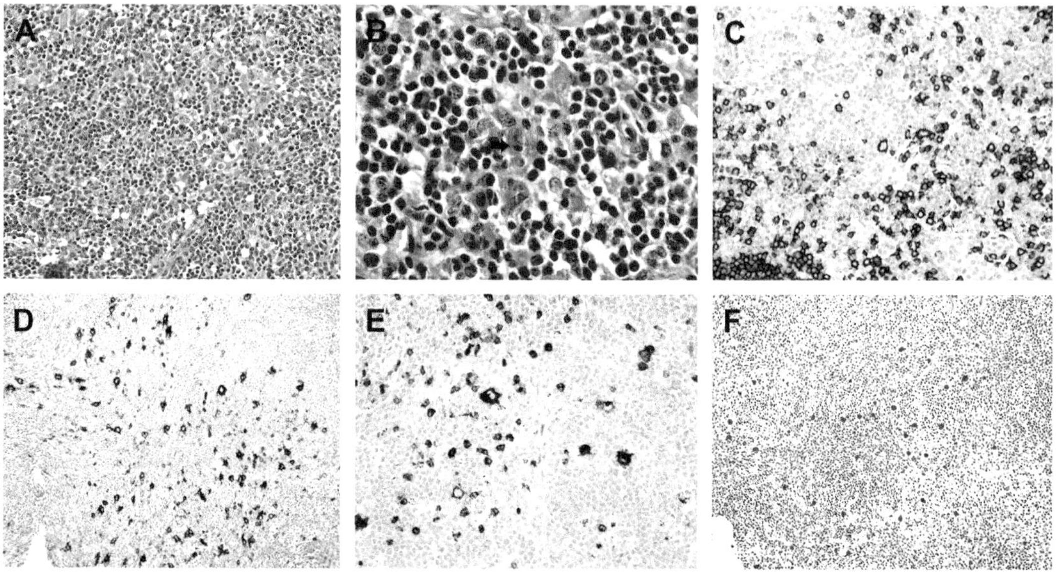

Fig. 10. Classic Hodgkin lymphoma, EBV-positive, iatrogenic/therapy-related (post-transplantation, solid organ). H&E-stained tissue sections of lymph node show nodal architectural effacement and involvement by a polymorphic infiltrate composed of small lymphocytes, plasma cells, histiocytes, eosinophils, and scattered and clustered Reed-Sternberg cells and variants (*arrow*) (*A*, *B*). A subset of Hodgkin cells expresses CD20 (*C*), and all express strong CD30 (*D*) and CD15 (*E*). EBER is positive in large Hodgkin cells (*F*). Hodgkin cells additionally showed dim to moderate expression of PAX5, were mostly negative for CD45 and negative for CD79a (not shown).

diffuse, related to the underlying *MYC* rearrangement present in most cases. HHV-8 and ALK must be negative, by definition, as positivity for either would support alternate diagnoses of extracavitary primary effusion lymphoma or ALK-positive LBCL, respectively.

PBL can usually be distinguished from multiple myeloma or anaplastic plasmacytoma based on

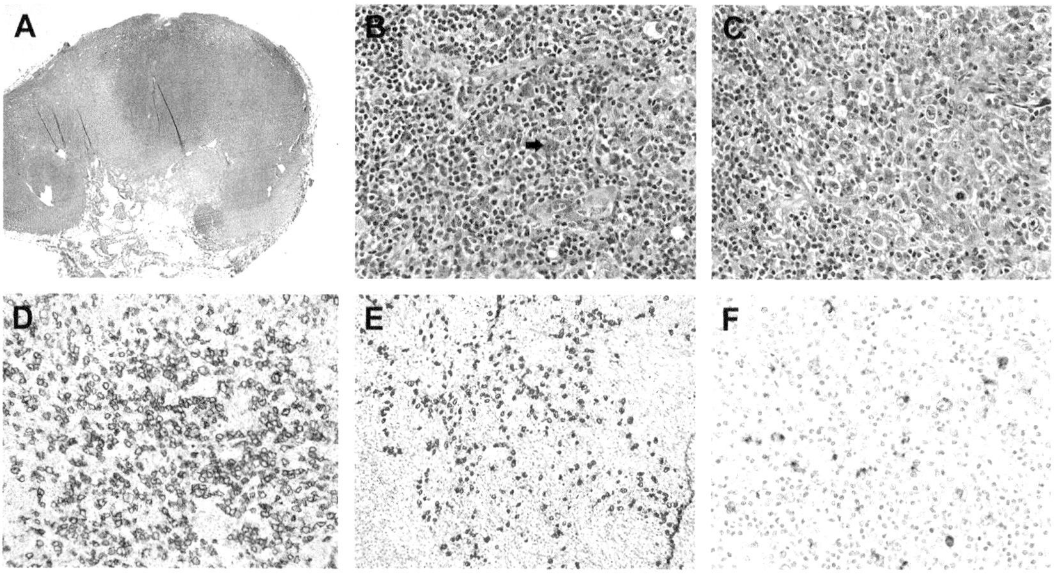

Fig. 11. Classic Hodgkin lymphoma, EBV-positive, HIV-associated. H&E-stained tissue sections of an excisional lymph node biopsy show nodal architectural effacement by a nodular lymphoid infiltrate with broad bands of collagen fibrosis (*A*). The polymorphic infiltrate is composed of scattered Reed-Sternberg cells and variants (*arrow*) admixed with small lymphocytes, eosinophils, rare plasma cells, and histiocytes (*B*). In some foci, lymphoma cells are present in clusters (*C*). Lymphoma cells express strong and diffuse CD30 (*D*) and are positive for EBER (*E*) and LMP1 (*F*).

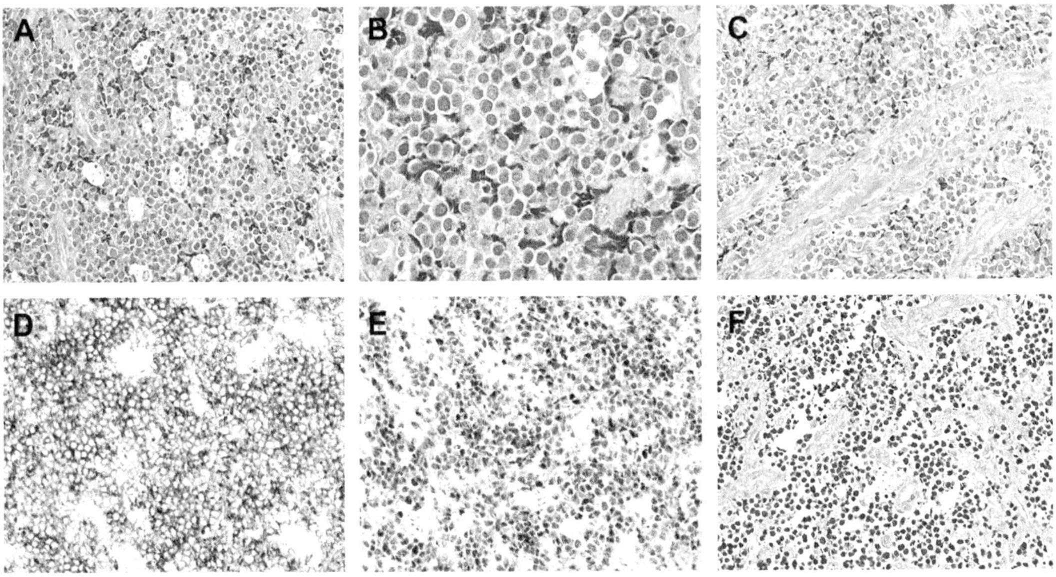

Fig. 12. Burkitt lymphoma, EBV-positive, iatrogenic/therapy-related (post-transplantation, multivisceral). Excisional biopsy of inguinal lymph node shows diffuse nodal effacement by an aggressive lymphoma composed of a monotonous population of medium-sized lymphoid cells with high nuclear-to-cytoplasmic ratios and frequent tingible body macrophages (*A–C*). Lymphoma cells express CD20 (*D*) and are diffusely positive for MYC protein (*E*) and EBER (*F*). Lymphoma cells were additionally diffusely positive for CD10 and BCL6 and negative for BCL2, MUM1, TdT, and CD34 (not shown). FISH studies were positive for *IGH:MYC* fusion and negative for *BCL2* and *BCL6* rearrangements (not shown).

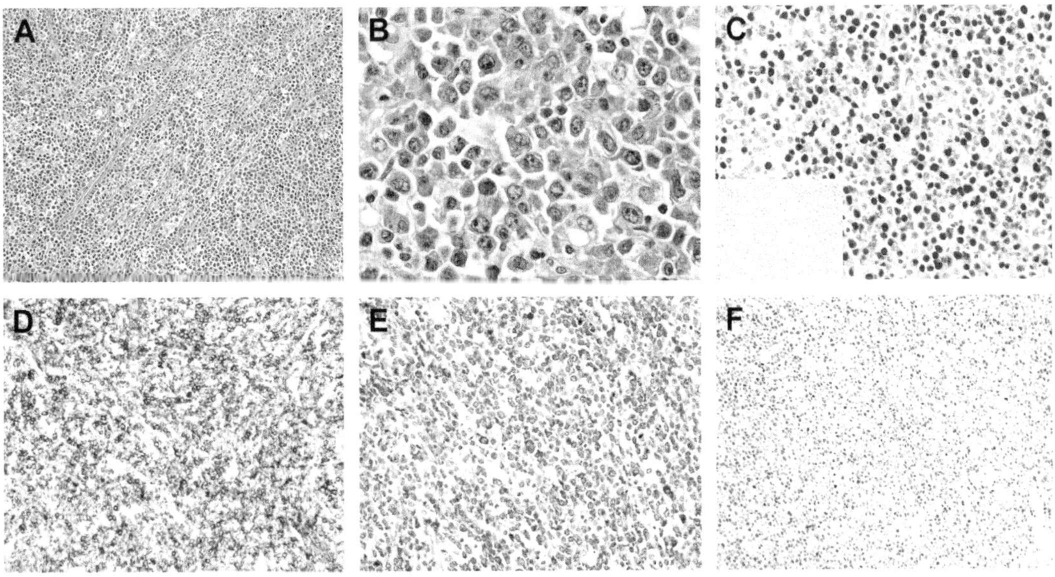

Fig. 13. Plasmablastic lymphoma, EBV-positive, HIV. Histologic sections of terminal ileum and cecum mass show extensive involvement by large cell lymphoma (*A*). Lymphoma cells have variable immunoblastic and plasmablastic morphology (*B*). Tumor cells are diffusely positive for EBER (*C*) and negative for HHV-8 (*C, inset*). Lymphoma cells express CD138 (*D*) and are kappa restricted by in situ hybridization (*E*) with diffuse expression of MYC protein (*F*). Lymphoma cells were additionally positive for MUM1, BCL2, and CD10 and negative for CD20, PAX5, BCL6, and pan-T-cell markers (not shown). FISH studies were positive for *IG::MYC* fusion and negative for *BCL2* and *BCL6* rearrangements (not shown).

the combination of EBV status, serum protein studies, bone marrow staging, and clinical history. In some cases, the distinction between PBL and anaplastic plasmacytoma may be very difficult, requiring extensive clinical correlation; this distinction may not be accomplished in rare cases. PBL are clinically aggressive, and survival is generally poor.

LOW-GRADE B-CELL LYMPHOMAS AND PLASMACYTOMAS, EPSTEIN-BARR VIRUS–POSITIVE, ARISING IN IMMUNE DEFICIENCY/DYSREGULATION

Example diagnosis: extranodal marginal zone lymphoma of mucosa-associated lymphoid tissue, EBV-positive, post-transplantation (solid organ).

Although less frequent than EBV-positive LBCL, EBV-positive low-grade B-cell lymphomas and plasmacytomas also occur. These most commonly include EBV-positive marginal zone lymphoma, lymphoplasmacytic lymphoma, and plasmacytoma; EBV-positive follicular lymphoma is also described, but the association with IDD is less well established.[35–38] These lymphomas have the same diagnostic criteria as they do in immune competent states, with the link to IDD status being EBV-positivity and clinical history. As with LBCLs, EBV-positive IDD-related low-grade B-cell lymphomas tend to have a postgerminal center immunophenotype, show frequent plasmacytic differentiation, and are composed of heavy chain class-switched cells.

DIFFUSE LARGE B-CELL LYMPHOMA ASSOCIATED WITH CHRONIC INFLAMMATION

Example diagnosis: DLBCL associated with chronic inflammation.

Small, enclosed anatomic spaces that are exposed to chronic antigenic stimulation (usually >10 years) may develop local immune dysregulation within the enclosed space, and CI-DLBCL may arise in this context. Pyothorax-associated DLBCL developing in the pleural cavity of patients with history of pyothorax resulting from treatment of tuberculosis is the classic example.[39] Other sites of involvement can include bones and joints where sources of inflammation include infection and orthopedic hardware. These lesions are symptomatic (painful), mass-forming, and are always EBV-positive.[39] CI-DLBCL are not conceptualized as IDD-related lymphomas in the sense that patients do not have systemic IDD.

Histologically, these lymphomas have typical DLBCL morphology and more frequently show immunoblastic or plasmablastic differentiation, related to the EBV association. Most tumors have a nongerminal center B-cell immunophenotype and EBV latency III. These neoplasms have features overlapping with FA-LBCL but must be distinguished from them because CI-DLBCL is clinically more aggressive. An infiltrative pattern, even if focal, and the presence of a mass favor CI-DLBCL.

FIBRIN-ASSOCIATED LARGE B-CELL LYMPHOMAS

Example diagnosis: fibrin-associated large B-cell lymphoma.

Similar to CI-DLBCL, FA-LBCL also arises in confined sites of chronic inflammation including cavities and cystic spaces. These lymphomas may also involve fibrin thrombi, and lymphoma cells are frequently present within fibrinoid material.[40] Patients may present with thromboembolic events, but the lymphoma is usually incidentally found and non–mass-forming. Most of the cases are EBV-positive, but patients do not have systemic IDD.[40] The local environment is believed to create a localized immune dysregulation that allows EBV to escape immune surveillance. Histologically, lymphoma cells have cytologic features typical of LBCL but are frequently associated with fibrin and have no significant inflammatory reaction. These lesions have a better prognosis than CI-DLBCL, thus the distinction is clinically relevant.[40]

BASICS OF GENETICS AND IMMUNE ESCAPE MECHANISMS IN EPSTEIN-BARR VIRUS - POSITIVE LYMPHOPROLIFERATIVE DISORDERS ARISING IN IMMUNE DEFICIENCY/DYSREGULATION

LBCLs occurring in IDD are usually activated B-cell (ABC) type tumors regardless of EBV status. This ABC status is linked to activation of NF-κB, either occurring by somatic mutation in EBV-negative tumors or via contribution of EBV-derived oncogenic mechanisms of LMP1 and LMP2A in EBV-positive tumors.[41–44] EBV-positive LBCLs occur at lower mutational burden rates per tumor compared with EBV-negative counterparts, as EBV itself provides oncogenic signals, in particular in latency II and III. EBV-positive DLBCL in PLWH are also enriched for *STAT3* mutations, as are PBL.[45,46]

DLBCL and CHL arising in IDD also show more frequent alterations in 9p24.1 (containing *PDL1*, *PDL2*, and *JAK2*) and tumor cells often express

PD-L1.[47,48] These abnormalities support that lymphomas and LPDs arising in IDD take advantage of activation of the PD-1/PD-L1 pathway that allows for immune escape of tumor cells via suppression of cytotoxic T-cell function. 9p24.1 abnormalities allowing for immune escape likely contribute to a unifying immune evasion oncogenic mechanism that characterize these tumors and could provide an avenue for a unified treatment approach.[18,49] Expression of PD-L1 and PD-L2 is detectable by immunohistochemistry in clinical practice and may assist with recognition of these lesions.

Chromosomal abnormalities including rearrangements of *MYC* and *BCL6* are also frequent in EBV-positive LBCLs arising in IDD, but *BCL2* translocations are uncommon unless related to an antecedent follicular lymphoma. *MYC* rearrangements are also present in approximately 80% of EBV-positive PBL, and mutations in JAK-STAT, MAPK/ERK, and NOTCH pathways are also frequent in these neoplasms.

THERAPEUTIC CONSIDERATIONS

In general, LPDs and lymphomas occurring in IDD may respond to less aggressive approaches compared with their counterpart lymphomas arising in patients with intact immunity. For this reason, a more guarded and tiered treatment approach is desired in lesions arising in IDD. This direct clinical implication makes recognition of LPDs as arising in the setting of IDD of significant importance. Because there are no objective histologic features or assays to determine immune status, suspicion of an underlying IDD requires recognition of histopathologic nuances of these lesions, including the presence of polymorphic B-cell infiltrates characterized by a range of morphology and maturation across the B-cell/plasma cell spectrum, admixed with immunoblasts and Hodgkin-like cells. EBV testing should be performed in these cases without hesitation! Open dialog between patients, clinicians, and pathologists is critical.

DISCLOSURE

The author has nothing to disclose.

REFERENCES

1. Tzellos S, Farrell PJ. Epstein-barr virus sequence variation-biology and disease. Pathogens 2012;1(2):156–74.
2. Kanda T, Yajima M, Ikuta K. Epstein-Barr virus strain variation and cancer. Cancer Sci 2019;110(4):1132–9.
3. Tsurumi T, Fujita M, Kudoh A. Latent and lytic Epstein-Barr virus replication strategies. Rev Med Virol 2005;15(1):3–15.
4. Morgan SM, Tanizawa H, Caruso LB, et al. The three-dimensional structure of Epstein-Barr virus genome varies by latency type and is regulated by PARP1 enzymatic activity. Nat Commun 2022;13(1):187.
5. Heslop HE. How I treat EBV lymphoproliferation. Blood 2009;114(19):4002–8.
6. Callan MF, Tan L, Annels N, et al. Direct visualization of antigen-specific CD8+ T cells during the primary immune response to Epstein-Barr virus In vivo. J Exp Med 1998;187(9):1395–402.
7. Yang J, Lemas VM, Flinn IW, et al. Application of the ELISPOT assay to the characterization of CD8(+) responses to Epstein-Barr virus antigens. Blood 2000;95(1):241–8.
8. Mancao C, Altmann M, Jungnickel B, et al. Rescue of "crippled" germinal center B cells from apoptosis by Epstein-Barr virus. Blood 2005;106(13):4339–44.
9. Levitskaya J, Coram M, Levitsky V, et al. Inhibition of antigen processing by the internal repeat region of the Epstein-Barr virus nuclear antigen-1. Nature 1995;375(6533):685–8.
10. Frappier L. Ebna1. *Curr Top Microbiol Immunol.* 2015;391:3–34.
11. Zimber-Strobl U, Strobl LJ. EBNA2 and Notch signalling in Epstein-Barr virus mediated immortalization of B lymphocytes. Semin Cancer Biol 2001;11(6):423–34.
12. Bargou RC, Emmerich F, Krappmann D, et al. Constitutive nuclear factor-kappaB-RelA activation is required for proliferation and survival of Hodgkin's disease tumor cells. J Clin Invest 1997;100(12):2961–9.
13. Kulwichit W, Edwards RH, Davenport EM, et al. Expression of the Epstein-Barr virus latent membrane protein 1 induces B cell lymphoma in transgenic mice. Proc Natl Acad Sci U S A 1998;95(20):11963–8.
14. Komano J, Maruo S, Kurozumi K, et al. Oncogenic role of Epstein-Barr virus-encoded RNAs in Burkitt's lymphoma cell line Akata. J Virol 1999;73(12):9827–31.
15. Medeiros LJ, Marques-Piubelli ML, Sangiorgio VFI, et al. Epstein-Barr-virus-positive large B-cell lymphoma associated with breast implants: an analysis of eight patients suggesting a possible pathogenetic relationship. Mod Pathol 2021;34(12):2154–67.
16. Alaggio R, Amador C, Anagnostopoulos I, et al. The 5th edition of the World Health Organization Classification of Haematolymphoid Tumours: Lymphoid Neoplasms. Leukemia 2022;36(7):1720–48.
17. Natkunam Y, Goodlad JR, Chadburn A, et al. EBV-Positive B-Cell Proliferations of Varied Malignant Potential: 2015 SH/EAHP Workshop Report-Part 1. Am J Clin Pathol 2017;147(2):129–52.

18. de Jong D, Roemer MG, Chan JK, et al. B-Cell and Classical Hodgkin Lymphomas Associated With Immunodeficiency: 2015 SH/EAHP Workshop Report-Part 2. Am J Clin Pathol 2017;147(2):153–70.
19. Natkunam Y, Gratzinger D, Chadburn A, et al. Immunodeficiency-associated lymphoproliferative disorders: time for reappraisal? Blood 2018;132(18):1871–8.
20. Hudnall SD, Ge Y, Wei L, et al. Distribution and phenotype of Epstein-Barr virus-infected cells in human pharyngeal tonsils. Mod Pathol 2005;18(4):519–27.
21. Ito Y, Makita S, Maeshima AM, et al. EBV-encoded RNA1-positive cells in the bone marrow specimens of patients with EBV-negative lymphomas and sarcomas. Pathol Int 2019;69(7):392–7.
22. Dojcinov SD, Venkataraman G, Raffeld M, et al. EBV positive mucocutaneous ulcer–a study of 26 cases associated with various sources of immunosuppression. Am J Surg Pathol 2010;34(3):405–17.
23. Prieto-Torres L, Erana I, Gil-Redondo R, et al. The Spectrum of EBV-Positive Mucocutaneous Ulcer: A Study of 9 Cases. Am J Surg Pathol 2019;43(2):201–10.
24. Kim CH, Chapman JR, Vega F. A case of EBV-associated blastic lymphoplasmacytic proliferation in an oesophageal ulcer with a self-limiting course: overlapping lesion between EBV mucocutaneous ulcer and polymorphic lymphoplasmacytic disorder. Histopathology 2019;74(6):964–6.
25. Nicolae A, Pittaluga S, Abdullah S, et al. EBV-positive large B-cell lymphomas in young patients: a nodal lymphoma with evidence for a tolerogenic immune environment. Blood 2015;126(7):863–72.
26. Murray PG, Young LS. An etiological role for the Epstein-Barr virus in the pathogenesis of classical Hodgkin lymphoma. Blood 2019;134(7):591–6.
27. Mueller N, Evans A, Harris NL, et al. Hodgkin's disease and Epstein-Barr virus. Altered antibody pattern before diagnosis. N Engl J Med 1989;320(11):689–95.
28. Levin LI, Chang ET, Ambinder RF, et al. Atypical prediagnosis Epstein-Barr virus serology restricted to EBV-positive Hodgkin lymphoma. Blood 2012;120(18):3750–5.
29. Connelly RR, Christine BW. A cohort study of cancer following infectious mononucleosis. Cancer Res 1974;34(5):1172–8.
30. Rosdahl N, Larsen SO, Clemmesen J. Hodgkin's disease in patients with previous infectious mononucleosis: 30 years' experience. Br Med J 1974;2(5913):253–6.
31. Hjalgrim H, Smedby KE, Rostgaard K, et al. Infectious mononucleosis, childhood social environment, and risk of Hodgkin lymphoma. Cancer Res 2007;67(5):2382–8.
32. Jarrett RF, Stark GL, White J, et al. Impact of tumor Epstein-Barr virus status on presenting features and outcome in age-defined subgroups of patients with classic Hodgkin lymphoma: a population-based study. Blood 2005;106(7):2444–51.
33. Carbone A, Gloghini A, Serraino D, et al. Immunodeficiency-associated Hodgkin lymphoma. Expert Rev Hematol 2021;14(6):547–59.
34. Atallah-Yunes SA, Murphy DJ, Noy A. HIV-associated Burkitt lymphoma. Lancet Haematol 2020;7(8):e594–600.
35. Mackrides N, Campuzano-Zuluaga G, Maque-Acosta Y, et al. Epstein-Barr virus-positive follicular lymphoma. Mod Pathol 2017;30(4):519–29.
36. Mackrides N, Chapman J, Larson MC, et al. Prevalence, clinical characteristics and prognosis of EBV-positive follicular lymphoma. Am J Hematol 2019;94(2):E62–4.
37. Gong S, Crane GM, McCall CM, et al. Expanding the Spectrum of EBV-positive Marginal Zone Lymphomas: A Lesion Associated With Diverse Immunodeficiency Settings. Am J Surg Pathol 2018;42(10):1306–16.
38. Gibson SE, Swerdlow SH, Craig FE, et al. EBV-positive extranodal marginal zone lymphoma of mucosa-associated lymphoid tissue in the post-transplant setting: a distinct type of posttransplant lymphoproliferative disorder? Am J Surg Pathol 2011;35(6):807–15.
39. Sukswai N, Lyapichev K, Khoury JD, et al. Diffuse large B-cell lymphoma variants: an update. Pathology 2020;52(1):53–67.
40. Boyer DF, McKelvie PA, de Leval L, et al. Fibrin-associated EBV-positive Large B-Cell Lymphoma: An Indolent Neoplasm With Features Distinct From Diffuse Large B-Cell Lymphoma Associated With Chronic Inflammation. Am J Surg Pathol 2017;41(3):299–312. https://doi.org/10.1097/PAS.0000000000000775. PMID: 28195879.
41. Morscio J, Dierickx D, Ferreiro JF, et al. Gene expression profiling reveals clear differences between EBV-positive and EBV-negative posttransplant lymphoproliferative disorders. Am J Transplant 2013;13(5):1305–16.
42. Montes-Moreno S, Odqvist L, Diaz-Perez JA, et al. EBV-positive diffuse large B-cell lymphoma of the elderly is an aggressive post-germinal center B-cell neoplasm characterized by prominent nuclear factor-kB activation. Mod Pathol 2012;25(7):968–82.
43. Vento-Tormo R, Rodriguez-Ubreva J, Lisio LD, et al. NF-kappaB directly mediates epigenetic deregulation of common microRNAs in Epstein-Barr virus-mediated transformation of B-cells and in lymphomas. Nucleic Acids Res 2014;42(17):11025–39.
44. Price AM, Tourigny JP, Forte E, et al. Analysis of Epstein-Barr virus-regulated host gene expression changes through primary B-cell outgrowth reveals delayed kinetics of latent membrane protein 1-

mediated NF-kappaB activation. J Virol 2012;86(20): 11096–106.
45. Satou A, Nakamura S. EBV-positive B-cell lymphomas and lymphoproliferative disorders: Review from the perspective of immune escape and immunodeficiency. Cancer Med 2021;10(19):6777–85.
46. Chapman JR, Bouska AC, Zhang W, et al. EBV-positive HIV-associated diffuse large B cell lymphomas are characterized by JAK/STAT (STAT3) pathway mutations and unique clinicopathologic features. Br J Haematol 2021;194(5):870–8.
47. Yoon H, Park S, Ju H, et al. Integrated copy number and gene expression profiling analysis of Epstein-Barr virus-positive diffuse large B-cell lymphoma. Genes Chromosomes Cancer 2015;54(6): 383–96.
48. Shiraiwa S, Kikuti YY, Carreras J, et al. 9p24.1 Genetic Alteration and PD-L1 Expression Are Characteristic of De Novo and Methotrexate-associated Epstein-Barr Virus-positive Hodgkin Lymphoma, But Not Methotrexate-associated Hodgkin-like Lesions. Am J Surg Pathol 2022;46(8):1017–24.
49. Chen BJ, Chapuy B, Ouyang J, et al. PD-L1 expression is characteristic of a subset of aggressive B-cell lymphomas and virus-associated malignancies. Clin Cancer Res 2013;19(13):3462–73.

Navigating the Heterogeneity of Follicular Lymphoma and its Many Variants

An Updated Approach to Diagnosis and Classification

Abner Louissaint Jr, MD, PhD

KEYWORDS

• Follicular lymphoma • International Consensus Classification • World health organization • Lymphoma

Key points

- Classic nodal follicular lymphoma (FL) represents the majority of FL cases and is characterized by follicular architecture, predominantly centrocytic composition, and BCL2 expression by germinal center B cells, driven by the hallmark t(14;18) (q32;q21) rearrangement.
- Several FL variants have been described that tend to present as localized nodal (eg, pediatric-type FL) or extranodal disease (eg, primary cutaneous follicle center lymphoma), lack *BCL2* gene rearrangements, and have generally excellent prognosis. These variants have mutational profiles that are different from those of classic nodal FL.
- The 5th edition of the World Health Organization (WHO) Classification of Haematolymphoid Tumors has moved from grading classic FL to applying a new system of subclassification, including classic FL, follicular large cell lymphoma, FL with predominantly diffuse growth pattern, and FL with unusual cytologic features. Grading is no longer required for diagnosis but remains optional.
- The 2022 International Consensus Classification of Mature Lymphoid Neoplasms has retained grading (eg, grade 1, 2, 3A, 3B) as described in the Revised 4th edition of the WHO Classification of Tumors of Haematopoietic and Lymphoid Tissues.

Follicular lymphoma (FL) is a lymphoid neoplasm composed of follicle center (germinal center) B cells, with varying proportions of centrocytes and centroblasts, that usually has a predominantly follicular architectural pattern. Over the past decade, our understanding of FL has evolved significantly, with new recognition of several recently defined FL variants characterized by distinct clinical presentations, behaviors, genetic alterations, and biology. This manuscript aims to review the heterogeneity of FL and its variants, to provide an updated guide on their diagnosis and classification, and to describe how approaches to the histologic subclassification of classic FL have evolved in current classification schemes.

OVERVIEW

Follicular lymphoma (FL) is a lymphoid neoplasm composed of follicle center (germinal center) B cells, with a varying proportion of centrocytes and centroblasts, that usually has a predominantly follicular architectural pattern. FL affects male and female adults with a median age of 55 to 60 years and is the second most common lymphoma worldwide,

Department of Pathology, Massachusetts General Hospital, 149 13th St, Charlestown, MA 02114, USA
E-mail address: alouissaint@partners.org

Surgical Pathology 16 (2023) 233–247
https://doi.org/10.1016/j.path.2023.02.001

accounting for 20% of all non-Hodgkin lymphomas. Most patients have a widespread nodal disease at diagnosis (up to two-thirds of patients have stage III to stage IV disease). Peripheral, mediastinal, and retroperitoneal nodes are often involved. Extranodal involvement occurs in up to 20% of cases, including the involvement of spleen and bone marrow. Other more common sites of non-nodal tissue involvement include gastrointestinal tract, soft tissue, breast, and ocular adnexa. Pure extranodal presentations and significant involvement of peripheral blood are uncommon.[1]

The neoplastic follicles in FL are comprised of centrocytes and centroblasts that are morphologically similar to those of normal follicle germinal centers. Although most cases of FL show a predominantly follicular pattern of growth, a small subset of cases show a predominantly diffuse proliferation of centrocytes and centroblasts. The genetic hallmark, and one of the main initiating events in FL, is the t(14;18)(q32;q21) rearrangement, involving the reciprocal rearrangement of *IGH* and *BCL2*. FL with *BCL2* rearrangements (*BCL2*-R-FL) represent 85% to 90% of FL cases.[2,3] These *BCL2* rearrangements result in constitutive overexpression of antiapoptotic protein BCL2. FL pathogenesis requires the additional accumulation of genetic alterations including multiple loss-of-function mutations in chromatin modifier genes such as *KMT2D, CREBBP, ARID1a, MEF2B, KMT2C*, and/or gain-of-function mutations in *EZH2*.[4–10]

Over the past decade, our understanding of FL has evolved significantly, with new recognition of several recently defined FL variants characterized by distinct clinical presentations, behaviors, genetic alterations, and biology. These variants tend to be negative for *BCL2* rearrangements and/or have primary extranodal presentation. There has also been a significant evolution in our understanding and interpretation of the histologic variations in classic nodal FL, including variations in architectural pattern and histologic grade (as defined by the number of centroblasts and centrocytes). This manuscript aimed to review the heterogeneity of FL and its variants, to provide an updated guide on their diagnosis and classification, and to describe how approaches to the histologic subclassification of classic FL have evolved in current classification schemes.

DISCUSSION

BCL2-NEGATIVE AND EXTRANODAL SUBTYPES OF FOLLICULAR LYMPHOMA

Several subtypes of FL have recently been characterized and are now recognized as biologically and clinically distinct diseases with unique clinical presentations, behaviors, genetics, and underlying pathogeneses. These lymphoma subtypes, which often lack *BCL2* rearrangements and/or are characterized by primary extranodal presentation, are described below. Fig. 1 outlines an approach to their diagnosis and workup.

Pediatric-type Follicular Lymphoma

Pediatric-type follicular lymphoma (PTFL) is a localized follicular proliferation of germinal center B cells occurring in the lymph nodes of children and young adults. Though there is no upper age cut-off for diagnosis, the disease predominantly occurs in pediatric and adolescent age groups.[11–13] PTFL is always localized and tends to involve young male patients (M:F ratio of 10:1). PTFL involves peripheral lymph nodes, most commonly in the head and neck, but can less commonly involve axillary and groin lymph nodes as well. Intrathoracic, intra-abdominal, and retroperitoneal lymph nodes are not involved. PTFL has a particularly excellent prognosis with a 5-year survival of >95%.[11,12,14–19] In contrast to classic FL, local excision of the node involved by PTFL appears to be curative. Retrospective studies have shown that young adults have similar excellent prognosis irrespective of therapy. Although extranodal presentation formally excludes PTFL in the World Health Organization (WHO) Classification, rare cases of FLs with morphologic and molecular features identical to those of PTFL have been described in the conjunctiva with similarly excellent prognosis.[20–22]

In addition to its clear clinical distinctions, PTFL is also genetically distinct from classic FL. PTFL lacks *BCL2* and *BCL6* rearrangements, whereas one or both rearrangements are present in greater than 85% of classic FL.[11,13,23–25] PTFL also lacks *IRF4* rearrangements that characterize large B-cell lymphoma with *IRF4* rearrangement (LBCL-*IRF4*-R).[26,27] Approximately 60% of PTFL cases harbor mutations in MAPK pathway genes (including *MAP2K1*), which are not present in classic FL. In addition, PTFL shows recurrent deletions and copy-neutral loss of heterozygosity at 1p36 as well as *IRF8* mutations in a subset of cases.[11,13,23–25,28,29] PTFL lacks mutations in chromatin-modifying genes and other genes commonly mutated in classic FL, such as *CREBBP, KTM2D, EP300,* and *ARID1A*. Both PTFL and classic FL harbor mutations in *TNFRSF14* in less than 50% of cases.[11,13,23–25]

Morphologically, PTFL cases are characterized by large expansile follicles and/or serpiginous follicles that at least partially efface nodal

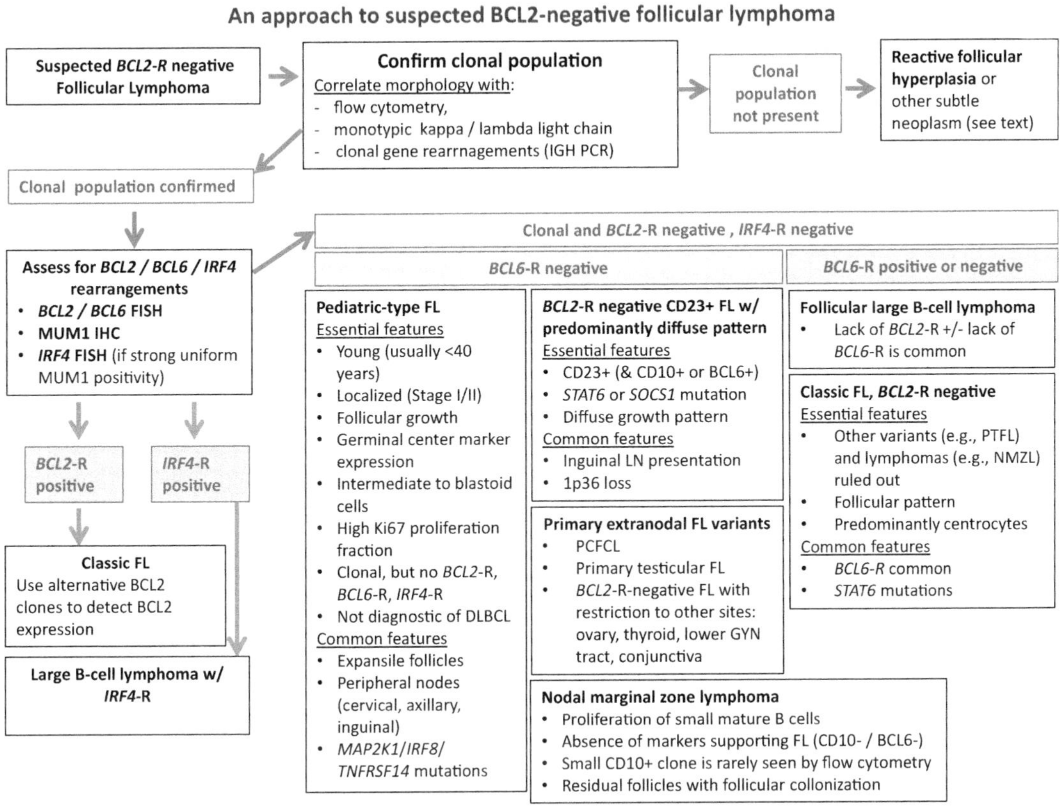

Fig. 1. Diagnostic algorithm for BCL2-negative follicular lymphoma. If morphology is suspicious for BCL2 negative FL (architectural effacement), it is often helpful to confirm the presence of a clonal B-cell population by flow cytometry, immunohistochemistry, or PCR for clonal IGH rearrangement. If a clonal population is not detected, reactive follicular hyperplasia or other reactive processes should be considered. If there is still a suspicion of lymphoma, consider the possibility of a subtle neoplastic process (eg, interfollicular classic Hodgkin lymphoma, angioimmunoblastic T-cell lymphoma). If there is a clonal B-cell proliferation, assessment for *BCL2*, *BCL6*, and *IRF4* rearrangements together with clinical and other molecular genetic features can help guide and narrow down the differential diagnosis, as shown in the figure. DLBCL, diffuse large B-cell lymphoma; FISH, fluorescence in situ hybridization; FL, follicular lymphoma; IHC, immunohistochemistry; NMZL, nodal marginal zone lymphoma, PCFCL, primary cutaneous follicle center lymphoma; PTFL, pediatric-type follicular lymphoma; R, rearranged; w/, with.

architecture. The presence of areas diagnostic of diffuse large B-cell lymphoma (DLBCL), defined by areas containing sheets of centroblasts, excludes the diagnosis of PTFL. The neoplastic cells of PTFL are often intermediate-sized “blastoid” cells that are not characteristic of centrocytes or centroblasts. Tingible-body macrophages are often present and evenly dispersed across follicles. Neoplastic cells are B cells (CD20+ PAX5+ CD79a+) that express germinal center markers (CD10+ BCL6+) but tend to lack BCL2 expression or occasionally have very faint BCL2 expression. In addition, PTFL usually has a relatively high proliferation fraction (>30%) by Ki67 staining compared with classic FL.[11,14,25,29–32]

The combination of expansile follicles with weak to absent BCL2 expression and high proliferation index (PI) in a patient younger than 40 years of age should warrant consideration of a diagnosis of PTFL. Rarely, patients older than 40 years may be diagnosed with PTFL. Whenever a diagnosis of PTFL is considered, FISH for *BCL2* and *BCL6* rearrangements should be performed, since the presence of either of these rearrangements excludes the possibility of PTFL. In addition, staging should be recommended, as the presence of advanced-stage disease would exclude PTFL. LBCL-*IRF4*-R is sometimes in the differential diagnosis as this lymphoma often occurs in Waldeyer ring in younger patients, is often localized, and tends to lack *BCL2* rearrangement.[26,27] However, in addition to *IRF4* rearrangement, LBCL-*IRF4*-R often harbors *BCL6* rearrangements, whereas PTFL lacks both *IRF4* and *BCL6* rearrangements.

LBCL-*IRF4*-R typically shows a mixture of FL grade 3A and DLBCL morphology.[26,27] In contrast, any area diagnostic of DLBCL excludes a diagnosis of PTFL. PTFL may also occasionally morphologically overlap with florid follicular hyperplasia. Cases of florid follicular hyperplasia with clonal CD10+ B cell populations detected by flow cytometry have been described most often in young boys.[33] PTFL can usually be distinguished from florid follicular hyperplasia with clonal B cells (FFHCBC) by the presence of architectural effacement that characterizes PTFL. However, the possibility that cases of FFHCBC and PTFL may reflect a biological continuum requires further careful study. There is some early data to suggest that expression of FOXP1 by germinal center B cells in PTFL may be helpful in distinguishing PTFL from reactive follicular hyperplasia, in which germinal center B cells are reported to lack FOXP1 expression.[25]

BCL2-R-negative and CD23-positive Follicle Center Lymphoma

This is a unique FL subtype characterized by a distinctive clinical presentation and histologic and molecular genetic features, including the characteristic absence of *BCL2* rearrangements. These patients typically present with painless localized (stage I-II) lymphadenopathy, most commonly in the inguinal area in greater than 75% of cases, but in non-inguinal lymph nodes can be involved. Histologically, these lymphomas are predominantly composed of centrocytes (grade 1 to 2 of 3 histology) usually growing in a diffuse pattern with scattered microfollicles and frequent interstitial sclerosis. However, some cases may retain follicular architecture (Figs. 2A–C). The neoplastic cells usually express germinal center markers CD10 and BCL6, are usually positive for CD23, and have variable expression of BCL2 (see Figs. 2B, D, F, G). These cases have recurrent deletions of 1p36 (involving *TNFRSF14*) and deletion at 16p (involving *CREBBP* and *SOCS1*) and/or *CREBBP* and *STAT6 or SOCS1* mutations.[34] This group of FL generally has an excellent prognosis.

Primary Cutaneous Follicle Center Lymphoma

PCFCL is a tumor of follicular center (germinal center) cells involving and localized to the skin. PCFCL makes up approximately 10% of all cutaneous lymphomas and 30% to 50% of primary cutaneous lymphomas arising in skin.[35,36] PCFCL presents clinically with plaques and/or tumors at a solitary cutaneous site, most commonly on the scalp, forehead, or trunk, but can present less commonly at other sites.[35–37] Most cases diagnosed as PCFCL have an indolent course and excellent prognosis, with a 5-year survival rate of 95%.[35,36,38,39] Multifocal skin lesions occur in approximately 15% of patients but are not associated with worse prognosis.[35–37] Progression to systemic disease or dissemination to extracutaneous sites is uncommon, even in the absence of therapy. Cutaneous relapses after therapy occur in approximately 30% of patients (often in the location of initial presentation) with excellent survival rates.[35–37] In contrast, cases of systemic FL with secondary cutaneous involvement have a worse prognosis than PCFCL, often requiring systemic therapy.

Cases of PCFCL that remain skin restricted have molecular features that are distinct from classic nodal FL, including absence of *BCL2* rearrangements and a marked reduction in the frequency of *CREBBP*, *KTM2D*, *EZH2,* and *EP300* mutations.[40–44] In contrast, cases of classic nodal FL with secondary cutaneous involvement tend to harbor *BCL2* rearrangements and multiple loss of function mutations in *CREBBP*, *KTM2D*, *EZH2,* and *EP300*.[45] Rare cases initially diagnosed as PCFCL based on morphology and absent extracutaneous involvement may later show extracutaneous spread and have a worse prognosis. These cases are more likely to harbor *BCL2* rearrangements and/or harbor mutations in *CREBBP, KTM2D, EZH2,* and *EP300* at diagnosis, suggesting that the underlying biology of these lesions is more similar to FL with secondary cutaneous involvement than PCFCL.[45]

PCFCL shows dermal infiltrates (often perivascular or periadnexal) with sparing of the epidermis. PCFCL can have a follicular, follicular, and diffuse, or completely diffuse growth pattern, and characteristically is composed predominantly of large centrocytes (irregular and angulated nuclei, but larger in size than typical classic nodal FL centrocytes) and admixed centroblasts.[38,46,47] The neoplastic B cells (CD20+, PAX5+, CD79a+) usually express the germinal center marker BCL6, but often have weak to absent expression of CD10, particularly in cases with a diffuse pattern.[35,48–50] Most cases do not express BCL2 or show faint staining, although some studies have reported BCL2 expression in a subset of cases.[35,37,43,49,51–54] The Ki67 proliferation fraction of PCFCL is generally high (>30%) and CD21 staining for follicular dendritic cell meshworks is often weak or sometimes negative. Although this combination of histologic features should raise suspicion of PCFCL, definitive diagnosis of PCFCL generally requires ruling out the presence of extracutaneous disease with adequate staging.

Fig. 2. BCL2-R negative, *CD23-positive follicle center lymphoma*. This lymphoma presented as isolated inguinal lymphadenopathy in a 39-year-old woman. There is mostly a follicular architecture composed predominantly of centrocytes, with focal microfollicular foci (*A*) and focal diffuse infiltration into fat (*E*). There are numerous CD20+ B cells that co-express BCL6 (*B*) and CD10 (*F*) present in follicles highlighted by CD21+ follicular dendritic cell meshworks (*C*); follicles lack BCL2 expression

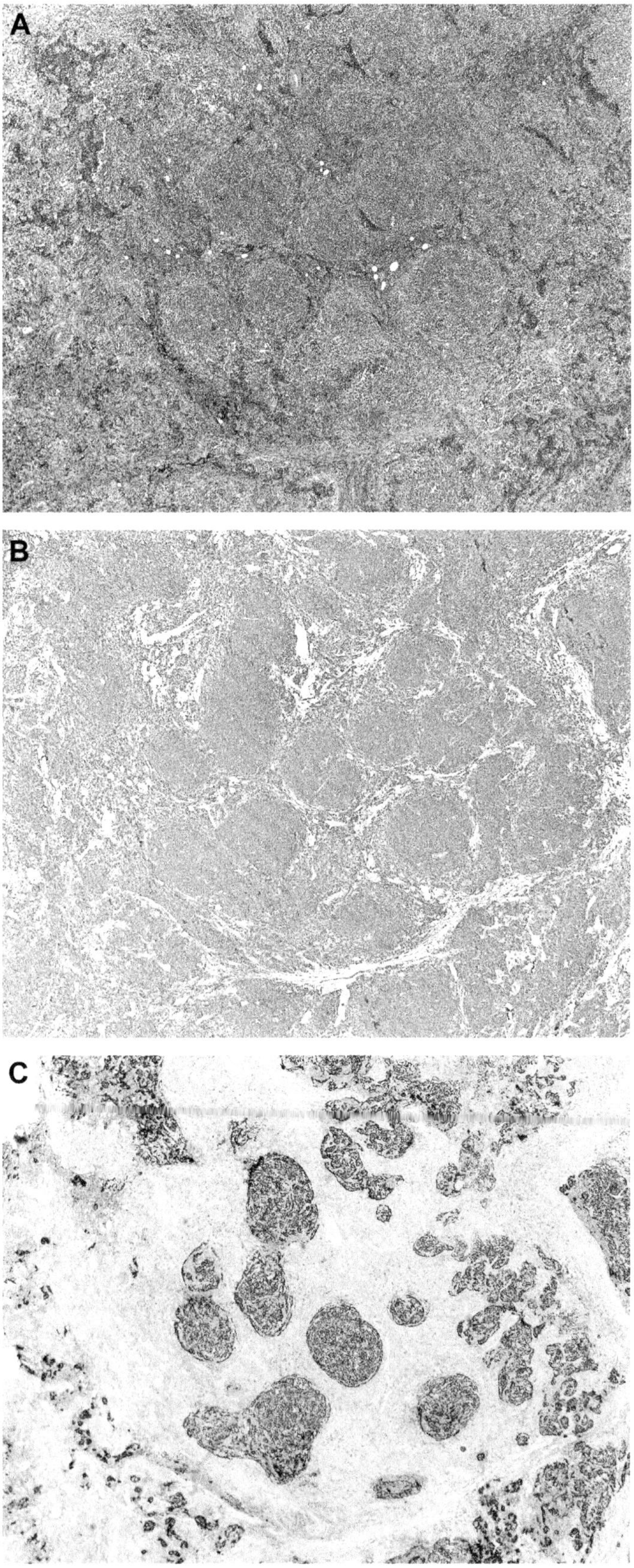

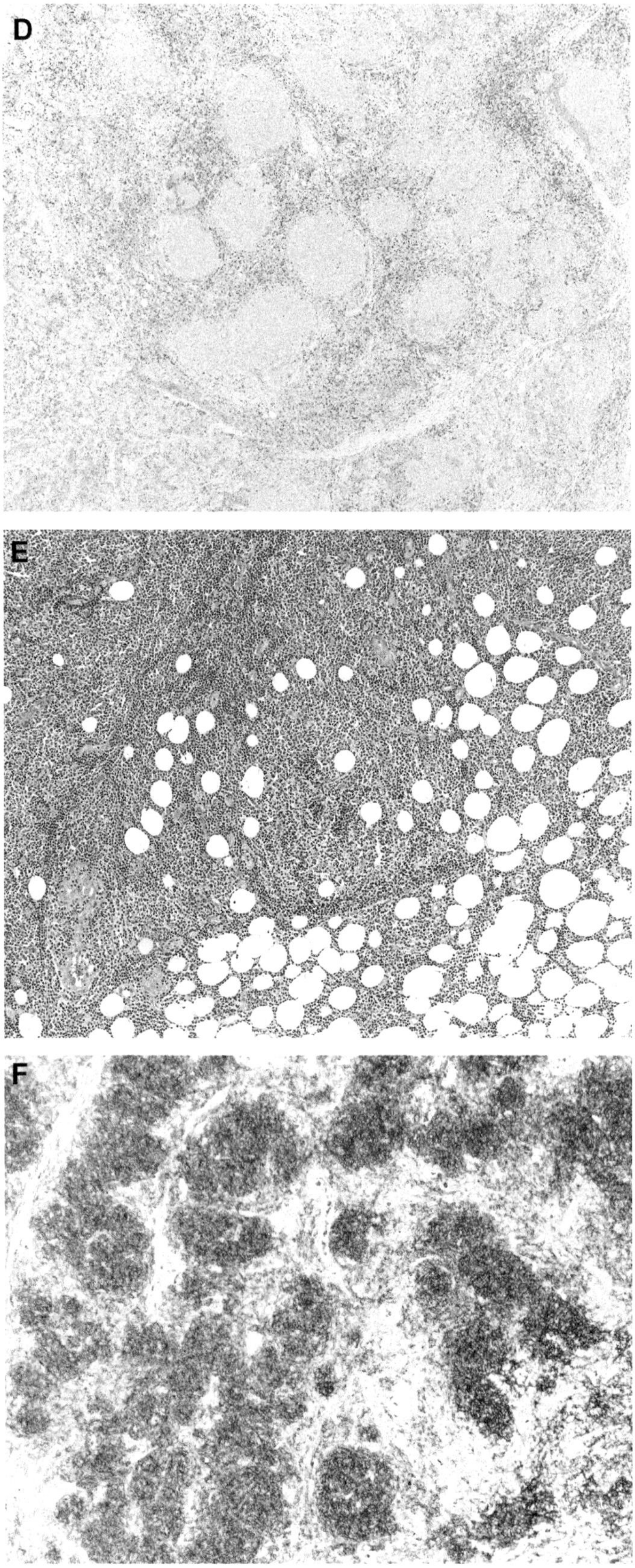

Fig. 2. (*D*). The neoplastic cells express CD23+

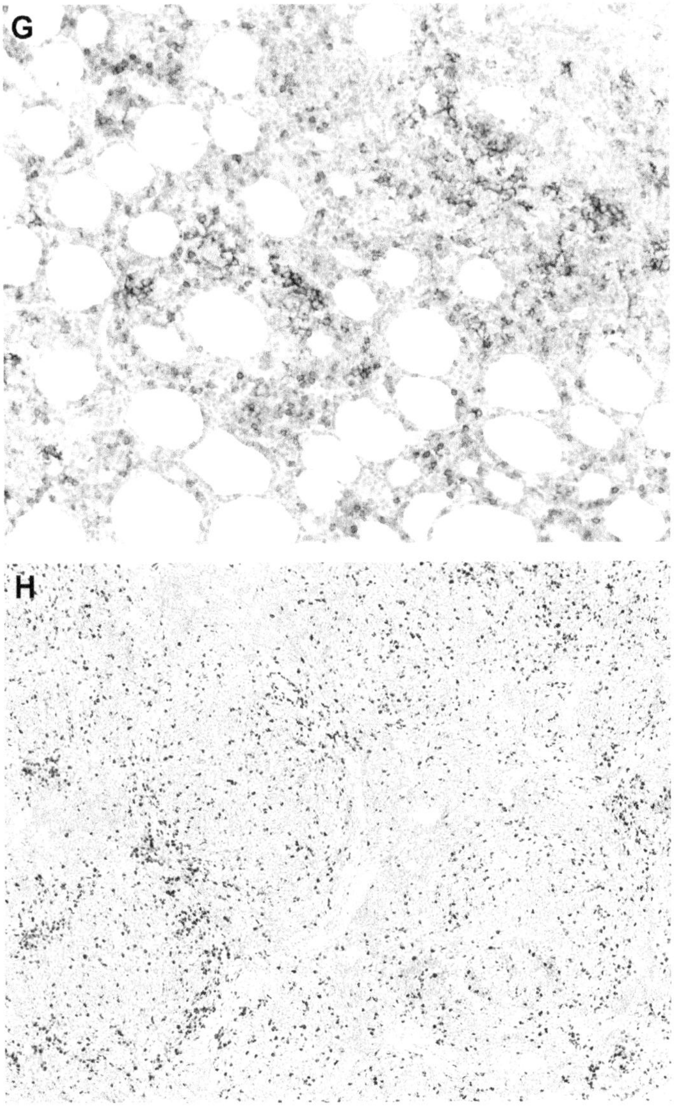

Fig. 2. (*G*, image shows expression in diffuse areas) and have a low Ki67 proliferation index (*H*). FISH showed an absence of *BCL2* and *BCL6* rearrangements and chromosomal microarray showed 1p copy neutral loss of heterozygosity (CN-LOH), involving *TNFRSF14*, *SESTRIN1*, *ARID1A,* and *RRAGC*, and 16p CN-LOH, involving *CREBBP* and *SOCS1*. The morphologic, immunophenotypic, and molecular genetic features are diagnostic of *BCL2*-R negative, CD23+ follicle center lymphoma, a newly recognized provisional variant in ICC 2022. (Photos courtesy of Dr Aliyah Sohani.)

The presence of any combination of the following–*BCL2* rearrangement, low proliferation fraction, or the presence of gene mutations listed above–should raise the possibility of systemic disease, and closer follow-up may be considered.

PCFCL with diffuse pattern must also be distinguished from primary cutaneous DLBCL, leg type, which can occasionally present a diagnostic challenge. Cases of primary cutaneous DLBCL, leg type have distinctive features, such as the expression of IgM, MUM1, and a non-germinal center phenotype. In addition, cases of primary cutaneous DLBCL, leg type harbor *MYD88* mutations and inactivation of *CDKN2A* and *CDKN2B* by 9p21.3 deletion or promoter hypermethylation, which are generally not found in PCFCL.[55–57]

PCFCL with follicular pattern can sometimes overlap morphologically with cutaneous follicular hyperplasia, which usually shows discrete reactive follicles with polarized germinal centers. In contrast to cutaneous follicular hyperplasia, follicles of PCFCL are generally more monotonous, lack polarization, and have attenuated mantle zones. Evidence of a clonal population by immunohistochemistry, in situ hybridization, or B-cell clonality PCR is helpful in ruling out a reactive process.[51,58]

Duodenal-type Follicular Lymphoma

Duodenal-type FL (DFL) is a clinically and biologically distinct variant of FL that shows primary involvement of the intestine in the absence of systemic involvement. Most cases show localized involvement of the duodenum, although other portions of the small intestine, and rarely the stomach and portions of the colorectum, may be involved.[59] DFL usually has a characteristic nodular mucosal appearance on endoscopy and a follicular architecture histologically.[60] The prognosis of DFL is excellent with very low mortality.[60,61]

Although DFL is genetically similar to classic nodal FL (with *BCL2* rearrangements, and mutations in *TNFRSF14, EZH2, KMT2D,* and/or *CREBBP*), DFL has less genetic complexity with a lower frequency of these mutations and much fewer cases with multiple mutations than classic nodal FL. There are significant differences in the gene expression profile of DFL compared with nodal FL that suggests that there may be a role for chronic inflammation and antigenic stimulation in the pathogenesis of DFL.[61]

DFL typically shows a follicular infiltrate that centers in the lamina propria of involved mucosa, comprised predominantly of cells with classic centrocytic morphology. The immunophenotype of neoplastic DFL B cells is similar to those of classic nodal FL (CD20+ PAX5+ CD79a + CD10+ BCL6+), typically with co-expression of BCL2. Follicular dendritic meshworks sometimes tend to be less well developed and/or pushed to periphery of follicles. The Ki67 proliferation fraction of DFL is usually low (<20%). *BCL2* rearrangements are present in the majority of DFL cases. The diagnosis of DFL is usually straightforward, although clinical staging may be needed to rule out intestinal involvement by systemic FL.

Other BCL2-negative Extranodal Follicular Lymphomas

Rare cases of FL show primary extranodal involvement without systemic disease.[62–64] As described above, the more common sites for primary extranodal involvement are skin and gastrointestinal tract. Primary testicular FL is rare; less than 20 cases have been reported in the literature in children and adults.[65–68] These cases tend to occur in younger male patients and lack *BCL2* rearrangements. On this basis, the 2022 International Consensus Classification of Mature Lymphoid Neoplasms (ICC 2022) classification has designated primary testicular FL as a provisional entity. Other reported sites for primary extranodal involvement by FL include thyroid,[69,70] conjuctiva,[20–22] ovary,[71] and lower female genital tract.[72] Primary extranodal involvement at these sites is rare but share some common features: most importantly, they often lack BCL2 expression as well as mutations in chromatin-modifying genes that are frequently mutated in classic nodal FL. *MAP2K1* mutations have been identified in a subset of conjunctival cases, reminiscent of pediatric-type FL. These cases of primary extranodal FL with absent *BCL2* rearrangements usually remain localized to the original extranodal site (stage I or stage II disease) and have excellent clinical outcomes like PTFL.[60,61]

OTHER PROGNOSTIC PARAMETERS IN CLASSIC NODAL FOLLICULAR LYMPHOMA

Over the past decades, several histologic, immunophenotypic, and other pathologic features have been evaluated for prognostic significance in nodal FL, including histologic grade, architectural pattern, extranodal location, Ki67 proliferation fraction, *BCL2* or *BCL6* rearrangement, and BCL2 expression. In addition to the FL variants that are now recognized because of these studies (and described in the sections above), there are other prognostic features worth mentioning that are reviewed below; some of these have resulted in recent modifications in FL classification and nomenclature (see **Fig. 1**).

BCL2-negative Nodal Follicular Lymphomas

BCL2-negative FLs comprise 10% to 15% of FL cases, and most lack underlying *BCL2* rearrangements (*BCL2*-R-negative FL). However, some BCL2-negative cases actually harbor *BCL2* rearrangements (*BCL2*-R-positive FL) but have mutation-related alterations in the BCL2 epitope that prevent standard BCL2 antibodies from binding, causing cases to appear to lack BCL2 expression. In these cases, alternative BCL2 antibodies may be used to show BCL2 expression.[73]

As described above, FL variants that lack *BCL2* rearrangements include PTFL, PCFCL, and BCL2-R-negative CD23+ follicle center lymphoma. Once these distinctive FL variants have been accounted for, there remains a nonspecific heterogeneous group of classic FL cases that lacks *BCL2* rearrangements. Recent studies have shown this remaining nonspecific group of nodal *BCL2*-R-negative FL to be quite molecularly heterogeneous molecularly.[74] A subset of these cases harbors *BCL6* rearrangements, t(3;14) (q27;q32), suggesting an alternative role for BCL6 in these cases.[75] Some cases share many features with classic FL, including *TNFRSF14* mutations, 1p36 alterations, and frequent mutations in epigenetic regulators, whereas other cases show fewer genetic alterations with an increased frequency of *STAT6* and *CREBBP* mutations.[74] This heterogenous group of *BCL2*-R-negative FL appears to have variable clinical presentation and behavior.

Low-Grade Follicular Lymphoma with Elevated Proliferation Fraction

The PI within neoplastic follicles as determined by Ki-67 immunohistochemistry has been shown to have some prognostic value in FL. Specifically, PI has been shown to correlate with histologic grade (as defined in the WHO 3rd, 4th, and revised 4th editions), with the higher histologic grade being associated with higher PI. In addition, cases of low-grade FL with discordantly high PI of ≥30% Ki67 staining within follicles appeared to behave more like high-grade FL in multiple retrospective studies.[76,77] Low-grade FL with high PI was associated with shorter 3-year and 5-year disease-specific survival than similarly low-grade FL with low PI.[76] In addition, in a prospective study of low-grade FL patients treated with anti-CD20-based biologic therapy, elevated Ki67 PI of ≥30% within neoplastic follicles was associated with inferior progression-free survival (PFS) and a higher risk of disease progression or relapse within 2 years (POD24).[78]

PROGNOSTIC SIGNIFICANCE OF HISTOLOGIC VARIATIONS IN FOLLICULAR LYMPHOMA

Architectural Patterns

Most cases of FL involving lymph nodes have characteristic effacement of nodal architecture by a proliferation of neoplastic follicles. The follicles are usually uniformly sized, closely packed, and evenly distributed throughout lymph node, and lack polarization, mantle zones, and a starry-sky pattern. Subcapsular and medullary sinuses are usually at least partially obliterated. Involvement of interfollicular regions of the lymph node, the areas in between neoplastic follicles, by neoplastic centrocytes is not uncommon. Although interfollicular involvement can be prominent in some cases of classic FL, there is no evidence that this finding impacts clinical behavior or prognosis.

Rare cases of FL composed predominantly of centrocytes have a purely (or almost entirely) diffuse pattern of growth. In the 3rd, 4th, and revised 4th editions of the WHO Classification, these cases have been referred to as "diffuse FL" or "FL with predominantly diffuse pattern." Importantly cases of lymphoma in which there is a proliferation composed predominantly of centroblasts or large cells are excluded from this category and should be classified as DLBCL. Some cases with a predominantly diffuse pattern seen on needle biopsy may represent cases of classic FL in which the follicular component has not been adequately sampled. Many well-sampled cases of FL with a predominantly diffuse pattern have CD23 expression, lack *BCL2* rearrangements, harbor *STAT6* and *CREBBP* mutations, and/or 1p36 deletions, and may be part of the discrete subtype of *BCL2*-R negative, CD23-positive follicle center lymphoma described above.[34] The clinical behavior and prognosis of predominantly diffuse FL lacking these features does not seem to differ from classic FL.

Centrocytes and Centroblasts

Cases of FL have variable numbers of centrocytes and centroblasts. Centrocytes are generally small cells with irregular, angulated nuclei. Centroblasts are relatively large with round, less irregular nuclei, often with vesicular chromatin and multiple nucleoli adjacent to nuclear membranes. Traditionally clinical aggressiveness of FL has been thought to increase with the number of centroblasts. For decades, cell counting methods based on the original "Mann and Berard" method in which the number of centroblasts is counted in 10 to 20 standard 0.159 mm^2 high-power fields (hpf) have been used to determine FL grade.[79,80] A grading system was developed in which cases with up to 5 centroblasts per hpf were defined as grade 1 (low-grade), 6 to 15 centroblasts as grade 2 (low-grade), and cases with >15 centroblasts as grade 3 (high-grade). In the 2017 WHO classification (revised 4th edition or WHO-HAEM4R), it was recognized that there is no prognostic difference between grade 1 and grade 2, and these were combined into a "low-grade" category. Approximately 80% of FL cases are low-grade (grade 1 to 2) and 20% are high-grade or grade 3, which is further subdivided into grade 3A (>15 centroblasts, but centrocytes still present) or grade 3B (pure population of centroblasts). It has also been recognized that there is a subset of FL cases with high-grade features and unconventional morphology, including large cleaved cells or small to medium-sized blastoid cells, designated "unconventional" high-grade FL (FL3U). FL3U has been shown to have higher MUM1 expression and Ki67 proliferation fraction, less frequent *BCL2* rearrangements, and more frequent *BCL6* rearrangements. FL3U in at least one study was associated with a worse outcome than FL grade 1 to 2.[81,82]

The reproducibility and prognostic significance of grading in FL has been a matter of debate over the past decades and similar issues have been raised in each of the past editions of the WHO classification.[83,84] Based on studies looking at the genetic features and clinical behavior of cases classified using this grading system, there is accumulating evidence that grade 3A FL may be more indolent and more closely related to low-grade FL.[81,85,86] In addition, there have been several clinical trials performed for targeted therapies that have shown no differences in outcome between FL grade 1 to 2 and FL grade 3A.[83,87–90] Finally, it has been shown that of all FL patients receiving first-line therapy, approximately 20% progress within 24 months (POD24), and these patients have a 5-year overall survival of 50% as opposed to the non-POD24 group with a 5-year overall survival of 90%; the latter group is comparable to a similar population without lymphoma. POD24 is currently the most significant and earliest predictor of overall survival in FL but shows no correlation with histologic grade.[91,92] There is also a similar accumulation of studies showing the frequent association of FL grade 3B with areas of DLBCL (cases of pure FL grade 3B are quite rare), suggesting that FL grade 3B is genetically and behaviorally more related to DLBCL. For these reasons, the current 5th edition WHO Classification has chosen to move from a grading system for FL to a novel system in which FL is subclassified into one of four categories: (1) Classic FL, (2) Diffuse FL, (3) FL with unusual features, and (4) Follicular large B-cell lymphoma (FLBCL; see below).[93]

THE CURRENT CLASSIFICATION OF FOLLICULAR LYMPHOMA

As described in the sections above, there have been several advances in our understanding of FL biology, behavior, and the characterization of several recently described variants of FL, often characterized by absent *BCL2* rearrangements and/or primary extranodal presentation. These advances have resulted in significant changes in the 5th edition of the WHO Classification of Haematolymphoid Tumors (WHO-HAEM5),[93] and the ICC 2022.[94] We outline the changes in both classifications below.

5th edition WHO Classification of Haematolymphoid Tumors (WHO-HAEM5)[93]: Given persistent questions regarding the reproducibility and the absence of data to support the distinction between FL grades 1, 2, and 3A, WHO-HAEM5 no longer requires grading as part of FL classification (though grading is considered optional if required by local clinical practice). In place of grading, WHO-HAEM5 introduces a new way of subtyping FL that distinguishes classic FL from the three other less frequent subtypes (Table 1).

1. Classic FL: classic FL represents the most common FL subtype in WHO-HAEM5 and includes most FL cases in which the neoplastic proliferation has a predominantly follicular architecture and is comprised predominantly of centrocytes with a variable admixture of centroblasts. This category includes cases previously called FL grade 1 to 2 and FL grade 3A.
2. FLBCL: In WHO-HAEM5, FLBCL is defined by the presence of a follicular pattern with follicles composed of sheets of centroblasts and absence of centrocytes. It replaces those cases previously known as FL grade 3B and represents the follicular counterpart of DLBCL, as reflected by its name. FLBCL is thought to be biologically more similar to DLBCL than classic FL, and frequently coexists with DLBCL. In fact, pure FLBCL is quite rare.
3. FL with predominantly diffuse growth pattern (dFL): In WHO-HAEM5, dFL includes cases of FL with a predominantly diffuse growth pattern. Some cases of classic FL may have a component of significant diffuse growth between follicles. Therefore, a diagnosis of dFL should not be made on limited biopsy samples. This subtype

Table 1
Correlation between 5th edition of the World Health Organization Classification of Haematolymphoid Tumors follicular lymphoma subtypes and International Consensus Classification 2022 follicular lymphoma grades

WHO-HAEM4R Grade	WHO-HAEM5 Subtype	ICC 2022 Grade
FL1-2, follicular pattern	Classic follicular lymphoma	FL1-2, follicular pattern
FL3A, follicular pattern	Classic follicular lymphoma	FL3A, follicular pattern
FL1-2, diffuse pattern	FL with a predominantly diffuse pattern	FL1-2, diffuse pattern
FL3B, follicular pattern	Follicular large B-cell lymphoma	FL3B, follicular pattern
N/A	FL with unusual cytologic features	N/A

Abbreviations: FL, follicular lymphoma; ICC, International Consensus Classification; N/A, not applicable; WHO-HAEM44, Revised 4th edition of the World Health Organization Classification of Haematopoietic and Lymphoid Tissues; WHO-HAEM5, 5th edition of the World Health Organization Classification of Haematolymphoid Tumors.

Table 2
Follicular Lymphoma variants recognized by 5th edition of the World Health Organization Classification of Haematolymphoid Tumors and International Consensus Classification 2022

WHO-HAEM4R Grade	WHO-HAEM5 Subtype	ICC 2022 Grade
Primary cutaneous follicle center lymphoma	Primary cutaneous follicle center lymphoma	Primary cutaneous follicle center lymphoma
Duodenal-type FL	Duodenal-type FL	Duodenal FL *(considered subtype of FL early lesion)*
Subtype of FL	Subtype of FL	Testicular lymphoma
Subtype of FL	Subtype of FL *(overlap with FL with predominantly diffuse pattern)*	*BCL2*-R negative, CD23+ follicle center lymphoma[a] *(includes FL with diffuse architecture)*

Abbreviations: BCL2-R, BCL2 rearrangement; FL, follicular lymphoma; ICC, International Consensus Classification; N/A, not applicable; WHO-HAEM44, Revised 4th edition of the World Health Organization Classification of Haematopoietic and Lymphoid Tissues; WHO-HAEM5, 5th edition of the World Health Organization Classification of Haematolymphoid Tumors.

[a] Provisional.

includes cases of predominantly diffuse FL originally described by Katzenberger and colleagues in 2009 that lacked *BCL2* rearrangements, had frequent 1p36 deletions, and presented as localized inguinal lymphadenopathy.[95] Recently, it has been shown that these cases often have CD23 expression and *STAT6* and *CREBBP* mutations, but sometimes lack 1p36 deletions and may have noninguinal presentations. This subtype overlaps with *BCL2*-R negative, CD23-positive follicle center lymphoma, a new provisional entity in recognized in ICC 2022, but there are some differences including the inclusion of molecularly similar cases with a predominantly follicular pattern (see below).

4. FL with unusual cytologic features: This category includes cases of FL with unusual morphology, including cases with predominantly medium-sized cells with immature or blastoid chromatin and cases with large cells with irregular nuclei ("large centrocytes"). These cases tend to have a high Ki67 proliferation fraction and may lack *BCL2* rearrangement. The prognostic impact of the rare cases in this category is not well categorized and requires further study.[81,82]

Outside of the FL category, WHO-HAEM5 recognizes the following FL variants described above as distinct entities: (1) primary cutaneous follicle center lymphoma, (2) pediatric-type FL, and (3) DFL, newly recognized by WHO-HAEM5 as a distinct entity for classification (**Table 2**).[93]

ICC 2022[94]: The ICC 2022 retains morphologic grading (grade 1 to 2, 3A, and 3B) as described above and in WHO-HAEM4 while recognizing the clinical distinction between grade 1 to 2 and grade 3A FL is debatable and needs further evaluation (see **Table 1**).

ICC 2022 recognizes the following FL variants as distinct entities: (1) primary cutaneous follicle center lymphoma, (2) pediatric-type FL, (3) testicular FL, designated by ICC 2022 as a distinct variant of FL in young boys, and (4) *BCL2*-R-negative CD23+ follicle center lymphoma, added as a provisional entity and recognized by ICC 2022 as an FL variant that lacks *BCL2* rearrangements, has CD23 expression, frequent *STAT6* mutations and frequently, but not always, involves the inguinal region (see **Table 2**, see **Fig. 2**).[94] Although these cases frequently have a diffuse growth pattern as originally described by Katzenberger in 2009,[95] this entity (as described by ICC 2022) also includes FL cases that retain a follicular growth pattern, but display other characteristic immunophenotypic and genetic alterations.[94]

SUMMARY

Our understanding of FL and the heterogenous group of biologically and clinically distinct FL variants have evolved significantly since the 3rd edition of WHO Classification. Progress in our understanding of our approach to FL has been driven by advances in the molecular characterization of these diseases, and our ability to identify new biomarkers that can define clinically distinct but rare subgroups with distinct clinical behavior. Over the past few decades, we have made significant progress in defining and characterizing FL variants with distinct clinical presentations (eg, pediatric-type, restriction to extranodal sites, localized disease) and pathologic features (eg, small blastoid cells, large centrocytes, *BCL2*-R-negative, and variations in the genetic alterations and frequencies). However, the overwhelming majority of FL cases diagnosed continue to have classic clinical presentation and behavior (eg, advanced stage nodal presentation in adult patients) and pathology (follicular proliferation comprised predominately of centrocytes associated with *BCL2* rearrangement). Over time, there has been an increasing recognition that traditional histologic grade (ie, grade 1 to 2, grade 3A) may not be a reliable method for determining clinical prognosis at diagnosis or predicting the likelihood of response to modern therapies. Given the heterogeneity in clinical outcomes in classic FL, there continues to be a dire need to identify reliable, prognostically impactful biomarkers for this disease.

CLINICS CARE POINTS

- For BCL2 negative FL harboring BCL2 rearangements, application of alternative BCL2 antibodies should be attempted to rule out possible mutation-related alterations in the BCL2 epitope that prevent standard BCL2 antibodies from binding.
- Once distinctive FL variants (PTFL, PCFCL, BCL2-R-negative CD23+ follicle center lymphoma have been ruled out, there remains a nonspecific heterogeneous group of classic FL cases that lacks BCL2 rearrangements.
- Although most cases of BCL2-R-negative CD23+ follicle center lymphoma frequently have a diffuse growth pattern as originally described by Katzenberger in 2009, some cases retain a follicular arcgitecture while displaying the other pathologic and molecular features of this entity.

DISCLOSURES

Dr A. Louissaint has no commercial or financial conflict of interest.

ACKNOWLEDGEMENTS

Aziz and Nur Hamzaogullari EndowementLymphoma Research Foundation.

REFERENCES

1. Jaffe ES, Harris NL, Swerdlow SH, et al. Follicular lymphoma. In: Swerdlow SH, Campo E, Harris NL, et al, editors. WHO classification of Tumours of haematopoietic and lymphoid tissues, revised. 4th edition. Lyon: IARC; 2017. p. 266–77.
2. Rowley JD. Chromosome studies in the non-Hodgkin's lymphomas: the role of the 14;18 translocation. J Clin Oncol 1988;6(5):919–25.
3. Leich E, Hoster E, Wartenberg M, et al. Similar clinical features in follicular lymphomas with and without breaks in the BCL2 locus. Leukemia 2016;30(4): 854–60.
4. Okosun J, Bodor C, Wang J, et al. Integrated genomic analysis identifies recurrent mutations and evolution patterns driving the initiation and progression of follicular lymphoma. Nat Genet 2014;46(2):176–81.
5. Zhang J, Dominguez-Sola D, Hussein S, et al. Disruption of KMT2D perturbs germinal center B cell development and promotes lymphomagenesis. Nat Med 2015;21(10):1190–8.
6. Kridel R, Chan FC, Mottok A, et al. Histological Transformation and Progression in Follicular Lymphoma: A Clonal Evolution Study. PLoS Med 2016; 13(12):e1002197.
7. Huet S, Szafer-Glusman E, Tesson B, et al. BCL2 mutations do not confer adverse prognosis in follicular lymphoma patients treated with rituximab. Am J Hematol 2017;92(6):515–9.
8. Huet S, Sujobert P, Salles G. From genetics to the clinic: a translational perspective on follicular lymphoma. Nat Rev Cancer 2018;18(4):224–39.
9. Dheilly E, Battistello E, Katanayeva N, et al. Cathepsin S Regulates Antigen Processing and T Cell Activity in Non-Hodgkin Lymphoma. Cancer Cell 2020;37(5):674–689 e612.
10. Bolen CR, Mattiello F, Herold M, et al. Treatment dependence of prognostic gene expression signatures in de novo follicular lymphoma. Blood 2021; 137(19):2704–7.
11. Oschlies I, Salaverria I, Mahn F, et al. Pediatric follicular lymphoma–a clinico-pathological study of a population-based series of patients treated within the Non-Hodgkin's Lymphoma–Berlin-Frankfurt-Munster (NHL-BFM) multicenter trials. Haematologica 2010;95(2):253–9.
12. Louissaint A Jr, Ackerman AM, Dias-Santagata D, et al. Pediatric-type nodal follicular lymphoma: an indolent clonal proliferation in children and adults with high proliferation index and no BCL2 rearrangement. Blood 2012;120(12):2395–404.
13. Louissaint A Jr, Schafernak KT, Geyer JT, et al. Pediatric-type nodal follicular lymphoma: a biologically distinct lymphoma with frequent MAPK pathway mutations. Blood 2016;128(8):1093–100.
14. Lorsbach RB, Shay-Seymore D, Moore J, et al. Clinicopathologic analysis of follicular lymphoma occurring in children. Blood 2002;99(6):1959–64.
15. Perkins SL, Gross TG. Pediatric indolent lymphoma–would less be better? Pediatr Blood Cancer 2011; 57(2):189–90.

16. McNamara C, Davies J, Dyer M, et al. Guidelines on the investigation and management of follicular lymphoma. Br J Haematol 2012;156(4):446–67.
17. Attarbaschi A, Beishuizen A, Mann G, et al. Children and adolescents with follicular lymphoma have an excellent prognosis with either limited chemotherapy or with a "Watch and wait" strategy after complete resection. Ann Hematol 2013; 92(11):1537–41.
18. Sorge C, Costa LJ, Taub JW, et al. Incidence and outcomes of rare paediatric non-hodgkin lymphomas. Br J Haematol 2019;184(5):864–7.
19. Attarbaschi A, Abla O, Arias Padilla L, et al. Rare non-Hodgkin lymphoma of childhood and adolescence: A consensus diagnostic and therapeutic approach to pediatric-type follicular lymphoma, marginal zone lymphoma, and nonanaplastic peripheral T-cell lymphoma. Pediatr Blood Cancer 2020;67(8):e28416.
20. Okudolo JO, Bagg A, Meghpara BB, et al. Conjunctival Pediatric-Type Follicular Lymphoma. Ophthalmic Plast Reconstr Surg 2020;36(2):e46–9.
21. Alnaim AF, Alhawsawi A, AlSomali A, et al. Conjunctival Pediatric-Type Follicular Lymphoma in a Young Male: A Case Report and Literature Review. Cureus 2022;14(2):e22023.
22. AlSemari MA, Maktabi A, AlSamnan MS, et al. Conjunctival Pediatric Follicular Lymphoma: Case Report and Literature Review. Ophthalmic Plast Reconstr Surg 2020;36(1):e14–5.
23. Martin-Guerrero I, Salaverria I, Burkhardt B, et al. Recurrent loss of heterozygosity in 1p36 associated with TNFRSF14 mutations in IRF4 translocation negative pediatric follicular lymphomas. Haematologica 2013;98(8):1237–41.
24. Schmidt J, Gong S, Marafioti T, et al. Genome-wide analysis of pediatric-type follicular lymphoma reveals low genetic complexity and recurrent alterations of TNFRSF14 gene. Blood 2016;128(8): 1101–11.
25. Agostinelli C, Akarca AU, Ramsay A, et al. Novel markers in pediatric-type follicular lymphoma. Virchows Arch 2019;475(6):771–9.
26. Salaverria I, Philipp C, Oschlies I, et al. Translocations activating IRF4 identify a subtype of germinal center-derived B-cell lymphoma affecting predominantly children and young adults. Blood 2011; 118(1):139–47.
27. Salaverria I, Martin-Guerrero I, Burkhardt B, et al. High resolution copy number analysis of IRF4 translocation-positive diffuse large B-cell and follicular lymphomas. Genes Chromosomes Cancer 2013;52(2):150–5.
28. Ozawa MG, Bhaduri A, Chisholm KM, et al. A study of the mutational landscape of pediatric-type follicular lymphoma and pediatric nodal marginal zone lymphoma. Mod Pathol 2016;29(10): 1212–20.
29. Schmidt J, Ramis-Zaldivar JE, Nadeu F, et al. Mutations of MAP2K1 are frequent in pediatric-type follicular lymphoma and result in ERK pathway activation. Blood 2017;130(3):323–7.
30. Swerdlow SH. Pediatric follicular lymphomas, marginal zone lymphomas, and marginal zone hyperplasia. Am J Clin Pathol 2004;122(Suppl):S98–109.
31. Quintanilla-Martinez L, Sander B, Chan JK, et al. Indolent lymphomas in the pediatric population: follicular lymphoma, IRF4/MUM1+ lymphoma, nodal marginal zone lymphoma and chronic lymphocytic leukemia. Virchows Arch 2016;468(2):141–57.
32. Koo M, Ohgami RS. Pediatric-type Follicular Lymphoma and Pediatric Nodal Marginal Zone Lymphoma: Recent Clinical, Morphologic, Immunophenotypic, and Genetic Insights. Adv Anat Pathol 2017;24(3):128–35.
33. Kussick SJ, Kalnoski M, Braziel RM, et al. Prominent clonal B-cell populations identified by flow cytometry in histologically reactive lymphoid proliferations. Am J Clin Pathol 2004;121(4):464–72.
34. Xian RR, Xie Y, Haley LM, et al. CREBBP and STAT6 co-mutation and 16p13 and 1p36 loss define the t(14;18)-negative diffuse variant of follicular lymphoma. Blood Cancer J 2020;10(6):69.
35. Senff NJ, Hoefnagel JJ, Jansen PM, et al. Reclassification of 300 primary cutaneous B-Cell lymphomas according to the new WHO-EORTC classification for cutaneous lymphomas: comparison with previous classifications and identification of prognostic markers. J Clin Oncol 2007;25(12):1581–7.
36. Zinzani PL, Quaglino P, Pimpinelli N, et al. Prognostic factors in primary cutaneous B-cell lymphoma: the Italian Study Group for Cutaneous Lymphomas. J Clin Oncol 2006;24(9):1376–82.
37. Kodama K, Massone C, Chott A, et al. Primary cutaneous large B-cell lymphomas: clinicopathologic features, classification, and prognostic factors in a large series of patients. Blood 2005;106(7):2491–7.
38. Santucci M, Pimpinelli N, Arganini L. Primary cutaneous B-cell lymphoma: a unique type of low-grade lymphoma. Clinicopathologic and immunologic study of 83 cases. Cancer 1991;67(9): 2311–26.
39. Grange F, Bekkenk MW, Wechsler J, et al. Prognostic factors in primary cutaneous large B-cell lymphomas: a European multicenter study. J Clin Oncol 2001;19(16):3602–10.
40. Vergier B, Belaud-Rotureau MA, Benassy MN, et al. Neoplastic cells do not carry bcl2-JH rearrangements detected in a subset of primary cutaneous follicle center B-cell lymphomas. Am J Surg Pathol 2004;28(6):748–55.
41. Gulia A, Saggini A, Wiesner T, et al. Clinicopathologic features of early lesions of primary cutaneous follicle center lymphoma, diffuse type: implications for early diagnosis and treatment. J Am Acad Dermatol 2011;65(5):991–1000.

42. Abdul-Wahab A, Tang SY, Robson A, et al. Chromosomal anomalies in primary cutaneous follicle center cell lymphoma do not portend a poor prognosis. J Am Acad Dermatol 2014;70(6):1010–20.
43. Pham-Ledard A, Cowppli-Bony A, Doussau A, et al. Diagnostic and prognostic value of BCL2 rearrangement in 53 patients with follicular lymphoma presenting as primary skin lesions. Am J Clin Pathol 2015;143(3):362–73.
44. Barasch NJK, Liu YC, Ho J, et al. The molecular landscape and other distinctive features of primary cutaneous follicle center lymphoma. Hum Pathol 2020;106:93–105.
45. Zhou XA, Yang J, Ringbloom KG, et al. Genomic landscape of cutaneous follicular lymphomas reveals 2 subgroups with clinically predictive molecular features. Blood Adv 2021;5(3):649–61.
46. Willemze R, Kerl H, Sterry W, et al. EORTC classification for primary cutaneous lymphomas: a proposal from the Cutaneous Lymphoma Study Group of the European Organization for Research and Treatment of Cancer. Blood 1997;90(1):354–71.
47. Burg G, Kempf W, Cozzio A, et al. WHO/EORTC classification of cutaneous lymphomas 2005: histological and molecular aspects. J Cutan Pathol 2005;32(10):647–74.
48. de Leval L, Harris NL, Longtine J, et al. Cutaneous b-cell lymphomas of follicular and marginal zone types: use of Bcl-6, CD10, Bcl-2, and CD21 in differential diagnosis and classification. Am J Surg Pathol 2001;25(6):732–41.
49. Mirza I, Macpherson N, Paproski S, et al. Primary cutaneous follicular lymphoma: an assessment of clinical, histopathologic, immunophenotypic, and molecular features. J Clin Oncol 2002;20(3):647–55.
50. Mohammadi MR, Akhondzadeh S. Schizophrenia: etiology and pharmacotherapy. Idrugs 2001;4(10):1167–72.
51. Cerroni L, Arzberger E, Putz B, et al. Primary cutaneous follicle center cell lymphoma with follicular growth pattern. Blood 2000;95(12):3922–8.
52. Child FJ, Russell-Jones R, Woolford AJ, et al. Absence of the t(14;18) chromosomal translocation in primary cutaneous B-cell lymphoma. Br J Dermatol 2001;144(4):735–44.
53. Aguilera NS, Tomaszewski MM, Moad JC, et al. Cutaneous follicle center lymphoma: a clinicopathologic study of 19 cases. Mod Pathol 2001;14(9):828–35.
54. Goodlad JR, Krajewski AS, Batstone PJ, et al. Primary cutaneous diffuse large B-cell lymphoma: prognostic significance of clinicopathological subtypes. Am J Surg Pathol 2003;27(12):1538–45.
55. Dijkman R, Tensen CP, Jordanova ES, et al. Array-based comparative genomic hybridization analysis reveals recurrent chromosomal alterations and prognostic parameters in primary cutaneous large B-cell lymphoma. J Clin Oncol 2006;24(2):296–305.
56. Menguy S, Gros A, Pham-Ledard A, et al. MYD88 Somatic Mutation Is a Diagnostic Criterion in Primary Cutaneous Large B-Cell Lymphoma. J Invest Dermatol 2016;136(8):1741–4.
57. Zhou XA, Louissaint A Jr, Wenzel A, et al. Genomic Analyses Identify Recurrent Alterations in Immune Evasion Genes in Diffuse Large B-Cell Lymphoma, Leg Type. J Invest Dermatol 2018;138(11):2365–76.
58. Goodlad JR, Krajewski AS, Batstone PJ, et al. Primary cutaneous follicular lymphoma: a clinicopathologic and molecular study of 16 cases in support of a distinct entity. Am J Surg Pathol 2002;26(6):733–41.
59. Takata K, Okada H, Ohmiya N, et al. Primary gastrointestinal follicular lymphoma involving the duodenal second portion is a distinct entity: a multicenter, retrospective analysis in Japan. Cancer Sci 2011;102(8):1532–6.
60. Schmatz AI, Streubel B, Kretschmer-Chott E, et al. Primary follicular lymphoma of the duodenum is a distinct mucosal/submucosal variant of follicular lymphoma: a retrospective study of 63 cases. J Clin Oncol 2011;29(11):1445–51.
61. Hellmuth JC, Louissaint A Jr, Szczepanowski M, et al. Duodenal-type and nodal follicular lymphomas differ by their immune microenvironment rather than their mutation profiles. Blood 2018;132(16):1695–702.
62. Weinberg OK, Ma L, Seo K, et al. Low stage follicular lymphoma: biologic and clinical characterization according to nodal or extranodal primary origin. Am J Surg Pathol 2009;33(4):591–8.
63. Shastri A, Janakiram M, Mantzaris I, et al. Sites of extranodal involvement are prognostic in patients with stage 1 follicular lymphoma. Oncotarget 2017;8(45):78410–8.
64. Andraos T, Ayoub Z, Nastoupil L, et al. Early Stage Extranodal Follicular Lymphoma: Characteristics, Management, and Outcomes. Clin Lymphoma Myeloma Leuk 2019;19(6):381–9.
65. Pileri SA, Sabattini E, Rosito P, et al. Primary follicular lymphoma of the testis in childhood: an entity with peculiar clinical and molecular characteristics. J Clin Pathol 2002;55(9):684–8.
66. Bacon CM, Ye H, Diss TC, et al. Primary follicular lymphoma of the testis and epididymis in adults. Am J Surg Pathol 2007;31(7):1050–8.
67. Pakzad K, MacLennan GT, Elder JS, et al. Follicular large cell lymphoma localized to the testis in children. J Urol 2002;168(1):225–8.
68. Finn LS, Viswanatha DS, Belasco JB, et al. Primary follicular lymphoma of the testis in childhood. Cancer 1999;85(7):1626–35.
69. Hamamoto Y, Kukita Y, Kitamura M, et al. Bcl-2-negative IGH-BCL2 translocation-negative follicular

lymphoma of the thyroid differs genetically and epigenetically from Bcl-2-positive IGH-BCL2 translocation-positive follicular lymphoma. Histopathology 2021;79(4):521–32.
70. Bacon CM, Diss TC, Ye H, et al. Follicular lymphoma of the thyroid gland. Am J Surg Pathol 2009;33(1):22–34.
71. Ozsan N, Bedke BJ, Law ME, et al. Clinicopathologic and genetic characterization of follicular lymphomas presenting in the ovary reveals 2 distinct subgroups. Am J Surg Pathol 2011;35(11):1691–9.
72. Saksena A, Jain A, Pack SD, et al. Follicle Center Lymphoma (FCL) of the Lower Female Genital Tract (LFGT): A Novel Variant of Primary Cutaneous Follicle Center Lymphoma (PCFCL). Am J Surg Pathol 2023;47(3):409–19.
73. Adam P, Baumann R, Schmidt J, et al. The BCL2 E17 and SP66 antibodies discriminate 2 immunophenotypically and genetically distinct subgroups of conventionally BCL2-"negative" grade 1/2 follicular lymphomas. Hum Pathol 2013;44(9):1817–26.
74. Nann D, Ramis-Zaldivar JE, Muller I, et al. Follicular lymphoma t(14;18)-negative is genetically a heterogeneous disease. Blood Adv 2020;4(22):5652–65.
75. Los-de Vries GT, Stevens WBC, van Dijk E, et al. Genomic and microenvironmental landscape of stage I follicular lymphoma, compared with stage III/IV. Blood Adv 2022;6(18):5482–93.
76. Samols MA, Smith NE, Gerber JM, et al. Software-automated counting of Ki-67 proliferation index correlates with pathologic grade and disease progression of follicular lymphomas. Am J Clin Pathol 2013;140(4):579–87.
77. Wang SA, Wang L, Hochberg EP, et al. Low histologic grade follicular lymphoma with high proliferation index: morphologic and clinical features. Am J Surg Pathol 2005;29(11):1490–6.
78. Sohani AR, Maurer MJ, Giri S, et al. Biomarkers for Risk Stratification in Patients With Previously Untreated Follicular Lymphoma Receiving Anti-CD20-based Biological Therapy. Am J Surg Pathol 2021;45(3):384–93.
79. Nathwani BN, Metter GE, Miller TP, et al. What should be the morphologic criteria for the subdivision of follicular lymphomas? Blood 1986;68(4):837–45.
80. Mann RB, Berard CW. Criteria for the cytologic subclassification of follicular lymphomas: a proposed alternative method. Hematol Oncol 1983;1(2):187–92.
81. Laurent C, Adelaide J, Guille A, et al. High-grade Follicular Lymphomas Exhibit Clinicopathologic, Cytogenetic, and Molecular Diversity Extending Beyond Grades 3A and 3B. Am J Surg Pathol 2021;45(10):1324–36.
82. El Behery R, Laurini JA, Weisenburger DD, et al. Follicular large cleaved cell (centrocytic) lymphoma: an unrecognized variant of follicular lymphoma. Hum Pathol 2018;72:180–90.
83. Rimsza LM, Li H, Braziel RM, et al. Impact of histological grading on survival in the SWOG S0016 follicular lymphoma cohort. Haematologica 2018;103(4):e151–3.
84. Kroft SH. Stratification of Follicular Lymphoma: Time for a Paradigm Shift? Am J Clin Pathol 2019;151(6):539–41.
85. Koch K, Hoster E, Ziepert M, et al. Clinical, pathological and genetic features of follicular lymphoma grade 3A: a joint analysis of the German low-grade and high-grade lymphoma study groups GLSG and DSHNHL. Ann Oncol 2016;27(7):1323–9.
86. Horn H, Kohler C, Witzig R, et al. Gene expression profiling reveals a close relationship between follicular lymphoma grade 3A and 3B, but distinct profiles of follicular lymphoma grade 1 and 2. Haematologica 2018;103(7):1182–90.
87. Marcus R, Davies A, Ando K, et al. Obinutuzumab for the First-Line Treatment of Follicular Lymphoma. N Engl J Med 2017;377(14):1331–44.
88. Hiddemann W, Barbui AM, Canales MA, et al. Immunochemotherapy With Obinutuzumab or Rituximab for Previously Untreated Follicular Lymphoma in the GALLIUM Study: Influence of Chemotherapy on Efficacy and Safety. J Clin Oncol 2018;36(23):2395–404.
89. Morschhauser F, Fowler NH, Feugier P, et al. Rituximab plus Lenalidomide in Advanced Untreated Follicular Lymphoma. N Engl J Med 2018;379(10):934–47.
90. Bachy E, Seymour JF, Feugier P, et al. Sustained Progression-Free Survival Benefit of Rituximab Maintenance in Patients With Follicular Lymphoma: Long-Term Results of the PRIMA Study. J Clin Oncol 2019;37(31):2815–24.
91. Freeman CL, Kridel R, Moccia AA, et al. Early progression after bendamustine-rituximab is associated with high risk of transformation in advanced stage follicular lymphoma. Blood 2019;134(9):761–4.
92. Casulo C, Dixon JG, Le-Rademacher J, et al. Validation of POD24 as a robust early clinical end point of poor survival in FL from 5225 patients on 13 clinical trials. Blood 2022;139(11):1684–93.
93. Alaggio R, Amador C, Anagnostopoulos I, et al. The 5th edition of the World Health Organization Classification of Haematolymphoid Tumours: Lymphoid Neoplasms. Leukemia 2022;36(7):1720–48.
94. Campo E, Jaffe ES, Cook JR, et al. The International Consensus Classification of Mature Lymphoid Neoplasms: a report from the Clinical Advisory Committee. Blood 2022;140(11):1229–53.
95. Katzenberger T, Kalla J, Leich E, et al. A distinctive subtype of t(14;18)-negative nodal follicular non-Hodgkin lymphoma characterized by a predominantly diffuse growth pattern and deletions in the chromosomal region 1p36. Blood 2009;113(5):1053–61.

Modern Classification and Management of Pediatric B-cell Leukemia and Lymphoma

Alexandra E. Kovach, MD[a,b,*], Gordana Raca, MD, PhD[b,c]

KEYWORDS

• B-lymphoblastic leukemia • Pediatric leukemia • WHO classification • Pediatric lymphoma • Anterior mediastinal mass • Hematogone hyperplasia • Lymphadenitis

Key points

- Several novel genetic subtypes of pediatric lymphoblastic leukemia, described since the 2017 World Health Organization (WHO) classification (Revised fourth edition), underlie modern risk stratification and clinical management.
- Some nomenclature changes in the 2023 WHO classification (fifth edition) affect primarily pediatric lymphomas.
- In specific clinicopathologic scenarios, pediatric lymphomas require evaluation of surgical margins.

ABSTRACT

Although pediatric hematopathology overlaps with that of adults, certain forms of leukemia and lymphoma, and many types of reactive conditions affecting the bone marrow and lymph nodes, are unique to children. As part of this series focused on lymphomas, this article (1) details the novel subtypes of lymphoblastic leukemia seen primarily in children and described since the 2017 World Health Organization classification and (2) discusses unique concepts in pediatric hematopathology, including nomenclature changes and evaluation of surgical margins in selected lymphomas.

OVERVIEW

B-cell lymphoid diseases in children are diverse and require special consideration. An explosion of genomic and clinical data has significantly expanded the recognized biological subtypes of B-lymphoblastic leukemia/lymphoma (B-ALL/LBL), the most common cancer of childhood. Genetic classification underlies prognosis, risk stratification, and clinical management approaches. Similarly, the understanding of optimal management of mature B-cell non-Hodgkin lymphomas in pediatric patients has developed to include toxicity-sparing protocols, that is, minimization of chemotherapy, given their generally excellent prognosis.

As such, this article is divided into 2 parts. Part I details subtypes of pediatric B-lymphoblastic leukemia newly described and/or added to the fifth edition of the World Health Organization (WHO) Classification of Haematolymphoid Tumours[1] and 2022 International Consensus Classification (ICC), and highlights the clinical laboratory methodologies best suited to their detection.[2] Part II contextualizes a discussion of mature non-Hodgkin lymphomas presenting in children into modern classification[1,2] and clinical management, emphasizing those scenarios where surgical

[a] Division of Laboratory Medicine, Department of Pathology and Laboratory Medicine, Children's Hospital Los Angeles, Los Angeles, CA, USA; [b] Clinical Pathology, Keck School of Medicine, University of Southern California, Los Angeles, CA 90027, USA; [c] Division of Genomic Medicine, Department of Pathology and Laboratory Medicine, Center for Personalized Medicine, Children's Hospital Los Angeles, Los Angeles, CA, USA
* Corresponding author. Children's Hospital Los Angeles 4650 Sunset Boulevard, MS 32, Los Angeles, CA 90027.
E-mail address: akovach@chla.usc.edu

Surgical Pathology 16 (2023) 249–266
https://doi.org/10.1016/j.path.2023.01.001

margin assessment (complete surgical excision) is used to minimize systemic therapies.

DETECTION OF NOVEL GENETIC SUBTYPES OF PEDIATRIC B-LYMPHOBLASTIC LEUKEMIA

Subclassification of B-lymphoblastic leukemia today relies on cytogenetic and, at times, molecular testing to identify the genetic driver, a genetic rearrangement that results in a fusion protein or a point mutation.[3] Conventional karyotype and standardized fluorescence in situ hybridization (FISH) panels are the mainstays of this evaluation. However, many novel subtypes of leukemia, particularly in pediatrics, are cryptic by these cytogenetic methods.[4] Techniques such as RNA sequencing (RNAseq) are increasingly being incorporated into accurate leukemia subclassification,[5–7] which underlies prognosis and optimal therapy.[8] There are a number of excellent reviews on minimal/measurable residual disease (MRD) evaluation by flow cytometry for pediatric, as well as adult, leukemia[9,10] beyond the scope of this review.

B-LYMPHOBLASTIC LEUKEMIA/LYMPHOMA WITH *TCF::HLF* REARRANGEMENT

t(17;19);*TCF3::HLF* rearrangement defines an uncommon aggressive subtype of pediatric B-ALL, with rare adult cases described.[11] Although this clinicopathologic entity has long been recognized, it was added for the first time to the WHO classification in the fifth edition (2023)[1] and the parallel ICC,[2] both for completeness and to draw distinction from t(1;19);*TCF3::PBX1* rearrangement. At clinical presentation, there can be striking hypercalcemia.[12] Prognosis is relatively poor, with or without hematopoietic stem cell transplantation but relatively high uniform CD19 expression raises the possibility of responsiveness to anti-CD19 chimeric antigen receptor T-cell (CAR-T) and other therapies.[13]

The pathogenic fusion protein has been shown to interfere with cell differentiation.[14] t(17;19) is often detectable by conventional karyotype. Importantly, *TCF3* break-apart FISH probes are not recommended because recognition of the fusion partner (*HLF*, *PBX1* or other) is crucial for prognostication. **Fig. 1** depicts confirmatory RNA analysis from leukemic bone marrow aspirate with a previously reported t(17;19) rearrangement on karyotype from a 12-year-old girl.

B-LYMPHOBLASTIC LEUKEMIA WITH *ETV6::RUNX1*-LIKE FEATURES

Gene expression profiling studies to elucidate the pathogenesis of leukemias previously classified as B-ALL not otherwise specified (NOS) have yielded novel B-ALL subtypes.[15] Most recently, cases with the protein signaling properties of B-ALL with *ETV6::RUNX1* rearrangement, the most common subtype of childhood B-ALL, but not harboring the *ETV6::RUNX1* have been termed B-ALL, *ETV6::RUNX1*-like and included in the

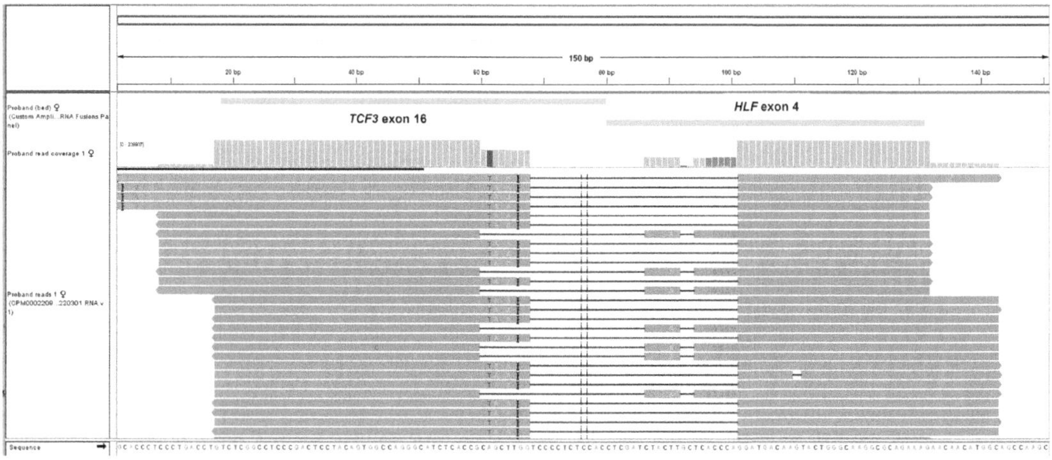

Fig. 1. B-ALL with t(17;19);*TCF3::HLF*. Institutional RNA analysis[111] was performed on formalin-fixed paraffin-embedded particle preparation (clot section) material from referred leukemic bone marrow aspirate with a t(17;19) rearrangement reported by karyotype. A *TCF3::HLF* fusion involving exons 16 and 4, respectively, was confirmed based on 241,473 supporting junction reads of 1,839,733 total mapped reads. Of note, inserted extra bases at the fusion junction are present, a common consequence of abnormal fusions.

new WHO classification[1] and as a provisional entity in the ICC.[2] The best clinical method for the detection of these cases,[4] and their epidemiology and clinical characteristics, will likely be refined in coming years. To date, these cases tend to occur in pediatric patients,[15] and show high rates of relapsed disease.[16]

B-LYMPHOBLASTIC LEUKEMIA WITH *BCR::ABL1*-LIKE (PH-LIKE) FEATURES

Similarly identified but described earlier, B-ALL with *BCR::ABL1*-like (Ph-like) features is a heterogeneous group of diseases with genetic rearrangements and mutations that lead to basal tumor signaling through tyrosine kinase and related pathways.[17,18] This group of diseases was discovered through gene expression signatures shared with B-ALL, *BCR::ABL1* (Ph+) but lacking the Philadelphia chromosome.[19] Ph-like B-ALL is enriched in young adult and Hispanic patients, especially B-ALL with *CRLF2* rearrangements,[20,21] and may be amenable to tyrosine kinase inhibitor therapy.[22] This category has been included in the WHO classification since 2017, where it was a provisional entity, and is now a formal entity.[1] There are many excellent references available on this complex topic.[2,19,20,23–27]

The following B-ALL subtypes are presented in the WHO fifth edition under the heading of "B-ALL/LBL with other defined genetic abnormalities"[1] and individually in the ICC.[2]

B-LYMPHOBLASTIC LEUKEMIA/LYMPHOMA WITH *DUX4* REARRANGEMENT

DUX4 rearrangement confers a relatively favorable prognosis in B-ALL.[15,28] This rearrangement is present in an estimated 4% to 7% of B-ALL,[29] predominantly in patients aged younger than 30 years.[30] It was identified by large-scale sequencing and in invariably associated with deletion of the *ERG* gene region.[31,32]

DUX4 has some unique immunophenotypic features: variability in CD10 expression, uniform CD371 (CLL-1) expression and CD2 expression in a subset of cases.[33] In B-ALL with variable CD10 expression, the differential diagnosis also includes *ZNF384* rearrangement (see later section)[34] and some cases of *KMT2A* rearrangement (although most *KMT2A*-rearranged B-ALL show absent CD10 expression).[35]

CD371 (CLL-1) expression by flow cytometry can be helpful into the diagnostic workup of B-ALL with variable CD10 expression, especially because *DUX4* rearrangement is cryptic by cytogenetics and may only be apparent by inference from *ERG* gene deletion from chromosome microarray or sequencing methods. CD371 is also a monocytic marker.[33,36] Indeed, *DUX4*-rearranged B-ALL may show mature monocytic differentiation, as can other B-ALL subtypes,[37] following induction chemotherapy or even subtly at presentation, which may complicate flow cytometric MRD assessment and raise a differential diagnosis with mixed phenotype acute leukemia (MPAL), B/Myeloid.[34] DUX4 expression by immunohistochemistry has also been reported as an additional screening tool at diagnosis.[38]

ZNF384 REARRANGEMENT IN B-LYMPHOBLASTIC LEUKEMIA/LYMPHOMA OR MIXED PHENOTYPE ACUTE LEUKEMIA, B/MYELOID

Genetic rearrangements involving *ZNF384* have been identified in cases presenting with immunophenotypic features of either B-ALL/LBL or MPAL, B/Myeloid, underlying the likely eventual classification of at least some leukemias by cyto/genetic features rather than immunophenotype.[4,16,28,34,39–44] The B-cell component (bilineal or biphenotypic cases are reported within MPAL) shows variable or decreased CD10 expression,[45] raising a differential diagnosis with *DUX4* rearrangement[15,28,34] and occasionally *KMT2A* rearrangement.[46] Identification is important because of both the propensity for lineage switch[40] and the relatively poor prognosis.

B-LYMPHOBLASTIC LEUKEMIA WITH *MEF2D* REARRANGEMENT

MEF2D rearrangement in B-ALL was described in 2016 by Gu and colleagues.[47] Representing an estimated 2% to 3% of B-ALL in a large cohort, and 5.3% of cases without known genetic drivers,[47] this rearrangement leads to constitutive pre-B-cell receptor signaling[48] and is becoming increasingly important to detect at diagnosis.[1,2] Aberrant CD5 expression is described as a sensitive and specific feature[45,47] of possible use in screening for triage of molecular testing,[45] as the *MEF2D* rearrangement is inapparent by conventional karyotype. In our experience, the rearrangement is detectable by RNAseq,[49] and all cases identified to date show uniform CD5 expression of at least moderate intensity by flow cytometry (Fig. 2).[45]

B-LYMPHOBLASTIC LEUKEMIA, *PAX5*alt

PAX5-altered (*PAX5*alt) B-ALL is characterized by a distinct expression profile and diverse

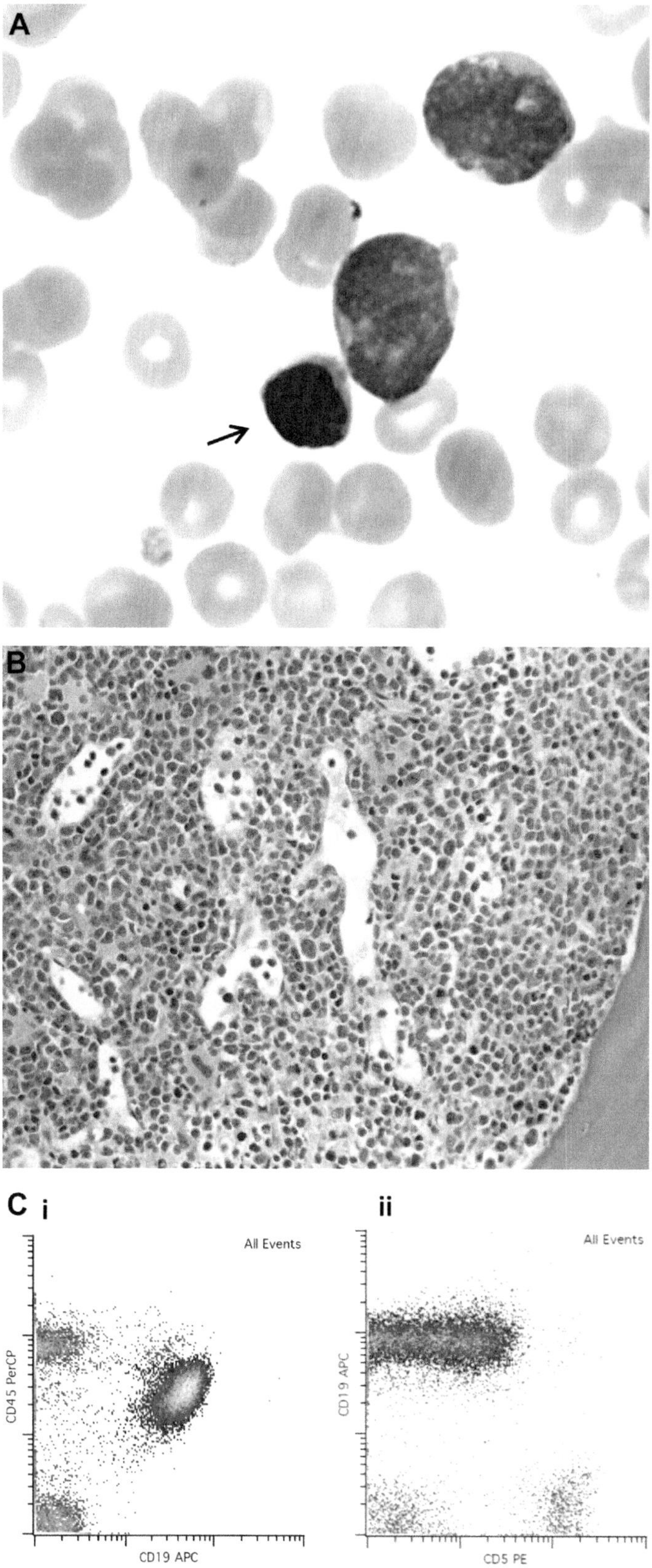

Fig. 2. B-ALL with *MEF2D* rearrangement. (*A*) Bone marrow aspirate (Wright-Giemsa stain, 1000× magnification) and (*B*) bone marrow core biopsy (H&E stain, 400× magnification) from a 13-year-old girl at diagnosis. Compared with a benign mature lymphocyte (*arrow*), the blasts are intermediate-sized, with scant cytoplasm and complex nuclear borders, consistent with lymphoblasts. (*C*) By flow cytometry of bone marrow aspirate material, the blasts, identified by dim CD45 compared with mature lymphocytes (i) express B-cell markers, including CD19 (i and ii), consistent with B-ALL, and coexpress CD5 with variably and to moderately bright intensity (ii).

abnormalities involving the *PAX5* (Paired Box 5) gene, which encodes a transcription factor serving as the master regulator of B-cell development and maintenance.[50–52] The *PAX5*alt-associated abnormalities include abnormal fusions with more than 20 partner genes (with *ETV6*, *NOL4L*, *AUTS2*, and *CBFA2T3* being the most common; Fig. 3), sequence mutations, focal and large deletions, and intragenic tandem multiplications (ITMs).[50] Sequence mutations that characterize this subtype are typically missense, occurring in the DNA-binding domain of the *PAX5*-encoded protein; secondary loss of the wild-type allele due to a deletion or copy-neutral loss of heterozygosity (CN-LOH) is observed in up to 40% of the cases.[50–52]

ITM is another *PAX5* abnormality seen in *PAX5*-alt B-ALL, and represents direct, in-frame, tandem insertion of multiple extra copies of the 5' portion (exons 2–5) of the gene.[53,54] In addition to being founding lesions in PAX5alt B-ALL, *PAX5* abnormalities (typically deletions and loss-of-function mutations) occur as secondary changes in up to one-third of B-ALL cases, across a range of genetic subtypes[55]; distinguishing between *PAX5* alterations as primary drivers versus secondary abnormalities can be challenging in the clinical setting. *PAX5*alt accounts for approximately 7% of B-ALL cases; it seems to be associated with an intermediate prognosis,[50] with its outcome possibly being modified by the presence of secondary *IKZF1* deletions.[30]

B-LYMPHOBLASTIC LEUKEMIA, *PAX5* p.P80R

The *PAX5* P80R subtype accounts for approximately 3% of B-ALL cases, and is defined by the presence of a specific c239C > G, p.Pro80Arg (P80R) missense variant, which replaces the proline residue at position 80 in the DNA-binding domain of the *PAX5*-encoded protein with arginine (Fig. 4).[50–52,56] There is a loss of the second wild-type *PAX5* allele through a deletion, CN-LOH, or truncating sequence mutation in the majority of the cases. The prognosis has been described as favorable to intermediate.[50,56]

B-LYMPHOBLASTIC LEUKEMIA WITH *NUTM1* REARRANGEMENT

Nuclear protein in testis midline carcinoma family 1 (*NUTM1*) rearrangements are a rare cause of pediatric B-ALL, occurring in less than 2% of the cases, almost exclusively in infants. *NUTM1* fusions with different partner genes have been observed (including *ACIN1*, *AFF1*, *ATAD5*, *BRD9*, *CHD4*, *CUX1*, *IKZF1*, *RUNX1*, *SLC12A6*, and *ZNF618*), resulting in an aberrant *NUTM1* expression.[57,58] The clinical significance of the *NUTM1* rearrangements in B-ALL stems from their association with an excellent prognosis, in contrast to infant B-ALL with *KMT2A* rearrangements and other genetic drivers.[57] Many *NUTM1* rearrangements are not detectable by karyotype analysis, necessitating FISH or molecular testing for these abnormalities in *KMT2A*-negative infant B-ALL.[59]

B-LYMPHOBLASTIC LEUKEMIA WITH *MYC* REARRANGEMENT

Rare neoplasms show the clinical, morphologic, and immunophenotypic features of B-ALL (young children [even infants[60]], leukemic presentation, lymphoblast morphology, and immunophenotype markers of immaturity [CD34 and/or TdT, dim to absent CD45, and absent surface light chain expression] and B-cell differentiation [CD19 with or without CD20 and/or cytoplasmic CD79a]) but the genetic features of Burkitt lymphoma: isolated C-*MYC* rearrangement[61,62] or *MYC* and *BCL2* rearrangements[63,64] (Fig. 5). Cures are reported with B-ALL-directed therapy. This is likely due to molecular underpinnings because B-ALL with *MYC* rearrangement has been shown to have characteristics of B-ALL and not of Burkitt lymphoma[65] and possibly a unique immunoglobulin class-switching mechanism.[66] In some cases, morphology may be closer to Burkitt lymphoma cells than to canonical lymphoblasts.[67] Before reconciliation in current classification schema, nomenclature has varied in this entity.[68] Such cases are best classified as B-ALL, and a WHO category of B-ALL with *MYC* rearrangement has been included in the WHO and ICC classifications in order to collect these cases.[1,2]

A related, arguably bettered studied scenario is that of TdT expression in high-grade B-cell lymphoma with *MYC* and *BCL2* and/or *BCL6* rearrangements ("double-hit" or "triple-hit" lymphoma[69–71]) or high-grade B-cell lymphoma, NOS.[72–75] Some of these high-grade B-cell lymphoma cases show blastoid morphology,[74] such that when coupled with TdT expression, a differential diagnosis with B-ALL is raised, especially ahead of FISH and/or molecular study results.[76] This dilemma has largely been resolved by several studies reporting TdT expression in confirmed "double-hit" lymphoma cases, with or without surface light chain expression, as well as gene expression studies,[72] such that the significance of TdT expression is uncertain and does not necessarily confer immaturity. Indeed, large B-cell lymphomas often downregulate light chain expression as well as CD45 expression, best appreciated by flow cytometry.[77] Of note, "double-hit" lymphoma

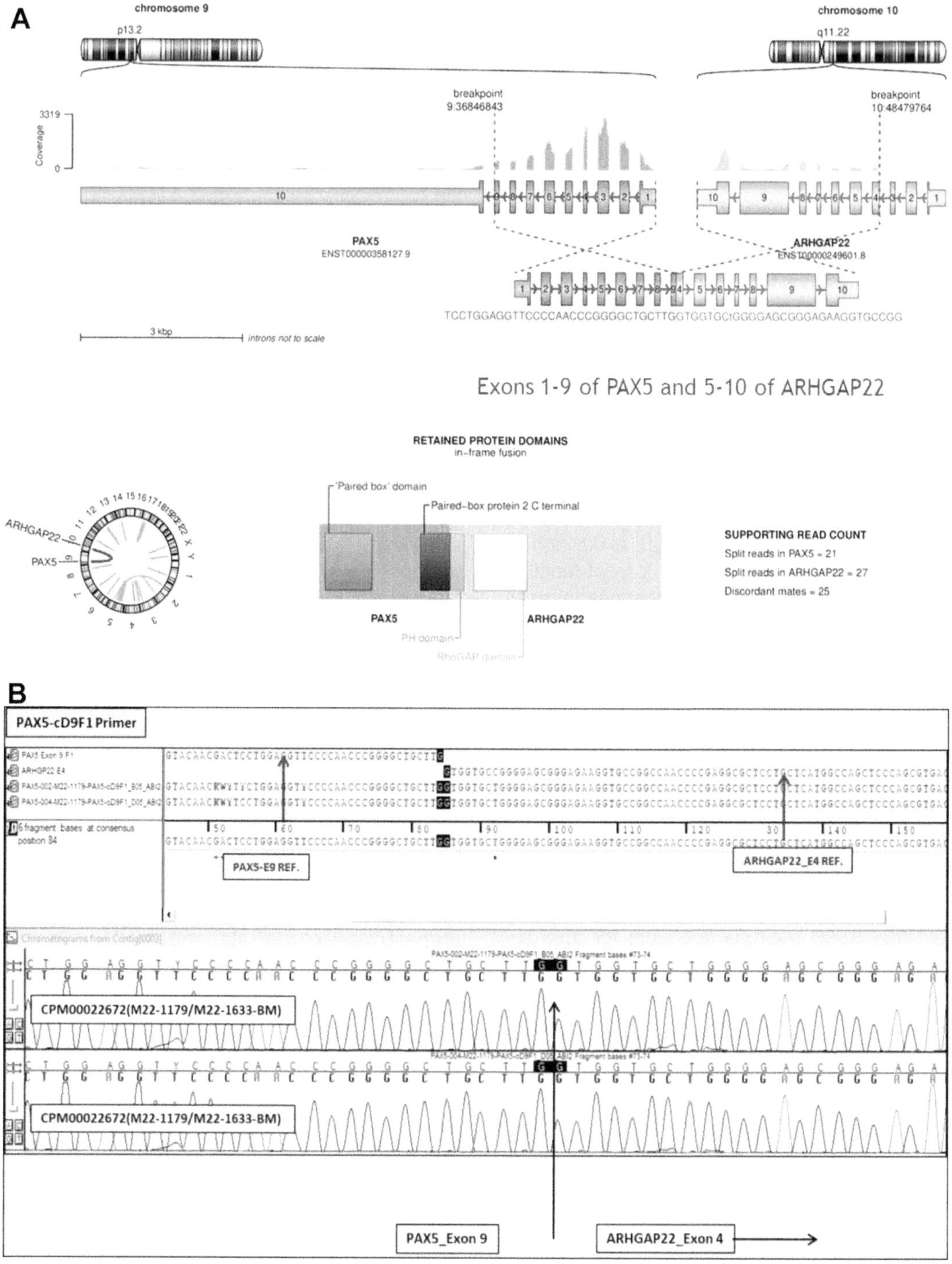

Fig. 3. *PAX5*alt subtype of B-ALL. *PAX5::ARHGAP22* fusion detected by RNAseq fusion assay in a case of *PAX5*alt B-ALL. (*A*) The fusion scheme and the scheme of the predicted fusion protein.[111] (*B*) Confirmation of the fusion by RT-PCR and Sanger sequencing of the junction fragment.

is rare in the pediatric population,[78] and most aggressive mature B-cell lymphomas in pediatric patients—including diffuse large B-cell lymphoma, Burkitt lymphoma, and rare cases of "double-hit" lymphoma—receive similar intensive multiagent chemotherapy regimens.[79]

LOW-STAGE PEDIATRIC MATURE B-CELL LYMPHOMAS: WHERE COMPLETE RESECTION MATTERS

Management of pediatric lymphoma includes some specific considerations.[80,81] In general, the assessment of surgical margins for resected lymphoma is not typical because lymphoma, such as most hematopoietic neoplasms, is considered by definition to represent systemic disease. However, some specific clinicopathologic scenarios of low-stage or otherwise localized lymphomas use the assessment of surgical margins to determine the eligibility for modern treatment protocols with limited, or even no, postsurgical (adjuvant) systemic therapy.[79,82] When feasible, such approaches are particularly attractive in children with curable lymphomas whose posttreatment life spans are largely ahead and as such reduction in long-term toxicities are especially desired.[82]

ILEOCECAL BURKITT LYMPHOMA

Terminal ileal or ileocecal Burkitt lymphoma is a stereotypical cause of intussusception in children aged older than 4 years in developed countries (compared with toddlers presenting with viral/idiopathic intussusception).[83,84] In this anatomic location, Burkitt and related high-grade B-cell lymphomas may also come to clinical attention, before the development of clinical intussusception or small bowel obstruction, with bleeding from a "polyp." Disease-free survival is excellent in the nonrelapsed setting.[85] Retrospective outcome studies have shown that the number of postsurgical chemotherapy cycles can be limited in patients with stage I or II disease per the International Pediatric Non-Hodgkin Lymphoma Staging System,[86,87] that is, lymphoma limited to the mass lesion, with negative ileocolectomy margins and involved or uninvolved regional lymph nodes, without a negative effect on disease-free survival and therefore sparing pediatric patients short-term and long-term toxicities.[85] This concept has long been present in the surgical literature[88,89] and today applies to other stage I completely resected aggressive B-cell lymphomas in pediatric patients as well.[82]

Fig. 6 depicts histologic sections from a terminal ileal "polyp" in a 5-year-old girl who presented with intermittent gastrointestinal bleeding and concern for intussusception. The lymphoma spanned 1.5 cm of a 2.5-cm segmental terminal ileal resection. The ileal and serosal margins were negative. No regional lymph nodes were sampled. The lymphoma was classified as stage II (primary abdomen with total resection), group A and treated without complication with limited cyclophosphamide vincristine, prednisolone, and doxorubicin (COPAD) chemotherapy with durable complete response.

The morphologic, immunophenotypic, and molecular spectrum of Burkitt lymphoma, including in the ileocecal region, is relatively narrow and well described elsewhere.[90,91] There are subsets of cases with relatively blastoid morphology rather than the canonical condensed chromatin with multiple nucleoli, and weak BCL2 expression (compared with the typically strong expression of interspersed nonneoplastic T cells) rather than an absent BCL2 expression that still meet diagnostic criteria for Burkitt lymphoma.[92,93] Rare cases without *MYC* rearrangement but with 11q deletion or other abnormality of this region,[87,94] termed Burkitt-like lymphoma with 11q aberration as a provisional entity in the revised fourth edition WHO classification,[95,96] has been renamed high-grade B-cell lymphoma with 11q aberration to parallel the nomenclature of other high-grade B-cell lymphomas.[1,97]

In the case depicted in Fig. 6, which had characteristic morphologic and immunophenotypic features of Burkitt lymphoma (with the exception of relatively strong BCL2 expression by immunohistochemistry), neither *MYC* rearrangement nor 11q aberration were detected by FISH studies; therefore, this lymphoma was classified as high-grade B-cell lymphoma, NOS.

NODULAR LYMPHOCYTE PREDOMINANT HODGKIN LYMPHOMA (NODULAR LYMPHOCYTE PREDOMINANT B-CELL LYMPHOMA)

Similarly, stage IA nodular lymphocyte predominant Hodgkin lymphoma (NLPHL) in children, usually involving cervical lymph node(s), is curable with excision alone.[98–100] Indeed, there are historical reports of excised cervical lymph nodes—from healthy patients with long disease-free clinical follow-up—originally diagnosed as reactive lymphoid hyperplasia with progressive transformation of germinal centers that in hindsight represent NLPHL. These data underlie the very indolent nature of this specific clinicopathologic scenario. Conglomerates of involved lymph nodes (stage II) and possibly histologically diffuse areas meeting criteria for T-cell/histiocyte-rich large B-cell lymphoma (THRLBCL, a diagnosis both controversial and rare in children), are not amenable to excision alone.[98]

Of note, NLPHL is undergoing a nomenclature change due to biologic reclassification as a non-Hodgkin lymphoma.[1,101] Although NLPHL histologically resembles classic Hodgkin lymphoma (CHL) in that the tumor cells are infrequent and scattered in a background of abundant nonneoplastic inflammatory cells, the tumor cells are B cells that retain B-cell antigen expression (unlike

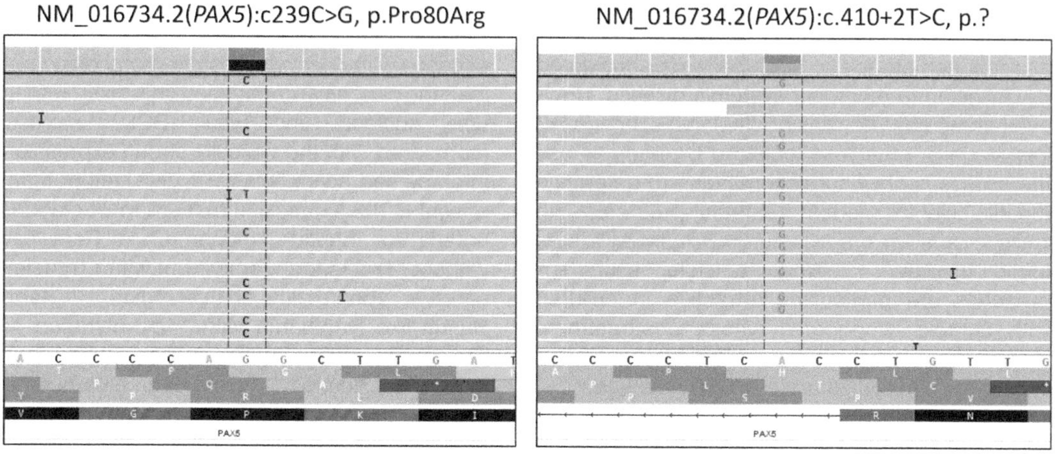

Fig. 4. *PAX5* P80R subtype of B-ALL. Screenshots from the Integrated Genome Viewer showing the p.Pro80Arg (P80R) variant and a truncating splice variant in the second *PAX5* allele in a case of *PAX5* P80R B-ALL.

CHL), originate within lymph node B-cell follicles, and share clinicopathologic properties at ends of a morphologic spectrum as closer to either follicular lymphoma or THRLBCL than to CHL.[102] For these reasons, "nodular lymphocyte predominant B-cell lymphoma" has been put forward as an alternate acceptable term in the fifth edition WHO classification[1] and has outright replaced NLPHL in the 2022 ICC of mature lymphoid neoplasms.[101] Ongoing study is elucidating the variant histologic patterns recognized in NLPHL[103] in relation to tumor microenvironment, suggesting that the disease progresses from the confines of the germinal center environment to the extrafollicular T-cell-rich zone.[104]

PEDIATRIC TESTICULAR FOLLICULAR LYMPHOMA

Primary follicular lymphoma of the testis in children is rare, clinically distinct from pediatric-type follicular lymphoma (PTFL) of the head-and-neck region,[105,106] and also somewhat biologically distinct from the primary testicular follicular lymphoma seen in adults. The histologic features include a variably sclerotic or pseudosarcomatous appearance, grade 3A cytology with frequent centroblasts admixed with centrocytes identifiable in noncompressed areas, inconspicuous to absent follicular dendritic cell meshworks, CD10 and BCL2 negativity by immunohistochemistry, and absence of *BCL2* rearrangement.[107–110] PTFL seen in cervical lymph nodes shares some of these histologic features, namely grade 3A cytology and absent *BCL2* rearrangement but CD10 tends to be expressed.[105,106]

Fig. 7 depicts a typical case of pediatric testicular follicular lymphoma in the orchiectomy specimen from 7-year-old boy. The testicular parenchyma was infiltrated by an abnormal fibroinflammatory process bounded by the tunica (see **Fig. 7**A) and sparing seminiferous tubules (see **Fig. 7**B). Throughout the tumor, the lymphoid cells were small to intermediate-sized with condensed nuclear chromatin and were associated with a delicate background fibroblastic response with myxoid stroma, mimicking a spindle-cell or other soft tissue neoplasm (see **Fig. 7**C). The lymphoid cells were CD20+ (see **Fig. 7**D), PAX5+, CD79a + B cells that coexpressed BCL6; were negative CD5, CD10, CD30, MUM1, BCL2, MYC, TdT, and Epstein Barr Virus (EBV)-encoded RNA (EBER); and had a high Ki67 proliferation fraction (approximately 80%–90%). Occasional tight follicular dendritic cell networks were seen scattered throughout the tumor, mainly at the periphery but the majority of the tumor did not show follicular dendritic cells. Admixed small T cells were frequent.

A variant of strong clinical significance was detected in *EZH2* by DNA sequencing of the tumor.[111] Given its rarity, the molecular features of primary follicular lymphoma of the testis in childhood are not well characterized; however, *EZH2* mutation is a common initiating event across follicular lymphoma.[112] With a negative spermatic cord margin (in this and virtually all cases because the lymphomas are well circumscribed in the testicular parenchyma), adjuvant therapy has been limited to a few chemotherapy cycles or observation alone (as was the case with the patient whose tumor is depicted in **Fig. 7**) with excellent disease-free survival.[113]

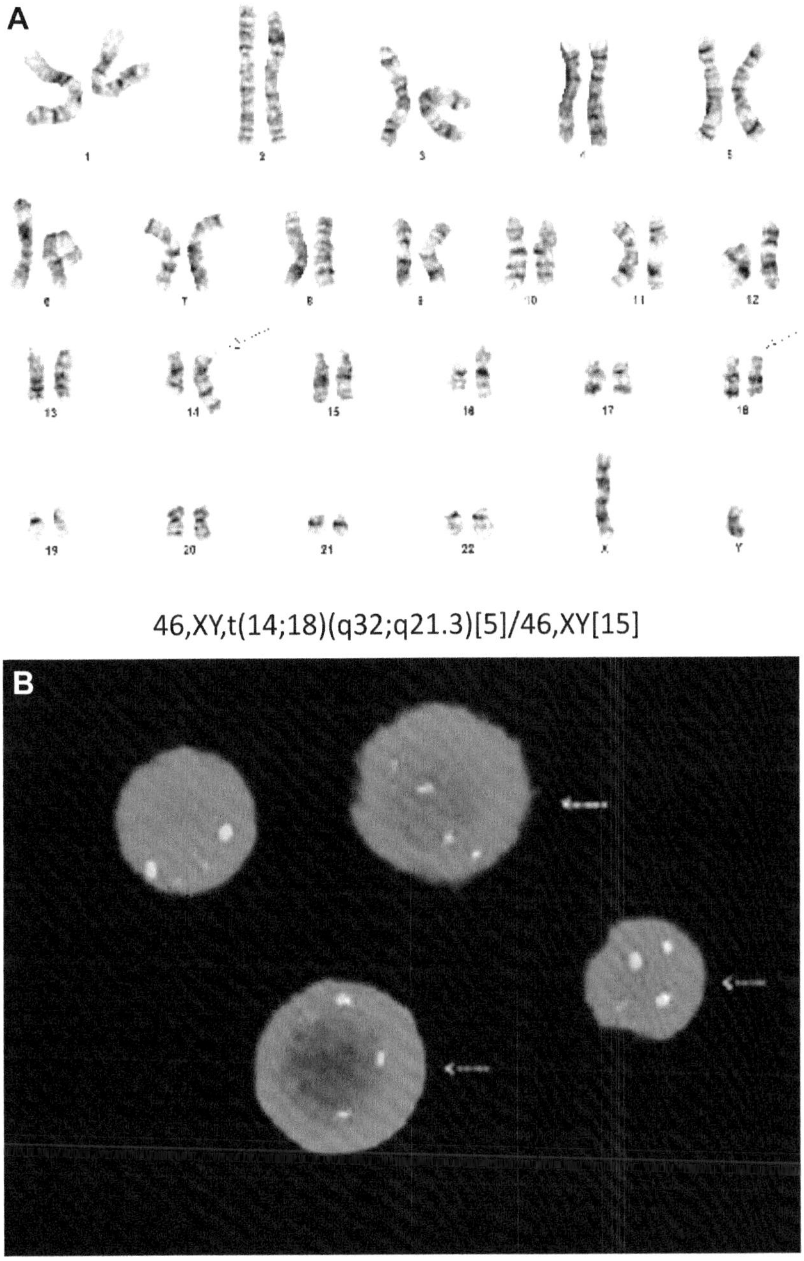

Fig. 5. B-ALL with *IGH::BCL2* rearrangement. (*A*) Karyotype shows a t(14;18) (*arrow*) involving the *IGH* locus at 14q32 and the *BCL2* locus at 18q21.3. (*B*) FISH with a dual-fusion probe was positive for an *IGH::BCL2* rearrangement (*arrowed cells*) in 65% (130/200) of interphase cells.

PEDIATRIC-TYPE FOLLICULAR LYMPHOMA AND PEDIATRIC NODAL MARGINAL ZONE LYMPHOMA

PTFL is a rare indolent clonal proliferation of *BCL2*-rearrangement-negative B cells typically presenting in a single head-and-neck lymph node of an adolescent male with recurrent *MAP2K* pathway mutations and *TNFRSF14* mutations.[105,106] Similarly, pediatric nodal marginal zone lymphoma (PNMZL) has a predilection for cervical lymph nodes, male sex, and adolescent age. Moreover, PNMZL is epidemiologically and biologically distinct from nodal marginal zone lymphoma presenting in adults.

A recent study of a large international cohort of PNMZL (n = 45) demonstrated overlapping genetic features with those of PTFL, namely 1p36/*TNFRSF14* alterations but limited additional copy number changes.[114] This and other studies have also highlighted overlapping morphologic features

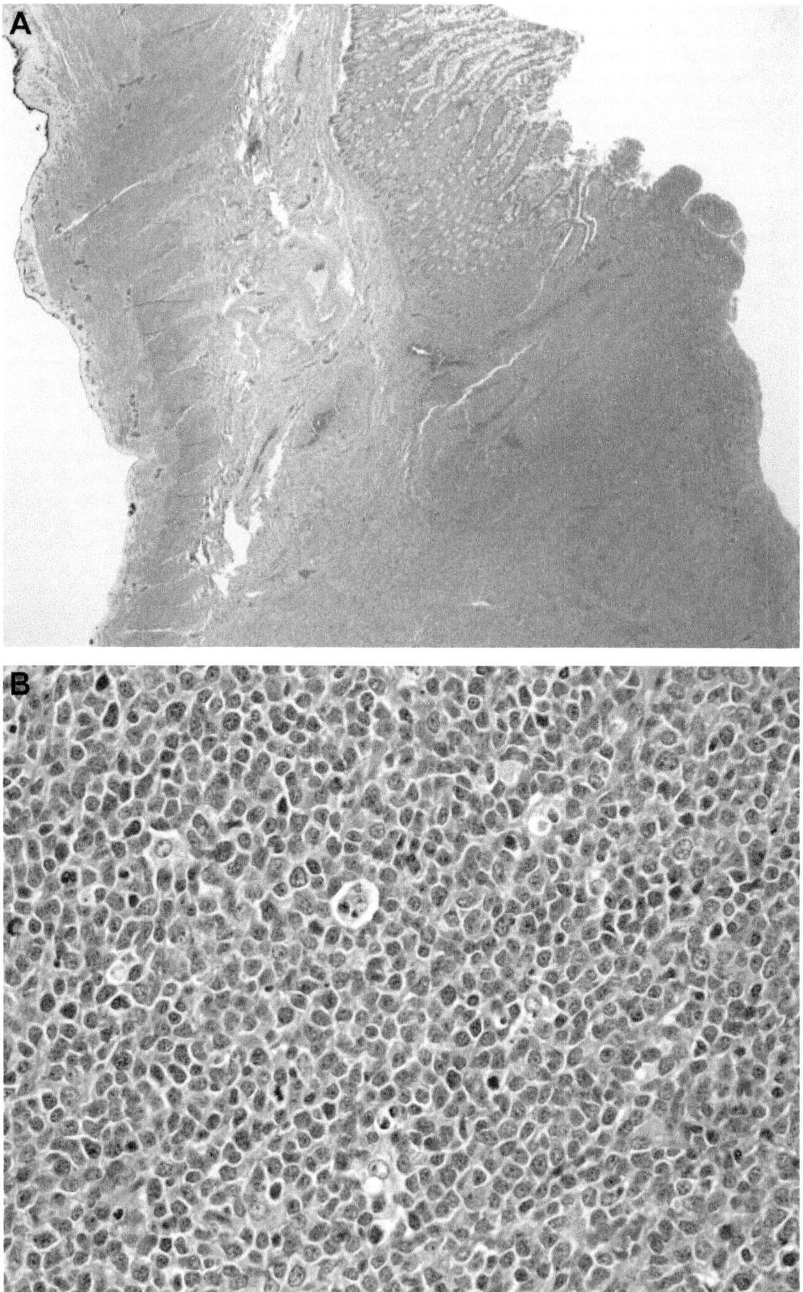

Fig. 6. Ileal high-grade B-cell lymphoma, NOS. (*A*) H&E, 20×. (*B–D*) 400× magnification as follows: (*B*) H&E,

between PNMZL and PTFL.[115] Indeed, marginal zone differentiation was identified in subsets of PTFL in prior cohorts.[105,106]

Given these data, the diagnostic category of PTFL with or without marginal zone differentiation has been proposed by the ICC to encompass these previously separated entities.[101] A proposed downgrading from "lymphoma" to "neoplasia" has also been recommended, to parallel the nomenclature used for "in situ follicular neoplasia" and "in situ mantle cell neoplasia," to better reflect the indolent clinical behavior of these lesions and avoid an implication of malignancy in otherwise young healthy patients.[116]

Although surgical margins are not utilized in these disorders per se, surgical excision is

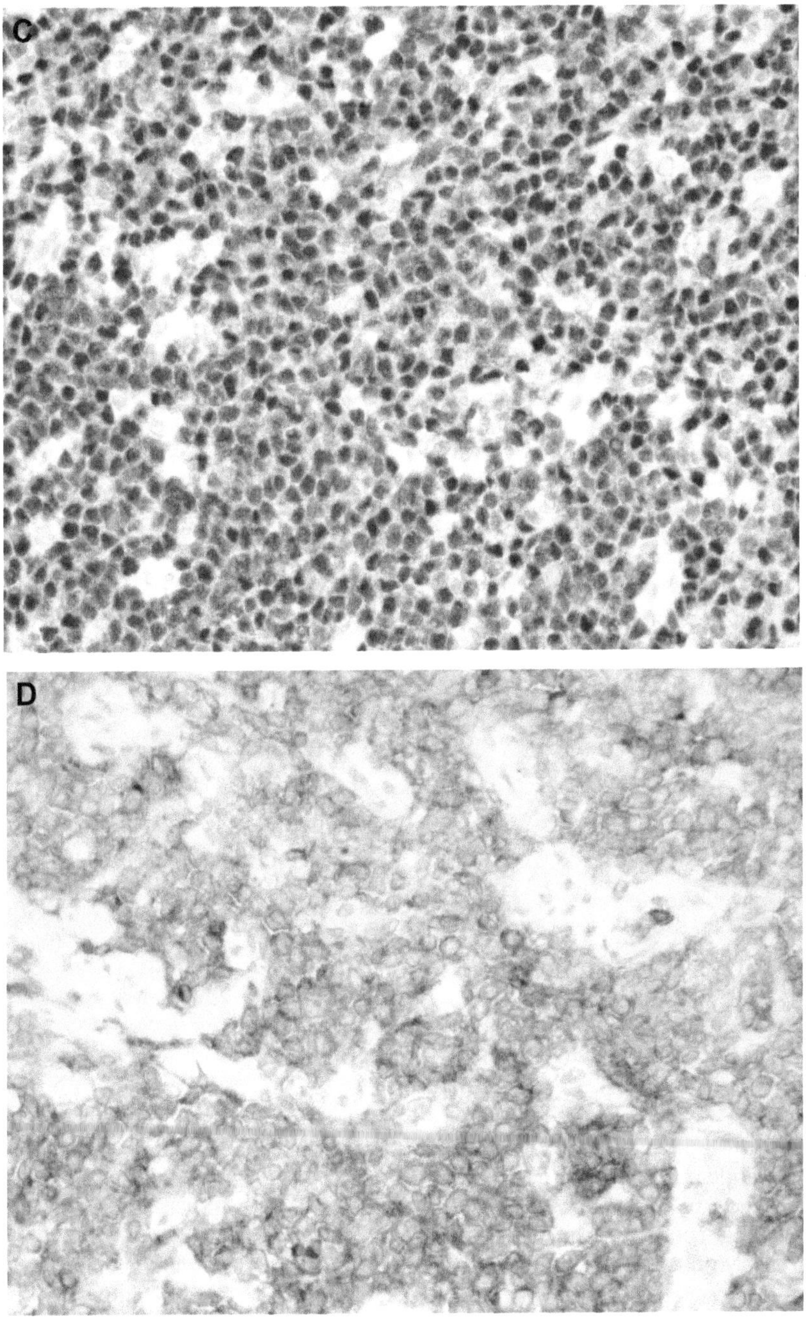

Fig. 6. (*continued*). (*C*) PAX5, and (*D*) CD10. Not shown: the lymphoma cells also expressed MYC and BCL2 (moderate), demonstrated a high Ki67 proliferation fraction (approaching 100%), and were negative for EBER (EBV-encoded RNA, in situ hybridization).

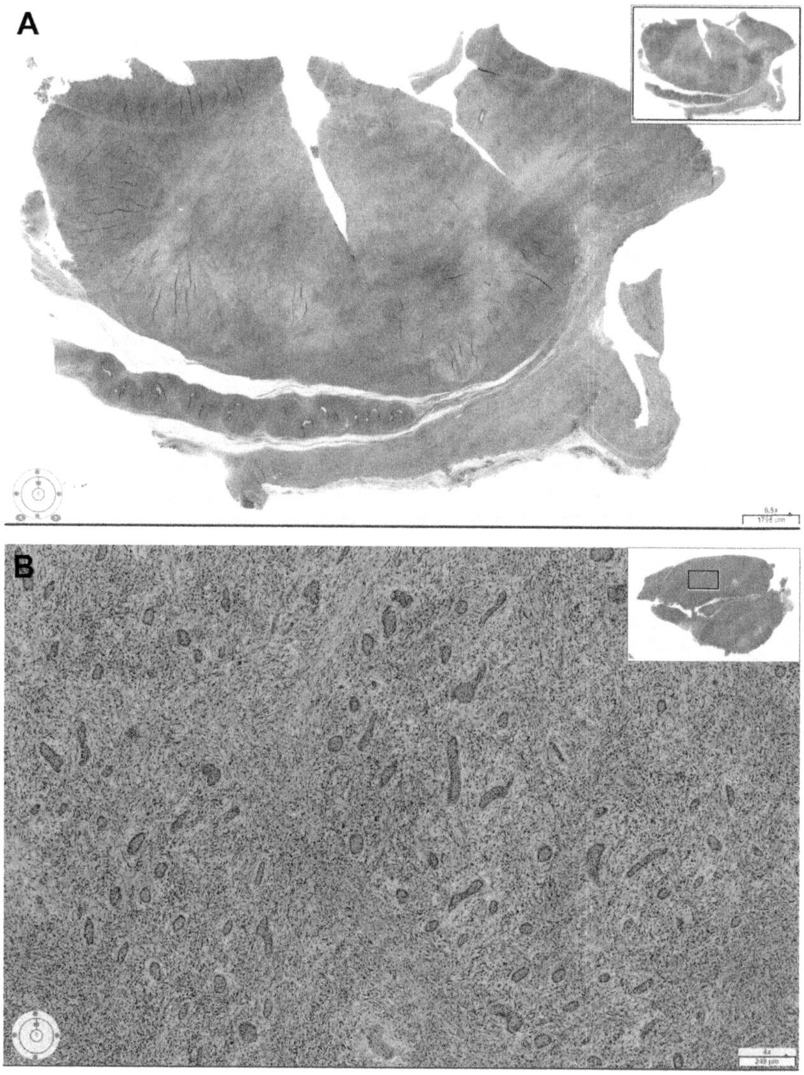

Fig. 7. Pediatric testicular follicular lymphoma. Digital whole-slide image from the radical orchiectomy specimen of a 4-year-old boy. H&E (*A*) 5×, (*B*) 40×, and

uniformly curative, emphasizing their indolent nature and supporting the recent proposal of reclassification to one disorder (PTFL with or without marginal zone differentiation) and to "neoplasia" from "lymphoma."

LARGE B-CELL LYMPHOMA WITH *IRF4* REARRANGEMENT

Although large B-cell lymphoma with *IRF4* rearrangement (LBCL *IRF4*-rearranged) is common in young patients with limited-stage disease and high cure rate,[117,118] decreasing or omitting adjuvant chemotherapy is thought to be riskier than in PTFL[79,95]; however, this concept may evolve so the entity is mentioned here. Similar to PTFL and PNMZL, surgical margins are not utilized per se, although complete excision for stage I disease is expected.

LBCL *IRF4*-rearranged is well described elsewhere.[117,118] The diagnosis should be pursued in the differential diagnosis of large B-cell lymphoma—with or without follicular growth pattern—in the head-and-neck region in children, particularly Waldeyer ring.[96] Interestingly, presentations of pediatric large B-cell lymphoma with *IRF4* rearrangement in ileocecal[119] and other[120] locations have been reported.

Commercial FISH probes are available, which can be used in parallel with FISH for *MYC*, *BCL2*, and *BCL6*. Alternatively, *IRF4* FISH can be pursued following negative results for *MYC* FISH. Of note, *TP53* alterations are common and CD5 may be expressed.[117,118]

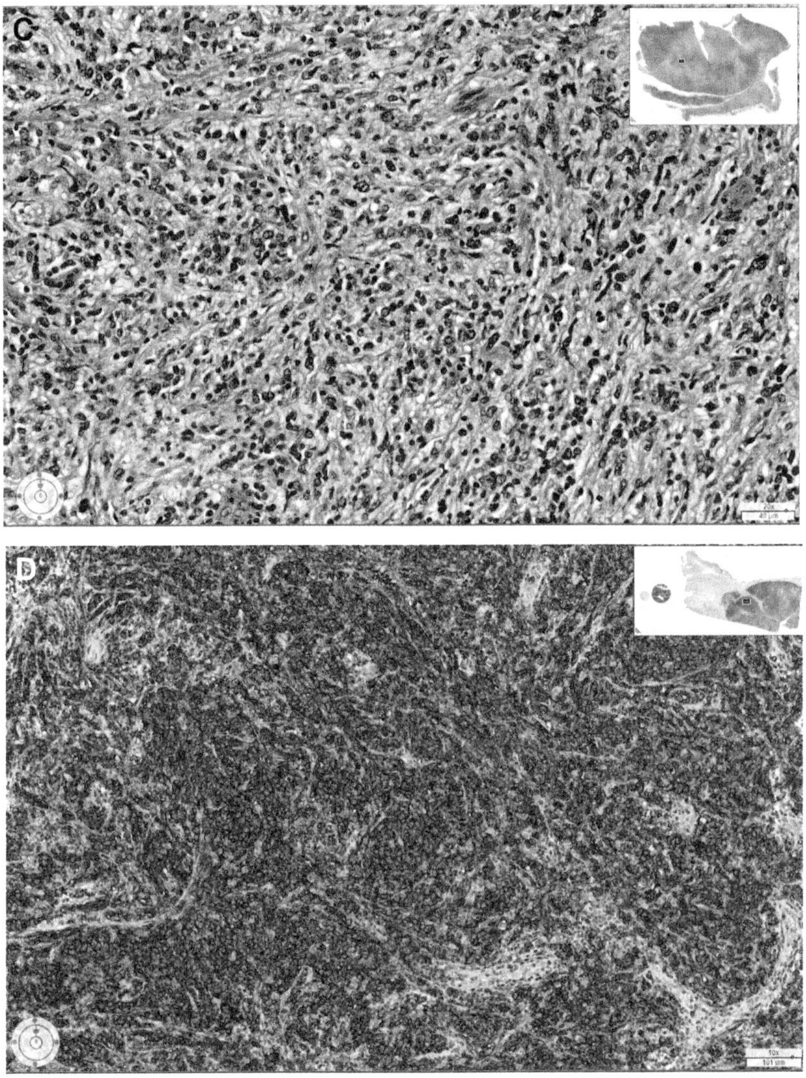

Fig. 7. (*continued*). (*C*) 200×. (*D*) CD20, 100×.

SUMMARY

Pediatric B-cell lymphoid neoplasia overlaps with adult diseases but the epidemiology and clinical presentations differ in important ways, arguably most crucially for optimal clinical management. Attention by the pathologist to genetic subclassification of B-ALL/LBL and to surgical considerations for unique low-stage mature B-cell lymphomas in pediatric patients often makes a difference in the patient's management, clinical course, and ultimate outcome.

DECLARATION OF INTERESTS

The authors have nothing to disclose.

REFERENCES

1. Alaggio R, Amador C, Anagnostopoulos I, et al. The 5th edition of the World Health Organization Classification of Haematolymphoid Tumours: Lymphoid Neoplasms. Leukemia 2022;36(7):1720–48.
2. Arber DA, Orazi A, Hasserjian RP, et al. International Consensus Classification of Myeloid Neoplasms and Acute Leukemias: integrating morphologic, clinical, and genomic data. Blood 2022;140(11):1200–28.
3. Iacobucci I, Kimura S, Mullighan CG. Biologic and therapeutic implications of genomic alterations in acute lymphoblastic Leukemia. J Clin Med 2021;10(17):3792.
4. Li J, Dai Y, Wu L, et al. Emerging molecular subtypes and therapeutic targets in B-cell precursor acute

lymphoblastic leukemia. Front Med 2021;15(3): 347–71.
5. Li JF, Dai YT, Lilljebjorn H, et al. Transcriptional landscape of B cell precursor acute lymphoblastic leukemia based on an international study of 1,223 cases. Proc Natl Acad Sci U S A 2018;115(50): E11711–20.
6. Brown LM, Lonsdale A, Zhu A, et al. The application of RNA sequencing for the diagnosis and genomic classification of pediatric acute lymphoblastic leukemia. Blood Adv 2020;4(5):930–42.
7. Tran TH, Langlois S, Meloche C, et al. Whole-transcriptome analysis in acute lymphoblastic leukemia: a report from the DFCI ALL Consortium Protocol 16-001. Blood Adv 2022;6(4):1329–41.
8. Brown P, Inaba H, Annesley C, et al. Pediatric acute lymphoblastic leukemia, version 2.2020, NCCN clinical practice guidelines in oncology. J Natl Compr Canc Netw 2020;18(1):81–112.
9. Chen X, Wood BL. Monitoring minimal residual disease in acute leukemia: technical challenges and interpretive complexities. Blood Rev 2017;31(2): 63–75.
10. Andreani G, Cilloni D. Strategies for minimal residual disease detection: current perspectives. Blood Lymphat Cancer 2019;9:1–8.
11. Panagopoulos I, Micci F, Thorsen J, et al. A novel TCF3-HLF fusion transcript in acute lymphoblastic leukemia with a t(17;19)(q22;p13). Cancer Genet 2012;205(12):669–72.
12. Inukai T, Hirose K, Inaba T, et al. Hypercalcemia in childhood acute lymphoblastic leukemia: frequent implication of parathyroid hormone-related peptide and E2A-HLF from translocation 17;19. Leukemia 2007;21(2):288–96.
13. Mouttet B, Vinti L, Ancliff P, et al. Durable remissions in TCF3-HLF positive acute lymphoblastic leukemia with blinatumomab and stem cell transplantation. Haematologica 2019;104(6):e244–7.
14. Fischer U, Forster M, Rinaldi A, et al. Genomics and drug profiling of fatal TCF3-HLF-positive acute lymphoblastic leukemia identifies recurrent mutation patterns and therapeutic options. Nat Genet 2015;47(9):1020–9.
15. Lilljebjorn H, Henningsson R, Hyrenius-Wittsten A, et al. Identification of ETV6-RUNX1-like and DUX4-rearranged subtypes in paediatric B-cell precursor acute lymphoblastic leukaemia. Nat Commun 2016;7:11790.
16. Jeha S, Choi J, Roberts KG, et al. Clinical significance of novel subtypes of acute lymphoblastic leukemia in the context of minimal residual disease-directed therapy. Blood Cancer Discov 2021;2(4):326–37.
17. Roberts KG, Li Y, Payne-Turner D, et al. Targetable kinase-activating lesions in Ph-like acute lymphoblastic leukemia. N Engl J Med 2014; 371(11):1005–15.
18. Roberts KG, Morin RD, Zhang J, et al. Genetic alterations activating kinase and cytokine receptor signaling in high-risk acute lymphoblastic leukemia. Cancer Cell 2012;22(2):153–66.
19. Pui CH, Roberts KG, Yang JJ, et al. Philadelphia chromosome-like acute lymphoblastic leukemia. Clin Lymphoma Myeloma Leuk 2017;17(8):464–70.
20. Harvey RC, Mullighan CG, Chen IM, et al. Rearrangement of CRLF2 is associated with mutation of JAK kinases, alteration of IKZF1, Hispanic/Latino ethnicity, and a poor outcome in pediatric B-progenitor acute lymphoblastic leukemia. Blood 2010;115(26):5312–21.
21. Raca G, Abdel-Azim H, Yue F, et al. Increased Incidence of IKZF1 deletions and IGH-CRLF2 translocations in B-ALL of Hispanic/Latino children-a novel health disparity. Leukemia 2021;35(8): 2399–402.
22. Reshmi SC, Harvey RC, Roberts KG, et al. Targetable kinase gene fusions in high-risk B-ALL: a study from the Children's Oncology Group. Blood 2017;129(25):3352–61.
23. Jain N, Roberts KG, Jabbour E, et al. Ph-like acute lymphoblastic leukemia: a high-risk subtype in adults. Blood 2017;129(5):572–81.
24. Mullighan CG. How advanced are we in targeting novel subtypes of ALL? Best Pract Res Clin Haematol 2019;32(4):101095.
25. Roberts KG, Gu Z, Payne-Turner D, et al. High frequency and poor outcome of philadelphia chromosome-like acute lymphoblastic leukemia in adults. J Clin Oncol 2017;35(4):394–401.
26. Roberts KG, Mullighan CG. The biology of B-Progenitor acute lymphoblastic leukemia. Cold Spring Harb Perspect Med 2020;10(7).
27. Roberts KG, Reshmi SC, Harvey RC, et al. Genomic and outcome analyses of Ph-like ALL in NCI standard-risk patients: a report from the Children's Oncology Group. Blood 2018;132(8): 815–24.
28. Lilljebjorn H, Fioretos T. New oncogenic subtypes in pediatric B-cell precursor acute lymphoblastic leukemia. Blood 2017;130(12):1395–401.
29. Rehn JA, O'Connor MJ, White DL, et al. DUX hunting-clinical features and diagnostic challenges associated with DUX4-rearranged leukaemia. Cancers 2020;12(10).
30. Li Z, Lee SHR, Chin WHN, et al. Distinct clinical characteristics of DUX4- and PAX5-altered childhood B-lymphoblastic leukemia. Blood Adv 2021; 5(23):5226–38.
31. Zhang J, McCastlain K, Yoshihara H, et al. Deregulation of DUX4 and ERG in acute lymphoblastic leukemia. Nat Genet 2016;48(12):1481–9.

32. Qian M, Xu H, Perez-Andreu V, et al. Novel susceptibility variants at the ERG locus for childhood acute lymphoblastic leukemia in Hispanics. Blood 2019; 133(7):724–9.
33. Schinnerl D, Mejstrikova E, Schumich A, et al. CD371 cell surface expression: a unique feature of DUX4-rearranged acute lymphoblastic leukemia. Haematologica 2019;104(8):e352–5.
34. Novakova M, Zaliova M, Fiser K, et al. DUX4r, ZNF384r and PAX5-P80R mutated B-cell precursor acute lymphoblastic leukemia frequently undergo monocytic switch. Haematologica 2021;106(8): 2066–75.
35. Hrusak O, Porwit-MacDonald A. Antigen expression patterns reflecting genotype of acute leukemias. Leukemia 2002;16(7):1233–58.
36. Daga S, Rosenberger A, Kashofer K, et al. Sensitive and broadly applicable residual disease detection in acute myeloid leukemia using flow cytometry-based leukemic cell enrichment followed by mutational profiling. Am J Hematol 2020;95(10):1148–57.
37. Novakova M, Zaliova M, Fiser K, et al. DUX4r, ZNF384r and PAX5-P80R mutated B-cell precursor acute lymphoblastic leukemia frequently undergo monocytic switch. Haematologica 2021;106(8): 2066–75.
38. Siegele BJ, Stemmer-Rachamimov AO, Lilljebjorn H, et al. N-terminus DUX4-immunohistochemistry is a reliable methodology for the diagnosis of DUX4-fused B-lymphoblastic leukemia/lymphoma (N-terminus DUX4 IHC for DUX4-fused B-ALL). Genes Chromosomes Cancer 2022;61(8):449–58.
39. Kimura S, Mullighan CG. Molecular markers in ALL: clinical implications. Best Pract Res Clin Haematol 2020;33(3):101193.
40. Alexander TB, Gu Z, Iacobucci I, et al. The genetic basis and cell of origin of mixed phenotype acute leukaemia. Nature 2018;562(7727):373–9.
41. Hirabayashi S, Butler ER, Ohki K, et al. Clinical characteristics and outcomes of B-ALL with ZNF384 rearrangements: a retrospective analysis by the Ponte di Legno Childhood ALL Working Group. Leukemia 2021;35(11):3272–7.
42. Liu YF, Wang BY, Zhang WN, et al. Genomic profiling of adult and pediatric B-cell acute lymphoblastic leukemia. EBioMedicine 2016;8:173–83.
43. Marincevic-Zuniga Y, Dahlberg J, Nilsson S, et al. Transcriptome sequencing in pediatric acute lymphoblastic leukemia identifies fusion genes associated with distinct DNA methylation profiles. J Hematol Oncol 2017;10(1):148.
44. Zaliova M, Stuchly J, Winkowska L, et al. Genomic landscape of pediatric B-other acute lymphoblastic leukemia in a consecutive European cohort. Haematologica 2019;104(7):1396–406.
45. Moe Takeda MW, D Bhojwani, Z Gu, BL. Wood, G Raca, Alexandra E. Kovach. Distinct immunophenotypic features of noval genetic subtypes of pediatric B-lymphoblastic leukemia are recognizable in a clinical setting and can help direct molecular testing. Paper presented at: Society for Pediatric Pathology (SPP); March 19, 2022, 2022; Los Angeles, CA.
46. Ohki K, Takahashi H, Fukushima T, et al. Impact of immunophenotypic characteristics on genetic subgrouping in childhood acute lymphoblastic leukemia: Tokyo Children's Cancer Study Group (TCCSG) study L04-16. Genes Chromosomes Cancer 2020;59(10):551–61.
47. Gu Z, Churchman M, Roberts K, et al. Genomic analyses identify recurrent MEF2D fusions in acute lymphoblastic leukaemia. Nat Commun 2016;7:13331.
48. Sadras T, Müschen M. MEF2D fusions drive oncogenic Pre-BCR signaling in B-ALL. Blood Cancer Discov 2020;1(1):18–20.
49. Gordana Raca AEK, Z Hu, V Yellapantula, D Ostrow, A Doan, J Ji, R Schmidt, JA. Biegel, Z Gu, D Bhojwani. Transcriptome Sequencing (RNA-Seq) Allows Comprehensive Genomic Characterization of Pediatric B-Lymphoblastic Leukemia (B-ALL) in the Clinical Setting Paper presented at: Association for Molecular Pathology (AMP); November 3, 2022, 2022; Phoenix, AZ.
50. Gu Z, Churchman ML, Roberts KG, et al. PAX5-driven subtypes of B-progenitor acute lymphoblastic leukemia. Nat Genet 2019;51(2):296–307.
51. Bastian L, Schroeder MP, Eckert C, et al. PAX5 biallelic genomic alterations define a novel subgroup of B-cell precursor acute lymphoblastic leukemia. Leukemia 2019;33(8):1895–909.
52. Jia Z, Gu Z. PAX5 alterations in B-cell acute lymphoblastic leukemia. Front Oncol 2022;12: 1023606.
53. Schwab C, Nebral K, Chilton L, et al. Intragenic amplification of PAX5: a novel subgroup in B-cell precursor acute lymphoblastic leukemia? Blood Adv 2017;1(19):1473–7.
54. Jean J, Kovach AE, Doan A, et al. Characterization of PAX5 intragenic tandem multiplication in pediatric B-lymphoblastic leukemia by optical genome mapping. Blood Adv 2022;6(11):3343–6.
55. Coyaud E, Struski S, Prade N, et al. Wide diversity of PAX5 alterations in B-ALL: a Groupe Francophone de Cytogenetique Hematologique study. Blood 2010;115(15):3089–97.
56. Passet M, Boissel N, Sigaux F, et al. PAX5 P80R mutation identifies a novel subtype of B-cell precursor acute lymphoblastic leukemia with favorable outcome. Blood 2019;133(3):280–4.
57. Boer JM, Valsecchi MG, Hormann FM, et al. Favorable outcome of NUTM1-rearranged infant and pediatric B cell precursor acute lymphoblastic leukemia in a collaborative international study. Leukemia 2021;35(10):2978–82.

58. Hormann FM, Hoogkamer AQ, Beverloo HB, et al. NUTM1 is a recurrent fusion gene partner in B-cell precursor acute lymphoblastic leukemia associated with increased expression of genes on chromosome band 10p12.31-12.2. Haematologica 2019;104(10):e455–9.
59. Pincez T, Landry JR, Roussy M, et al. Cryptic recurrent ACIN1-NUTM1 fusions in non-KMT2A-rearranged infant acute lymphoblastic leukemia. Genes Chromosomes Cancer 2020;59(2):125–30.
60. Gagnon MF, Sill D, Meyer R, et al. Frequency of double-hit cytogenetics and MYC rearrangement partners in pediatric (<18) and yound adult (18-30) patients: a 10-year Mayo Clinic review. Paper presented at: 21st European Association of Haematopathology (EAHP) Congress; September 20, 2022, 2022; Florence, Italy.
61. Tchinda J, Volpert S, Berdel WE, et al. Novel three-break rearrangement and cryptic translocations leading to colocalization of MYC and IGH signals in B-cell acute lymphoblastic leukemia. Cancer Genet Cytogenet 2006;165(2):180–4.
62. Testoni N, Zaccaria A, Martinelli G, et al. t(8;14)(q11;q32) in acute lymphoid leukemia: description of two cases. Cancer Genet Cytogenet 1993;67(1):55–8.
63. Kelemen K, Holden J, Johnson LJ, et al. Immunophenotypic and cytogenetic findings of B-lymphoblastic leukemia/lymphoma associated with combined IGH/BCL2 and MYC rearrangement. Cytometry B Clin Cytom 2017;92(4):310–4.
64. Uchida A, Isobe Y, Uemura Y, et al. De novo acute lymphoblastic leukemia-like disease of high grade B-cell lymphoma with MYC and BCL2 and/or BCL6 rearrangements: a case report and literature review. BMC Clin Pathol 2017;17:21.
65. Wagener R, López C, Kleinheinz K, et al. IG-MYC (+) neoplasms with precursor B-cell phenotype are molecularly distinct from Burkitt lymphomas. Blood 2018;132(21):2280–5.
66. Burmeister T, Molkentin M, Schwartz S, et al. Erroneous class switching and false VDJ recombination: molecular dissection of t(8;14)/MYC-IGH translocations in Burkitt-type lymphoblastic leukemia/B-cell lymphoma. Mol Oncol 2013;7(4):850–8.
67. Li Y, Gupta G, Molofsky A, et al. B Lymphoblastic Leukemia/Lymphoma With Burkitt-like Morphology and IGH/MYC Rearrangement: Report of 3 Cases in Adult Patients. Am J Surg Pathol 2018;42(2): 269–76.
68. Yoon J, Yun JW, Jung CW, et al. Molecular characteristics of terminal deoxynucleotidyl transferase negative precursor B-cell phenotype Burkitt leukemia with IGH-MYC rearrangement. Genes Chromosomes Cancer 2020;59(4):255–60.
69. Snuderl M, Kolman OK, Chen YB, et al. B-cell lymphomas with concurrent IGH-BCL2 and MYC rearrangements are aggressive neoplasms with clinical and pathologic features distinct from Burkitt lymphoma and diffuse large B-cell lymphoma. Am J Surg Pathol 2010;34(3):327–40.
70. Tomita N, Tokunaka M, Nakamura N, et al. Clinicopathological features of lymphoma/leukemia patients carrying both BCL2 and MYC translocations. Haematologica 2009;94(7):935–43.
71. Knezevich S, Ludkovski O, Salski C, et al. Concurrent translocation of BCL2 and MYC with a single immunoglobulin locus in high-grade B-cell lymphomas. Leukemia 2005;19(4):659–63.
72. Bhavsar S, Liu YC, Gibson SE, et al. Mutational landscape of TdT+ large B-cell lymphomas supports their distinction from B-lymphoblastic neoplasms: a multiparameter study of a rare and aggressive entity. Am J Surg Pathol 2022;46(1):71–82.
73. Hamdan H, Luu L, Opsahl M, et al. Genomic profile of TdT(positive) MYC/BCL2 rearranged high-grade B-cell lymphoma supporting its diagnosis as mature aggressive lymphoma. Cytometry B Clin Cytom 2022;102(6):448–50.
74. Khanlari M, Medeiros LJ, Lin P, et al. Blastoid high-grade B-cell lymphoma initially presenting in bone marrow: a diagnostic challenge. Mod Pathol 2022;35(3):419–26.
75. Ok CY, Medeiros LJ, Thakral B, et al. High-grade B-cell lymphomas with TdT expression: a diagnostic and classification dilemma. Mod Pathol 2019; 32(1):48–58.
76. Moench L, Sachs Z, Aasen G, et al. Double- and triple-hit lymphomas can present with features suggestive of immaturity, including TdT expression, and create diagnostic challenges. Leuk Lymphoma 2016;57(11):2626–35.
77. Axler OPA. Immunophenotyping of mature B-cell lymphomas. In: Porwit ABM, editor. Multiparameter flow cytometry in the diagnosis of hematologic malignancies. Cambridge, UK: Cambridge University Press; 2018. p. 105–27.
78. Oschlies I, Klapper W, Zimmermann M, et al. Diffuse large B-cell lymphoma in pediatric patients belongs predominantly to the germinal-center type B-cell lymphomas: a clinicopathologic analysis of cases included in the German BFM (Berlin-Frankfurt-Munster) Multicenter Trial. Blood 2006; 107(10):4047–52.
79. Barth M, Xavier AC, Armenian S, et al. Pediatric aggressive mature B-Cell lymphomas, version 3.2022, NCCN clinical practice guidelines in oncology. J Natl Compr Canc Netw 2022;20(11): 1267–75.
80. Minard-Colin V, Brugieres L, Reiter A, et al. Non-Hodgkin lymphoma in children and adolescents: progress through effective collaboration, current knowledge, and challenges ahead. J Clin Oncol 2015;33(27):2963–74.

81. Sandlund JT, Martin MG. Non-Hodgkin lymphoma across the pediatric and adolescent and young adult age spectrum. Hematology Am Soc Hematol Educ Program 2016;2016(1):589–97.
82. Matthew Barth ACX, Armenian S, Audino AN, et al. Pediatric Aggressive Mature B-Cell Lymphomas. NCCN Clinical Practice Guidelines in Oncology (NCCN Guidelines) 2022. Available at: https://www.nccn.org/professionals/physician_gls/pdf/ped_b-cell.pdf. Accessed October 13, 2022.
83. Bussell HR, Kroiss S, Tharakan SJ, et al. Intussusception in children: lessons learned from intestinal lymphoma as a rare lead-point. Pediatr Surg Int 2019;35(8):879–85.
84. Naeem B, Ayub A. Primary pediatric non-hodgkin lymphomas of the gastrointestinal tract: a population-based analysis. Anticancer Res 2019;39(11):6413–6.
85. Egan G, Goldman S, Alexander S. Mature B-NHL in children, adolescents and young adults: current therapeutic approach and emerging treatment strategies. Br J Haematol 2019;185(6):1071–85.
86. Rosolen A, Perkins SL, Pinkerton CR, et al. Revised international pediatric non-hodgkin lymphoma staging system. J Clin Oncol 2015;33(18):2112–8.
87. Murphy SB. Classification, staging and end results of treatment of childhood non-Hodgkin's lymphomas: dissimilarities from lymphomas in adults. Semin Oncol 1980;7(3):332–9.
88. Shamberger RC, Weinstein HJ. The role of surgery in abdominal Burkitt's lymphoma. J Pediatr Surg 1992;27(2):236–40.
89. Gupta H, Davidoff AM, Pui CH, et al. Clinical implications and surgical management of intussusception in pediatric patients with Burkitt lymphoma. J Pediatr Surg 2007;42(6):998–1001, [discussion: 1001].
90. Ferry JA. Burkitt's lymphoma: clinicopathologic features and differential diagnosis. Oncol 2006;11(4):375–83.
91. Hecht JL, Aster JC. Molecular biology of Burkitt's lymphoma. J Clin Oncol 2000;18(21):3707–21.
92. Hummel M, Bentink S, Berger H, et al. A biologic definition of Burkitt's lymphoma from transcriptional and genomic profiling. N Engl J Med 2006;354(23):2419–30.
93. Rimsza L, Pittaluga S, Dirnhofer S, et al. The clinicopathologic spectrum of mature aggressive B cell lymphomas. Virchows Arch 2017;471(4):453–66.
94. Grygalewicz B, Woroniecka R, Rymkiewicz G, et al. The 11q-Gain/Loss Aberration Occurs Recurrently in MYC-Negative Burkitt-like Lymphoma With 11q Aberration, as Well as MYC-Positive Burkitt Lymphoma and MYC-Positive High-Grade B-Cell Lymphoma, NOS. Am J Clin Pathol 2017;149(1):17–28.
95. Au-Yeung RKH, Arias Padilla L, Zimmermann M, et al. Experience with provisional WHO-entities large B-cell lymphoma with IRF4-rearrangement and Burkitt-like lymphoma with 11q aberration in paediatric patients of the NHL-BFM group. Br J Haematol 2020;190(5):753–63.
96. Mason EF, Kovach AE. Update on pediatric and young adult mature lymphomas. Clin Lab Med 2021;41(3):359–87.
97. Gonzalez-Farre B, Ramis-Zaldivar JE, Salmeron-Villalobos J, et al. Burkitt-like lymphoma with 11q aberration: a germinal center-derived lymphoma genetically unrelated to Burkitt lymphoma. Haematologica 2019;104(9):1822–9.
98. Appel BE, Chen L, Buxton AB, et al. Minimal treatment of low-risk, pediatric lymphocyte-predominant hodgkin lymphoma: a report from the children's oncology group. J Clin Oncol 2016;34(20):2372–9.
99. Klekawka T, Balwierz W, Brozyna A, et al. Nodular lymphocyte predominant Hodgkin lymphoma: experience of polish pediatric leukemia/lymphoma study group. Pediatr Hematol Oncol 2021;38(7):609–19.
100. Bessen SY, Gardner JA, Chen EY. When is surgical resection alone appropriate treatment for pediatric nodular lymphocyte-predominant Hodgkin lymphoma? SAGE open medical case reports 2021;9, 2050313x211022422.
101. Campo E, Jaffe ES, Cook JR, et al. The international consensus classification of mature lymphoid neoplasms: a report from the clinical advisory committee. Blood 2022;140(11):1229–53.
102. Hartmann S, Eichenauer DA. Nodular lymphocyte predominant Hodgkin lymphoma: pathology, clinical course and relation to T-cell/histiocyte rich large B-cell lymphoma. Pathology 2020;52(1):142–53.
103. Fan Z, Natkunam Y, Bair E, et al. Characterization of variant patterns of nodular lymphocyte predominant hodgkin lymphoma with immunohistologic and clinical correlation. Am J Surg Pathol 2003;27(10):1346–56.
104. Panayi C, Akarca A, Vitale L, et al. Deciphering the microenvironment of NLPHL by multispectral immunofluorescence and digital image analysis generates biomarkers relevant to diagnostic and prognostic stratification. 21st European Association of Haematopathology (EAHP) Congress; September 19, 2022, 2022; Florence, Italy.
105. Liu Q, Salaverria I, Pittaluga S, et al. Follicular lymphomas in children and young adults: a comparison of the pediatric variant with usual follicular lymphoma. Am J Surg Pathol 2013;37(3):333–43.
106. Louissaint A Jr, Schafernak KT, Geyer JT, et al. Pediatric-type nodal follicular lymphoma: a

biologically distinct lymphoma with frequent MAPK pathway mutations. Blood 2016;128(8):1093–100.
107. Pileri SA, Sabattini E, Rosito P, et al. Primary follicular lymphoma of the testis in childhood: an entity with peculiar clinical and molecular characteristics. J Clin Pathol 2002;55(9):684–8.
108. Finn LS, Viswanatha DS, Belasco JB, et al. Primary follicular lymphoma of the testis in childhood. Cancer 1999;85(7):1626–35.
109. Pakzad K, MacLennan GT, Elder JS, et al. Follicular large cell lymphoma localized to the testis in children. J Urol 2002;168(1):225–8.
110. Lones MA, Raphael M, McCarthy K, et al. Primary follicular lymphoma of the testis in children and adolescents. J Pediatr Hematol Oncol 2012;34(1):68–71.
111. Hiemenz MC, Ostrow DG, Busse TM, et al. OncoKids: a comprehensive next-generation sequencing panel for pediatric malignancies. J Mol Diagn 2018;20(6):765–76.
112. Bödör C, Grossmann V, Popov N, et al. EZH2 mutations are frequent and represent an early event in follicular lymphoma. Blood 2013;122(18):3165–8.
113. Heller KN, Teruya-Feldstein J, La Quaglia MP, et al. Primary follicular lymphoma of the testis: excellent outcome following surgical resection without adjuvant chemotherapy. J Pediatr Hematol Oncol 2004;26(2):104–7.
114. Salmeron-Villalobos J, Egan C, Borgmann V, et al. A unifying hypothesis for PNMZL and PTFL: morphological variants with a common molecular profile. Blood Adv 2022;6(16):4661–74.
115. Lim S, Lim KY, Koh J, et al. Pediatric-Type Indolent B-Cell Lymphomas With Overlapping Clinical, Pathologic, and Genetic Features. Am J Surg Pathol 2022;46(10):1397–406.
116. Jaffe ES. Pediatric nodal marginal zone lymphoma (PNMZL) shares a common molecular profile with pediatric-type follicular lymphoma (PTFL). European Association of Hematopathology (EAHP); September 20, 2022, 2022; Florence, Italy.
117. Pittaluga S, Harris NL, Siebert R, et al. Large B-cell lymphoma with IRF4 rearrangement. In: Swerdlow SH, Campo E, Harris NL, et al, editors. WHO classification of tumours of haematopoietic and lymphoid tissues. Revised. 4th ed. Lyon: International Agency for Research on Cancer; 2017. p. 280–1.
118. Salaverria I, Philipp C, Oschlies I, et al. Translocations activating IRF4 identify a subtype of germinal center-derived B-cell lymphoma affecting predominantly children and young adults. Blood 2011;118(1):139–47.
119. Wang D, Ahn J. Ileocoloc intussusception and atypical FISH signal pattern in a pediatric patient with large B-cell lymphoma with IRF4 rearrangement. 21st European Association of Haematopathology (EAHP) Congress; September 21, 2022, 2022; Florence, Italy.
120. Chisholm KM, Mohlman J, Liew M, et al. IRF4 translocation status in pediatric follicular and diffuse large B-cell lymphoma patients enrolled in Children's Oncology Group trials. Pediatr Blood Cancer 2019;66(8):e27770.

Current Concepts in Nodal Peripheral T-Cell Lymphomas

Naoki Oishi, MD, PhD[a], Andrew L. Feldman, MD[b,*]

KEYWORDS

- Peripheral T-cell lymphoma • Anaplastic large cell lymphoma • T-follicular helper cell lymphoma
- Epstein-Barr virus–positive nodal T/NK-cell lymphoma

Key points

- The diagnosis and classification of peripheral T-cell lymphoma (PTCL) is based on a combination of clinical features, morphology, immunophenotype, viral positivity, and genetics.
- There are 4 anaplastic large cell lymphoma (ALCL) entities: primary cutaneous, breast implant–associated, (systemic) anaplastic lymphoma kinase (ALK)-positive, and ALK-negative; ALK-negative ALCL has further genetic heterogeneity, including distinct subgroups with *DUSP22* and/or *TP63* rearrangements.
- The spectrum of PTCL with T-follicular helper (TFH) phenotype has been expanded beyond angioimmunoblastic T-cell lymphoma and a new entity of nodal TFH cell lymphoma established, requiring immunohistochemistry for TFH markers and possibly genetic studies for diagnosis.
- Epstein-Barr virus–positive nodal T/natural killer(NK)-cell lymphoma (EBV+ nTNKL) is a new entity, and Epstein-Barr encoding region in situ hybridization is recommended in evaluating nodal cytotoxic PTCLs.
- PTCL, not otherwise specified, remains a diagnosis of exclusion: ALCL, TFH lymphoma, EBV + nTNKL, adult T-cell leukemia/lymphoma, and other extranodal entities must be ruled out by immunohistochemical workup and clinicopathologic correlation.

ABSTRACT

This review summarizes the current understanding of mature T-cell neoplasms predominantly involving lymph nodes, including ALK-positive and ALK-negative anaplastic large cell lymphomas, nodal T-follicular helper cell lymphoma, Epstein-Barr virus–positive nodal T/NK-cell lymphoma, and peripheral T-cell lymphoma (PTCL), not otherwise specified. These PTCLs are clinically, pathologically, and genetically heterogeneous, and the diagnosis is made by a combination of clinical information, morphology, immunophenotype, viral positivity, and genetic abnormalities. This review summarizes the pathologic features of common nodal PTCLs, highlighting updates in the fifth edition of the World Health Organization classification and the 2022 International Consensus Classification.

Peripheral T-cell lymphomas (PTCLs) comprise a clinically, pathologically, and genetically heterogeneous group of neoplasms of mature T lymphocytes. Two recently published classification systems, the fifth edition of the World Health Organization classification of hematological malignancy (WHO-HAEM5) and the 2022 International Consensus Classification (ICC), are conceptually

[a] Department of Pathology, University of Yamanashi, 1110 Shimokato, Chuo, Yamanashi 409-3898, Japan; [b] Department of Laboratory Medicine and Pathology, Mayo Clinic, 200 First Street Southwest, Rochester, MN 55905, USA

* Corresponding author.

E-mail address: feldman.andrew@mayo.edu

Surgical Pathology 16 (2023) 267–285
https://doi.org/10.1016/j.path.2023.01.011

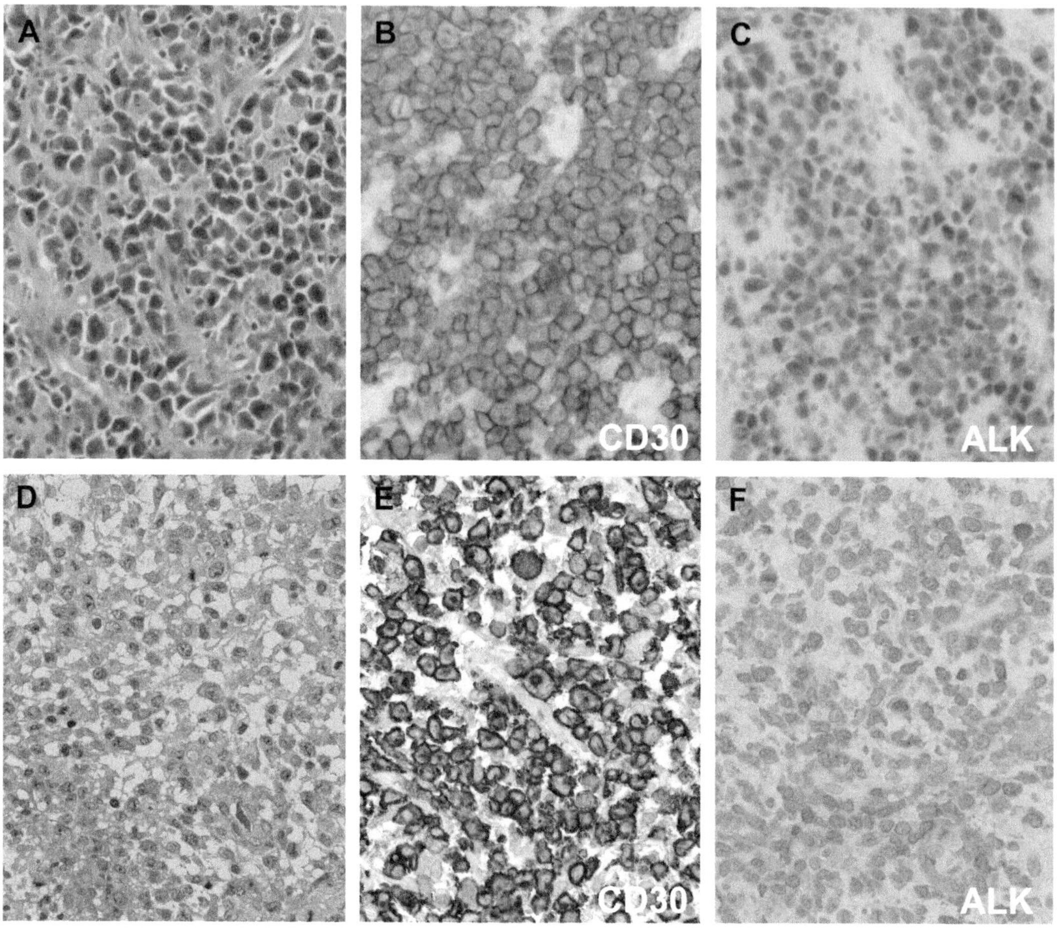

Fig. 1. ALK+ ALCL. Case 1 (*A–C*): this case exhibits proliferation of pleomorphic large cells (*A*) with CD30 (*B*) and nuclear and cytoplasmic ALK expression (*C*), suggesting *NPM1::ALK*. Case 2 (*D–F*): this case shows proliferation of medium-sized hallmark cells (*D*) with CD30 (*E*) and cytoplasmic ALK (*F*).

similar, although minor differences exist.[1,2] Classification of PTCL incorporates clinical presentation, morphology, immunophenotype, and genetics. In this review, we discuss the current understanding of nodal PTCLs and their diagnosis.

ANAPLASTIC LARGE CELL LYMPHOMA

INTRODUCTION

Anaplastic large cell lymphomas (ALCLs) represent a heterogeneous group of T-cell neoplasms showing distinct morphology and uniform CD30 expression.[3] WHO-HAEM5 and 2022 ICC define 4 forms of ALCL: anaplastic lymphoma kinase (ALK)+, ALK−, primary cutaneous (pc), and breast implant–associated (BIA).[1,2] ALK+ and ALK− ALCL are systemic diseases, whereas pcALCL and BIA-ALCL are usually localized. Here, the authors discuss nodal ALK+ and ALK− ALCL.

MICROSCOPIC FEATURES

In nodal ALCL, the normal lymph node architecture is usually effaced by a diffuse proliferation of neoplastic cells, which may spare residual reactive follicles.[3] Sinusoidal infiltration of the tumor cells is common. At least some neoplastic cells have large kidney- or horseshoe-shaped nuclei and are called hallmark cells. Other cells may have immunoblastic features or may be multinucleated or contain wreathlike, multilobated nuclei. A subset of small- to medium-sized tumor cells may be present. Several histologic patterns of ALK+ ALCL have been described, including common, lymphohistiocytic, small cell, and Hodgkin-like.

Most ALCLs show diffuse, uniform CD30 expression in the membrane and Golgi zone. Most ALCLs express CD4 and cytotoxic molecules such as TIA1 and granzyme B. Loss of pan-T-cell markers, especially CD3, is frequent;

sometimes all pan-T-cell markers are lost, resulting in a "null" phenotype. ALK+ ALCL harbors chromosomal rearrangements (R) involving *ALK* on 2p23, leading to the aberrant expression of ALK fusion proteins that can be detected by ALK immunohistochemistry (Fig. 1). The subcellular localization depends on the fusion, including *NPM1::ALK* (nuclear and cytoplasmic), *CLTC::ALK* (granular cytoplasmic), *MSN::ALK* (membranous), and others (diffuse cytoplasmic).[3,4] Immunohistochemistry is usually sufficient to detect *ALK*-R; in equivocal cases, confirmatory fluorescence in situ hybridization (FISH) can be performed.

ALK− ALCL with *DUSP22*-R shows distinct morphology and immunophenotype: the neoplastic cells are relatively small compared with other ALCLs, and "doughnut" cells containing nuclear pseudoinclusions are frequently seen.[5] They typically are positive by immunohistochemistry for LEF1 and negative for phospho-STAT3^{Y705} and cytotoxic markers (Fig. 2).[6–8]

MOLECULAR FEATURES

In ALK+ ALCL, *ALK*-R generates constitutively active ALK fusion proteins that activate MAPK and JAK/STAT pathways.[9] *NPM1::ALK* derived from t(2;5) (p23;q35) is most common. Other partners include *TPM3*, *ATIC*, *TFG*, *TPM4*, *MYH9*, *RNF213*, *TRAF1*, *CLTC*, and *MSN*.[3,4] Abnormalities other than *ALK*-R include mutations in *TP53* and *NOTCH1* pathway genes.[10]

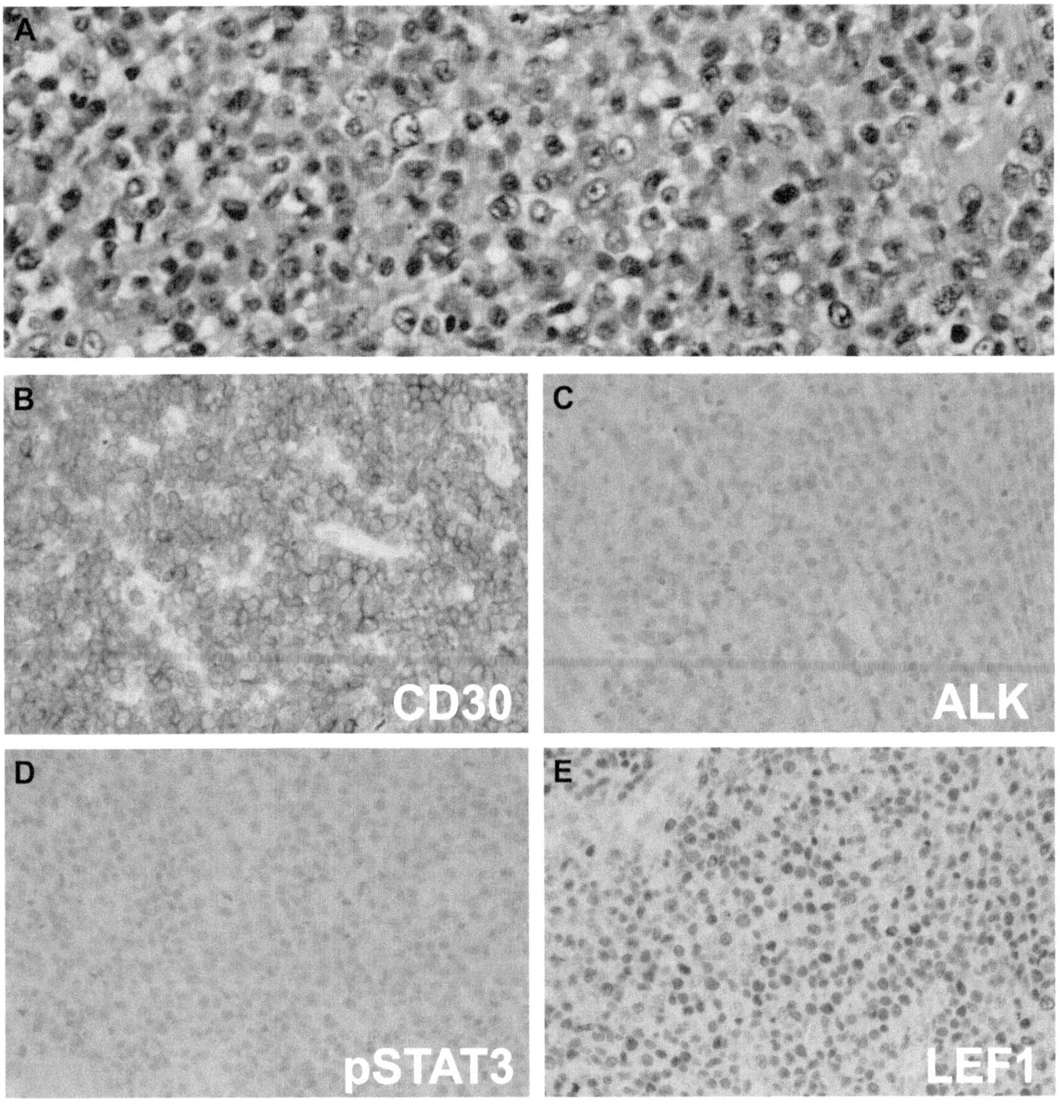

Fig. 2. ALK− ALCL with *DUSP22*-R. A diffuse proliferation of medium-sized lymphocytes is seen (*A*). Tumor cells are positive for CD30 (*B*) but negative for ALK (*C*) and phospho-STAT3^{Y705} (*D*). LEF1 is positive (*E*).

The molecular abnormalities in ALK– ALCL are more heterogeneous than in ALK+ ALCL. *DUSP22*-R involving 6p25.3 is seen in up to 30% of cases,[11] as well as in some pcALCLs and lymphomatoid papulosis, but is absent in BIA-ALCL.[12–15] ALCLs with *DUSP22*-R share unique molecular features, including absence of JAK/STAT3 pathway activation, absent expression of PD-L1, high expression of HLA class II, DNA hypomethylation, and frequent *MSC*^{E116K} mutations.[16–18]

TP63-R involving 3q28 is seen in 5% to 8% of ALK– ALCLs.[19] *TP63*-R leads to the expression of fusion transcripts, among which *TBL1XR1::TP63* corresponding to inv(3) (q26q28) is most common.[19] *TP63*-R is also found in rare pcALCLs, PTCL-not otherwise specified (NOS), mycosis fungoides, and diffuse large B-cell lymphoma.[20] *DUSP22*-R and *TP63*-R have not been reported in association with *ALK*-R; however, rare ALK– ALCLs harboring both *TP63*-R and *DUSP22*-R exist.[21] ALK– ALCL with *TP63*-R is highly aggressive, although its molecular pathogenesis remains unclear. Approximately 50% of ALK– ALCLs lack *ALK*-R, *DUSP22*-R, and *TP63*-R (ie, "triple-negative").[8]

Several genetic abnormalities in ALK– ALCL result in JAK/STAT pathway activation, including activating mutations (*JAK1*, *JAK3*, and *STAT3*) and tyrosine kinase gene fusions (*STAT3::JAK2*, *NFKB2::TYK2*, and *NCOR2::ROS1*).[22,23] Granzyme B and PD-L1/CD274, transcriptional targets of STAT3, are highly expressed in most cases.[8,24,25] ROS1 is a receptor tyrosine kinase (RTK) with structural homology to ALK, and the ROS1 fusion protein leads to aberrant activation of JAK/STAT and MAPK signaling.[26] Thus, some non-ALK RTK fusions have functions analogous to *ALK*-R, although they remain classified within ALK- ALCL; further studies are warranted to examine their sensitivity to RTK inhibitors.

The gold standard for genetic subtyping of ALK– ALCL is FISH; however, immunohistochemistry may be informative in some settings. *DUSP22*-R is associated with expression of CCR8[27] and LEF1[7] and absent expression of cytotoxic molecules such as TIA1.[8] For *TP63*-rearranged ALK-ALCLs, immunohistochemistry for p63 is highly sensitive although not specific; therefore, it can be used to screen cases for the need for *TP63* FISH.[28] An immunohistochemical algorithm incorporating ALK, LEF1, TIA1, and p63 has been proposed for genetic subtyping of ALCL (**Fig. 3**).[6]

DIFFERENTIAL DIAGNOSIS

If expression of CD30 and ALK is confirmed, the diagnosis of ALK+ ALCL is usually straightforward. Other hematolymphoid neoplasms with *ALK*-R include ALK+ large B-cell lymphoma (LBCL) and ALK+ histiocytosis. ALK+ LBCL is a B-cell neoplasm with plasmablastic morphology and immunophenotype.[29] In contrast to ALCL, ALK+ LBCL typically lacks CD30 and expresses

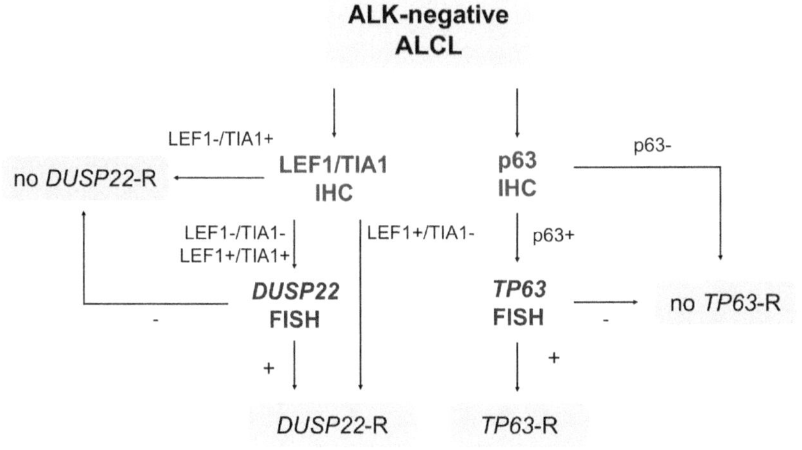

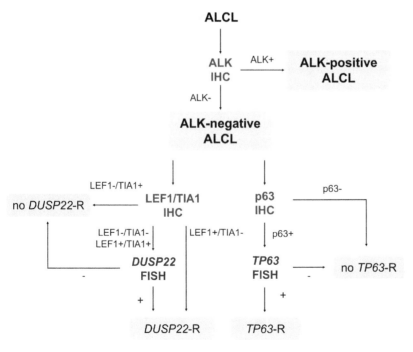

Fig. 3. Immunohistochemical algorithm for genetic subtyping of ALCL based on staining for ALK, LEF1, TIA1, and p63.[6] IHC, immunohistochemistry; R, rearrangement.

CD138, CD38, and immunoglobulin light chain. ALK+ histiocytosis is positive for macrophage/histiocyte markers (CD68, CD163, CD14, and CD4) but negative for CD30.[30,31] Because ALK can be positive in nonhematologic ALK+ neoplasms (eg, pulmonary adenocarcinoma), nodal metastasis should be excluded by immunohistochemistry and clinicopathologic correlation.

Classic Hodgkin lymphoma (CHL) also needs to be distinguished from ALCL. CHL shows variable numbers of CD30-positive Hodgkin/Reed-Sternberg (HRS) cells, typically with large eosinophilic nucleoli and perinucleolar halos, features unusual in ALCL. Reflecting their B-cell origin, HRS cells weakly express PAX5, which is rare in ALCL.[32] CD15 expression, often present in CHL, also can be seen in ALCL. Other lineage markers that can be aberrantly expressed in ALCL include cytokeratins, CD33, and CD13.[33]

Nodal involvement by pcALCL or BIA-ALCL must be differentiated from ALK− ALCL based on clinical history. Carbonic anhydrase-9 expression may aid in the diagnosis of nodal involvement of BIA-ALCL.[34,35]

PROGNOSIS

Genetic subtyping of ALCL has prognostic significance.[8,18,36] ALK+ ALCL generally has a more favorable prognosis than most ALK− ALCLs and other PTCLs, with 5-year overall survival (OS) rates of 70% to 80%.[8] Among ALK− ALCLs, most ALCL with *DUSP22*-R have favorable outcomes with 5-year OS rates of 80% to 90%, similar to ALK+ ALCL,[8,18,36] although cases with high-risk clinical features have been reported.[37] ALCL with *TP63*-R is highly aggressive with dismal prognosis.[8,36] Triple-negative ALCLs show a prognosis intermediate between ALCL with *DUSP22*-R and ALCL with *TP63*-R.[8]

CLINICS CARE POINTS

- ALCL comprises a heterogeneous group of CD30-positive T-cell lymphomas, with 2 systemic forms (ALK+ and ALK−).
- ALK− ALCL comprises biologically and prognostically distinct genetic subgroups, including *DUSP22*-R, *TP63*-R, and triple-negative; immunohistochemistry may aid with genetic subtyping.
- Virtually all PTCL subtypes may express CD30 to a varying extent; when diagnosing ALK− ALCL, confirm diffuse, uniform CD30 expression and carefully rule out other PTCLs and CHL.

T-FOLLICULAR HELPER CELL LYMPHOMA

INTRODUCTION

The prototypical T-follicular helper cell lymphoma (TFHL) is angioimmunoblastic T-cell lymphoma (AITL), which was shown to have a phenotype and gene expression signature similar to normal TFH cells.[38] The revised fourth edition of the WHO classification (WHO-HAEM4R) introduced an umbrella category of TFHLs that included AITL, follicular T-cell lymphoma, and nodal PTCL with TFH phenotype. Both the 2022 ICC and WHO-HAEM5 now consider TFHL a single entity with 3 subtypes: angioimmunoblastic-type, follicular-type, and NOS (**Table 1**).[1,2]

MICROSCOPIC FEATURES

AITL effaces the normal nodal architecture. The neoplastic cells are small- to medium-sized lymphocytes, often with pale, clear cytoplasm (**Fig. 4**); they may exhibit minimal atypia and be difficult to identify without immunohistochemistry. The background comprises a polymorphous mixture of small lymphocytes, immunoblasts (sometimes showing HRS-like features), histiocytes, and eosinophils. Proliferation of arborizing high endothelial venules (HEVs) and follicular dendritic cells (FDCs) is seen. Subcapsular sinuses are often patent and overtly dilated. The neoplastic cells are positive for CD4 and often show preserved expression of CD2, CD3, and CD5 with loss or diminished expression of CD7. At least 2 TFH markers such as CD10, BCL6, CXCL13, ICOS, and PD1 are positive. Typically, there are intermingled B-immunoblasts expressing CD20, CD79a, and PAX5, often associated with Epstein-Barr virus (EBV) infection. The proliferation of FDCs is highlighted by immunohistochemistry for CD21, CD23, and CD35. Small numbers of TdT+ T lymphoblasts, so-called indolent TdT+ lymphoblastic proliferation, is seen in about two-thirds of AITLs.[39]

Follicular-type TFHL (TFHL-F) is a nodal TFHL with a predominantly follicular pattern lacking characteristic features of AITL. The lymph node architecture is effaced by a nodular or follicular proliferation of medium-sized lymphocytes expressing TFH markers (**Fig. 5**). Two distinct histologic patterns are recognized, one resembling follicular lymphoma (FL-like pattern) and one showing large nodules reminiscent of progressive transformation of germinal centers (PTGC-like pattern).[40] Similar to AITL, EBV-positive B-immunoblasts are frequently found; however, proliferation of HEVs and FDCs is absent or minimal.

Table 1
Nodal peripheral T-cell lymphomas and their nomenclature in WHO-HAEM4R, WHO-HAEM5, and the 2022 International Consensus Classification

WHO-HAEM4R	WHO-HAEM5	2022 ICC
Anaplastic large cell lymphoma		
Anaplastic large cell lymphoma, ALK-positive	ALK-positive anaplastic large cell lymphoma	Anaplastic large cell lymphoma, ALK-positive
Anaplastic large cell lymphoma, ALK-negative	ALK-negative anaplastic large cell lymphoma	Anaplastic large cell lymphoma, ALK-negative
EBV-positive NK/T-cell lymphomas		
Included as a variant of peripheral T-cell lymphoma, NOS	EBV-positive nodal T- and NK-cell lymphoma	Primary nodal EBV-positive T/NK-cell lymphoma
Angioimmunoblastic T-cell lymphoma and other nodal lymphomas of T-follicular helper cell origin	**Nodal T-follicular helper (TFH) cell lymphoma**	**Follicular helper T-cell lymphoma**
Angioimmunoblastic T-cell lymphoma	Nodal TFH cell lymphoma, angioimmunoblastic-type	Follicular helper T-cell lymphoma, angioimmunoblastic type (angioimmunoblastic T-cell lymphoma)
Follicular T-cell lymphoma	Nodal TFH cell lymphoma, follicular-type	Follicular helper T-cell lymphoma, follicular-type
Nodal peripheral T-cell lymphoma with TFH phenotype	Nodal TFH cell lymphoma, NOS	Follicular helper T-cell lymphoma, NOS
Other peripheral T-cell lymphomas		
Peripheral T-cell lymphoma, NOS	Peripheral T-cell lymphoma, NOS	Peripheral T-cell lymphoma, NOS

Abbreviations: EBV, Epstein-Barr virus; NOS, not otherwise specified; WHO-HAEM4R, revised fourth edition of the World Health Organization Classification of Tumors of Hematopoietic and Lymphoid Tissues; WHO-HAEM5, fifth edition of the World Health Organization Classification of Hematolymphoid Tumors.

Nodal CD4+ THFLs that lack features of AITL and TFHL-F are designated TFHL-NOS. The nodal architecture is usually effaced by a proliferation of medium- to large-sized CD4+ lymphocytes expressing at least 2 TFH markers (Fig. 6). TFHL-NOS may express fewer TFH markers than AITL. Nevertheless, expression of TFH markers is not rare among nodal CD4+ PTCLs, and one study showed that 41% of previously diagnosed PTCL-NOS were reclassified into TFHL-NOS after reevaluation based on expression of more than or equal to 2 TFH markers.[41]

MOLECULAR FEATURES

The 3 subtypes of TFHL have overlapping mutational profiles and gene expression signatures. Frequently mutated genes include *RHOA*, *TET2*, *DNMT3A*, and *IDH2*. *RHOA*^{G17V} is seen in 50% to 70% of AITL and 50% to 60% of TFHL-F and TFHL-NOS.[42–44] RHOA^{G17V} lacks canonical GTP-binding capacity and specifically binds to VAV1, augmenting its adaptor function and accelerating T-cell receptor (TCR) signaling.[45] In mouse models, *RHOA*^{G17V} expression in CD4+ T cells led to TFH differentiation, increased proliferation associated with ICOS upregulation, and activation of PI3K and MAPK signaling.[46] Pathologically, *RHOA*^{G17V} is associated with accentuated AITL features such as FDC proliferation and expression of more TFH markers.[47,48]

TFHLs frequently harbor mutations in the epigenetic modifier genes *TET2*, *IDH2*, and *DNMT3A*.[44,49,50] These are also found in healthy, especially elderly, individuals with clonal hematopoiesis,[51] suggesting a possible multistep pathogenesis of TFHL.[52] These mutations are also found in PTCLs without TFH phenotype, but the frequency is higher in TFHLs. For example, loss-of-function *TET2* mutations are found in up to

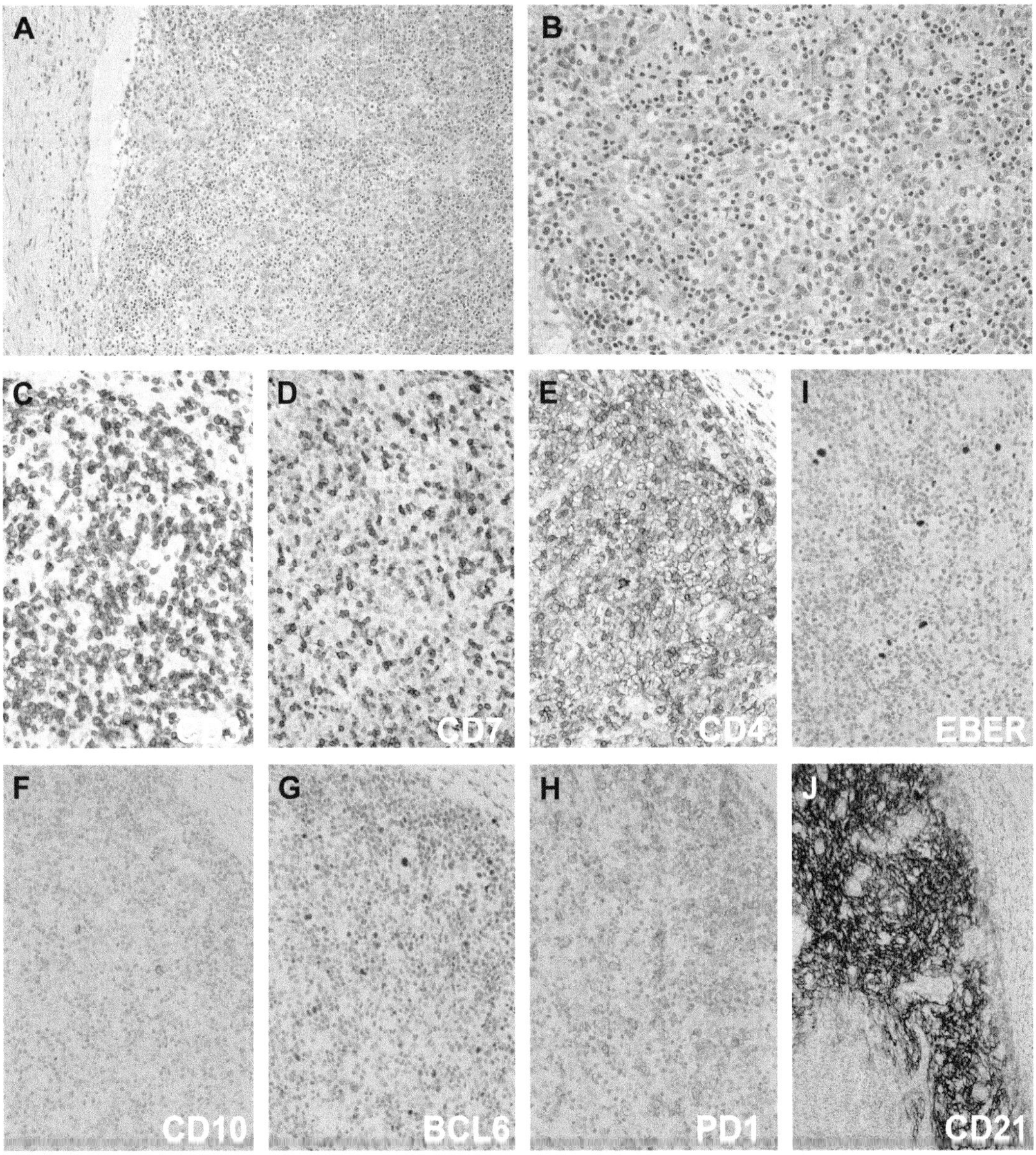

Fig. 4. Nodal TFHL, angioimmunoblastic-type (AITL). (*A, B*) The lymph node architecture is effaced by a polymorphous infiltrate of medium-sized cells with pale, clear cytoplasm, small lymphocytes, plasma cells, and immunoblasts. Vessels are prominent, and the subcapsular sinus is dilated (*A, left*). Neoplastic cells are positive for CD3 (*C*) but negative for CD7 (*D*). Tumor cells are positive for CD4 (*E*), focally positive for CD10 (*F*), and partially positive for BCL6 (*G*) and PD1 (*H*). Scattered B-immunoblasts are positive for EBER (*I*). Proliferation of follicular dendritic cells is highlighted by CD21 (*J*).

83% of AITL, 75% of TFHL-F, and 64% of TFHL-NOS.[42] Notably, occasional patients have both myeloid neoplasms and TFHL bearing the same epigenetic modifier gene mutations, for example, *TET2*, suggesting clonal hematopoiesis as the precursor to both malignancies.[53]

A chromosomal translocation, t(5;9) (q33;q22), resulting in *ITK::SYK*, is identified in approximately 40% of TFHL-F.[40,54] *ITK::SYK* is not entirely specific and is rarely seen in AITL.[55] Tyrosine kinase gene fusions, including *ITK::FER* and *RLTPR::FES*, have also been reported.[56]

DIFFERENTIAL DIAGNOSIS

Although the integration of PTCLs of TFH origin into a single entity with 3 subtypes is well justified by molecular data, the practical diagnosis and

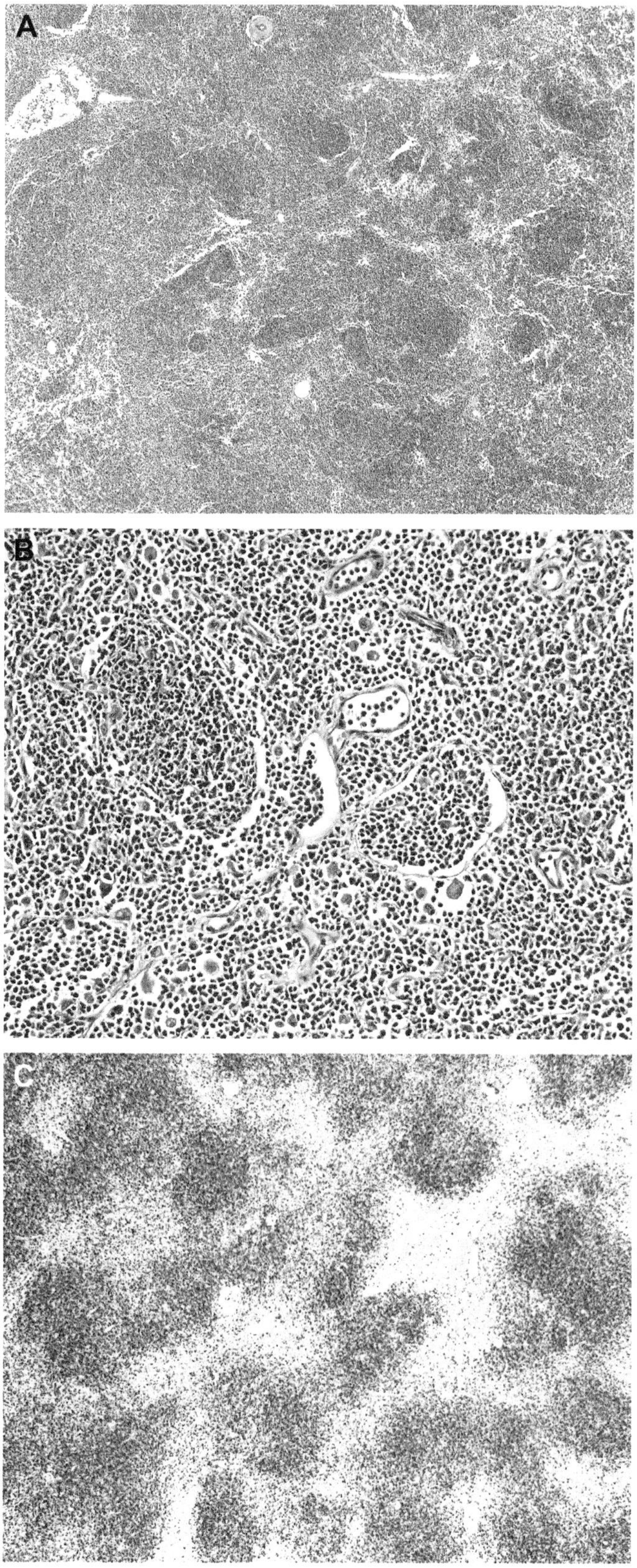

Fig. 5. Nodal TFHL, follicular-type (TFHL-F). (*A*) The lymph node architecture is effaced by an atypical follicular proliferation of small to medium-sized cells with irregular, hyperchromatic nuclei present in a mildly hypervascular background (*B*). The atypical follicles contain a predominance of T cells positive for CD5 (*C*) and CD4

Fig. 5. (*D*) with many fewer CD8-positive T cells (*D, inset*). The T-cell–rich follicles coexpress ICOS (*E*) and PD1 (*F*)

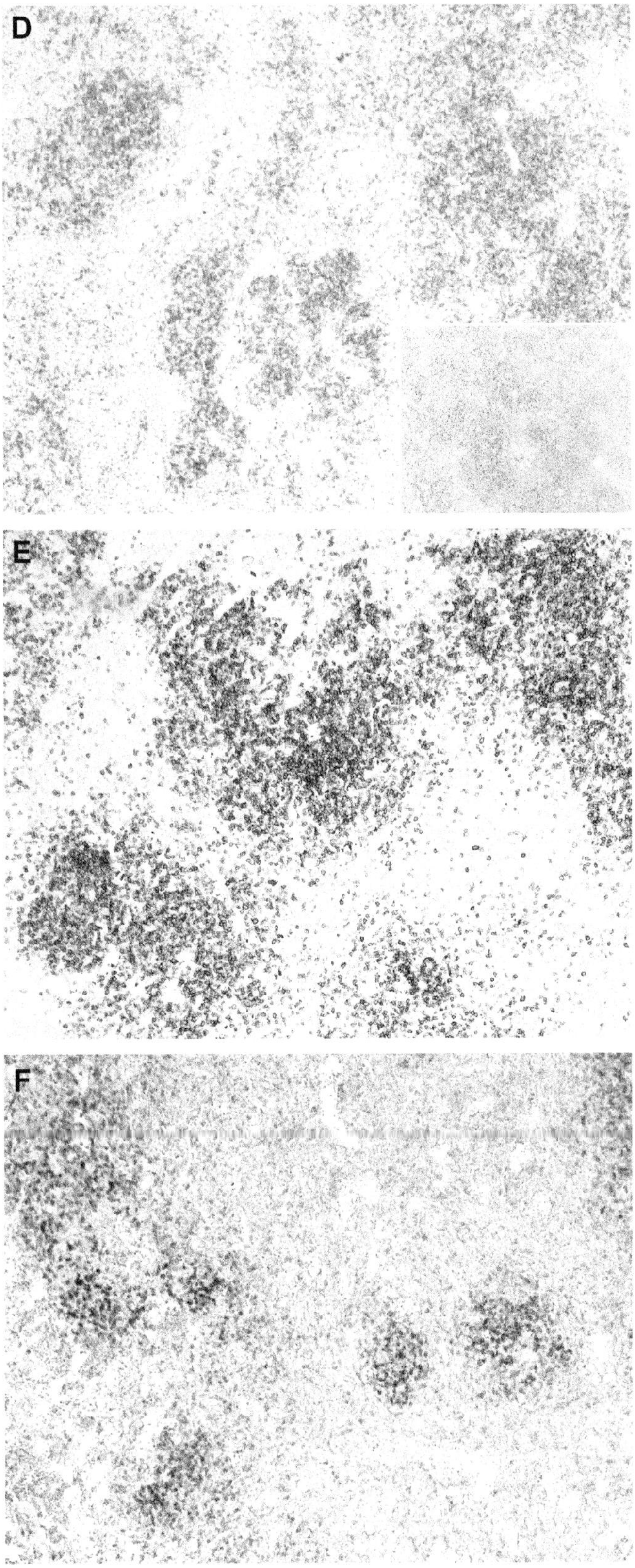

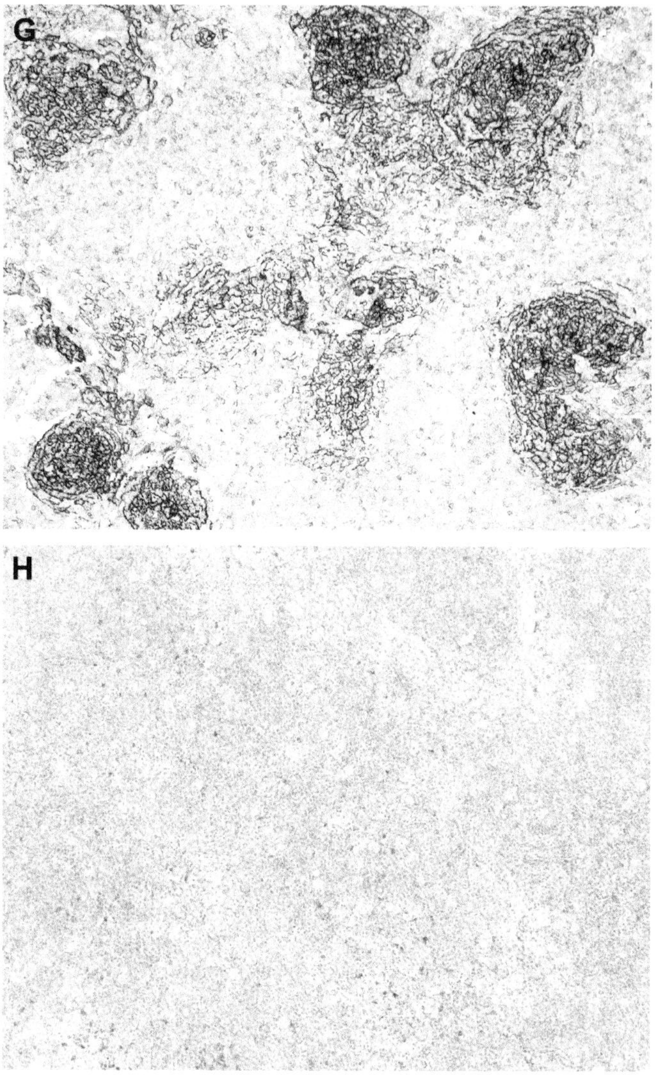

Fig. 5. and are encompassed by CD21-positive follicular dendritic cell meshworks (*G*). Follicles contain only rare CD20-positive small B cells (*H*). (Photos courtesy of Dr Aliyah Sohani, Boston, MA.)

subtyping of TFHLs is sometimes challenging. For instance, the extent of HEV and FDC proliferation and number of EBV-positive B-immunoblasts are variable and may be subjective, and there is potential interobserver discordance in distinction of AITL from TFHL-NOS. Distinction of TFHL from PTCL-NOS also remains challenging, particularly due to ambiguity in the definition of TFH phenotype by immunohistochemistry. AITL should be positive for CD4; otherwise, it is best classified as PTCL-NOS. Among TFH markers, including CD10, BCL6, CXCL13, ICOS, PD1, SAP1, and CXCR5, the sensitivity and specificity for TFHL vary considerably. CD10 and CXCL13 have high specificity but low sensitivity, whereas PD1 and ICOS have high sensitivity but low specificity.[41] Moreover, the extent and intensity of immunostaining are variable, and well-defined criteria for positivity have not been established. In one study, a significant impact on the number of cases classified as TFHL was observed comparing 4- and 5-marker panels and changing the minimum TFH marker positivity from 2 to 3.[41] Therefore, the proportions of TFHL and PTCL-NOS may vary depending on local practice patterns.

It is important to recognize that TFH markers may be positive in extranodal T-cell lymphomas and lymphoproliferative disorders (LPDs) but such cases should not be regarded as TFHL. For example, primary cutaneous small/medium CD4+ T-cell LPD often expresses PD1, ICOS, and, less frequently, CXCL13 and BCL6[57] but remains a distinct entity. In addition, reactive PD1+ T-cell populations may be expanded in B-cell lymphomas, particularly nodal marginal zone lymphoma.[58] These T cells lack cytologic atypia,

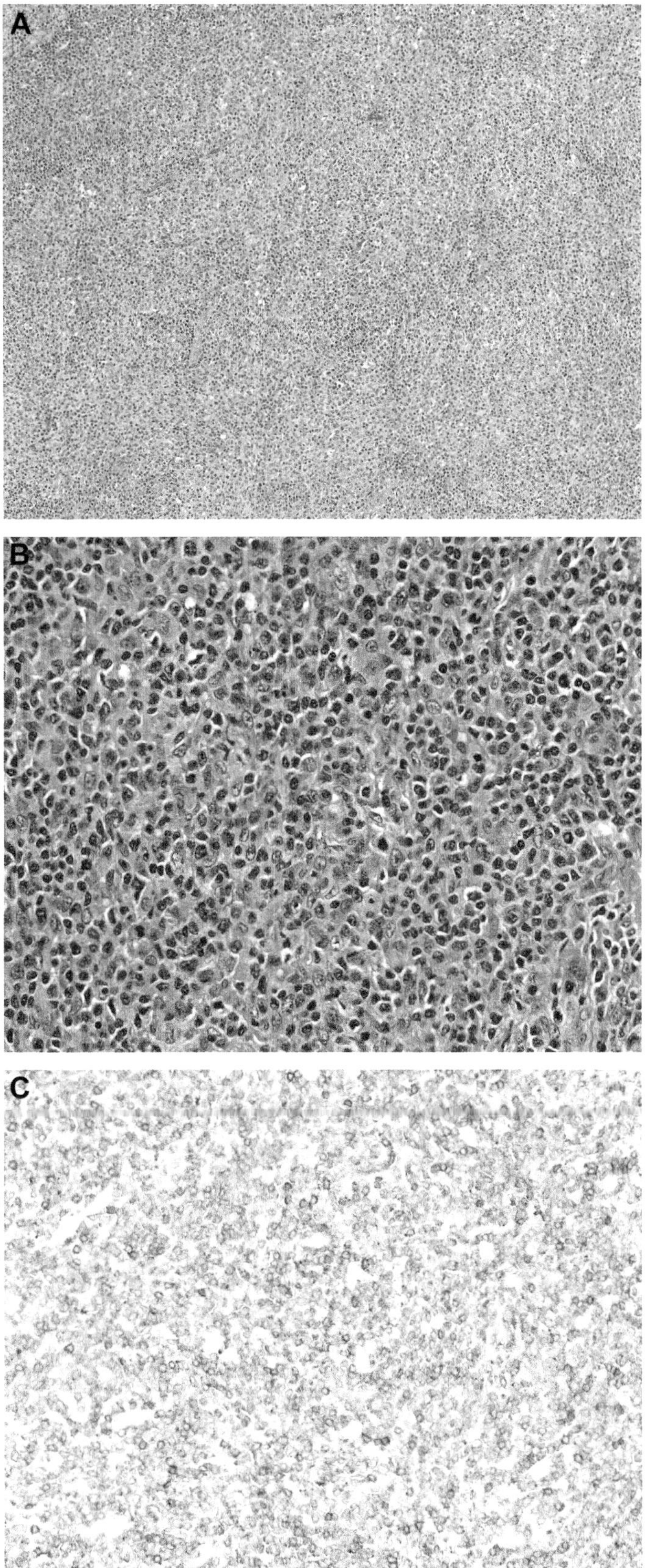

Fig. 6. Nodal TFHL, not otherwise specified (NOS). (*A*) The lymph node architecture is effaced by a diffuse proliferation of medium- to large-sized cells with irregular nuclei and vesicular chromatin; scattered eosinophils are present in the background (*B*). The atypical cells are diffusely positive for CD3 (*C*), CD4

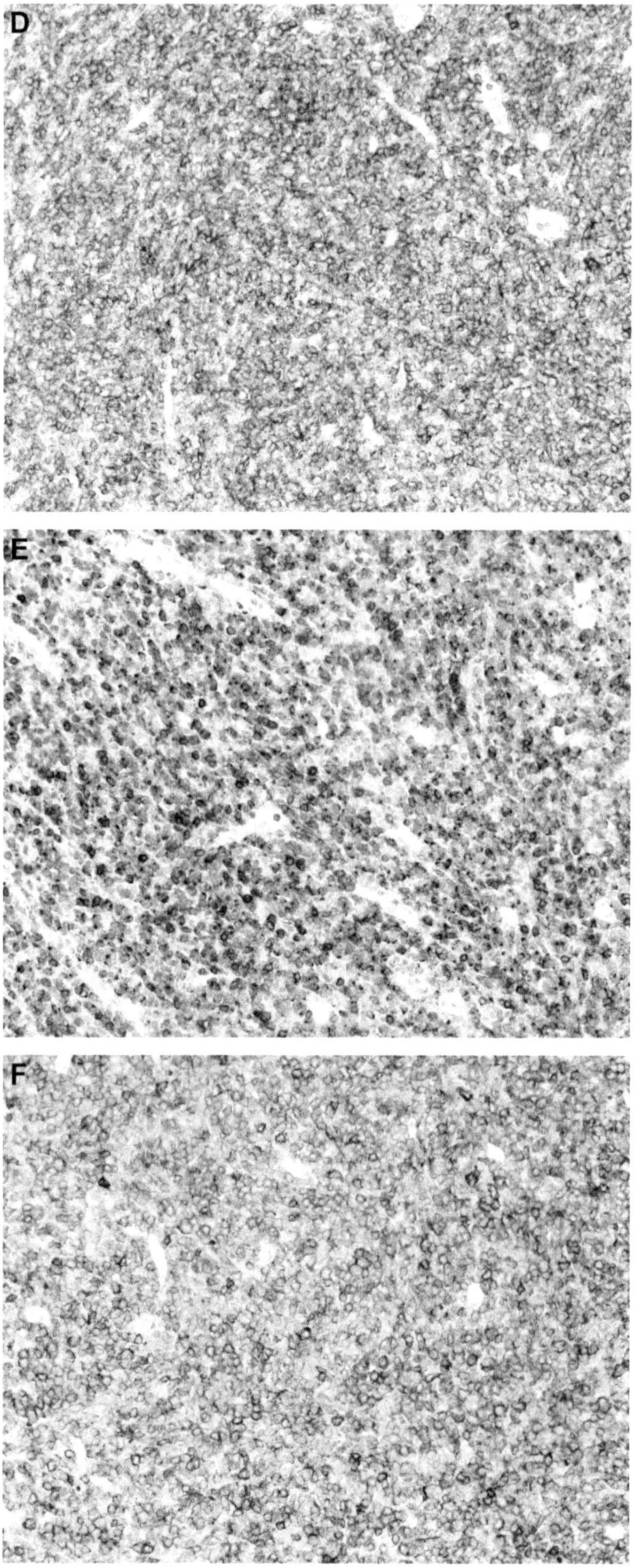

Fig. 6. (*D*) with coexpression of CD10 (*E*), ICOS (*F*), and BCL6 in a subset

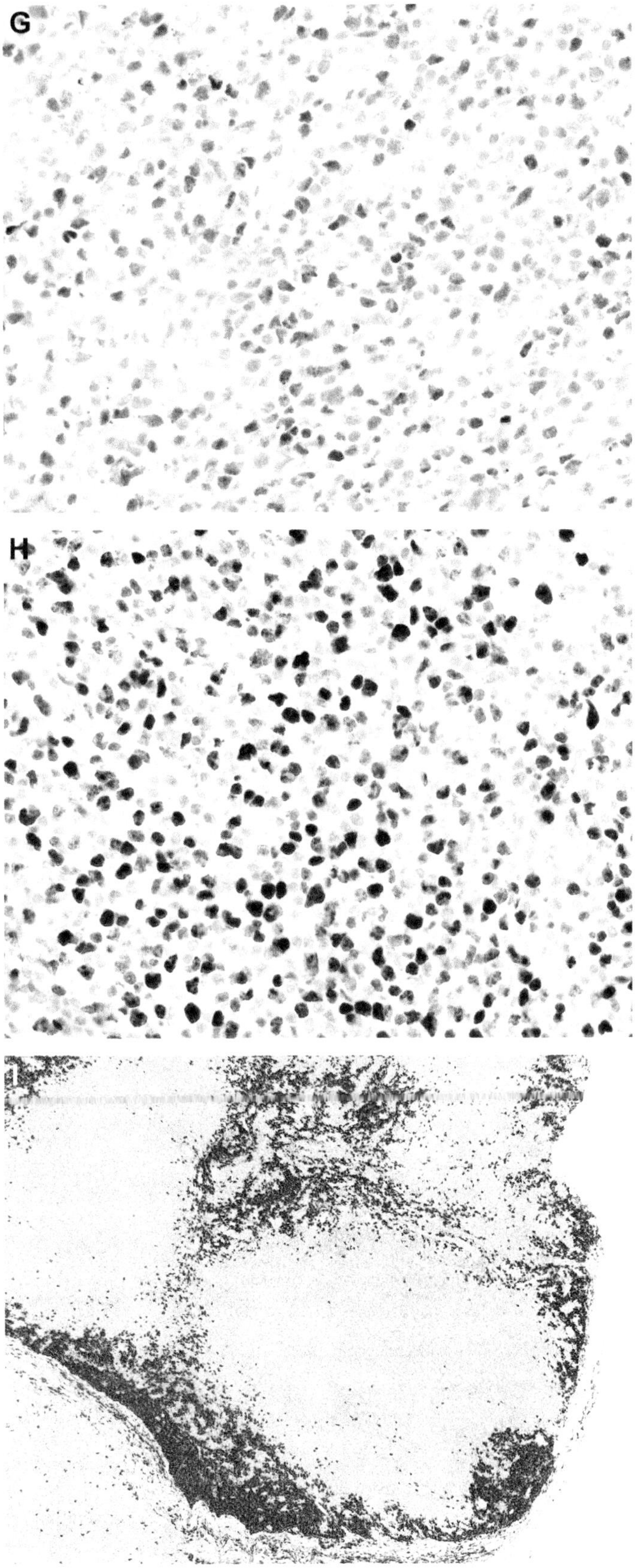

Fig. 6. (*G*). The Ki67 proliferation index is moderately elevated at 30% to 40% (*H*). A stain for CD20 highlights compressed B-cell follicles in the cortex (*I*). CD21-positive follicular dendritic cell meshworks are confined to B-cell follicles and do not extend into T-cell–rich areas

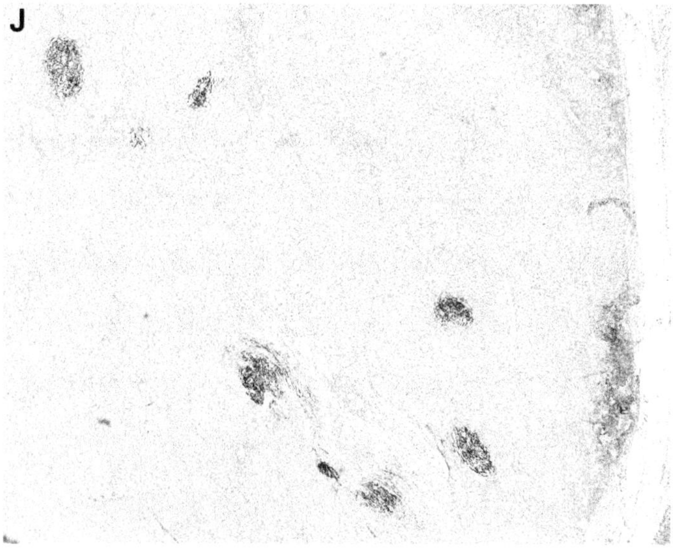

Fig. 6. (*J*). (Photos courtesy of Dr Aliyah Sohani, Boston, MA.)

phenotypic aberrancy, and clonal TCR gene rearrangements, supporting the diagnosis of B-cell lymphoma with reactive TFH expansion.

PROGNOSIS

The overall prognosis of patients with TFHL is poor. Three-year OS of AITL is approximately 50%.[59] Because of the low frequency and recent recognition of TFHL-F and TFHL-NOS, prognostic data are limited. One retrospective study showed that TFH phenotype predicted response to histone deacetylase inhibitors in relapsed/refractory PTCLs, suggesting the importance of correctly classifying TFHLs in routine pathologic diagnosis.[60]

CLINICS CARE POINTS

- Given the clinicopathologic and molecular overlap of PTCLs of TFH origin, a new entity of TFHL was established, which includes AITL, TFHL-F, and TFHL-NOS as pathological subtypes.
- A panel of TFH markers (eg, CD10, BCL6, PD1, CXCL13, and ICOS) is recommended in the classification of CD4+ PTCLs even when there are no histologic features of AITL or a TFHL-F.
- Genetic analysis for TFHL-related mutations, especially *RHOA*^{G17V}, may aid the differential diagnosis.

PRIMARY NODAL EPSTEIN-BARR VIRUS–POSITIVE T/NK-CELL LYMPHOMA

INTRODUCTION

Most EBV-positive T/NK-cell lymphomas arise in extranodal sites such as the upper aerodigestive tract and represent extranodal NK/T-cell lymphoma (ENKTL), nasal type. Primary nodal EBV-positive T/NK-cell lymphomas (EBV+ nTNKLs) are much rarer and were classified as a variant of PTCL-NOS in WHO-HAEM4R. However, there is growing evidence that EBV+ nTNKLs have clinicopathologic and immunophenotypic features distinct from both ENKTL and PTCL-NOS and are often associated with immunodeficiency. Most EBV+ nTNKLs have been reported from East Asia, similar to ENKTL. Patients typically present with lymphadenopathy with or without extranodal involvement but lacking nasal involvement, advanced-stage disease, and B symptoms.[61] The neoplastic cells originate more often from T cells rather than NK cells. Therefore, both 2022 ICC and WHO-HAEM5 define EBV+ nTNKL as a new distinct entity (see **Table 1**).[1,2]

MICROSCOPIC FEATURES

EBV+ nTNKL typically shows effacement of the lymph node architecture by a proliferation of medium- to large-sized lymphocytes (**Fig. 7**). Interfollicular infiltration of neoplastic cells also may be seen. Unlike ENKTL, angiocentric infiltration and necrosis are rare.[61] Neoplastic cells prototypically exhibit centroblastic morphology resembling diffuse large B-cell lymphoma.

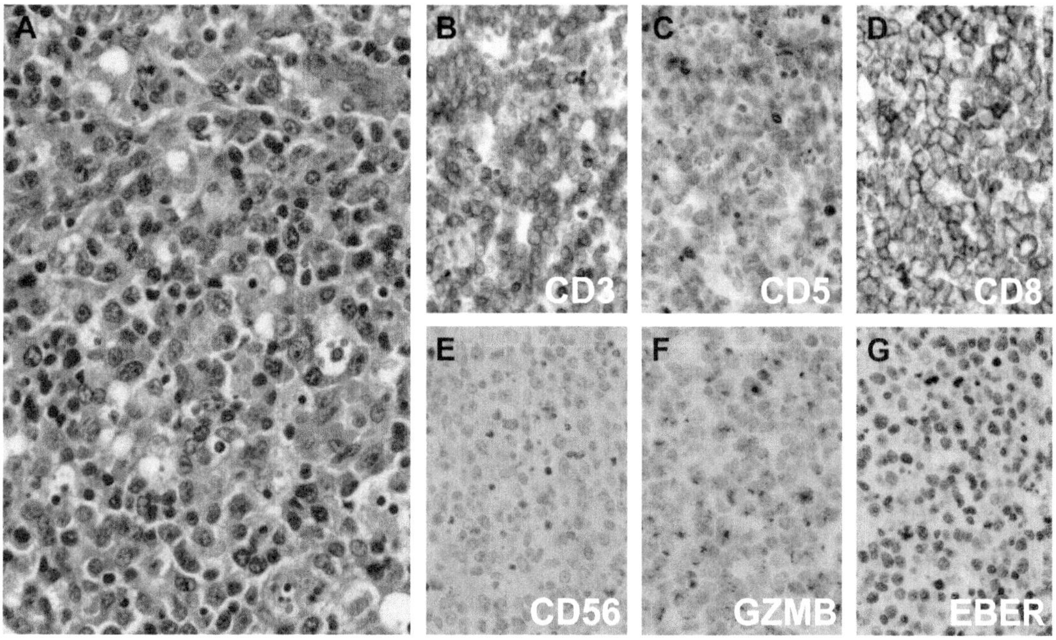

Fig. 7. EBV-positive nodal T/NK-cell lymphoma. (*A*) A diffuse proliferation of medium- to large-sized atypical lymphocytes is seen. The neoplastic cells express CD3 (*B*), CD5 (weak, *C*), and CD8 (*D*). CD56 is negative (*E*). Tumor cells are positive for granzyme B (*F*) and EBER (*G*, ISH).

Immunophenotypically, EBV+ nTNKL is positive for pan-T-cell markers and cytotoxic molecules, usually CD4−/CD8+ with frequent loss of CD5.[62] In situ hybridization for EBV-encoded small RNAs (EBER ISH) is positive by definition; they usually demonstrate a type 2 EBV latency pattern. EBV+ nTNKL is predominantly of T-cell origin based on TCR protein expression and/or clonal rearrangement of TCR genes. EBV+ nTNKL of NK-cell lineage, lacking TCR protein expression and clonal TCR gene rearrangements, accounts for less than 20% of cases.[62]

MOLECULAR FEATURES

EBV+ nTNKL has frequent mutations of *TET2* (64%), *PIK3CD* (33%), *DDX3X* (20%), and *STAT3* (19%), partially overlapping with ENKTL.[63] However, despite its highly aggressive behavior, EBV+ nTNKL demonstrates lower genomic instability than ENKTL or PTCL-NOS. Gene expression profiling has revealed upregulation of genes related to cytotoxic activation, JAK/STAT signaling, and immune-related pathways, including *CD274* encoding PD-L1, suggesting an immune-evasive phenotype of the neoplastic cells.[64]

DIFFERENTIAL DIAGNOSIS

Distinction from PTCL-NOS in lymph node specimens requires an index of suspicion and EBV studies. Among EBV+ lymphomas, EBV+ nTNKL must be distinguished from secondary nodal involvement by ENKTL based on clinical history and staging. A cytotoxic T-cell immunophenotype (CD4−/CD8+/CD56−) is more common in EBV+ nTNKL.[61] The differential diagnosis also includes chronic active EBV infection (CAEBV). Although occasional EBV+ nTNKLs arise in patients with history of CAEBV, suggesting an at least partially shared pathogenesis,[61] EBV+ nTNKL is primarily a nodal disease affecting the elderly, whereas CAEBV is a disease of childhood with frequent extranodal involvement.

PROGNOSIS

Patients with EBV+ nTNKL typically have advanced stage disease and poor outcomes compared with those with ENKTL or PTCL-NOS. Median OS is 2.5 to 8.9 months.[61,64]

CLINICS CARE POINTS

- EBV+ nTNKL is a new entity in the 2022 ICC and WHO-HAEM5 classifications and should be diagnosed with clinicopathologic correlation to exclude nodal involvement by ENKTL.
- EBER ISH should be performed when evaluating nodal PTCLs with a cytotoxic immunophenotype.

PERIPHERAL T-CELL LYMPHOMA, NOT OTHERWISE SPECIFIED

INTRODUCTION

PTCL-NOS is a heterogeneous category of nodal and extranodal mature T-cell lymphomas that cannot be assigned to a specific PTCL entity. Therefore, it is a diagnosis of exclusion. EBV+ nTNKL is now excluded from this category in both 2022 ICC and WHO-HAEM5.[1,2] In addition, WHO-HAEM5 newly recognizes primary cutaneous PTCL-NOS within the family of primary cutaneous T-cell lymphomas, distinct from the systemic/nodal form of PTCL-NOS discussed here.

MICROSCOPIC FEATURES

Nodal PTCL-NOS may show a paracortical pattern or diffuse architectural effacement. The neoplastic T cells have a wide spectrum of cytologic features. They are most often medium-sized lymphocytes exhibiting irregular nuclear contours; however, some cases contain predominantly small T cells. There are usually abundant background inflammatory cells including eosinophils, plasma cells, and small lymphocytes. Epithelioid histiocytes can be numerous, so-called Lennert lymphoma (lymphoepithelioid lymphoma). Occasional cases contain scattered HRS-like and/or EBV-positive B-immunoblasts, which are often CD30-positive.

The neoplastic T cells in PTCL-NOS exhibit a mature T-cell phenotype. Aberrant loss or diminished expression of one or more pan-T-cell markers (CD2, CD3, CD5, CD7, and TCR) is seen in up to 80% of cases.[65] PTCL-NOS predominantly shows a CD4+/CD8− immunophenotype,[65] and immunohistochemistry for TFH markers is recommended to exclude TFHL in these cases.[2] Cytotoxic molecules such as TIA1, granzyme B, and perforin are positive in a subset of PTCL-NOS; these cases are commonly CD8+ and sometimes CD56+. Nodal PTCLs with a cytotoxic phenotype require clinicopathological correlation and EBER ISH to exclude secondary nodal involvement by an extranodal PTCL, nodal involvement by ENKTL, and EBV+ nTNKL. Primary nodal EBV-negative cytotoxic PTCLs currently remain within the spectrum of PTCL-NOS but might be considered a distinct PTCL subtype in the future based on unique molecular features discussed later.

MOLECULAR FEATURES

Because PTCL-NOS is a diagnosis of exclusion, molecular alterations are heterogeneous. However, 2 distinct molecular subtypes have been recognized by gene expression profiling: PTCL-GATA3 and PTCL-TBX21.[66] PTCL-GATA3 shows a gene expression profile similar to Th2 cells, high expression of *GATA3* and its target genes, *CCR4*, *IL17RA*, *CXCR7*, and greater copy number alterations (CNAs).[66,67] PTCL-TBX21 shows high expression of *TBX21* and *EOMES* and their target genes, *CXCR3*, *IL2RB*, *CCL3*, and *IFNG*, and has fewer CNAs and more frequent mutations in genes associated with DNA methylation.[66–68] PTCL-TBX21 has a Th1-like gene expression profile, but some cytotoxic PTCL-NOS also cluster with this group. PTCL-GATA3 has poorer OS rates than PTCL-TBX21.[66] Classification of PTCL-GATA3 and PTCL-TBX21 using immunohistochemistry for GATA3, CCR4, TBX21, and CXCR3 has been proposed.[69]

The genomic landscape of PTCL-NOS is highly heterogeneous and complex. Recurrently mutated genes include those associated with TCR pathway (*PLCG1* and *CARD11*), JAK/STAT pathway (*JAK3*, *STAT3*, and *SOCS1*), cell cycle (*TP53*, *CDKN2A*, and *ATM*), and DNA methylation (*TET2* and *DNMT3A*).[67,70] *TP53* and *CDKN2A* mutations and/or deletions are associated with poorer outcomes.[67,70] PTCLs with *DNMT3A* mutations define a cytotoxic subset within PTCL-TBX21 with inferior survival.[68] Fusion genes involving *FER* and *VAV1* have been reported.[71]

DIFFERENTIAL DIAGNOSIS

PTCL-NOS is a diagnosis of exclusion, requiring comprehensive phenotyping and careful clinicopathologic correlation to rule out adult T-cell leukemia/lymphoma (ATLL), ALCL, TFHL, EBV+ nTNKL, and nodal involvement by extranodal PTCLs such as enteropathy-associated T-cell lymphoma and cutaneous PTCLs.

PROGNOSIS

PTCL-NOS is generally an aggressive lymphoma with poor response to therapy, frequent relapses, and short OS. PTCL-GATA3 subtype, expression of cytotoxic molecules, increased transformed cells, and *TP53* and/or *CDKN2A* alterations have been associated with inferior OS.[66,68,70]

CLINICS CARE POINTS

- PTCL-NOS is a diagnosis of exclusion; before designating as "NOS", exclude other PTCL subtypes including ATLL, ALCL, TFHL, EBV+ nTNKL, and nodal involvement by extranodal PTCLs.

- Molecular profiling has demonstrated phenotypically and prognostically distinct subgroups in PTCL-NOS: PTCL-TBX21 with a Th1-like signature and more favorable prognosis and PTCL-GATA3 with a Th2-like signature and poorer prognosis.
- Primary nodal EBV-negative cytotoxic PTCLs remain within the spectrum of PTCL-NOS but show distinct features including inferior survival and frequent *DNMT3A* mutations.

DISCLOSURE

A.L. Feldman receives research funding from Seattle Genetics and is an inventor of technology discussed in this article for which Mayo Clinic holds an unlicensed patent. N. Oishi has nothing to disclose.

REFERENCES

1. Alaggio R, Amador C, Anagnostopoulos I, et al. The 5th edition of the world health organization classification of haematolymphoid tumours: lymphoid neoplasms. Leukemia 2022;36(7):1720–48.
2. Campo E, Jaffe ES, Cook JR, et al. The international consensus classification of mature lymphoid neoplasms: a report from the clinical advisory Committee. Blood 2022;140(11):1229–53.
3. Xing X, Feldman AL. Anaplastic large cell lymphomas: ALK positive, ALK negative, and primary cutaneous. Adv Anat Pathol 2015;22(1):29–49.
4. Tsuyama N, Sakamoto K, Sakata S, et al. Anaplastic large cell lymphoma: pathology, genetics, and clinical aspects. J Clin Exp Hematop 2017;57(3):120–42.
5. King RL, Dao LN, McPhail ED, et al. Morphologic Features of ALK-negative Anaplastic Large Cell Lymphomas With DUSP22 Rearrangements. Am J Surg Pathol 2016;40(1):36–43.
6. Feldman AL, Oishi N, Ketterling RP, et al. Immunohistochemical Approach to Genetic Subtyping of Anaplastic Large Cell Lymphoma. Am J Surg Pathol 2022;1–10.
7. Ravindran A, Feldman AL, Ketterling RP, et al. Striking association of lymphoid enhancing factor (LEF1) overexpression and DUSP22 rearrangements in anaplastic large cell lymphoma. Am J Surg Pathol 2021;45(4):550–7.
8. Parilla Castellar ER, Jaffe ES, Said JW, et al. ALK-negative anaplastic large cell lymphoma is a genetically heterogeneous disease with widely disparate clinical outcomes. Blood 2014;124(9):1473–80.
9. Chiarle R, Voena C, Ambrogio C, et al. The anaplastic lymphoma kinase in the pathogenesis of cancer. Nat Rev Cancer 2008;8(1):11–23.
10. Larose Hugo, Prokoph Nina, Matthews Jamie D, et al. Whole Exome Sequencing reveals NOTCH1 mutations in anaplastic large cell lymphoma and points to Notch both as a key pathway and a potential therapeutic target. Haematologica 2020;106(6):1693–704.
11. Feldman AL, Dogan A, Smith DI, et al. Discovery of recurrent t(6;7)(p25.3;q32.3) translocations in ALK-negative anaplastic large cell lymphomas by massively parallel genomic sequencing. Blood 2011;117(3):915–9.
12. Oishi N, Brody GS, Ketterling RP, et al. Genetic subtyping of breast implant–associated anaplastic large cell lymphoma. Blood 2018;132(5):544–7.
13. Karai LJ, Kadin ME, Hsi ED, et al. Chromosomal rearrangements of 6p25.3 define a new subtype of lymphomatoid papulosis. Am J Surg Pathol 2013;37(8):1173–81.
14. Wada DA, Law ME, Hsi ED, et al. Specificity of IRF4 translocations for primary cutaneous anaplastic large cell lymphoma: a multicenter study of 204 skin biopsies. Mod Pathol 2011;24(4):596–605.
15. Onaindia A, Montes-Moreno S, Rodríguez-Pinilla SM, et al. Primary cutaneous anaplastic large cell lymphomas with 6p25.3 rearrangement exhibit particular histological features. Histopathology 2015;66(6):846–55.
16. Luchtel RA, Dasari S, Oishi N, et al. Molecular profiling reveals immunogenic cues in anaplastic large cell lymphomas with DUSP22 rearrangements. Blood 2018;132(13):1386–98.
17. Luchtel RA, Zimmermann MT, Hu G, et al. Recurrent MSCE116K mutations in ALK-negative anaplastic large cell lymphoma. Blood 2019;133(26):2776–89.
18. Onaindia A, de Villambrosía SG, Prieto-Torres L, et al. DUSP22 -rearranged anaplastic lymphomas are characterized by specific morphological features and a lack of cytotoxic and JAK/STAT surrogate markers. Haematologica 2019;104(4):e158–62.
19. Vasmatzis G, Johnson SH, Knudson RA, et al. Genome-wide analysis reveals recurrent structural abnormalities of TP63 and other p53-related genes in peripheral T-cell lymphomas. Blood 2012;120(11):2280–9.
20. Chavan RN, Bridges AG, Knudson RA, et al. Somatic rearrangement of the TP63 gene preceding development of mycosis fungoides with aggressive clinical course. Blood Cancer J 2014;4(10):e253.
21. Karube K, Feldman AL. "Double-hit" of DUSP22 and TP63 rearrangements in anaplastic large cell lymphoma, ALK-negative. Blood 2020;135(9):700.
22. Crescenzo R, Abate F, Lasorsa E, et al. Convergent mutations and kinase fusions lead to oncogenic STAT3 activation in anaplastic large cell lymphoma. Cancer Cell 2015;27(4):516–32.
23. Fitzpatrick MJ, Massoth LR, Marcus C, et al. JAK2 Rearrangements Are a Recurrent Alteration in CD30+ Systemic T-Cell Lymphomas With Anaplastic Morphology. Am J Surg Pathol 2021;45(7):895–904.

24. Shen J, Li S, Medeiros LJ, et al. PD-L1 expression is associated with ALK positivity and STAT3 activation, but not outcome in patients with systemic anaplastic large cell lymphoma. Mod Pathol 2019;1. https://doi.org/10.1038/s41379-019-0336-3.
25. Atsaves V, Tsesmetzis N, Chioureas D, et al. PD-L1 is commonly expressed and transcriptionally regulated by STAT3 and MYC in ALK-negative anaplastic large-cell lymphoma. Leukemia 2017;31(7):1633–7.
26. Drilon A, Jenkins C, Iyer S, et al. ROS1-dependent cancers — biology, diagnostics and therapeutics. Nat Rev Clin Oncol 2021;18(1):35–55.
27. Xing X, Flotte TJ, Law ME, et al. Expression of the Chemokine Receptor Gene, CCR8, is Associated With DUSP22 Rearrangements in Anaplastic Large Cell Lymphoma. Appl Immunohistochem Mol Morphol 2015;23(8):580–9.
28. Wang X, Boddicker RL, Dasari S, et al. Expression of p63 protein in anaplastic large cell lymphoma: implications for genetic subtyping. Hum Pathol 2017;64:19–27.
29. Valera A, Colomo L, Martínez A, et al. ALK-positive large B-cell lymphomas express a terminal B-cell differentiation program and activated STAT3 but lack MYC rearrangements. Mod Pathol 2013;26(10):1329–37.
30. Kemps PG, Picarsic J, Durham BH, et al. ALK-positive histiocytosis: a new clinicopathologic spectrum highlighting neurologic involvement and responses to ALK inhibition. Blood 2022;139(2):256–80.
31. Nguyen TT, Kreisel FH, Frater JL, et al. Anaplastic large-cell lymphoma with aberrant expression of multiple cytokeratins masquerading as metastatic carcinoma of unknown primary. J Clin Oncol 2013;31(33):e443–5.
32. Feldman AL, Law ME, Inwards DJ, et al. PAX5-positive T-cell anaplastic large cell lymphomas associated with extra copies of the PAX5 gene locus. Mod Pathol 2010;23(4):593–602.
33. Bovio IM, Allan RW. The expression of myeloid antigens CD13 and/or CD33 is a marker of ALK+ anaplastic large cell lymphomas. Am J Clin Pathol 2008;130(4):628–34.
34. Oishi N, Hundal T, Phillips JL, et al. Molecular profiling reveals a hypoxia signature in breast implant-associated anaplastic large cell lymphoma. Haematologica 2021;106(6):1714–24.
35. Oishi N, Feldman AL. CA9 expression in breast implant-associated anaplastic large cell lymphoma presenting in a lymph node. Histopathology 2022;81(2):270–2.
36. Pedersen MB, Hamilton-Dutoit SJ, Bendix K, et al. DUSP22 and TP63 rearrangements predict outcome of ALK-negative anaplastic large cell lymphoma: a Danish cohort study. Blood 2017;130(4):554–7.
37. Hapgood G, Ben-Neriah S, Mottok A, et al. Identification of high-risk DUSP22-rearranged ALK-negative anaplastic large cell lymphoma. Br J Haematol 2019;186(3):e28–31.
38. de Leval L, Rickman DS, Thielen C, et al. The gene expression profile of nodal peripheral T-cell lymphoma demonstrates a molecular link between angioimmunoblastic T-cell lymphoma (AITL) and follicular helper T (TFH) cells. Blood 2007;109(11):4952–63.
39. Ohgami RS, Zhao S, Ohgami JK, et al. TdT+ T-lymphoblastic populations are increased in castleman disease, in castleman disease in association with follicular dendritic cell tumors, and in angioimmunoblastic T-cell lymphoma. Am J Surg Pathol 2012;36(11):1619–28.
40. Huang Y, Moreau A, Dupuis J, et al. Peripheral T-cell lymphomas with a follicular growth pattern are derived from follicular helper T cells (TFH) and may show overlapping features with angioimmunoblastic T-cell lymphomas. Am J Surg Pathol 2009;33(5):682–90.
41. Basha BM, Bryant SC, Rech KL, et al. Application of a 5 marker panel to the routine diagnosis of peripheral T-cell lymphoma with T-follicular helper phenotype. Am J Surg Pathol 2019;43(9):1282–90.
42. Dobay MP, Lemonnier F, Missiaglia E, et al. Integrative clinicopathological and molecular analyses of angioimmunoblastic T-cell lymphoma and other nodal lymphomas of follicular helper T-cell origin. Haematologica 2017;102(4):e148–51.
43. Miyoshi H, Sakata-Yanagimoto M, Shimono J, et al. RHOA mutation in follicular T-cell lymphoma: clinicopathological analysis of 16 cases. Pathol Int 2020;70(9):12981.
44. Sakata-Yanagimoto M, Enami T, Yoshida K, et al. Somatic RHOA mutation in angioimmunoblastic T cell lymphoma. Nat Genet 2014;46(2):171–5.
45. Fujisawa M, Sakata-Yanagimoto M, Nishizawa S, et al. Activation of RHOA–VAV1 signaling in angioimmunoblastic T-cell lymphoma. Leukemia 2018;32(3):694–702.
46. Cortes JR, Ambesi-Impiombato A, Couronné L, et al. RHOA G17V induces T follicular helper cell specification and promotes lymphomagenesis. Cancer Cell 2018;33(2):259–73.e7.
47. Nagao R, Kikuti YY, Carreras J, et al. Clinicopathologic analysis of angioimmunoblastic T-cell lymphoma with or without RHOA G17V mutation Using formalin-fixed paraffin-embedded sections. Am J Surg Pathol 2016;40(8):1041–50.
48. Ondrejka SL, Grzywacz B, Bodo J, et al. Angioimmunoblastic T-cell lymphomas With the RHOA p.Gly17Val mutation have classic clinical and pathologic features. Am J Surg Pathol 2016;40(3):335–41.
49. Palomero T, Couronné L, Khiabanian H, et al. Recurrent mutations in epigenetic regulators, RHOA and

FYN kinase in peripheral T cell lymphomas. Nat Genet 2014;46(2):166–70.
50. Scourzic L, Couronné L, Pedersen MT, et al. DNMT3AR882H mutant and Tet2 inactivation cooperate in the deregulation of DNA methylation control to induce lymphoid malignancies in mice. Leukemia 2016;30(6):1388–98.
51. Chiba S. Dysregulation of TET2 in hematologic malignancies. Int J Hematol 2017;105(1):17–22.
52. Sakata-Yanagimoto M. Multistep tumorigenesis in peripheral T cell lymphoma. Int J Hematol 2015; 102(5):523–7.
53. Tiacci E, Venanzi A, Ascani S, et al. High-risk clonal hematopoiesis as the origin of AITL and NPM1 -mutated AML. N Engl J Med 2018;379(10):981–4.
54. Streubel B, Vinatzer U, Willheim M, et al. Novel t(5;9)(q33;q22) fuses ITK to SYK in unspecified peripheral T-cell lymphoma. Leukemia 2006;20(2): 313–8.
55. Attygalle AD, Feldman AL, Dogan A. ITK/SYK translocation in angioimmunoblastic T-cell lymphoma. Am J Surg Pathol 2013;37(9):1456–7.
56. Debackere K, van der Krogt J-A, Tousseyn T, et al. FER and FES tyrosine kinase fusions in follicular T-cell lymphoma. Blood 2020;135(8):584–8.
57. Wang L, Rocas D, Dalle S, et al. Primary cutaneous peripheral T-cell lymphomas with a T-follicular helper phenotype: an integrative clinical, pathological and molecular case series study. Br J Dermatol 2022. https://doi.org/10.1111/bjd.21791.
58. Egan C, Laurent C, Alejo JC, et al. Expansion of PD1-positive T cells in nodal marginal zone lymphoma. Am J Surg Pathol 2020;44(5):657–64.
59. Tokunaga T, Shimada K, Yamamoto K, et al. Retrospective analysis of prognostic factors for angioimmunoblastic T-cell lymphoma: a multicenter cooperative study in Japan. Blood 2012;119(12): 2837–43.
60. Ghione P, Faruque P, Mehta-Shah N, et al. T follicular helper phenotype predicts response to histone deacetylase inhibitors in relapsed/refractory peripheral T-cell lymphoma. Blood Adv 2020;4(19):4640–7.
61. Kato S, Yamashita D, Nakamura S. Nodal EBV+ cytotoxic T-cell lymphoma: a literature review based on the 2017 WHO classification. J Clin Exp Hematop 2020;60(2):30–6.
62. Kato S, Asano N, Miyata-Takata T, et al. T-cell receptor (TCR) phenotype of nodal Epstein-Barr virus (EBV)-positive cytotoxic T-cell lymphoma (CTL): a clinicopathologic study of 39 cases. Am J Surg Pathol 2015;39(4):462–71.
63. Wai CMM, Chen S, Phyu T, et al. Immune pathway upregulation and lower genomic instability distinguish EBV-positive nodal T/NK-cell lymphoma from ENKTL and PTCL-NOS. Haematologica 2022. https://doi.org/10.3324/haematol.2021.280003.
64. Ng S-B, Chung T-H, Kato S, et al. Epstein-Barr virus-associated primary nodal T/NK-cell lymphoma shows a distinct molecular signature and copy number changes. Haematologica 2018;103(2):278–87.
65. Went P, Agostinelli C, Gallamini A, et al. Marker expression in peripheral T-cell lymphoma: a proposed clinical-pathologic prognostic score. J Clin Oncol 2006;24(16):2472–9.
66. Iqbal J, Wright G, Wang C, et al. Gene expression signatures delineate biologic and prognostic subgroups in peripheral T-cell lymphoma. Blood 2014; 123(19):2915–24.
67. Heavican TB, Bouska A, Yu J, et al. Genetic drivers of oncogenic pathways in molecular subgroups of peripheral T-cell lymphoma. Blood 2019;133(15):1664–76.
68. Herek TA, Bouska A, Lone WG, et al. DNMT3A mutations define a unique biological and prognostic subgroup associated with cytotoxic T-cells in PTCL-NOS. Blood 2022. https://doi.org/10.1182/blood.2021015019.
69. Amador C, Greiner TC, Heavican TB, et al. Reproducing the molecular subclassification of peripheral T-cell lymphoma-NOS by immunohistochemistry. Blood 2019;134(24):2159–70.
70. Watatani Y, Sato Y, Miyoshi H, et al. Molecular heterogeneity in peripheral T-cell lymphoma, not otherwise specified revealed by comprehensive genetic profiling. Leukemia 2019;33(12):2867–83.
71. Boddicker RL, Razidlo GL, Dasari S, et al. Integrated mate-pair and RNA sequencing identifies novel, targetable gene fusions in peripheral T-cell lymphoma. Blood 2016;128(9):1234–45.

Hodgkin Lymphoma and Its Differential Diagnosis

New Twists on an Old Challenge

Aliyah R. Sohani, MD

KEYWORDS

- Classic Hodgkin lymphoma • Differential diagnosis • EBV-positive mucocutaneous ulcer
- Infectious mononucleosis • Nodular lymphocyte-predominant Hodgkin lymphoma
- Mediastinal gray-zone lymphoma • Primary mediastinal large B-cell lymphoma
- Nodal T-follicular helper cell lymphoma

Key points

- The differential diagnosis of classic Hodgkin lymphoma (CHL) includes the reactive Epstein-Barr virus (EBV)-driven entities of acute infectious mononucleosis and EBV-positive mucocutaneous ulcer.
- Primary mediastinal large B-cell lymphoma and mediastinal gray-zone lymphoma are related neoplastic entities that should be considered in the differential diagnosis of CHL with predominantly mediastinal involvement; they differ from CHL and from one another in terms of their morphology, immunophenotype, and prognosis.
- Nodular lymphocyte-predominant Hodgkin lymphoma (NLPHL) is an uncommon mature B-cell neoplasm that is classified historically in the category of Hodgkin lymphomas; it has varying immunoarchitectural patterns that relate to prognosis and background non-neoplastic T cells exhibit a characteristic immunophenotype but may show cytologic atypia in some cases.
- Progressive transformation of germinal centers (PTGC) is a pattern of reactive lymphoid hyperplasia that may exist with admixed reactive follicles, and that may precede, follow, or co-exist with NLPHL; cases of florid PTGC may be difficult to distinguish from NLPHL.
- Neoplastic entities in the differential diagnosis of NLPHL include T-cell/histiocyte-rich large B-cell lymphoma and nodal T-follicular helper cell lymphoma with large B cells; the vast differences in prognostic and therapeutic implications among these diagnoses necessitate careful morphologic evaluation, clinical correlation, and consideration of ancillary molecular genetic testing.

ABSTRACT

Hodgkin lymphoma is a B-cell neoplasm that typically presents with localized, nodal disease. Tissues are characterized by few large neoplastic cells, usually comprising less than 10% of tissue cellularity, present in a background of abundant nonneoplastic inflammatory cells. This inflammatory microenvironment, although key to the pathogenesis, can make diagnosis a challenge because reactive conditions, lymphoproliferative diseases, and other lymphoid neoplasms may mimic Hodgkin lymphoma and vice versa. This review provides an overview of the classification of Hodgkin lymphoma, its differential diagnosis, including emerging and recently recognized entities, and strategies to resolve challenging dilemmas and avoid diagnostic pitfalls.

OVERVIEW

The initial description of Hodgkin lymphoma, arguably one of the most well-known eponymous

Department of Pathology, Massachusetts General Hospital, Harvard Medical School, 55 Fruit Street, WRN 219, Boston, MA 02114, USA
E-mail address: arsohani@mgh.harvard.edu

Surgical Pathology 16 (2023) 287–346
https://doi.org/10.1016/j.path.2023.02.002

disease terms used in pathology and medicine today, is attributed to Dr Thomas Hodgkin, who, as the Morbid Anatomist and Museum Curator of Guy's Hospital, London, described a peculiar set of findings of lymphadenopathy and splenomegaly in a series of 7 autopsies in a paper presented to the Medical and Surgical Society of London in 1832.[1] The term "Hodgkin's disease" was coined 1 year before Hodgkin's death by Dr Samuel Wilks, another British pathologist, who independently published a series of postmortem cases in 1865 and realizing them to represent the same syndrome, credited his predecessor with the discovery.[1] During Hodgkin's time, the microscope was rarely used in autopsy pathology; instead, findings were documented by gross descriptions, and specimens were preserved and cataloged. Although Samuel Wilks was one of the first to use the microscope to study Hodgkin disease and noted the characteristic giant cells present in involved lymph nodes and spleens, it was several years later that Drs Carl Sternberg (1898) and Dorothy Reed (1902) provided more detailed descriptions of these neoplastic cells, which eventually came to bear their names.[1] In 1927, histologic examination of Hodgkin's original cases was finally undertaken on formalin-fixed tissues that he had cataloged and preserved in the Guy's Hospital and Museum nearly a century before. The microscopic findings were enlightening but perhaps not so surprising: of Hodgkin's original 7 cases, only 3 cases actually resembled Hodgkin lymphoma, 2 of which could be confirmed by immunophenotyping.[1] The others were examples of non-Hodgkin lymphoma or forms of chronic infection, namely syphilis or tuberculosis.

Ironically, nearly 200 years after the original description of Hodgkin lymphoma, despite current histologic, immunophenotypic, and molecular diagnostic techniques, the same differential diagnosis of infection, non-Hodgkin lymphoma, or another unusual lymphoproliferative process are frequently encountered when evaluating a diagnostically challenging case. The focus of this review is to provide a broad overview of the classification of Hodgkin lymphoma, its differential diagnosis, including emerging and recently recognized diagnostic entities, and strategies to help resolve challenging dilemmas and avoid diagnostic pitfalls.

Hodgkin lymphoma is a B-cell neoplasm with distinct features that merit separate classification from other B-cell lymphomas. It typically presents with nodal involvement and localized disease, and most commonly affects younger individuals, including children, adolescents, and young adults. Tissues are characterized by rare to few large neoplastic cells, usually comprising less than 10% of the tissue cellularity, that are present in a background of abundant nonneoplastic inflammatory cells.[2] It is now well established that this inflammatory microenvironment is key to the pathogenesis of Hodgkin lymphoma, which perhaps more than any other neoplasm usurps the host's immune response in ensuring tumor cell survival. T cells hold the starring role in this process and can often be found in close proximity to the large, neoplastic cells.

Since 2004, the World Health Organization (WHO) Classification of Tumours of Haematopoietic and Lymphoid Tissues has divided Hodgkin lymphoma into 2 categories: classic Hodgkin lymphoma (CHL) comprises 90% of cases and is divided into 4 subtypes (nodular sclerosis, mixed cellularity, lymphocytic rich, and lymphocyte depleted), whereas nodular lymphocyte-predominant Hodgkin lymphoma (NLPHL) represents about 10% of cases.[2] Although the proposed International Consensus Classification published in 2022 reclassifies NLPHL as a B-cell non-Hodgkin lymphoma, the current 5th edition of the WHO Classification of Haematolymphoid Tumours maintains NLPHL in the broad category of Hodgkin lymphoma, and this review will follow that historical precedent for ease of discussion.[3,4] NLPHL, CHL, and its various subtypes differ in terms of clinical characteristics, morphology, immunophenotype, cellular background, and frequency of EBV infection; these features form the basis of their distinction from one another.[2]

CLASSIC HODGKIN LYMPHOMA AND ITS DIFFERENTIAL DIAGNOSIS

The typical low-power histology of nodular sclerosis CHL is characterized by the presence of a thickened, sclerotic capsule and thick fibrous bands emanating from the capsule in a trabecular distribution that completely or partially surround nodules of inflammatory cells (Fig. 1A). The cellularity comprises small lymphocytes, occasional histiocytes and plasma cells, a conspicuous population of granulocytes, including eosinophils, and scattered neoplastic Reed-Sternberg cells, the classic form of which is binucleate with prominent eosinophilic nucleoli (Fig. 1B–D). There are usually many mononuclear variants with similar features, characterized by large nuclei with prominent nucleoli approaching the size of a small lymphocyte, para-nucleolar chromatin clearing, nuclear membrane irregularities, and moderate cytoplasm. Mononuclear and binucleate forms

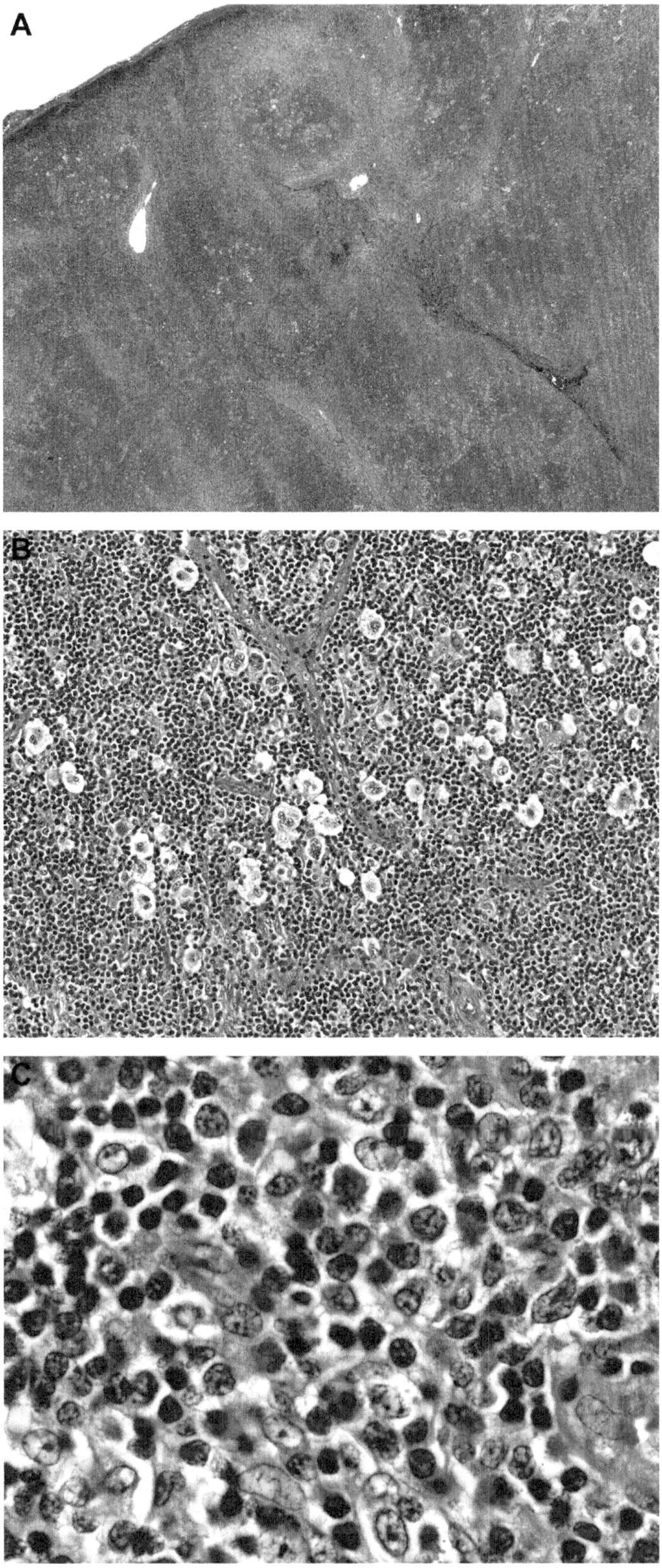

Fig. 1. CHL. (*A*) Low magnification demonstrates nodal architectural effacement by fibrous bands encircling cellular nodules (H&E, 20x). (*B*) Numerous Hodgkin/Reed-Sternberg cells are present in lacunar spaces in a background of small lymphocytes and scattered eosinophils (H&E, 200x). (*C*) Mononuclear Reed-Sternberg cell variants (Hodgkin cells) with prominent nucleoli and vesicular chromatin in a background of numerous eosinophils (H&E, 400x).

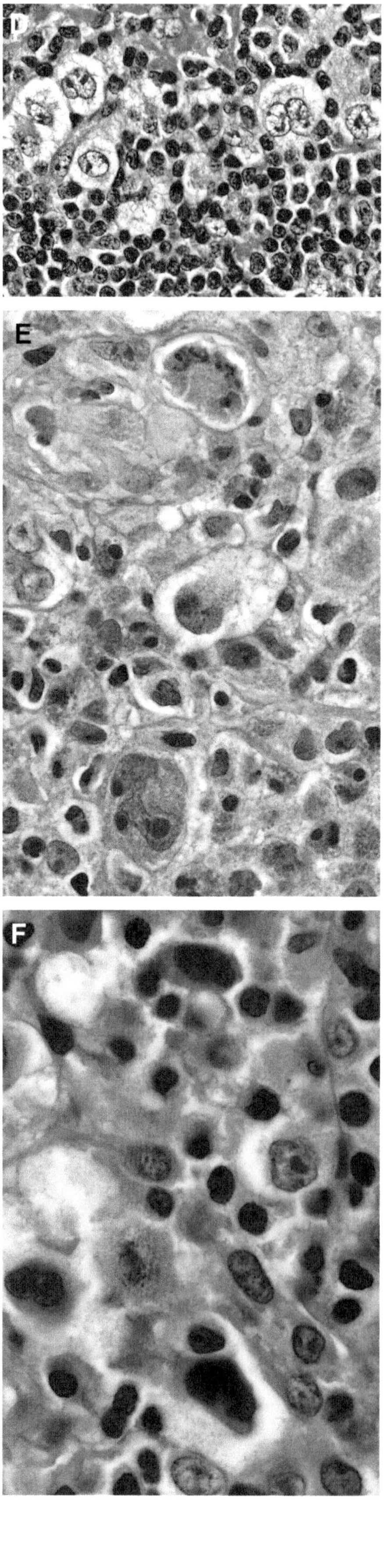

Fig. 1. (*D*) Classic binucleate Reed-Sternberg cells with prominent eosinophilic nucleoli, paranuclear chromatin clearing, and irregular nuclear membranes. (*E, F*) Reed-Sternberg cell variants include multinucleated forms (*E*, *bottom*), wreath cells (*E*, *top*), and mummified cells (*F*, *top* and *bottom*).

Fig. 1. (*G*), CD15 in membranous and Golgi pattern (*H*), and PAX5, which is weak in comparison to small B cells (*I*).

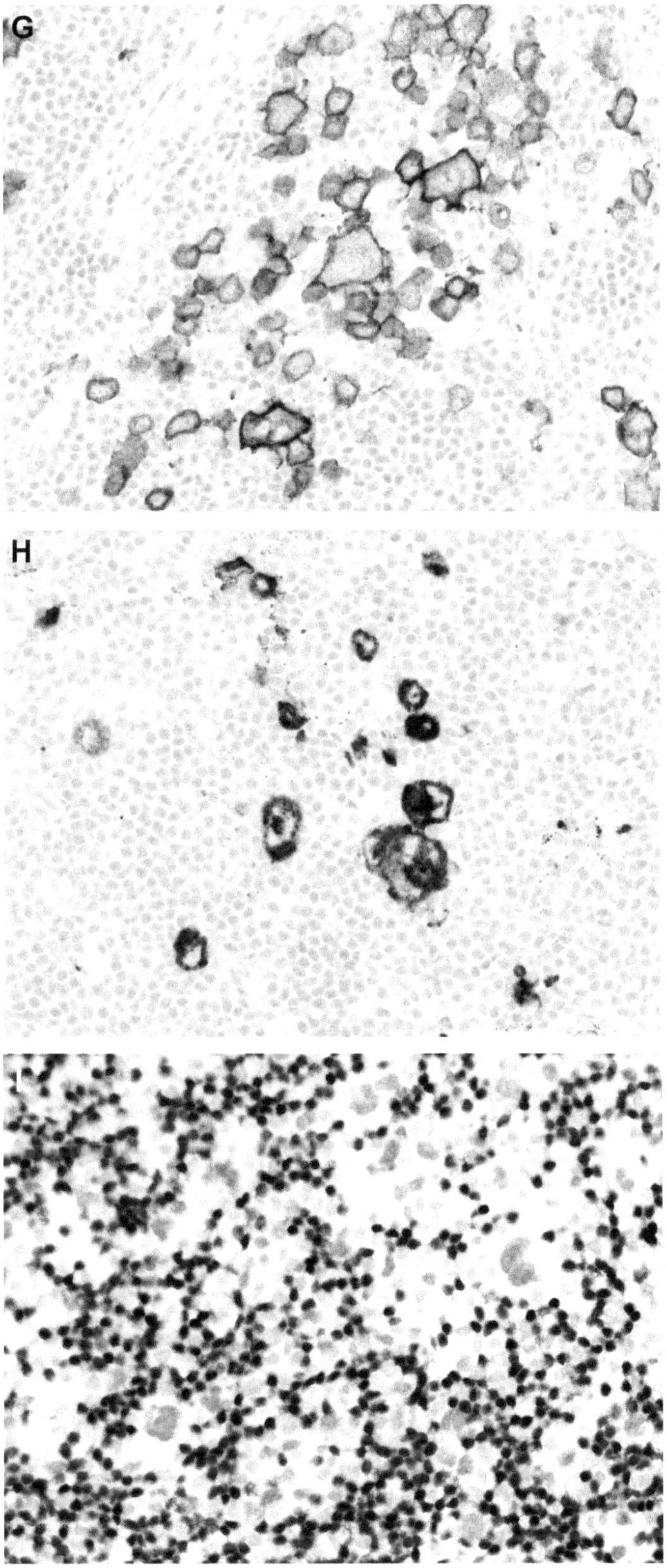

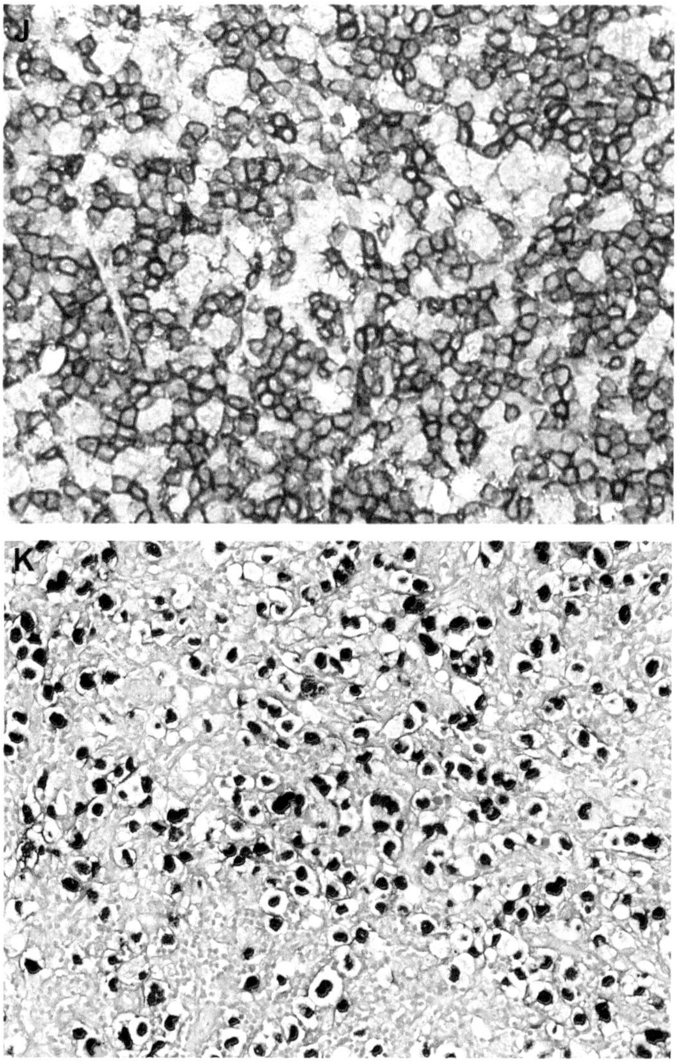

Fig. 1. (*J*) CD3 stains numerous T cells immediately surrounding neoplastic Reed-Sternberg cells with loose rosette formation. (*K*) In situ hybridization for EBER shows positive staining of neoplastic Reed-Sternberg cells.

are together termed Hodgkin/Reed-Sternberg cells. Other variant cells include multinucleated cells, wreath cells in which the nuclei are arranged in the shape of a ring around a central space, and mummified cells with degenerated-appearing nuclei and scant cytoplasm (Fig. 1E, F). In nodular sclerosis CHL, Hodgkin/Reed-Sternberg cells frequently reside in cleared-out spaces caused by retraction artifact from surrounding tissue, an appearance known as lacunar cells.[5] The mixed cellularity subtype of CHL has a higher incidence in low-/middle-income countries and is characterized by the same mixed background cell population of granulocytes, plasma cells, and small lymphocytes, but conspicuous fibrous bands are lacking.[6]

By immunohistochemistry, the large Hodgkin/Reed-Sternberg cells are positive for CD30 and CD15, with the latter ideally demonstrating strong membranous staining with accentuation in the Golgi region (Fig. 1G, H). In some cases, CD15 staining is weaker, more variable, and restricted to the Golgi, or with less-specific granular cytoplasmic staining. PAX5 is positive, but with weak staining compared with background small B cells, reflecting disruption of the B-cell transcription apparatus (Fig. 1I). Neoplastic cells are usually negative for CD20, but positive staining for CD20, usually weak or in a subset of cells, may be seen in 30% to 40% of cases. These stains form the basic diagnostic armamentarium in CHL, but additional stains may be helpful in cases with weak or negative CD15 or very weak PAX5 expression. These include MUM1, strongly expressed by Hodgkin/Reed-Sternberg cells; other B-cell–specific transcription factors, such as OCT2 and BOB1, for which expression is lost on Hodgkin/Reed-Sternberg cells; and CD45, which is typically negative, although its interpretation may be hampered by the abundance of background nonneoplastic cells. Most CHL subtypes show abundant nonneoplastic T cells, identifiable by a pan–T-cell antigen, such as CD2, CD3, or CD5. In most cases, T cells are closely associated with Hodgkin/Reed-Sternberg cells, although rosette formation is not as conspicuous as in NLPHL (Fig. 1J).[2] Finally, assessment of Epstein-Barr virus (EBV) status by in situ hybridization for EBV-encoded RNA (EBER), although not required for diagnosis, may be helpful in many circumstances: it can help to support the diagnosis of CHL in difficult cases in which the differential diagnosis includes entities that are either EBV-negative, such as mediastinal gray-zone lymphoma (MGZL) and primary mediastinal large B-cell lymphoma (PMBL), or for which EBV positivity is vanishingly rare, such as NLPHL (Fig. 1K, Table 1).[7] In other instances, it may raise the possibility of an EBV-driven reactive process mimicking CHL.

ACUTE EPSTEIN-BARR VIRUS INFECTION (ACUTE INFECTIOUS MONONUCLEOSIS)

An important aspect of carefully evaluating suspected cases of CHL is acquiring a strong awareness of how reactive lymphadenopathies may resemble it morphologically in order to avoid misdiagnosing malignancy and subjecting a patient to unnecessary cytotoxic chemotherapy. Reactive entities mimicking CHL include cases of reactive lymphoid hyperplasia characterized by a marked paracortical expansion with a prominent population of reactive immunoblasts, some of which may show cytologic atypia resembling that of Hodgkin/Reed-Sternberg cells. Causes of paracortical hyperplasia with a florid immunoblastic reaction include dermatopathic lymphadenitis and drug-induced lymphoid hyperplasia, as seen with phenytoin or other anticonvulsants. The one most important to be aware of and likely to cause diagnostic difficulty with CHL is that of acute EBV infection or acute infectious mononucleosis.

Such cases of infectious mononucleosis are usually characterized by marked distortion of the lymph node architecture with an interfollicular expansion consisting of a polymorphous infiltrate of small lymphocytes, plasmacytoid lymphocytes, and plasma cells, as well as large cells with prominent nucleoli and vesicular chromatin, consistent with immunoblasts (Fig. 2A–D). Scattered mitotic figures, occasional apoptotic bodies, and foci of necrosis are often present (see Fig. 2B, D). Some immunoblasts may exhibit cytologic atypia in the form of irregular, multilobated nuclei; however, features of classic Reed-Sternberg cells are lacking (see Fig. 2B, C). In a similar vein, the polymorphous nature of the inflammatory cell infiltrate is distinct from that of CHL in terms of the inconspicuous nature of eosinophils and neutrophils. Importantly, even in cases with a markedly expanded paracortex, there are almost always some preserved areas with patent sinuses and reactive-appearing follicles that merge with more abnormal areas (see Fig. 2A). Although necrosis and ulceration may be present, particularly in tonsillar specimens, there is typically minimal fibrosis.[8]

Immunohistochemistry and in situ hybridization are helpful in distinguishing acute infectious mononucleosis from CHL. The immunoblasts are CD20-positive B cells that typically coexpress CD30 and MUM1 but lack CD15 (Fig. 2E, F). Although both acute infectious mononucleosis and CHL are characterized by EBV-positive cells, there is more variability in the size of positive cells in acute EBV infection, with staining of both small- to medium-sized and large cells (Fig. 2G). Other helpful and reassuring features in acute infectious mononucleosis are that the immunoblasts usually retain pan–B-cell marker expression, such as OCT2 and BOB1, and demonstrate polytypic expression of kappa and lambda immunoglobulin light chains (Fig. 2H, I). Although it may be tempting to stain for immunoglobin light chains by in situ hybridization, the author's experience is that light chain staining on immunoblasts is usually better demonstrated by immunohistochemistry.[8] In addition, assessment of background T cells may be helpful, as these are predominantly CD8-positive in acute infectious mononucleosis, in contrast to CHL, which shows CD4 excess in background T cells; this feature may be evident by flow cytometry, and the inverted CD4:CD8 ratio should not lead to a misdiagnosis of peripheral T-cell lymphoma.

This differential diagnosis underscores the importance of correlating with other clinical and laboratory findings, if available. Serologic studies demonstrating evidence of acute EBV infection (positive EBV antiviral capsid antigen immunoglobulin M [IgM] antibody) or the presence of characteristic atypical reactive lymphocytes on peripheral smear can be reassuring corollary findings that are helpful in avoiding a misdiagnosis of CHL (Fig. 2J, K).[8] It is also important to note what ancillary studies may be misleading: given

Table 1
Differentiating nodular sclerosis classic Hodgkin lymphoma from its mimics

Feature	Nodular Sclerosis CHL	MGZL	PMBL	Acute EBV Infection	EBV-Positive MCU
Age, sex	Peak incidence 15–35 y, slight female predominance	Adolescents and young adults, M > F	Young adults, 20s–30s, M < F	Younger individuals but wide age range	Older or immunosuppressed
Localization	Mediastinum, with or without bulky disease			Peripheral lymph nodes, tonsil	*Extranodal*: oral cavity or gastrointestinal tract
Architecture and cellular composition	Nodular with fibrous bands, neutrophils, eosinophils, small lymphocytes, plasma cells, histiocytes, scattered HRS cells	Numerous large cells, pleomorphic, or lacunar features, focal fibrous bands	Diffuse sheets of large cells, clear cytoplasm (some HRS-like), compartmentalizing fibrosis	Small lymphocytes, plasmacytoid lymphocytes, plasma cells, immunoblasts (some HRS-like)	Plasma cells, histiocytes, eosinophils, small lymphocytes (dense T-cell rim at base), scattered HRS-like large cells
Large-cell phenotype (all are $MUM1^{+}$)	$CD45^{-}$/weak, $CD30^{+}$, $CD15^{+/-}$, PAX5 weak, OCT2/BOB1 loss, CD20 $^{-/+}$ (weak, subset), usually negative for CD79a, CD19, BCL6	CD45, PAX5, OCT2/BOB1 usually +, BCL6 variable *LBCL-like*: $CD30^{+}$, $CD15^{+}$, pan–B-cell antigen loss *CHL-like*: $CD20^{+}$, $CD19^{+}$, $CD79a^{+}$, $BCL6^{+}$, $CD30^{+}$, $CD15^{+/-}$	$CD45^{+}$, $CD20^{+}$, $PAX5^{+}$, OCT2/$BOB1^{+}$, kappa or lambda light chain negative, $CD79a^{+}$/weak, $CD30^{+/-}$, CD15 $^{-}$/focal	$CD20^{+}$, $CD30^{+}$, $CD15^{-}$, $PAX5^{+}$, OCT2/$BOB1^{+}$, polytypic kappa and lambda light chain expression	$CD20^{+}$/weak, $PAX5^{+}$, $CD30^{+}$, $CD15^{+/-}$, $OCT2^{+}$, BOB1 variable, CD79a often positive
EBV association	10%–25% of cases have EBV^{+} large HRS cells	Negative	Negative	Positive, variably sized	Positive, variably sized

Abbreviations: F, female; HRS, Hodgkin/Reed-Sternberg cells; M, male.

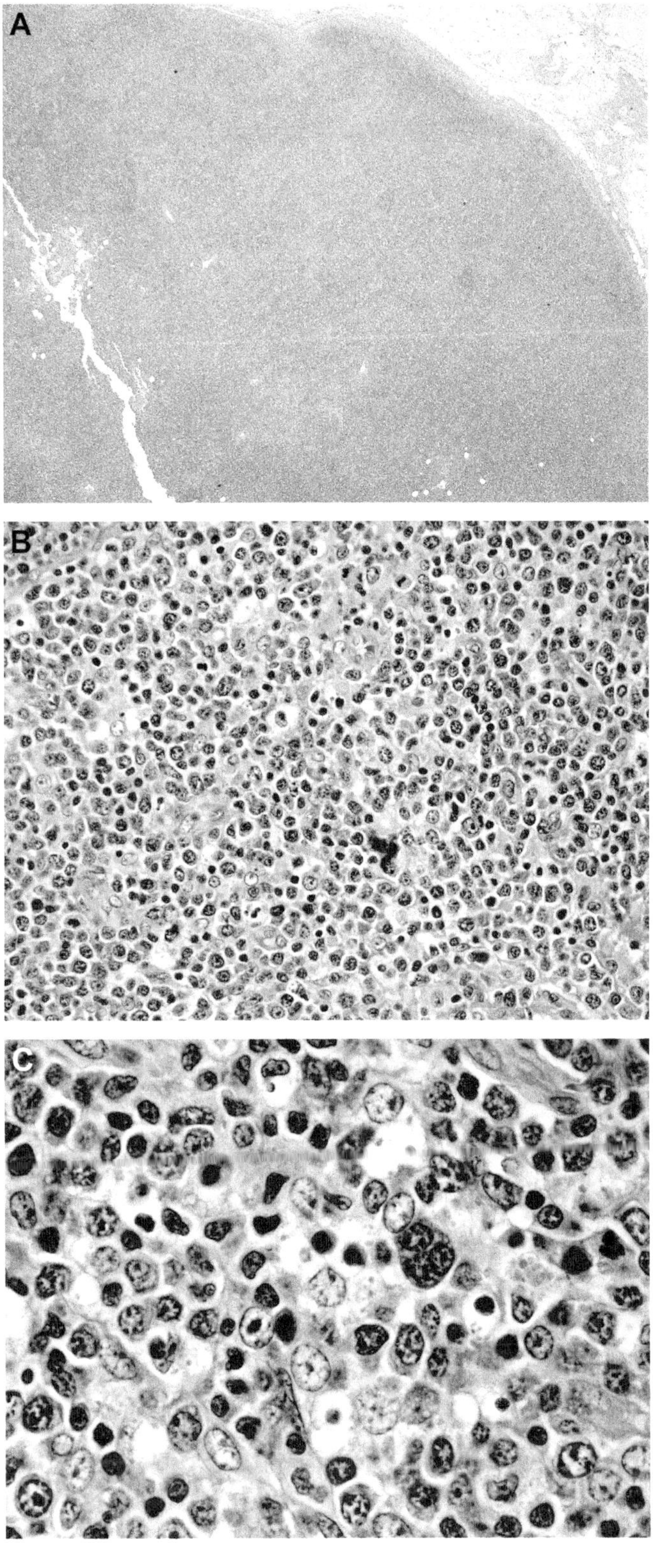

Fig. 2. Acute EBV infection (acute infectious mononucleosis). (*A*) The lymph node architecture is distorted by a marked paracortical expansion. However, sinuses are patent; the capsule is intact without extension of the lymphoid infiltrate into perinodal fat, and small reactive-appearing follicles are present subjacent to the capsule, indicating retention of the normal lymph node framework (H&E, 20x). (*B–D*) The paracortical infiltrate comprises a spectrum of small lymphocytes, plasmacytoid lymphocytes, plasma cells, and immunoblasts, including occasional forms with cytologic atypia (*B*, H&E, 200x) and multinucleation (*C*, H&E, 400x). Scattered mitotic figures (*B*, *D*) and apoptotic bodies

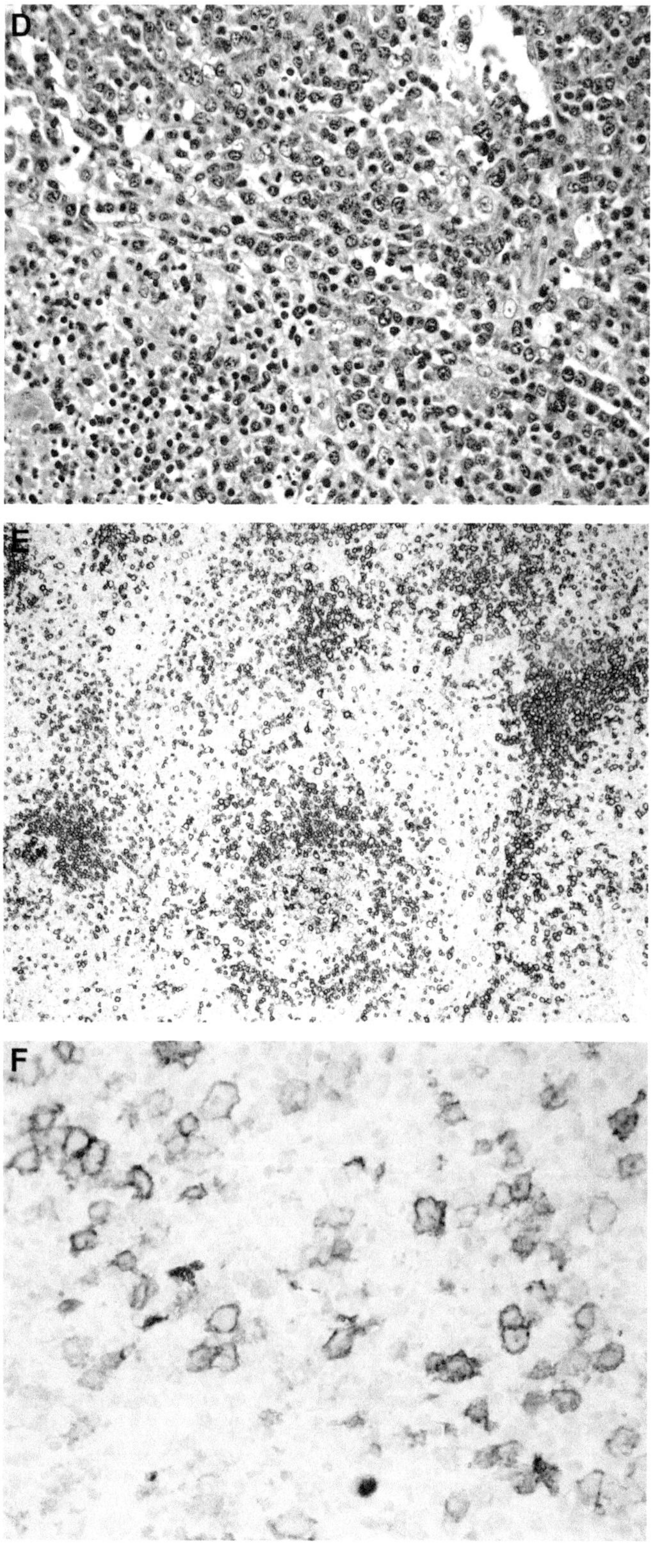

Fig. 2. (*D*) are present, including focal areas of incipient necrosis (*D, lower left*). However, eosinophils and neutrophils are inconspicuous; there is no significant fibrosis, and classic Reed-Sternberg cells are not seen. (*E, F*) A CD20 stain highlights loose aggregates of mature B cells and is positive in the larger immunoblasts (*E*), a subset of which coexpresses CD30 (*F*).

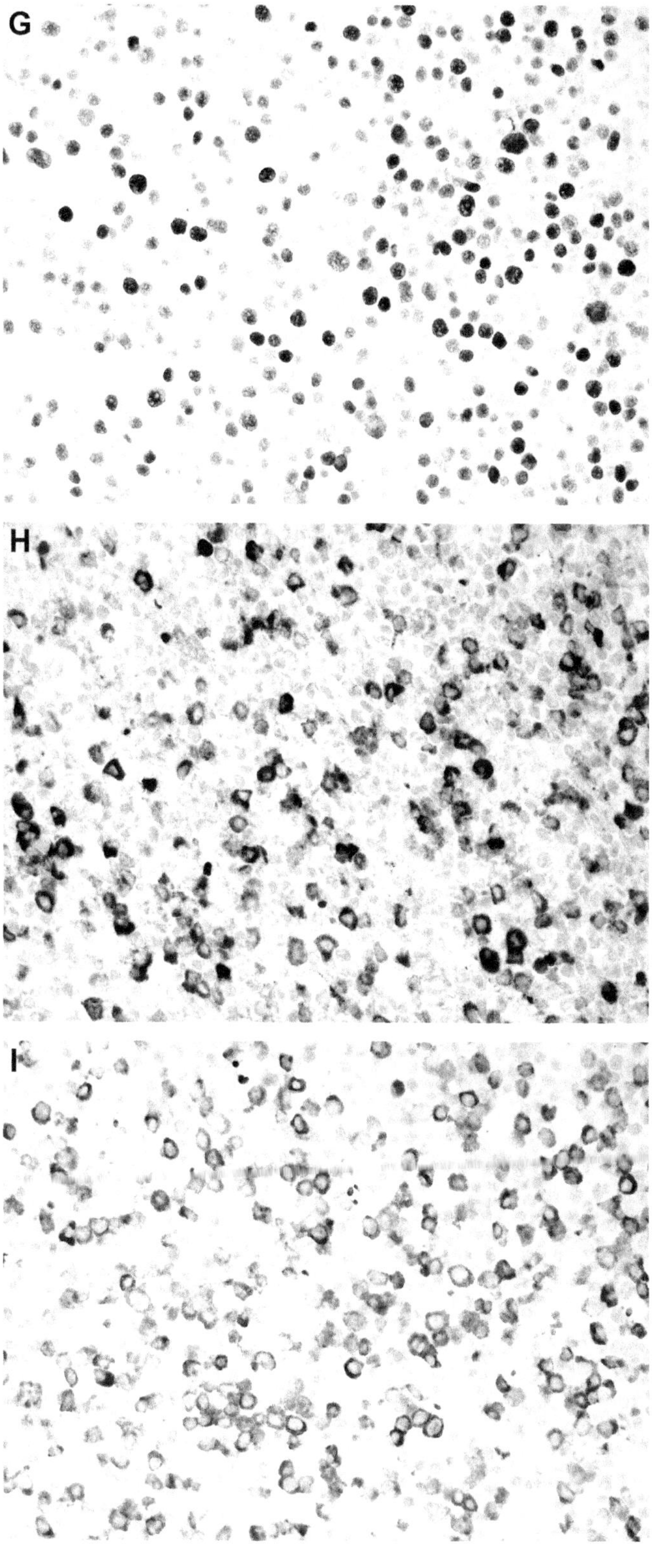

Fig. 2. (*G*) Numerous cells are positive for EBV by EBER in situ hybridization. Note the variability in nuclear size highlighted by the stain. (*H, I*) Immunoblasts are polytypic for kappa (*H*) and lambda (*I*) light chains by immunohistochemistry.

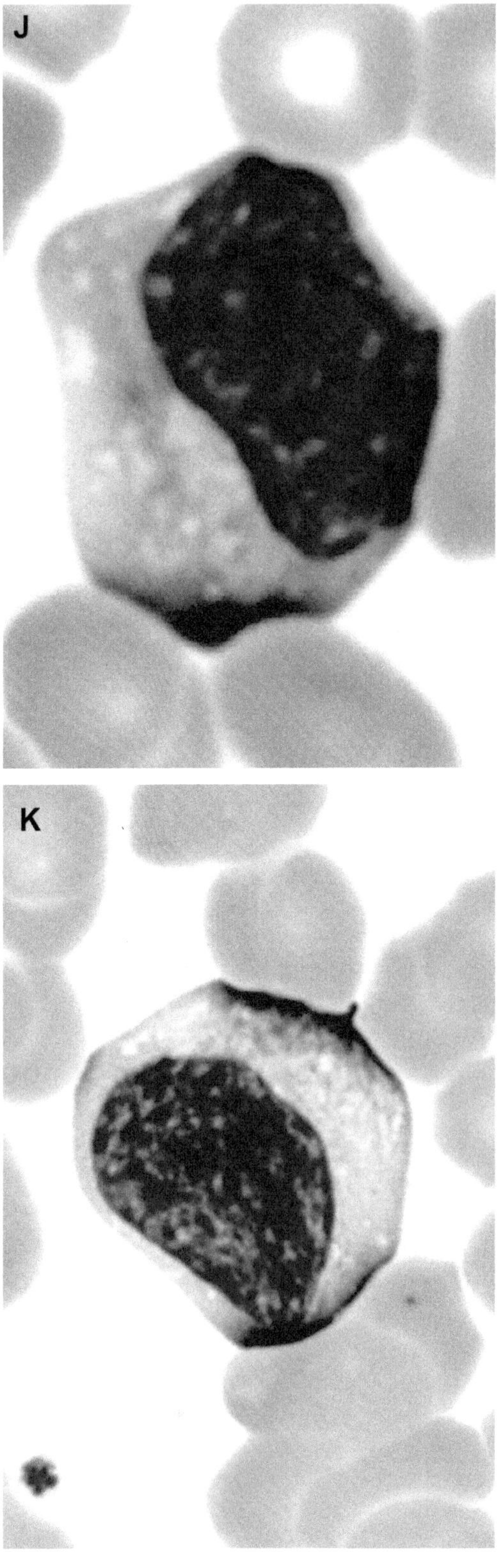

Fig. 2. (*J, K*) Peripheral blood smear from the same patient demonstrating circulating atypical reactive lymphocytes with irregular nuclei, clumped chromatin, and abundant basophilic cytoplasm with peripheral basophilic accentuation.

the floridly reactive nature of the proliferating B and T cells induced by the virus, polymerase chain reaction (PCR) for *IGH* or *TRG* gene rearrangement studies may unearth an oligoclonal pattern reflecting a restricted immune repertoire, but this finding should not be overinterpreted as evidence for a B-cell non-Hodgkin lymphoma or peripheral T-cell lymphoma.

EPSTEIN-BARR VIRUS–POSITIVE MUCOCUTANEOUS ULCER

EBV-positive mucocutaneous ulcer (MCU) is not a lymphoma but an EBV-associated lymphoproliferative disorder that develops in the setting of immune deficiency and dysregulation, which may be age-related, iatrogenic, virally induced, or congenital. Lesions are typically sharply circumscribed and involve isolated or focal areas of the oral mucosa or gastrointestinal tract, all of which are highly unusual locations for CHL (Fig. 3A).[9,10]

Histologic examination demonstrates surface erosion or ulceration with an underlying mixed inflammatory cell infiltrate containing scattered large cells with prominent nucleoli in a background of smaller lymphocytes and frequent granulocytes (Fig. 3B, C). Occasional large cells may be highly atypical, reminiscent of Hodgkin/Reed-Sternberg cells (see Fig. 3C inset). There is often a prominent vascular component with angiocentricity and angioinvasion (Fig. 3D). By immunohistochemistry, the large, atypical cells are positive for CD45, CD30, MUM1, CD20, and PAX5 and typically retain expression of OCT2 and BOB1 (Fig. 3E–H). Up to one-half of cases may show positivity for CD15 (Fig. 3I). On generous biopsies that are well-oriented, a dense rim of small T cells is typically present at the base of the inflammatory focus, which is most readily appreciated on a pan–T-cell antigen stain, such as CD3 or CD5 (Fig. 3K). Similar to acute infectious mononucleosis, EBV by EBER in situ hybridization shows positive staining on both large and small cells, and background T cells show a predominance of CD8 expression over CD4 (Fig. 3J, L, M).[9,10]

As is the case with acute EBV infection, the diagnosis of EBV-positive MCU can be supported further by correlation with other available clinical and laboratory findings. Regional lymph nodes, if enlarged, typically show reactive changes on biopsy, and the absence of systemic disease is required to make this diagnosis. Underscoring the localized, extranodal nature of the lesion, EBV viral load is negative in the setting of EBV-positive MCU, in contrast to high EBV viral load seen with an EBV-driven lymphoma. In cases with limited tissue or lacking supportive clinical, imaging, or laboratory data, a definitive diagnosis of EBV-positive MCU may not be possible, and describing the findings with a differential diagnosis is appropriate and will serve the patient better than making an outright diagnosis of lymphoma.

PRIMARY MEDIASTINAL LARGE B-CELL LYMPHOMA

PMBL is a large B-cell neoplasm with distinct clinicopathologic features and is therefore considered a separate entity from diffuse large B-cell lymphoma, not otherwise specified (DLBCL-NOS). This rare lymphoma comprises 2% to 4% of non-Hodgkin lymphoma. There is a female predominance with a median age of 35 years at presentation. Patients typically present with a bulky mediastinal mass with frequent invasion of adjacent structures; however, bone marrow or nonmediastinal lymph node involvement is uncommon. Extranodal disease may be seen at the time of relapse, with involvement of the central nervous system or more unusual sites, such as kidneys, adrenal glands, liver, or gonads.[11]

Morphologically, the tumor is composed of a diffuse infiltrate of large, atypical cells with abundant pale cytoplasm and irregular, sometimes multilobated nuclei surrounded by thin bands of compartmentalizing fibrosis (Fig. 4A–C). Some of the large cells may show more pleomorphic nuclear features resembling Hodgkin/Reed-Sternberg cells (see Fig. 4C). On immunohistochemical analysis, tumor cells are positive for CD45 and pan–B-cell antigens (CD19, CD20, PAX5, CD79a, OCT2, BOB1) and typically show a nongerminal center B-cell phenotype with positivity for MUM1 and negative staining for CD10 (Fig. 4D–F). Many cases are positive for CD23 and CD30, the latter often weaker or more variable compared with CHL (Fig. 4G, H).[11] Additional helpful immunohistochemical features include positivity for CD200 and MAL (Fig. 4I, J).[12,13]

PMBL and CHL also share a genetic transcription profile with activation of NF-kappaB and JAK-STAT signaling pathways. Combined expression of TRAF1 and nuclear cREL, targets of NK-kappaB antiapoptotic signaling, has been found by immunohistochemistry in more than 80% of CHL and 50% of PMBL, but only rarely in DLBCL-NOS (Fig. 4K, L).[14] Genetic aberrations shared by PMBL and CHL include 9p24 amplifications resulting in increased JAK-STAT activity and PDL1/PDL2 upregulation, as well as *CIITA* translocations at 16p13, both of which are implicated in

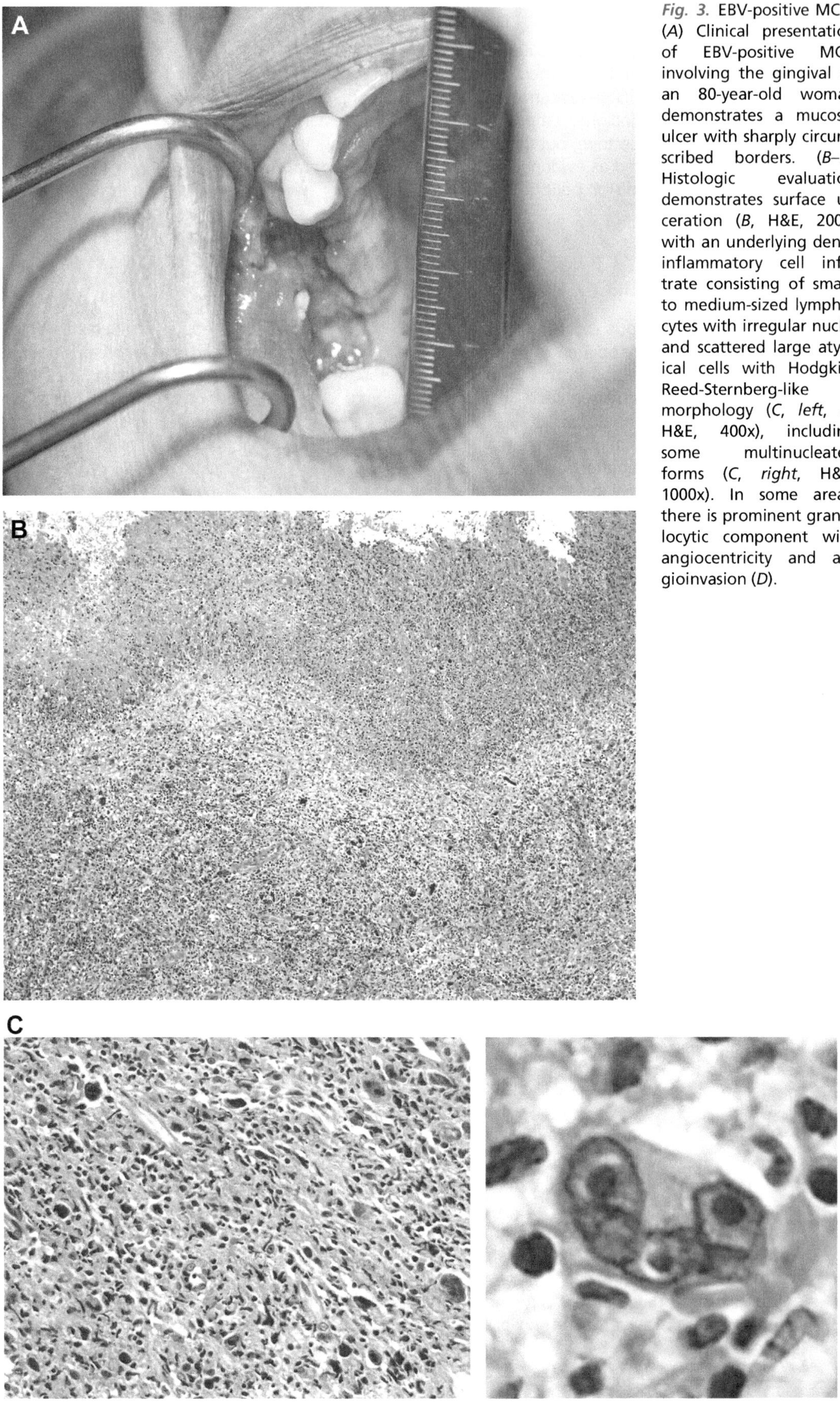

Fig. 3. EBV-positive MCU. (*A*) Clinical presentation of EBV-positive MCU involving the gingival of an 80-year-old woman demonstrates a mucosal ulcer with sharply circumscribed borders. (*B–D*) Histologic evaluation demonstrates surface ulceration (*B*, H&E, 200x) with an underlying dense inflammatory cell infiltrate consisting of small-to medium-sized lymphocytes with irregular nuclei and scattered large atypical cells with Hodgkin/Reed-Sternberg-like morphology (*C*, *left*, *D*, H&E, 400x), including some multinucleated forms (*C*, *right*, H&E, 1000x). In some areas, there is prominent granulocytic component with angiocentricity and angioinvasion (*D*).

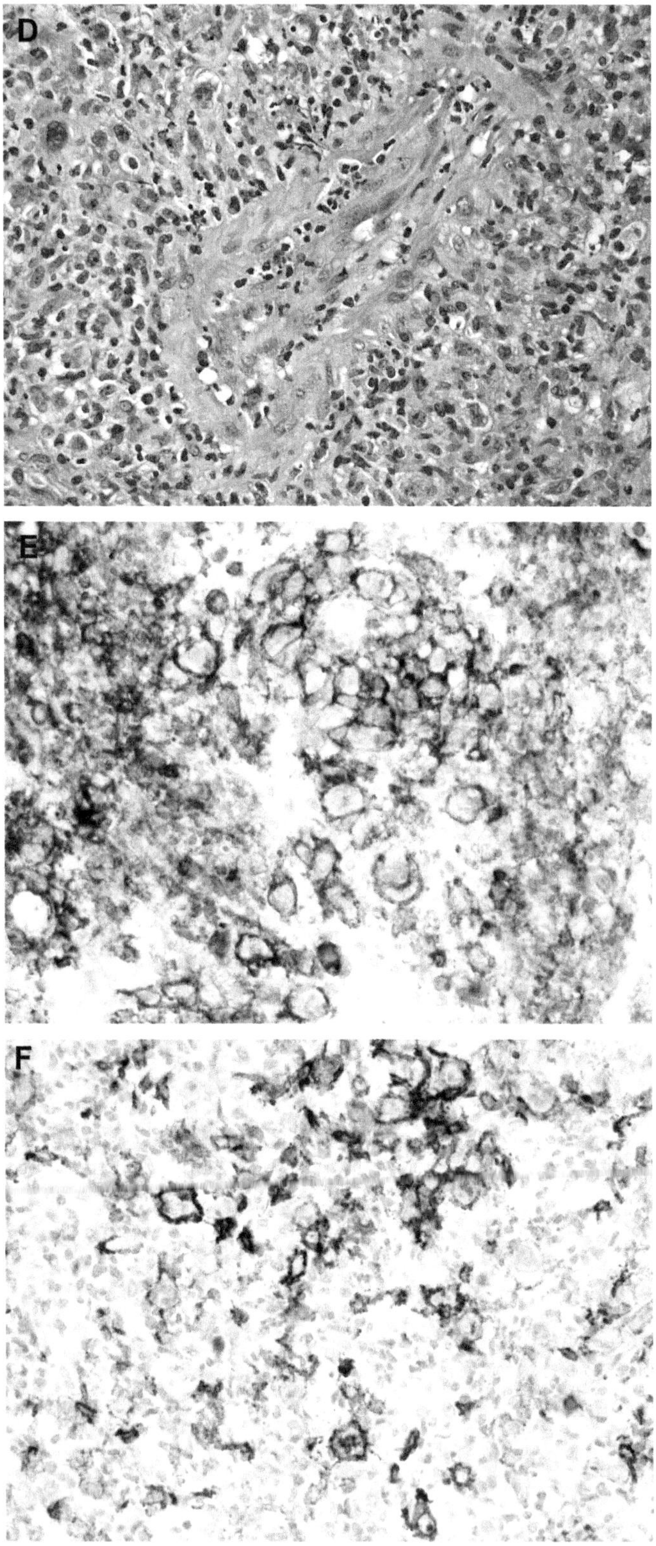

Fig. 3. (*E–I*) The large cells are positive for CD45 (*E*), CD20 (*F*),

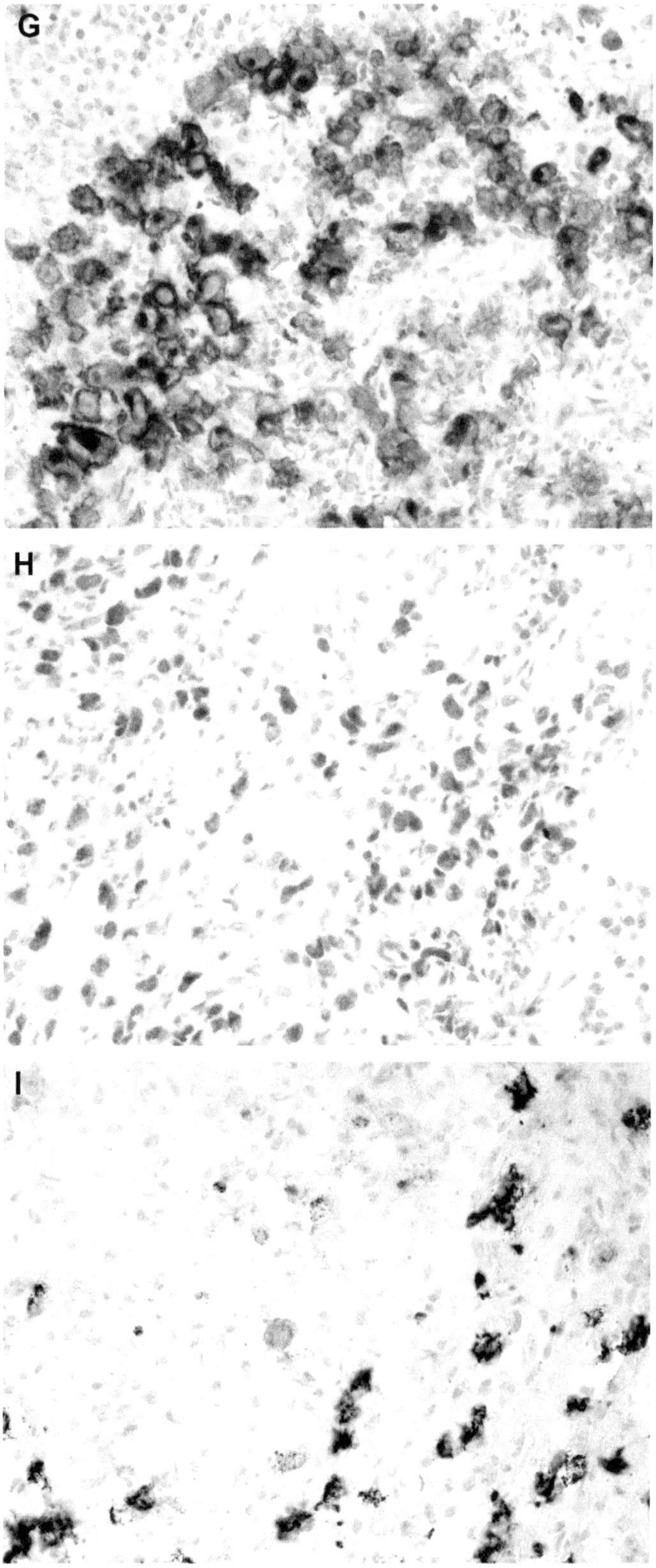

Fig. 3. (*G*), and PAX5 (*H*), with focal, weak staining for CD15 (*I*) by immunohistochemistry.

Fig. 3. (*J*) EBER in situ hybridization is positive in cells of variable size. (*K–M*) The base of the lesion contains a prominent rim of small T cells (*K*, CD3) with an inverted CD4:CD8 ratio (*L*, CD4; and *M*, CD8).

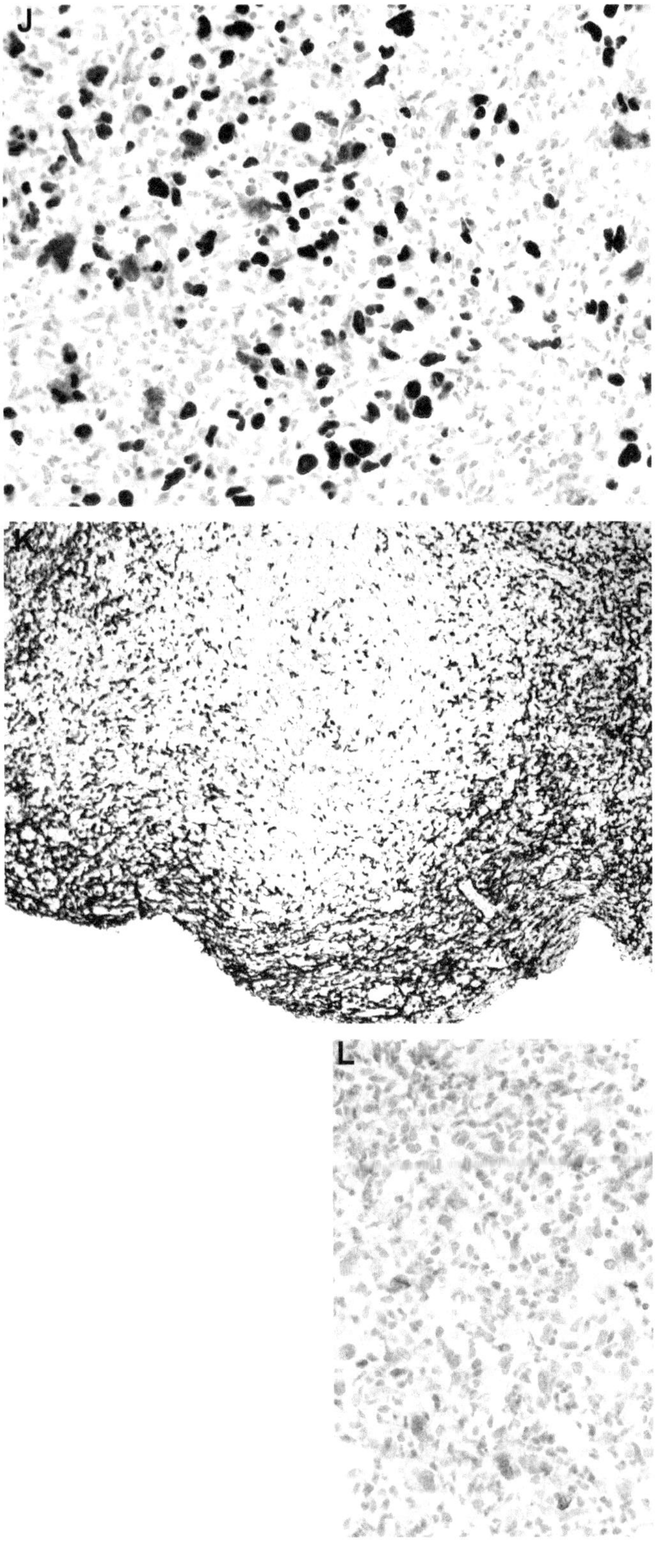

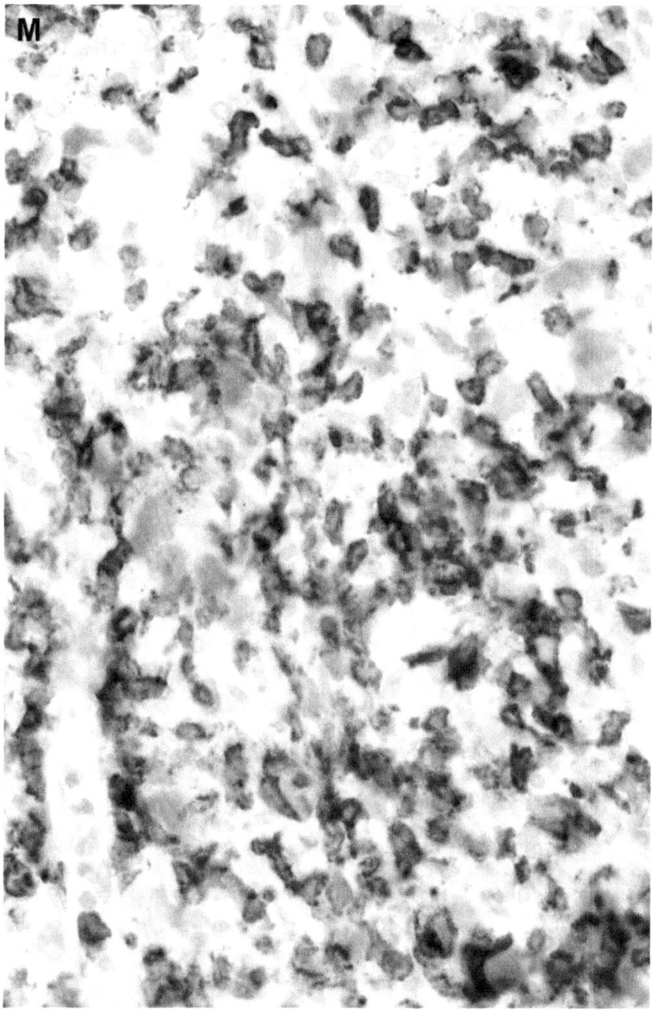

Fig. 3. *M,* CD8).

tumor-mediated immune evasion in both entities. Somatic mutations involving *PTPN1* have also been identified in both PMBL and CHL.[15] Therefore, PMBL shows more clinicopathologic and biologic overlap with CHL, particularly the nodular sclerosis subtype, than it does with DLBCL-NOS, likely reflecting a common cell of origin presumed to be a thymic medullary B cell.

Interestingly, although most cases of PMBL are negative for CD15, some CD15 positivity has been reported in up to a third of cases in some series. CD15 positivity is typically seen as Golgi or membranous staining in only rare large cells, although in some cases, most tumor cells exhibit CD15 positivity in a paranuclear dotlike Golgi pattern (Fig. 4M–P). A relatively large study of patients with PMBL uniformly treated with R-CHOP found CD15 expression to be an isolated feature without an adverse prognosis.[15] The same study also found that other markers of potential prognostic significance in DLBCL-NOS, including cell-of-origin as determined by the Hans algorithm, MYC positivity, double-expressor phenotype (MYC/BCL2 double-positivity), or Ki67 proliferation index, did not hold prognostic significance in PMBL. In contrast, the combination of high MUM1 and low PDL1 expression was found to be an adverse prognostic factor for both progression-free and overall survival, identifying potential biomarkers for risk stratification in PMBL that require confirmation in larger, prospective studies.[15]

Despite the overlapping clinical, morphologic, and immunophenotypic features detailed above stemming from their shared underlying biology, distinguishing PMBL from CHL is usually relatively straightforward owing to the diffuse nature of the

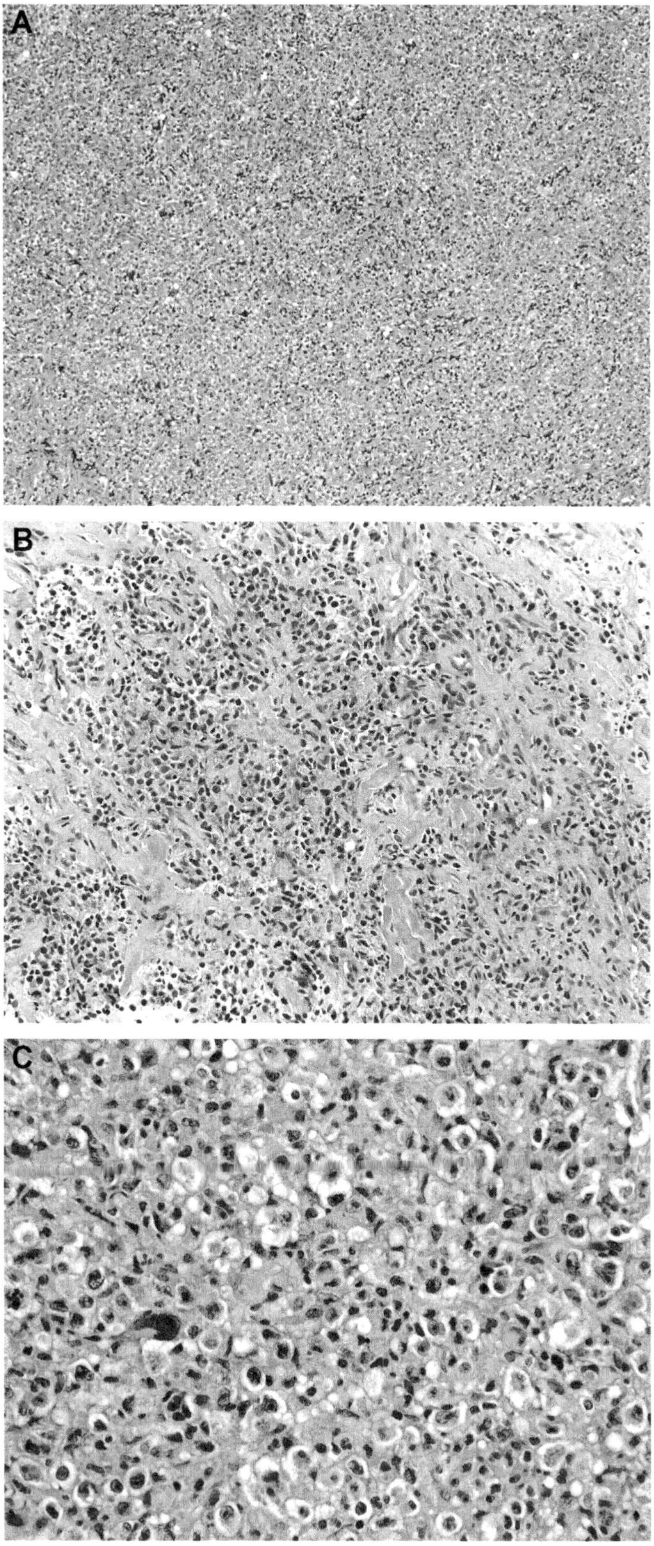

Fig. 4. PMBL. (*A, B*) PMBL is characterized by a diffuse infiltrate of large, atypical cells present in background of fibrosis, which is often composed of thin bands intervening between clusters of atypical lymphocytes (A, H&E, 40x; *B*, compartmentalizing fibrosis, H&E, 200x). (*C*) The neoplastic cells have large, irregular to lobated nuclei, prominent nucleoli, and moderately abundant pale eosinophilic cytoplasm (H&E, 400x). Occasional cells have features reminiscent of Hodgkin/Reed-Sternberg cells, including scattered bizarre or anaplastic forms and surrounding clear lacunar spaces. (*D–F*) The neoplastic cells are strongly and diffusely positive for CD45

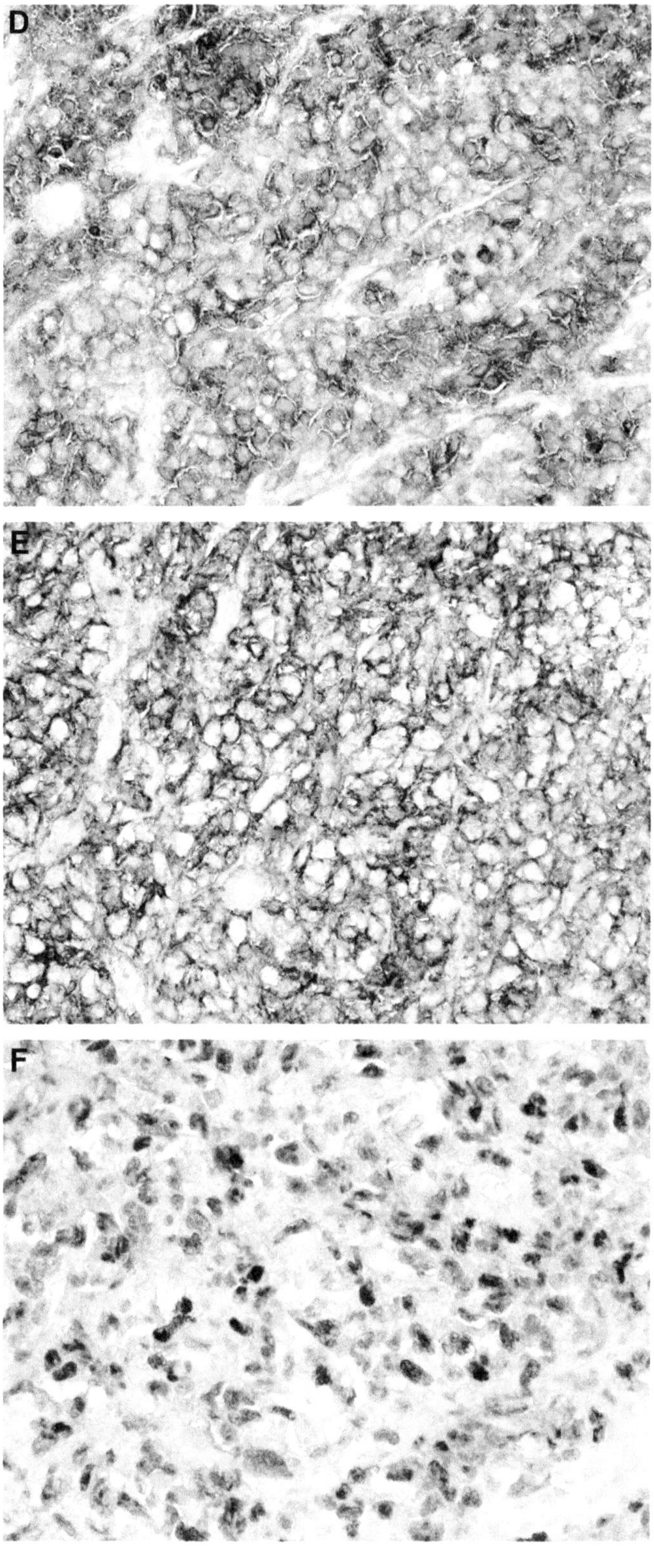

Fig. 4. (*D*), CD20 (*E*), and MUM1 (*F*).

Fig. 4. (*G*) CD23 is frequently coexpressed. (*H*) CD30 is often positive, often weak, and variable compared with CHL.

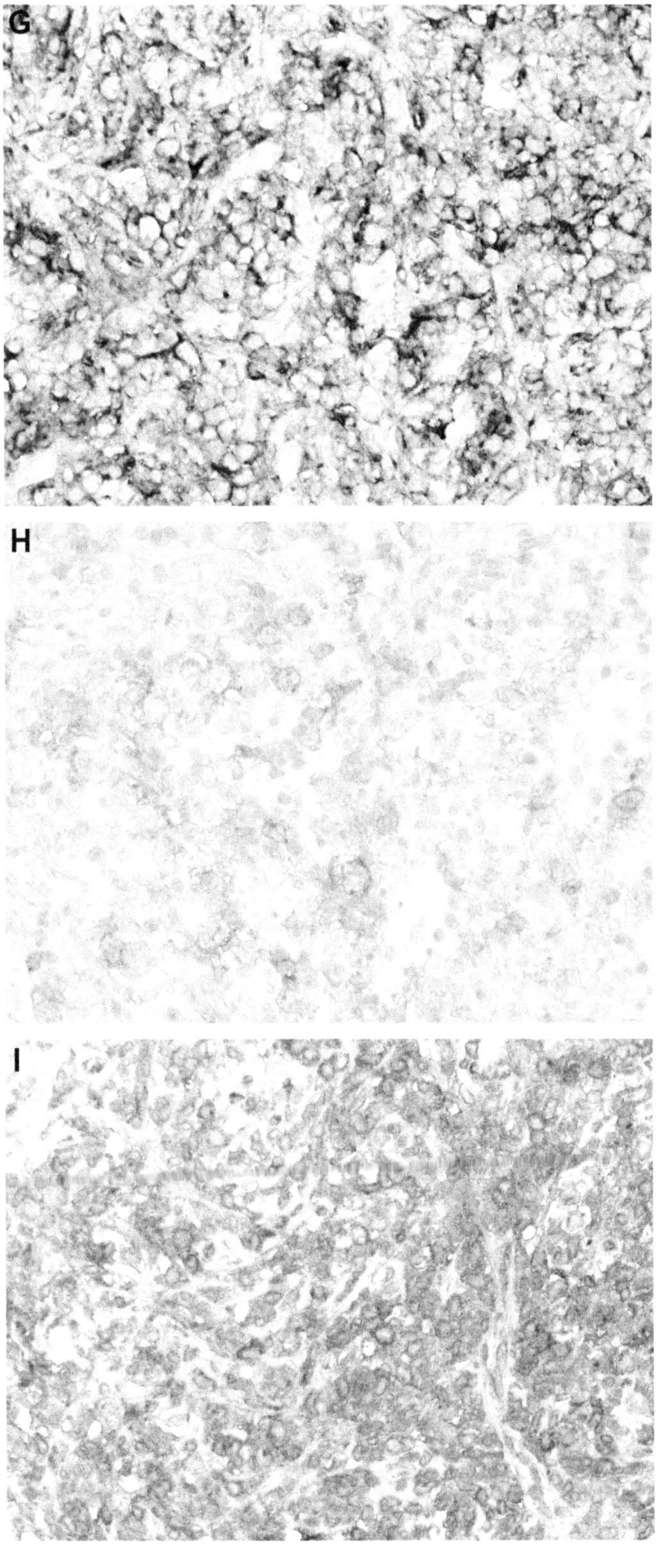

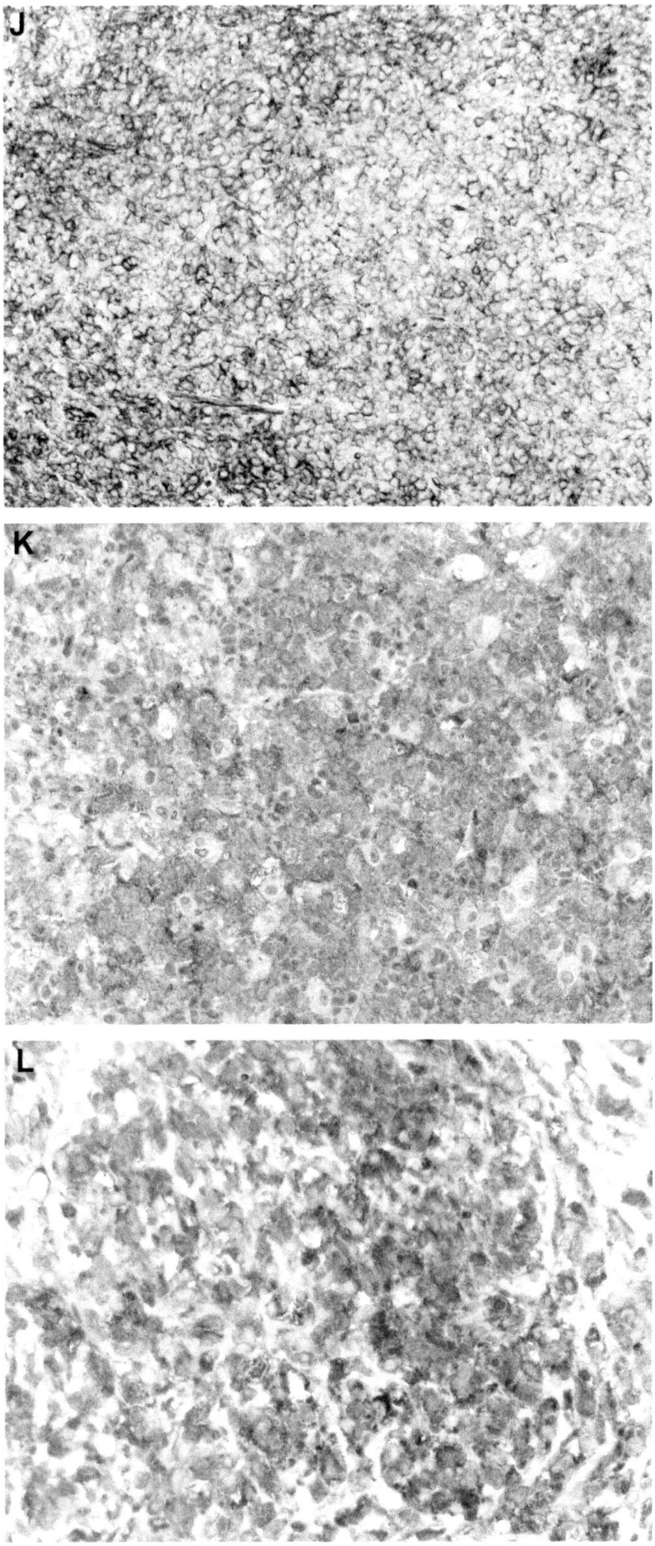

Fig. 4. (*I–L*) Stains useful in distinguishing PMBL from DLBCL-NOS include MAL (*I*) and CD200 (*J*), both cytoplasmic stains, as well as the combined expression of cytoplasmic TRAF (*K*) and nuclear cREL (*L*).

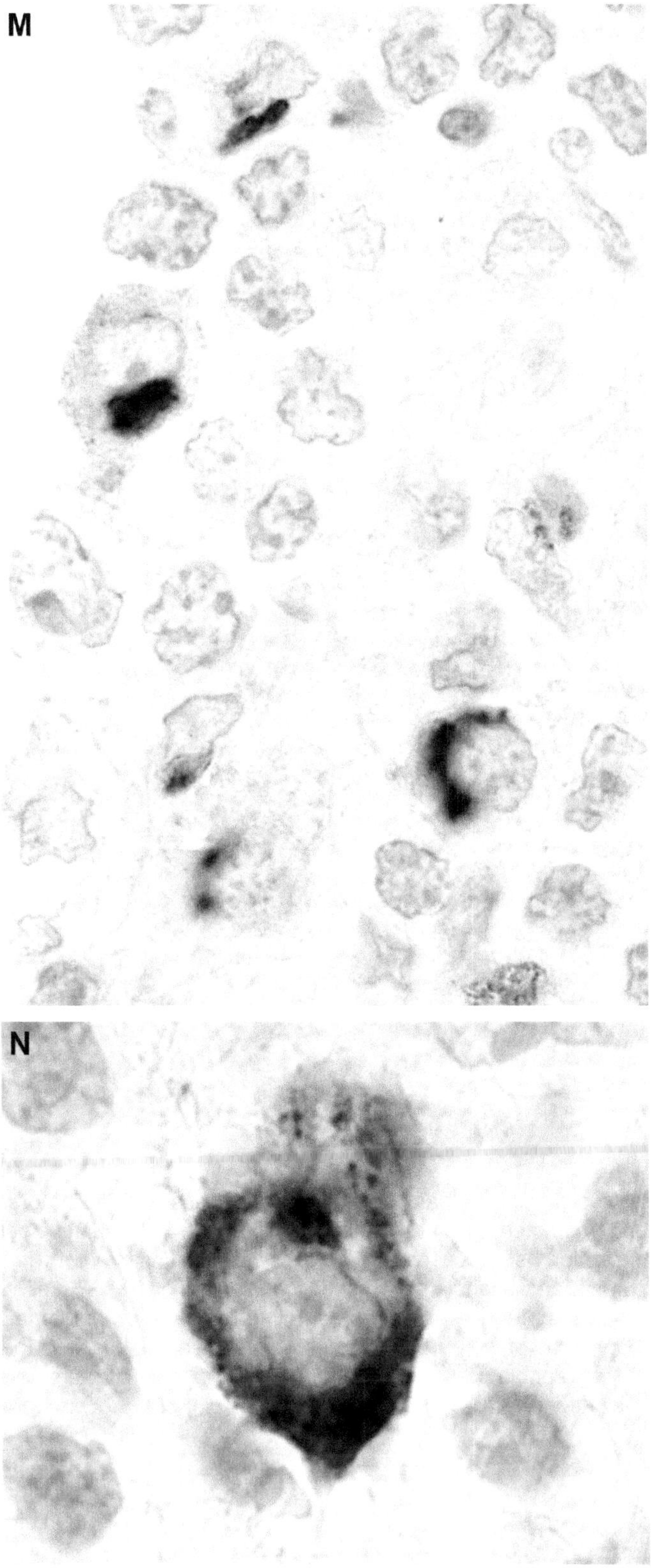

Fig. 4. (*M–P*) CD15 is infrequently expressed, often in a granular cytoplasmic pattern with Golgi accentuation. In cases with CD15 positivity, it is usually seen in a small subset of cells

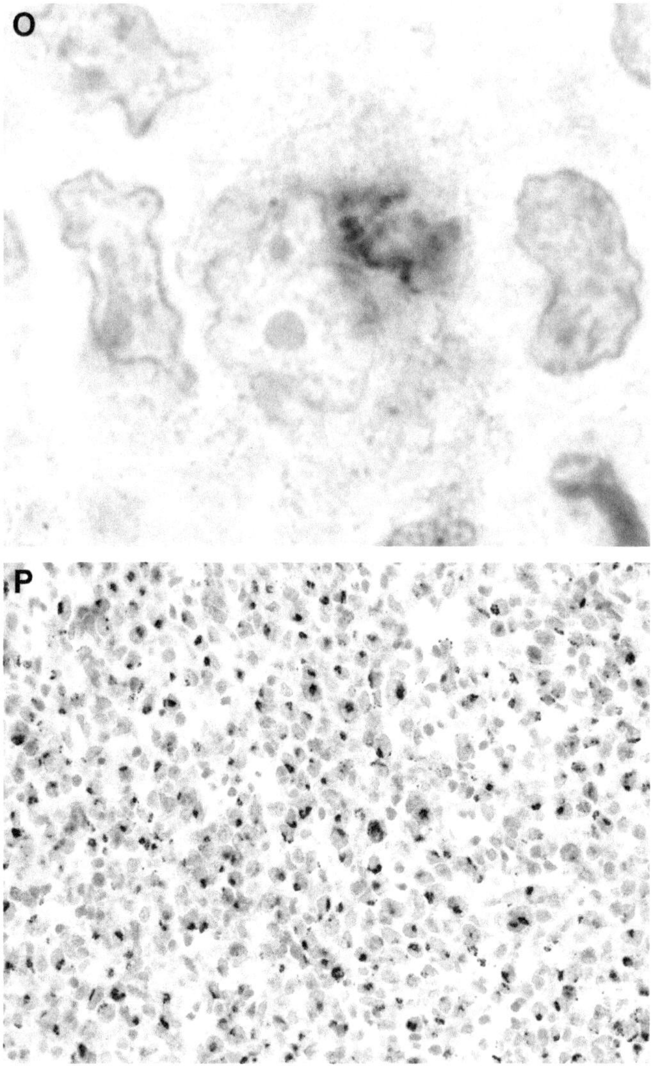

Fig. 4. (*M–O*) but may be rarely expressed by the majority of cells in otherwise typical cases of PMBL (*P*).

large cell infiltrate, pan–B-cell marker expression, and restricted pattern of fibrosis in PMBL. An exception is in cases with dense mediastinal fibrosis and associated crushed cellular artifact, which may require extensive sampling to identify focal areas of well-preserved cellularity amenable to morphologic and immunohistochemical evaluation.[16]

MEDIASTINAL GRAY-ZONE LYMPHOMA

MGZL is related to both PMBL and nodular sclerosis CHL and represents a rare group of mediastinal lymphomas with transitional features between the 2 entities.[4,17] With the release of the 5th edition of the WHO Classification of Haematolymphoid Tumors, MGZL replaces the previously used terminology of "B-cell lymphoma, unclassifiable, with features intermediate between diffuse large B-cell lymphoma and classic Hodgkin lymphoma."[4,18] Cases show more numerous large cells than typical CHL, present in prominent clusters or sheets in a relatively sparse inflammatory background. Fibrous bands and lacunar cells may be seen. Like PMBL and CHL, MGZL is more common in young people but affects men more than women. It is clinically more aggressive than either CHL or PMBL; therefore, this diagnosis has important prognostic implications. However, it is important to note that weak, variable, or even moderate staining for CD20 in an otherwise typical case of CHL should not raise concern for a

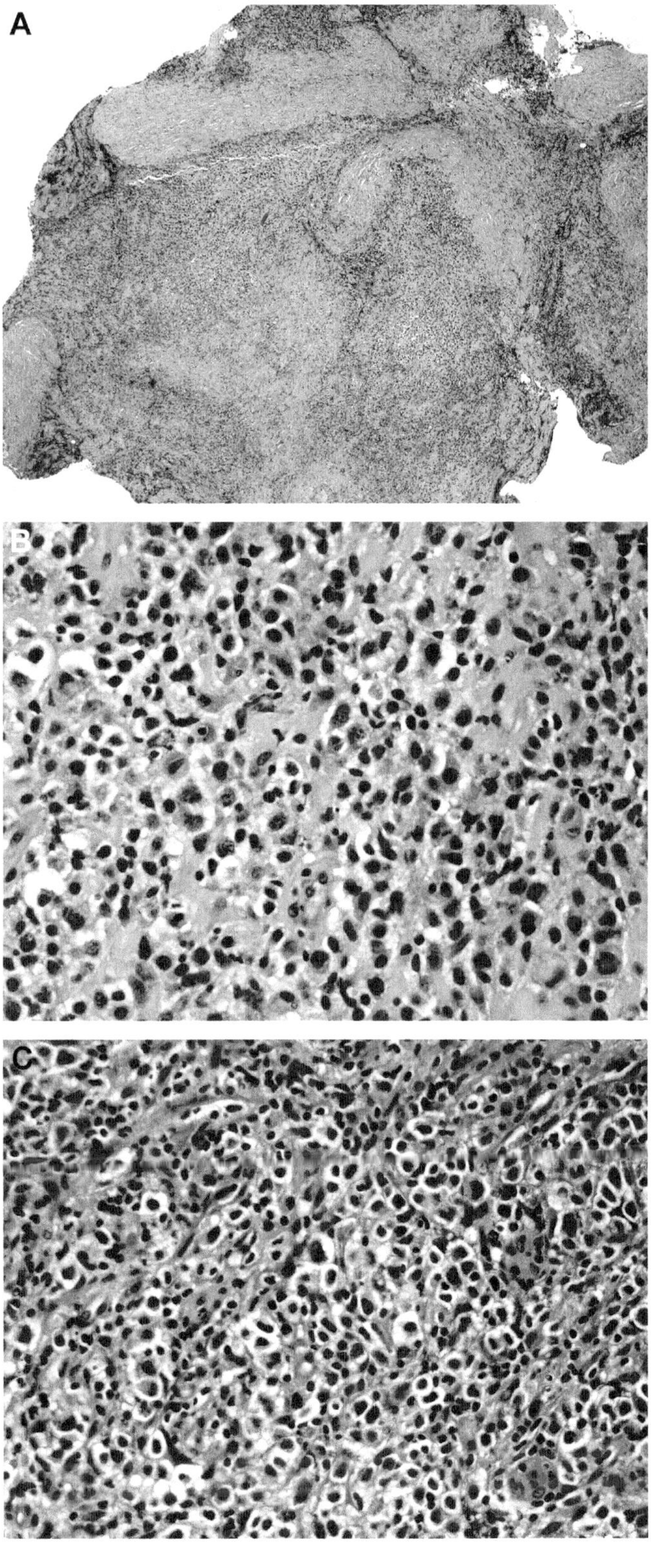

Fig. 5. MGZL, large cell lymphoma-like morphology with loss of normal B-cell program. (*A*, H&E, 20x) On low magnification, there is a dense lymphoid infiltrate with prominent fibrous bands partially encircling nodules. (*B, C*, H&E, 400x) On higher magnification, there is a predominance of large atypical cells with irregular hyperchromatic nuclei, some of which appear to lie within lacunar spaces (*C, H&E*, 400x).

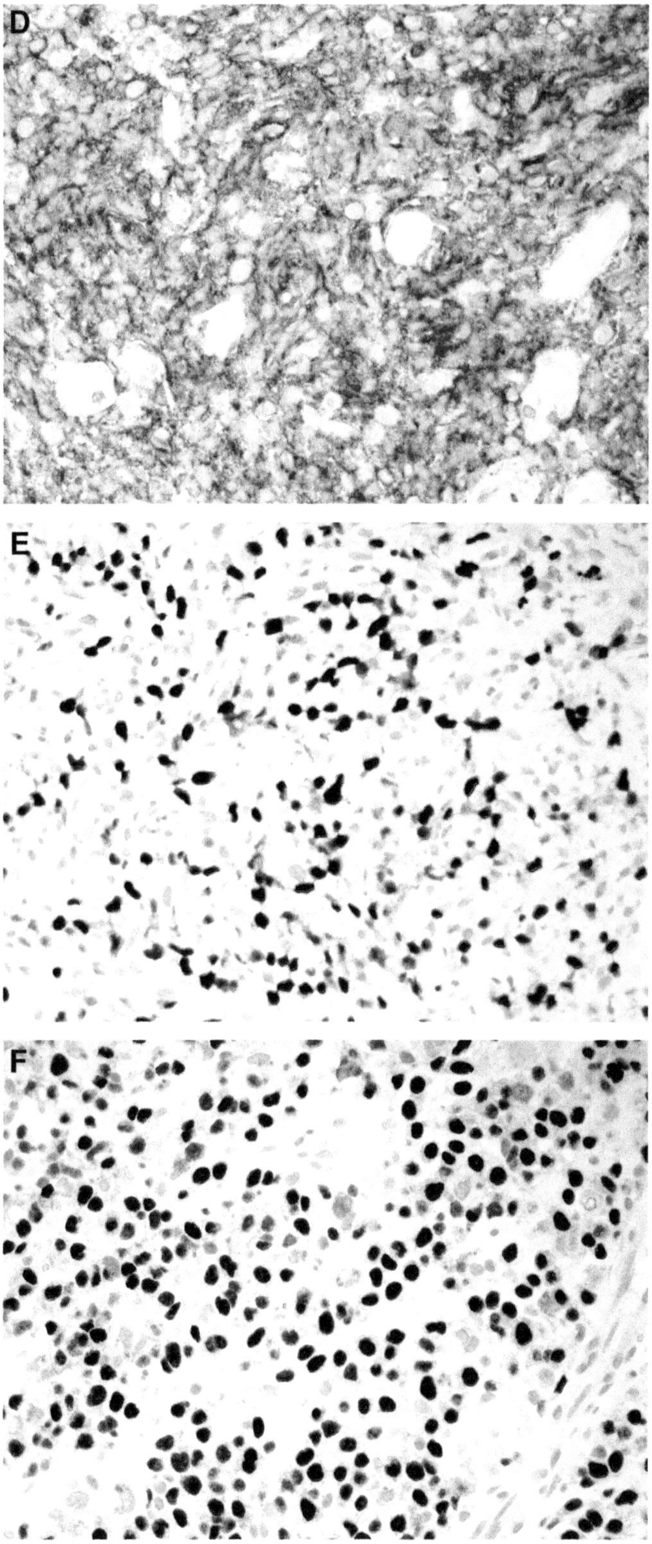

Fig. 5. (*D*), PAX5 (*E*), OCT2 (*F*),

Fig. 5. and BOB1 (*G*), but have diminished staining for other components of the B-cell program, including weak staining for CD79a (*H*) and negative staining for CD20 (*I*).

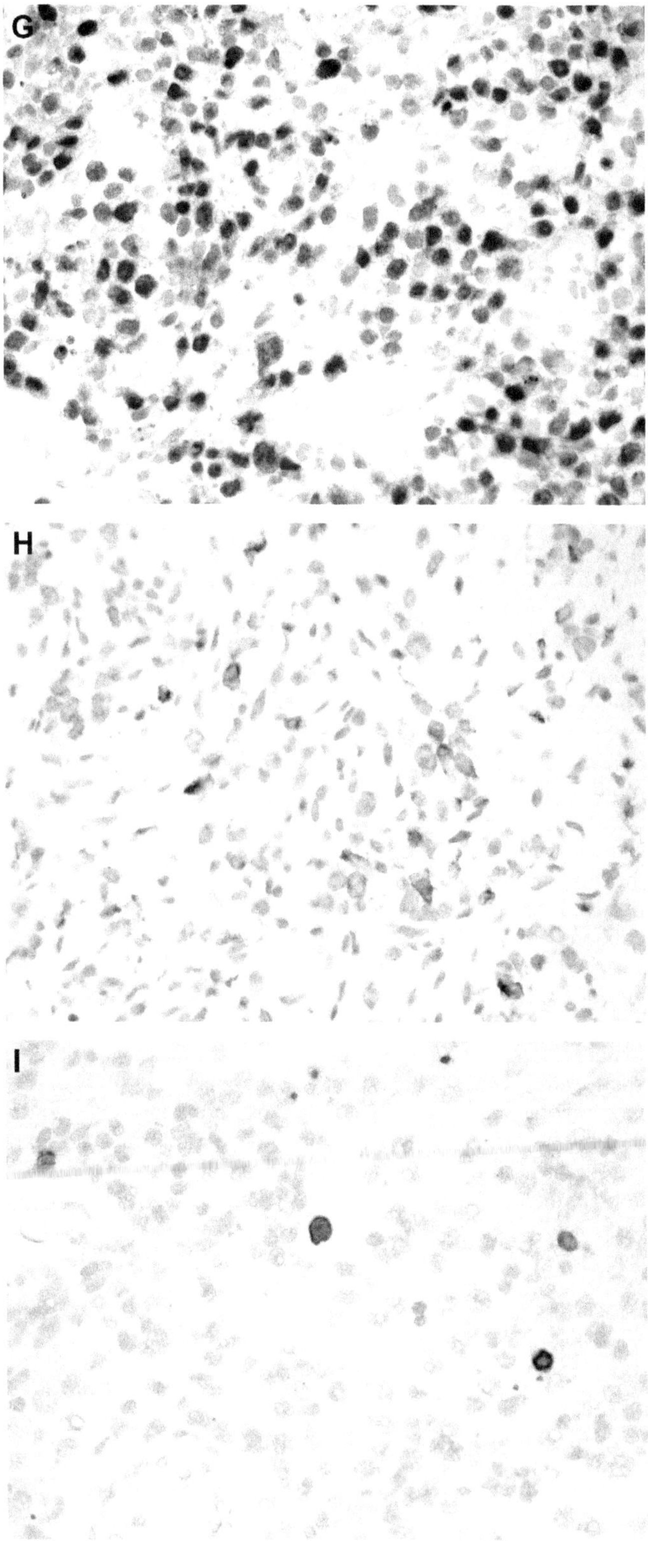

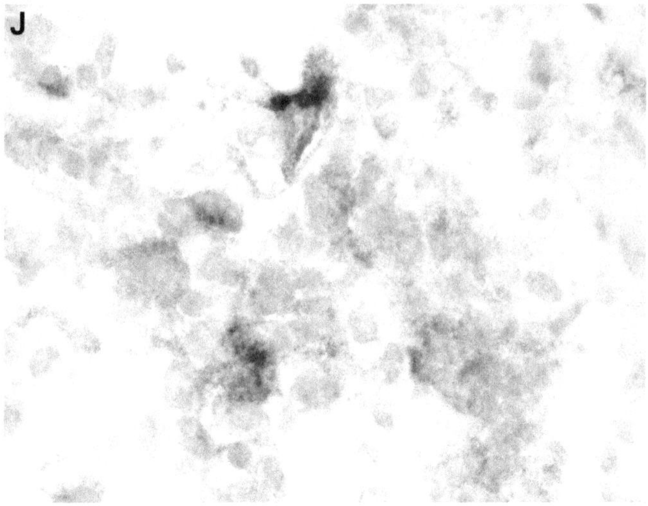

Fig. 5. (*J*) CD30 shows focal weak staining of large cells, and CD15 was negative (not shown).

diagnosis of MGZL, as this is a well established feature in a subset of CHL.[2]

By contrast, the diagnosis of MGZL should be considered in 2 broad scenarios. In the more common scenario, seen in about three-quarters of cases, the morphology is large cell lymphoma-like or PMBL-like with sheeting of large cells, but the immunophenotype is more like CHL with loss of CD20, diminished staining for other pan–B-cell antigens, and expression of markers seen on Hodgkin/Reed-Sternberg cells, such as CD30 and/or CD15 (**Fig. 5**). Despite the numerous large cells, such cases may contain other morphologic features reminiscent of nodular sclerosis CHL, such as fibrous bands and lacunar cell morphology (see **Fig. 5**A, C). In the less common scenario, seen in the remaining one-quarter of cases, the morphology is more CHL-like with scattered large atypical cells, but there is greater-than-expected retention of the B-cell program with expression of multiple B-cell antigens, including strong CD20 expression, retained expression of both OCT2 and BOB1, and expression of pan–B-cell stains not typically expressed by CHL, such as CD19 and/or CD79a (**Fig. 6**).[18]

NODULAR LYMPHOCYTE-PREDOMINANT HODGKIN LYMPHOMA AND ITS DIFFERENTIAL DIAGNOSIS

NLPHL differs from the nodular sclerosis and mixed cellularity subtypes of CHL in several ways, beginning with its clinical presentation: it is characterized by a male predominance with a higher median age of presentation. Although all age groups may be affected, most patients are diagnosed in the fifth decade. NLPHL typically presents with localized disease involving peripheral lymph nodes, such as the cervical, axillary, and inguinal regions; mediastinal, abdominal, or retroperitoneal disease is relatively uncommon. The clinical course is indolent with good therapeutic responses; however, some patients may have late relapses more than 5 years following their original diagnosis, or rarely, in less than 5% of cases, may progress to large B-cell lymphoma.[19]

From a histologic standpoint, NLPHL is characterized by few neoplastic Hodgkin/Reed-Sternberg variant cells, termed lymphocyte-predominant cells, in a background of reactive small B cells, T-follicular helper cells, and follicular dendritic cells, indicating a relationship to B-cell follicles. There are several immunoarchitectural variants described based on differences in the distribution of lymphocyte-predominant cells and overall pattern and composition of background immune cells; these patterns are important to recognize because they relate to prognosis.[20] The most common pattern is the classic B-cell–rich nodular pattern, also known as pattern A, characterized by expanded, back-to-back follicles composed of an admixture of small lymphocytes, follicular dendritic cells, histiocytes, and scattered large atypical lymphocyte-predominant cells that often give the nodules a moth-eaten appearance at low power (**Fig. 7**A, B). Cytologically, the lymphocyte-predominant cells are large with irregular,

Fig. 6. MGZL, Hodgkin lymphoma-like morphology with abnormal retention of B-cell program. (*A*) Low magnification shows complete nodal architectural effacement by an atypical lymphohistiocytic infiltrate (H&E, 100x). (*B–E*) High magnification shows scattered large atypical mononuclear cells with Hodgkin-like features, including irregular nuclear membranes, prominent eosinophilic nucleoli, para-nucleolar chromatin clearing (*B*, H&E, 400x). The large arypical cells show strong positivity for CD30 (*C*, 400x) and MUM1

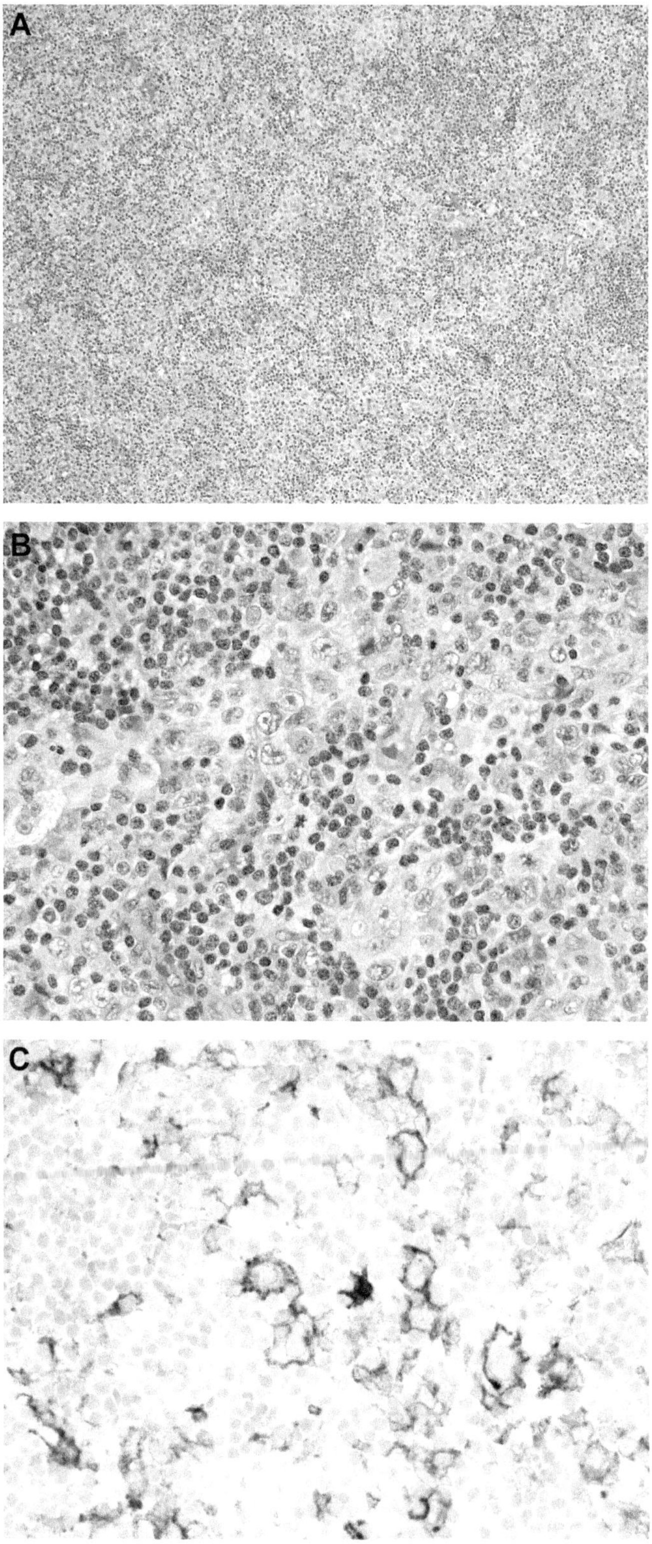

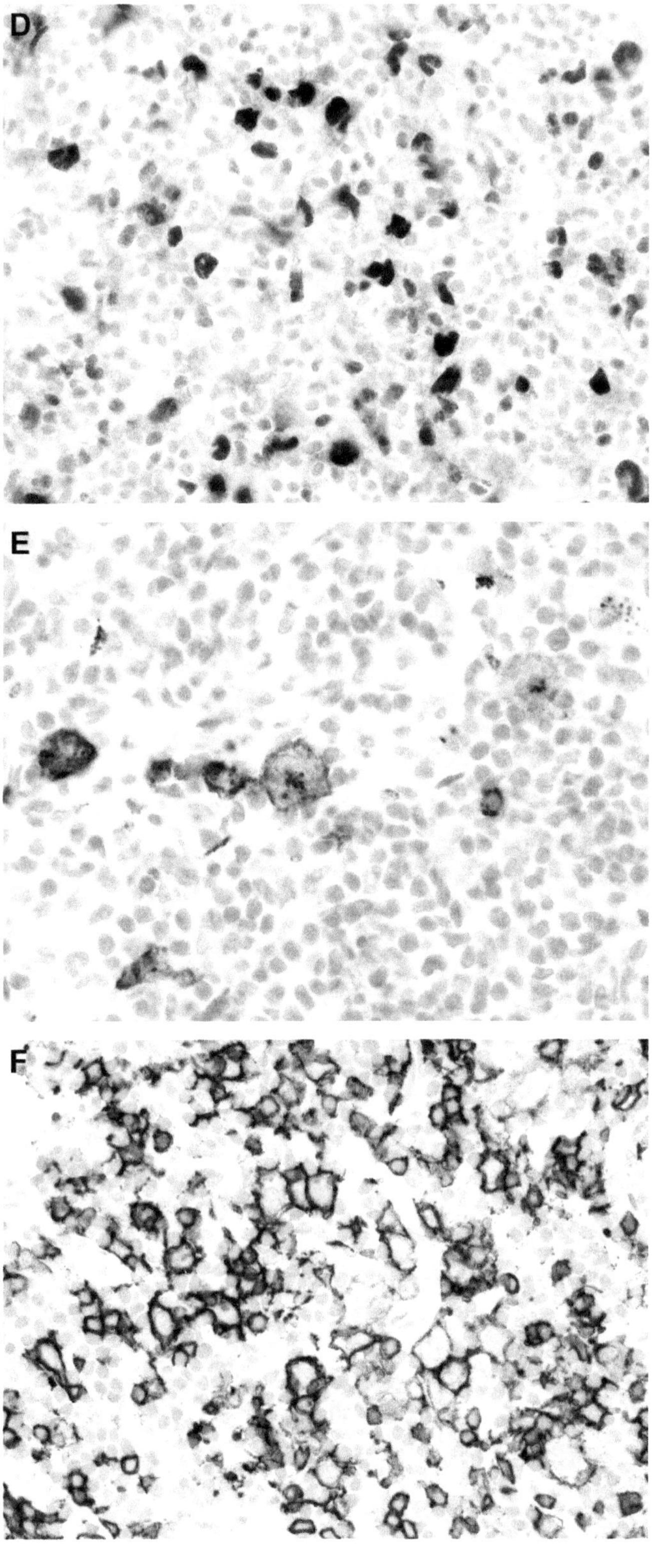

Fig. 6. (*D*) with focal expression of CD15 (*E*). (*F–J*) However, there is extensive staining for numerous B-cell markers, including CD20 (*F*),

Fig. 6. CD19 (*G*), OCT2 (*H*), and BOB1 (*I*),

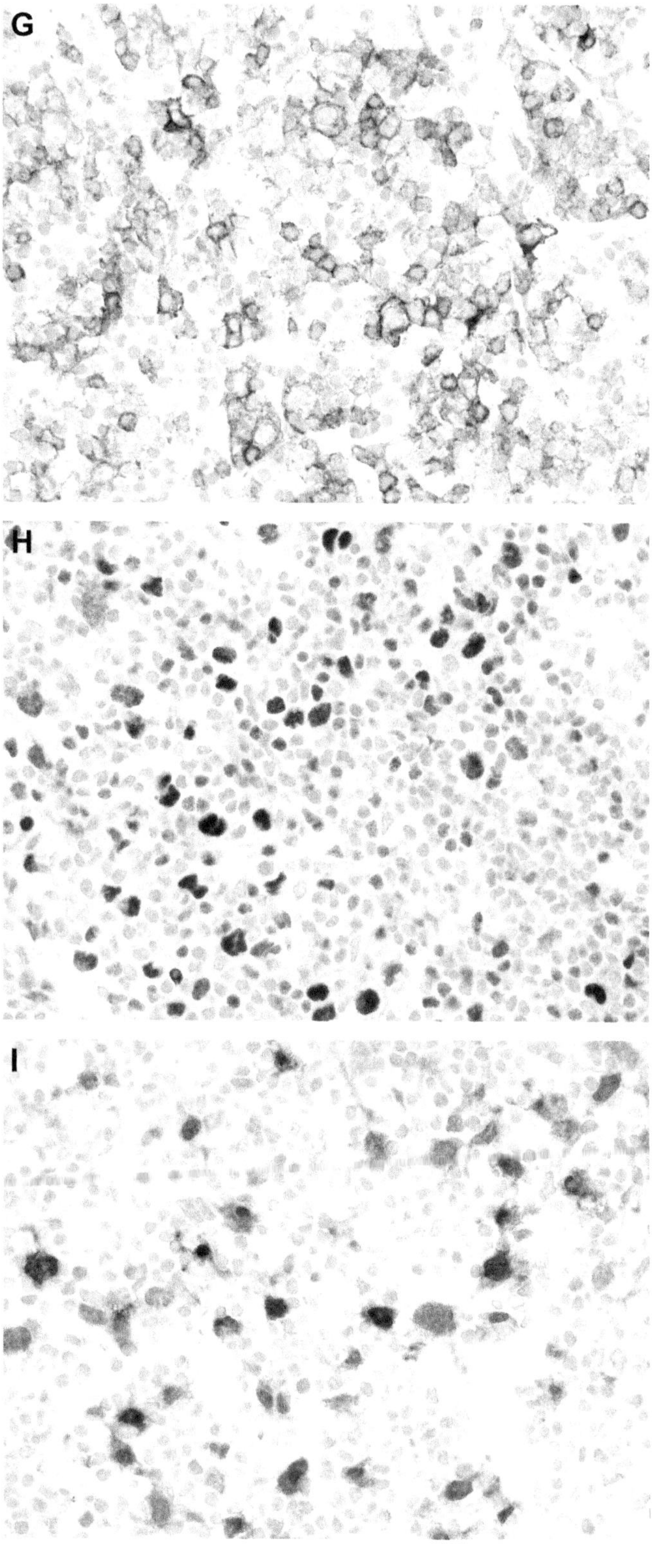

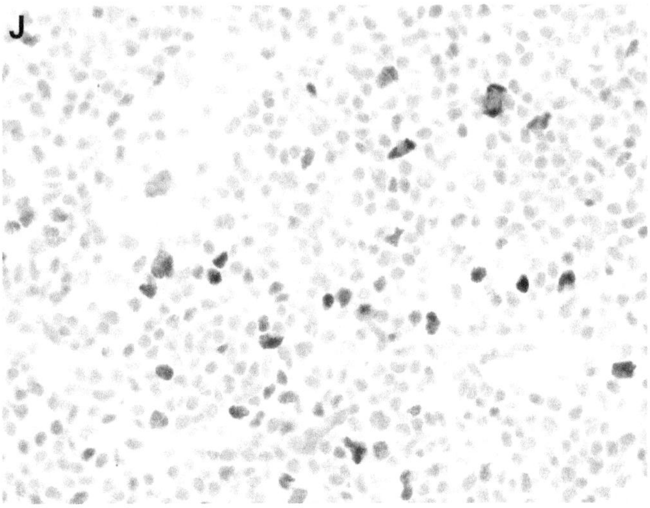

Fig. 6. and strong staining for BCL6 in a subset of cells (*J*).

multilobated nuclei, pale chromatin, one or more prominent nucleoli, and moderately abundant pale cytoplasm, a nuclear shape reminiscent of a popped kernel of corn; hence, "popcorn cell" is sometimes used to describe these cells (Fig. 7C, D). On immunohistochemical analysis, the atypical nodules are characterized by expanded follicular dendritic cell meshworks that are best highlighted with antibody to CD21 (Fig. 7E). Within the individual nodules, both the large lymphocyte-predominant cells and small B cells typically express the full B-cell program, including CD20, PAX5, and OCT2; PAX5 is usually expressed at a level comparable to that of small B cells, whereas OCT2 is typically quite strong on lymphocyte-predominant cells (Fig. 7F–H); the latter stain can be helpful in supporting the diagnosis in cases with diminished staining for CD20 and other pan–B-cell markers.[19,21] The small B cells are positive for CD23 and IgD, indicative of mantle zone B cells that have permeated the preexisting follicle structure. CD30 and CD15 are typically negative on lymphocyte-predominant cells, with positivity for these markers only infrequently reported.[22,23] The neoplastic cells are typically positive for BCL6, indicative of germinal center B-cell derivation, and are often surrounded by rosettes of T-follicular helper cells, themselves positive for BCL6 or other T-follicular helper cell antigens, such as CD57, PD1, or ICOS (Fig. 7I–K).[19] When subject to flow cytometric analysis, about half of NLPHL cases are found to contain $CD4^{+}$/CD8dim double-positive T cells, a reactive T-cell subset with preserved pan–T-cell antigen expression that has been shown to be negative for TdT and CD1a with polyclonal T-cell receptor gene rearrangement (Fig. 7L).[24,25]

In addition to the classic B-cell–rich nodular pattern (pattern A), 5 additional variant patterns have been described in NLPHL, designated patterns B through F. These patterns are best identified by routine evaluation of hematoxylin-and-eosin–stained (H&E) slides combined with key immunohistochemical markers, namely CD20 for lymphocyte-predominant cells and CD21 or an alternate follicular dendritic cell marker to highlight this background immune cell component. The serpiginous/interconnected pattern (pattern B) is similar to pattern A, but instead of forming discrete nodules, the B-cell–rich areas are coalescent (see Fig. 7E). In pattern C (prominent extranodular lymphocyte-predominant cells), the neoplastic cells are found in increased numbers outside of B-cell–rich nodules (see Fig. 7G). Both patterns D and E are T-cell–rich patterns, rather than B-cell–rich patterns, with pattern D being T-cell–rich nodular (with discernible follicular dendritic cell meshworks by immunohistochemistry) and pattern E being T-cell-rich diffuse or T-cell/histiocyte-rich large B-cell lymphoma (THRLBCL)-like and lacking a background follicular dendritic cell component. Pattern F is the rarest of the 6 patterns and is a diffuse B-cell–rich pattern devoid of background follicular dendritic cells. In large descriptive studies of NLPHL, most cases typically exhibit pattern A, the classic B-cell–rich nodular pattern, as a pure or

Table 2
Differentiating nodular lymphocyte-predominant Hodgkin lymphoma from its mimics

Feature	NLPHL	PTGC	THRLBCL	Lymphocyte-Rich CHL	Nodal TFH Cell Lymphoma
Age, sex	30s–50s, M > F 2.5–3:1	Children and young adults, M > F	Middle-aged or elderly, M > F	30s–50s, M > F 2:1	Middle-aged or elderly, M > F
Localization	Peripheral lymph nodes; mediastinal disease uncommon	Peripheral lymph nodes, typically single site, cervical/axillary most common	Widespread lymphadenopathy; spleen, BM, retroperitoneum often involved	Commonly involves peripheral lymph nodes; mediastinal and bulky disease uncommon	Widespread lymphadenopathy, B symptoms, skin rash
Architecture	Nodular (at least in part) and diffuse	Nodular	Diffuse	Nodular (common) and diffuse (rare)	Vaguely nodular
Background cellularity	Lymphocytes and histiocytes, FDCs at least focally, TFH rosettes, $CD4^+$/CD8dim T cells	Mantle zone B cells, FDCs, adjacent reactive follicles, scattered TFH cells, $CD4^+$/CD8dim T cells, $IgG4^+$ plasma cells	Lymphocytes and histiocytes, no FDCs	Lymphocytes, fewer histiocytes, small germinal centers may be present	Prominent vessels, expanded FDCs encompassing atypical T cells, focal mixed inflammation
Neoplastic cell phenotype	CD20/CD79a/$PAX5^-$, strong OCT2, $BCL6^+$, $CD30^-$, $CD15^-$	N/A; residual centroblasts have B-cell phenotype, $BCL6^+$, but lack cytologic atypia	CD20/$PAX5^+$, $BCL6^+$, $CD30^-$, $CD15^-$	$CD30^+$, $CD15^{+/-}$, PAX5 weak, OCT2/BOB1 loss, $CD20^{-/+}$	Surface CD3dim/–, $CD4^+$, TFH phenotype (positive for CD10, BCL6, PD1, ICOS, CXCL13)
EBV association	Very rare in LP cells; EBV^+ bystander cells	Negative; may have EBV^+ bystander cells	Negative (positive cases classified as EBV^+ DLBCL NOS)	Intermediate between nodular sclerosis and mixed cellularity subtypes (25%–40% of cases)	Large B cells may be EBV-positive (AITL) or EBV-negative (follicular type or NOS)

Abbreviations: AITL, angioimmunoblastic T-cell lymphoma; BM, bone marrow; FDCs, follicular dendritic cells; N/A, not applicable; TFH, T-follicular helper.

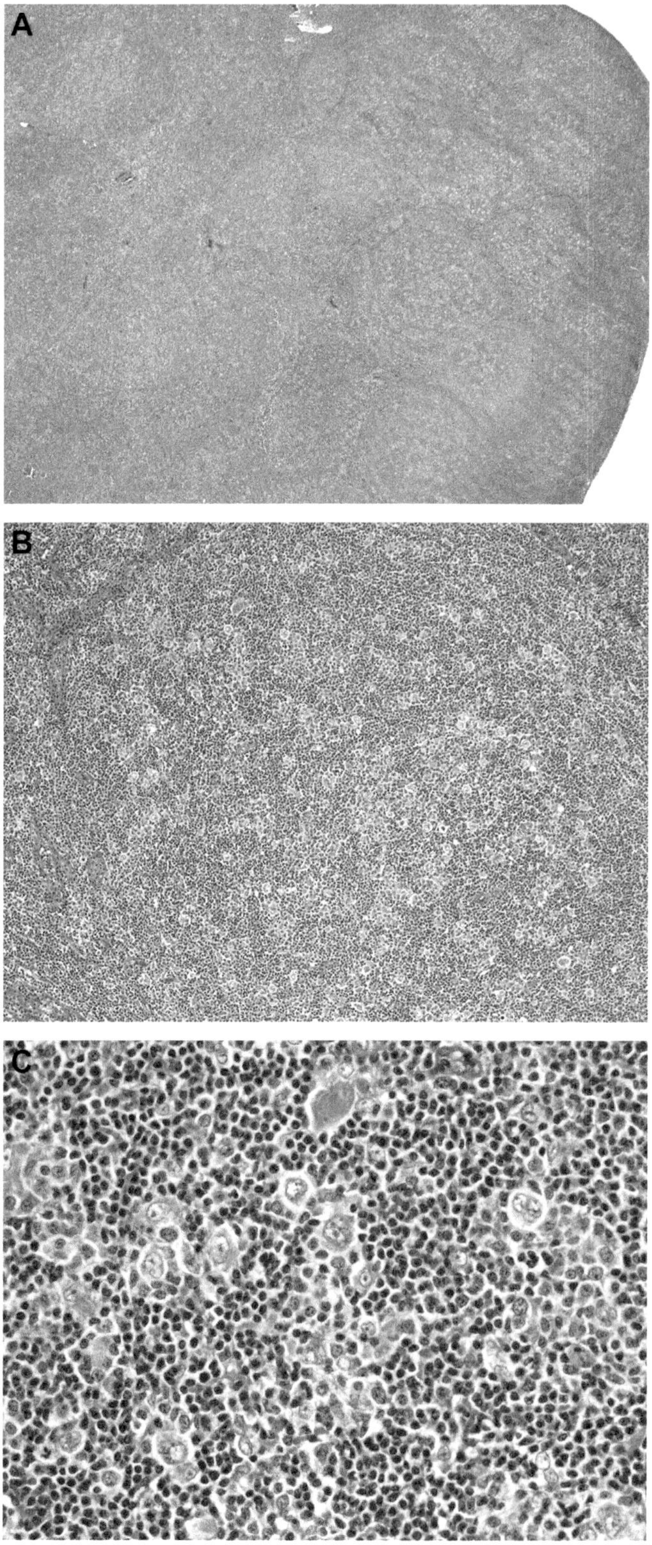

Fig. 7. Nodular lymphocyte-predominant Hodgkin lymphoma. (*A, B*) Low magnification of the classic B-cell–rich nodular pattern (pattern A) of NLPHL shows architectural effacement by expanded round or oval nodules that contain a predominance of small lymphocytes and scattered paler-staining follicular dendritic cells, histiocytes, and lymphocyte-predominant cells, yielding a so-called moth-eaten appearance on H&E-stained sections (*A*, 20x; *B*, 200x).

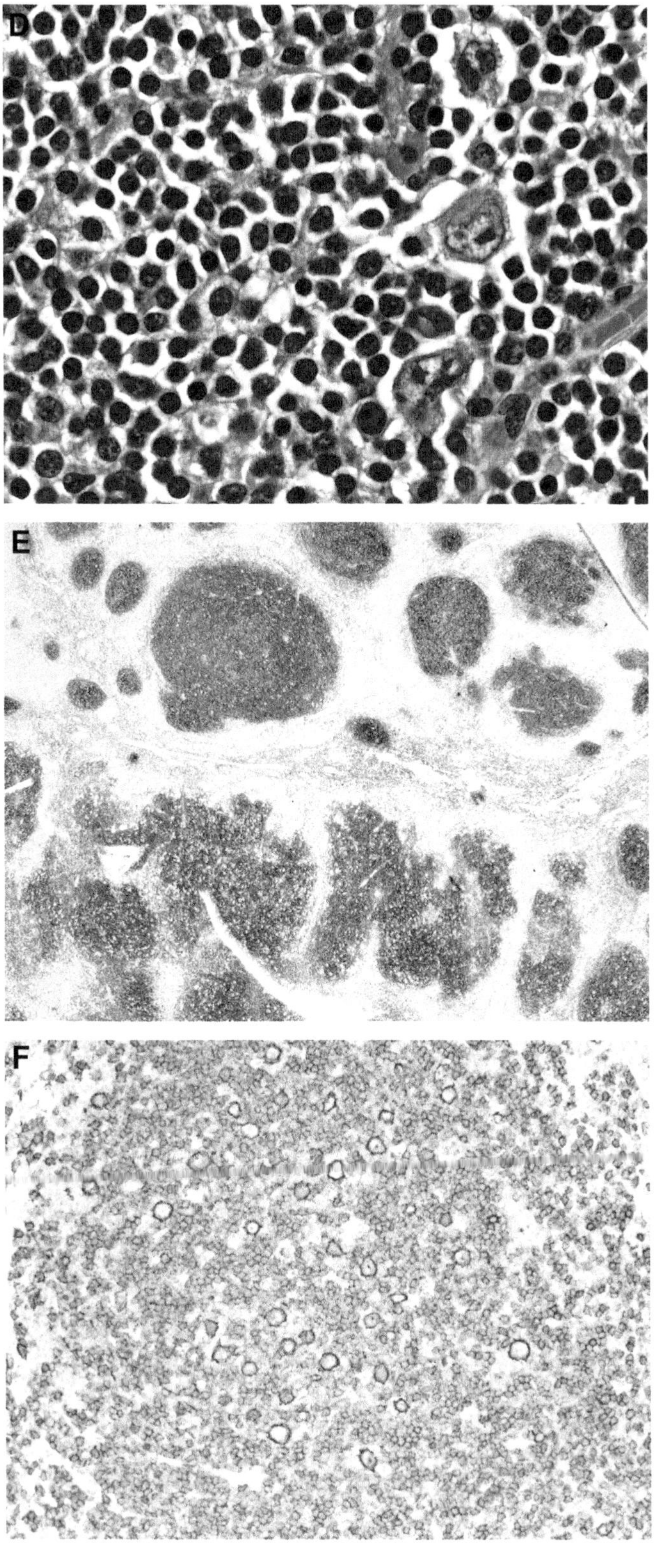

Fig. 7. (*C, D*) On higher magnification, the large lymphocyte-predominant cells contain irregular to multilobated nuclei, prominent nucleoli surrounded by pale chromatin, and moderately abundant cytoplasm; the nuclear shape is sometimes reminiscent of popcorn. (*E*) CD21 highlights expanded follicular dendritic cell aggregates encompassing the abnormal enlarged follicles. Note that this image shows both pattern A nodules (*top*) and serpiginous/interconnected nodules characteristic of pattern B (*bottom*). (*F, G*) The large lymphocyte-predominant cells are strongly and uniformly positive for CD20 and are present in a background of nodules rich in small B cells, representing mantle zone B cells that have infiltrated the preexisting follicle. Shown are examples of pattern A (*F*)

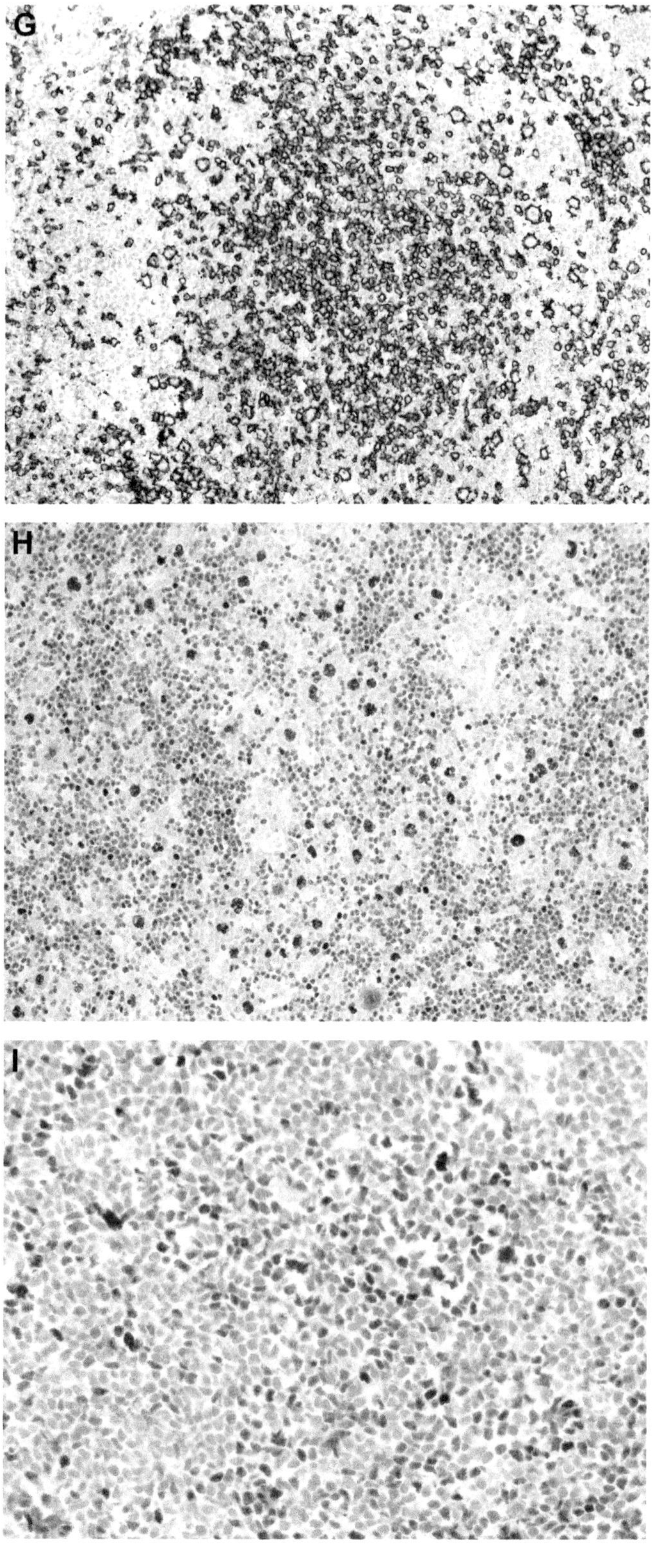

Fig. 7. and pattern C with prominent extranodular lymphocyte-predominant cells (*G*). (*H*) The lymphocyte-predominant cells characteristically show strong expression of OCT2 compared with background small mantle zone B cells. (*I*) BCL6 is expressed by both lymphocyte-predominant cells, indicating their germinal center derivation, as well as surrounding small T cells, reflecting their T-follicular helper cell phenotype.

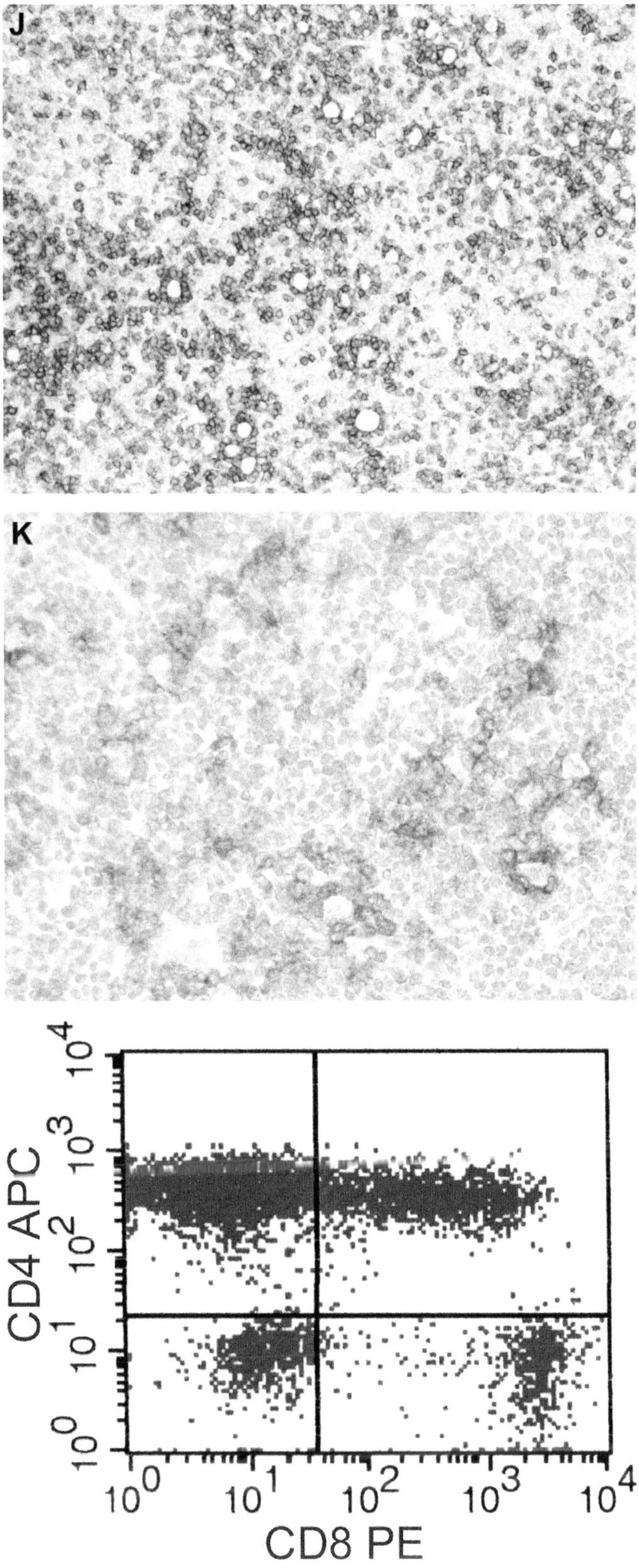

Fig. 7. (*J, K*) The T cells coexpress PD1 (*J*) and ICOS (*K*) and form conspicuous rosettes around the negatively stained lymphocyte-predominant cells. (*L*) A double-positive T-cell population coexpressing CD4 and dim CD8 may be seen in about half of cases of NLPHL by flow cytometry (*upper right quadrant*, CD4 versus CD8 gated on lymphocytes based on CD45 and side scatter plots not shown).

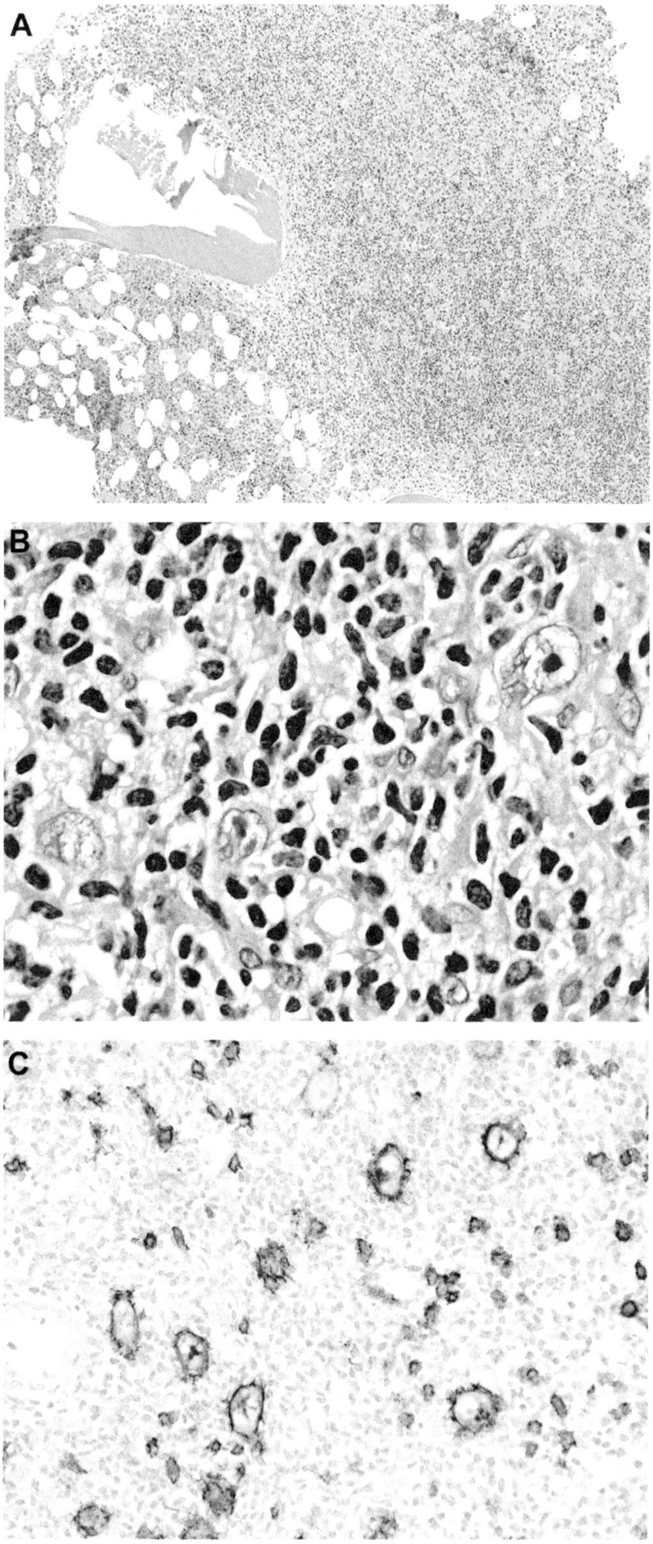

Fig. 8. Transformation of NLPHL to large B-cell lymphoma showing varying histology at different sites. (*A*) In this example of NLPHL with bone marrow involvement, there are large lymphoid aggregates partially replacing the marrow seen on low magnification (H&E, 40x). (*B*) On high magnification, the aggregates are composed of mostly small, mature lymphocytes with scattered large, atypical cells with multilobated nuclei, prominent nucleoli, and pale chromatin, consistent with lymphocyte-predominant cells (H&E, 1000x). (*C*) The large atypical cells are strongly positive for CD20; note the presence of scattered small B cells in the background, which would be unusual for de novo THRLBCL (400x).

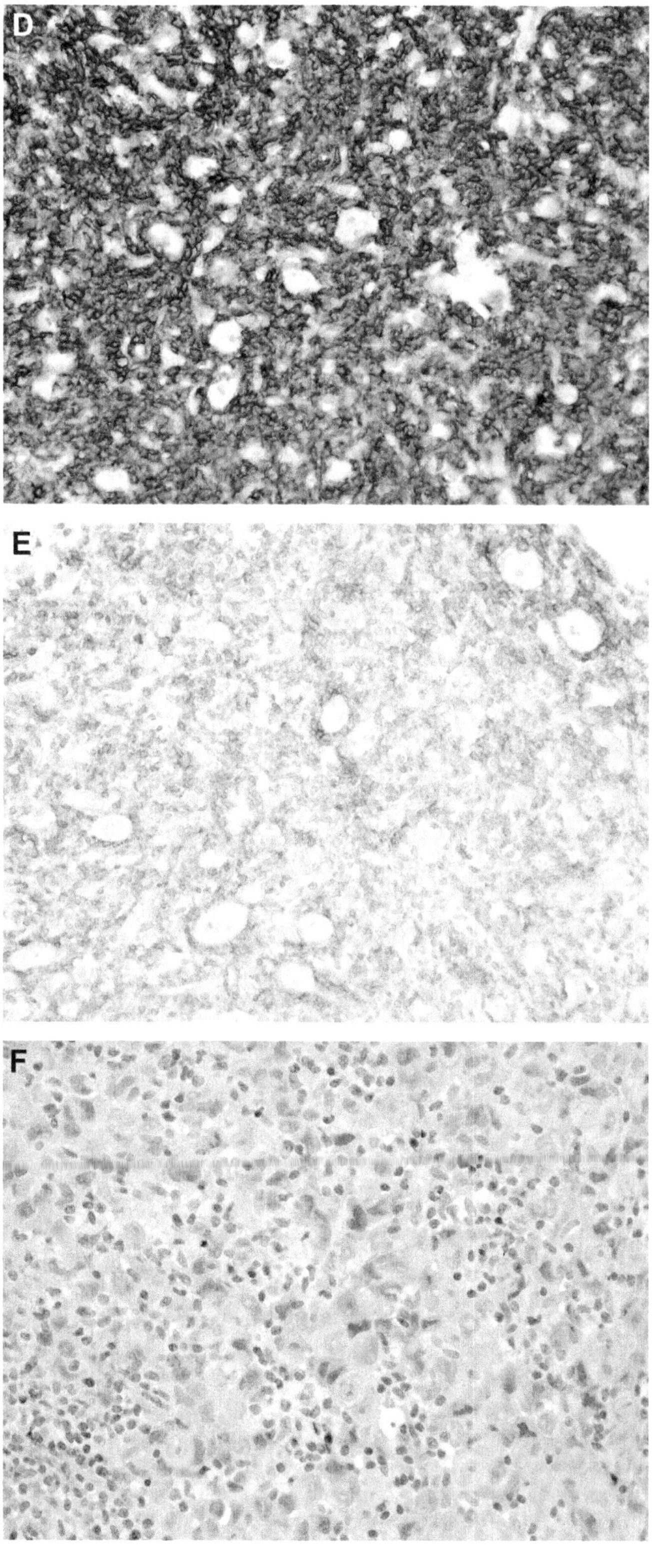

Fig. 8. (*D*) Most of the background small lymphocytes are CD3-positive T cells. (*E*) The T cells show significant coexpression of PD1 with prominent rosetting of the large cells, features that would also be unusual in de novo THRLBCL. In a patient with a history of NLPHL, these features are diagnostic of progression to large B-cell lymphoma in the form of THRLBCL. (*F*) Biopsy of an abdominal mass taken 1 week later from the same patient demonstrates a predominance of large atypical cells with irregular to multilobated nuclei and prominent nucleoli.

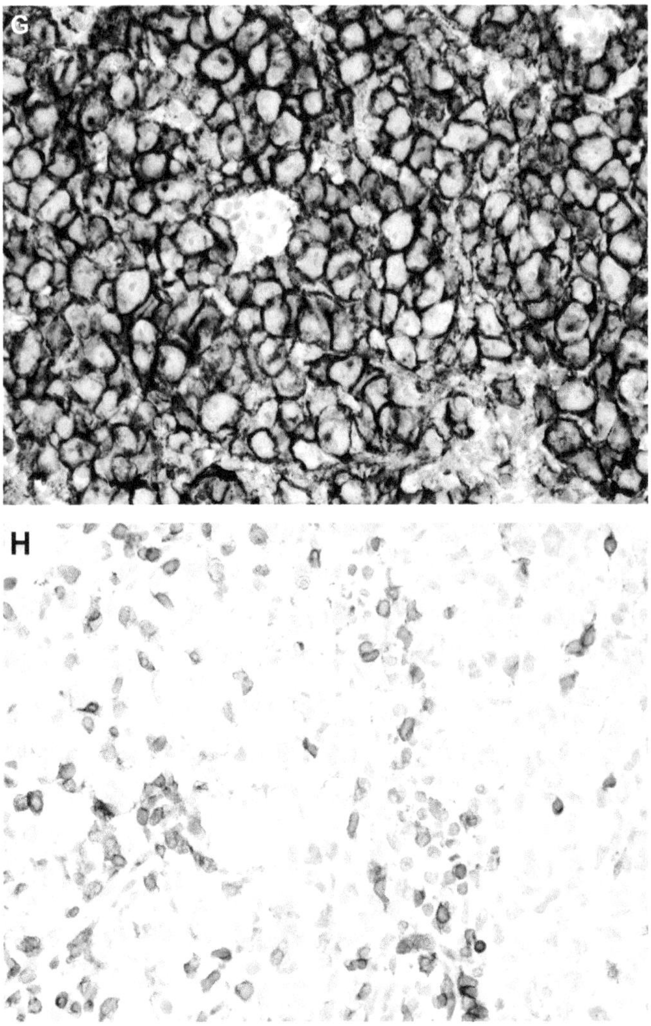

Fig. 8. (*G, H*) The large cells are diffusely positive for CD20 (*G*) with few background CD3-positive T cells (*H*), findings diagnostic of transformation to large B-cell lymphoma resembling conventional DLBCL.

predominant pattern with one or more of patterns B through F as a minor component, although occasionally one of these latter patterns predominates.[20]

Among these immunoarchitectural variants, patterns C, D, and E are all characterized by the presence of lymphocyte-predominant cells in a T-cell–rich background and have been variably associated with more advanced disease, a higher risk of recurrence, and a higher risk of progression to DLBCL, and their presence, even if a minor component, should be mentioned in the pathology report.[20] Importantly, pattern E, the T-cell–rich diffuse or THRLBCL-like pattern, needs to be distinguished from de novo THRLBCL by the presence of at least a focal B-cell–rich or nodular component, which might not always be discernible in a core biopsy or limited specimen (**Table 2**). Furthermore, identification of pure pattern E in a patient with a prior history of NLPHL is diagnostic of progression to THRLBCL (**Fig. 8**A–E).[4,17] Immunohistochemistry is of limited utility in this differential diagnosis as pattern E of NLPHL, de novo THRLBCL, and THRLBCL progression from NLPHL by definition all lack background follicular dendritic meshworks, may contain a paucity of small B cells, and may show variable staining in terms of T-cell subsets and T-follicular helper cell or histiocytic components. The large neoplastic B cells of de novo THRLBCL may have a lymphocyte-predominant or Hodgkin/Reed-Sternberg-like morphology or may resemble more conventional centroblasts or immunoblasts; however, their immunophenotype, including

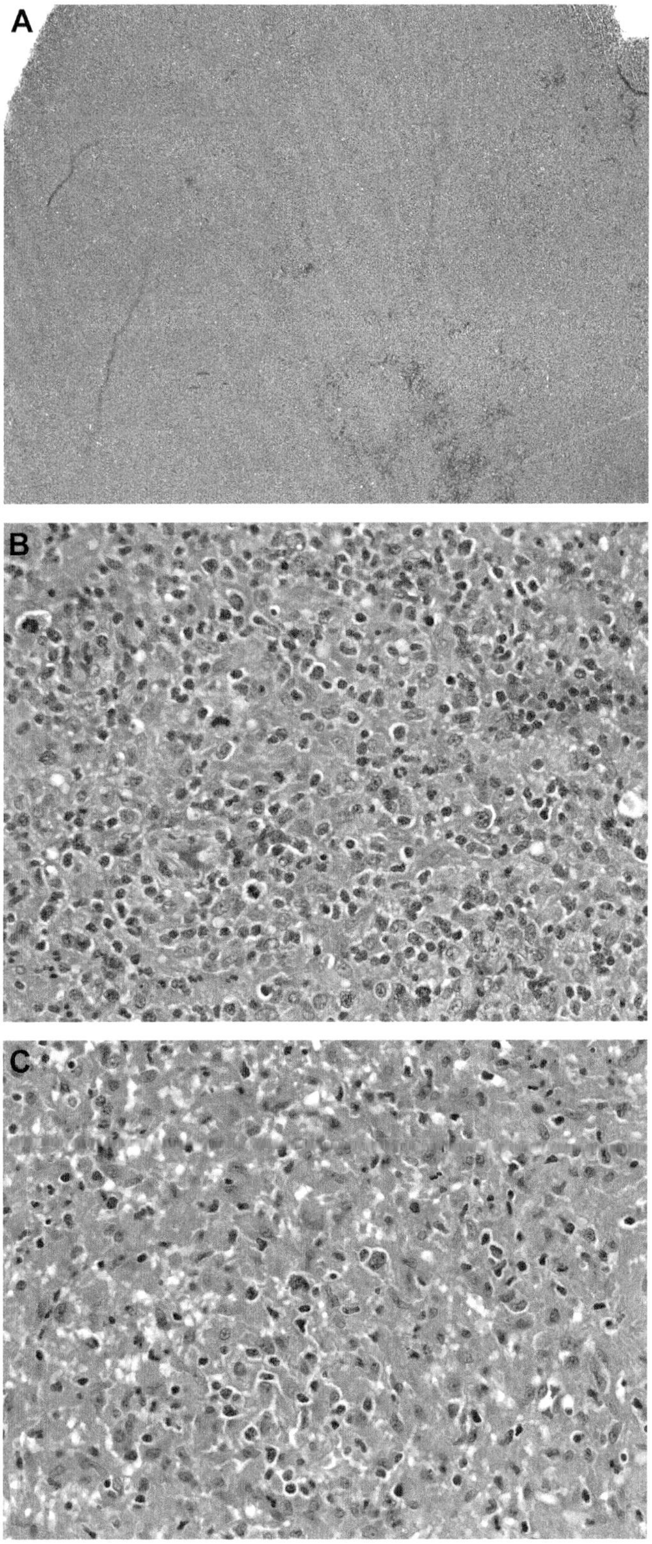

Fig. 9. T-cell/histiocyte-rich large B-cell lymphoma. (*A*) On low magnification, the lymph node architecture is completely effaced by a diffuse lympho-histiocytic infiltrate without any discernible nodularity (H&E, 20x). (*B, C*) Scattered large atypical cells are present in a predominant background composed of an admixture of nonneoplastic small lymphocytes and histiocytes (H&E, 200x); the latter are relatively abundant compared with NLPHL and predominate in some areas (*C*).

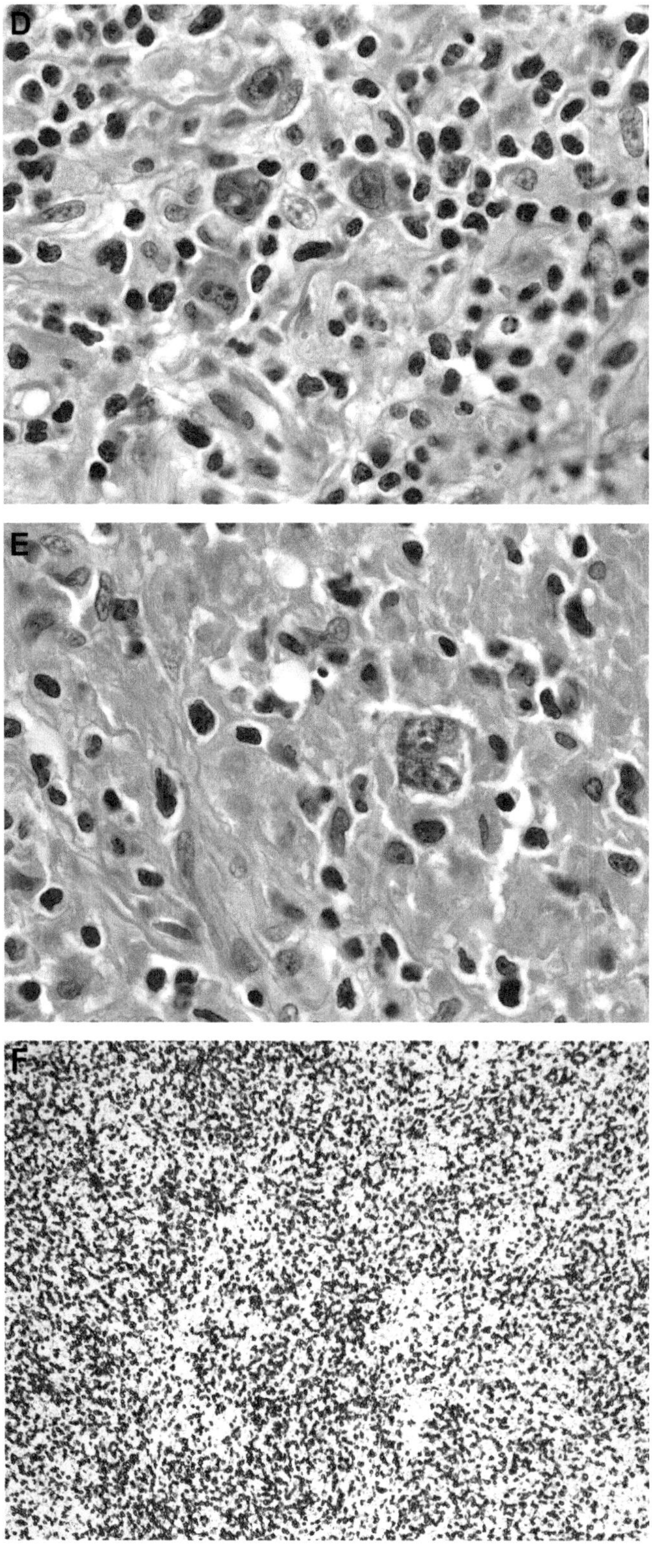

Fig. 9. (*D, E*) On high magnification, the large neoplastic cells may resemble centroblasts or immunoblasts, or have more variable morphology with irregular nuclei or binucleation reminiscent of lymphocyte-predominant cells or Hodgkin/Reed-Sternberg cells. (*F*). CD3 stains numerous background T cells.

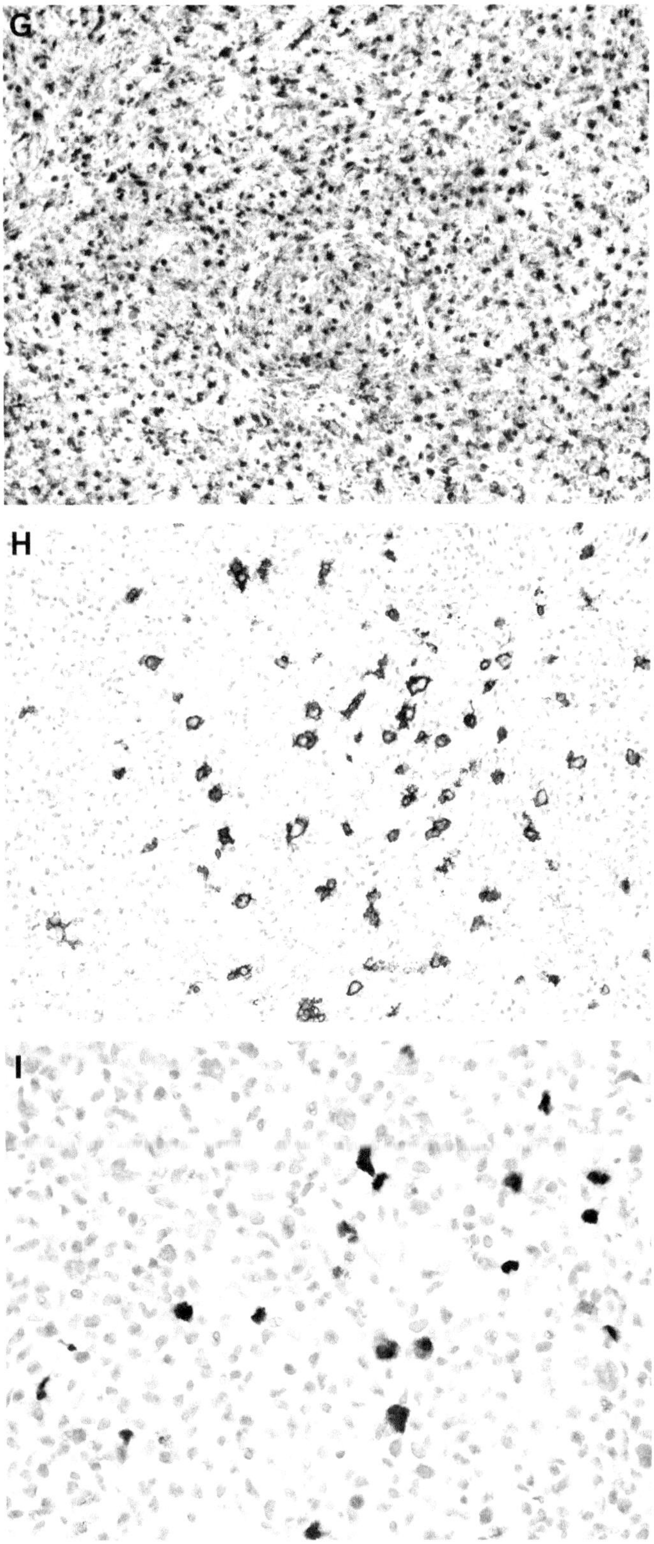

Fig. 9. (*G*) CD68 is positive in frequent background histiocytes. (*H–J*) The large neoplastic cells are positive for CD20 (*H*), PAX5 (*I*),

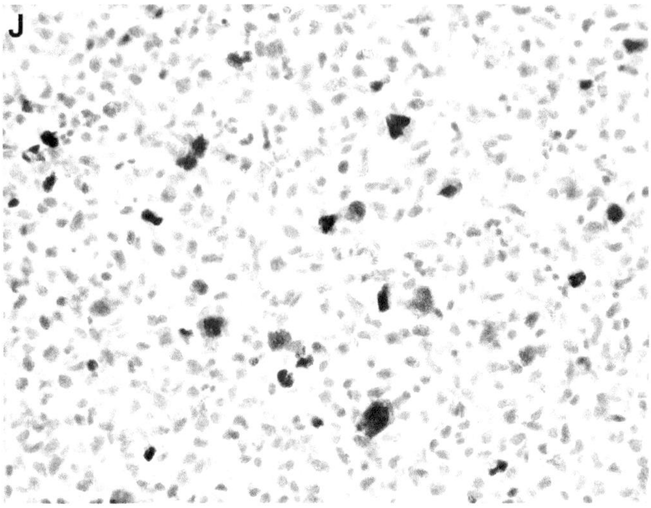

Fig. 9. and BCL6 (*J*) and negative for CD30 and EBV by EBER staining (not shown). Similar morphologic features to those seen here may be seen as a pattern E component of NLPHL; such cases should have at least a focal B-cell–rich or nodular component by immunohistochemistry with a B-cell or follicular dendritic cell marker, respectively, in order to make the diagnosis of NLPHL harboring a variant T-cell–rich pattern. On the other hand, if similar features to those seen here were identified in a well-sampled biopsy from a patient with a history of NLPHL, the findings would be diagnostic of progression to THRLBCL (see Fig. 8A–E).

expression of CD20, PAX5, and BCL6 and absence of CD30, CD15, and EBV, is identical to the neoplastic cells of NLPHL (Fig. 9). Although most patients with de novo THRLBCL have advanced clinical presentations with involvement of the reticuloendothelial system, including the bone marrow, liver, and spleen, the same may be true with THRLBCL progression from NLPHL or rare cases of NLPHL with a predominant T-cell–rich background that presents with advanced-stage disease.[4,17] These issues underscore the challenges inherent in diagnosing NLPHL and some of the entities in its differential diagnosis on limited material and the need for extensive sampling of excisional biopsy or resection specimens for routine microscopic evaluation.[4] On the other hand, NLPHL progression to large B-cell lymphoma may also take the form of a tumor rich in large B cells resembling DLBCL-NOS; this form of transformation may be more straightforward to diagnose (Fig. 8F–H).

LYMPHOCYTE-RICH CLASSIC HODGKIN LYMPHOMA

Although T-cell–rich patterns of NLPHL may raise the differential diagnosis of THRLBCL, the conventional B-cell–rich nodular pattern more closely resembles the lymphocyte-rich subtype of CHL histologically, as both are centered on B-cell follicles (Fig. 10A–F). The 2 neoplasms also overlap terms of clinical features and sites of involvement (see Table 2). Immunohistochemistry is the mainstay technique used to distinguish between the 2, as the neoplastic cells of lymphocyte-rich CHL, as with other CHL subtypes, are positive for CD30 and CD15, show weak staining for PAX5, and exhibit variable loss of pan–B-cell markers (Fig. 10F–H). In lymphocyte-rich CHL, the neoplastic cells are often present at the periphery of expanded follicles in the mantle zone region.[26] Positivity for EBV in the neoplastic cells is also a helpful feature supporting a diagnosis of lymphocyte-rich CHL, but does not entirely exclude the possibility of NLPHL, as the finding of EBV-positive lymphocyte-predominant cells has been reported in rare cases of NLPHL originating from both high-income countries and low-/middle-income countries.[7,27] Although cases of EBV-positive NLPHL resemble typical NLPHL with strong expression of OCT2 and overall retention of a B-cell phenotype, they are reported to show a higher frequency of CD30 expression by lymphocyte-predominant cells.[28,29] Therefore, extensive immunophenotypic evaluation may be needed to establish the correct diagnosis in this unusual circumstance.

PROGRESSIVE TRANSFORMATION OF GERMINAL CENTERS

Another consideration in the differential diagnosis of NLPHL is an unusual pattern of reactive nodal hyperplasia known as progressive transformation

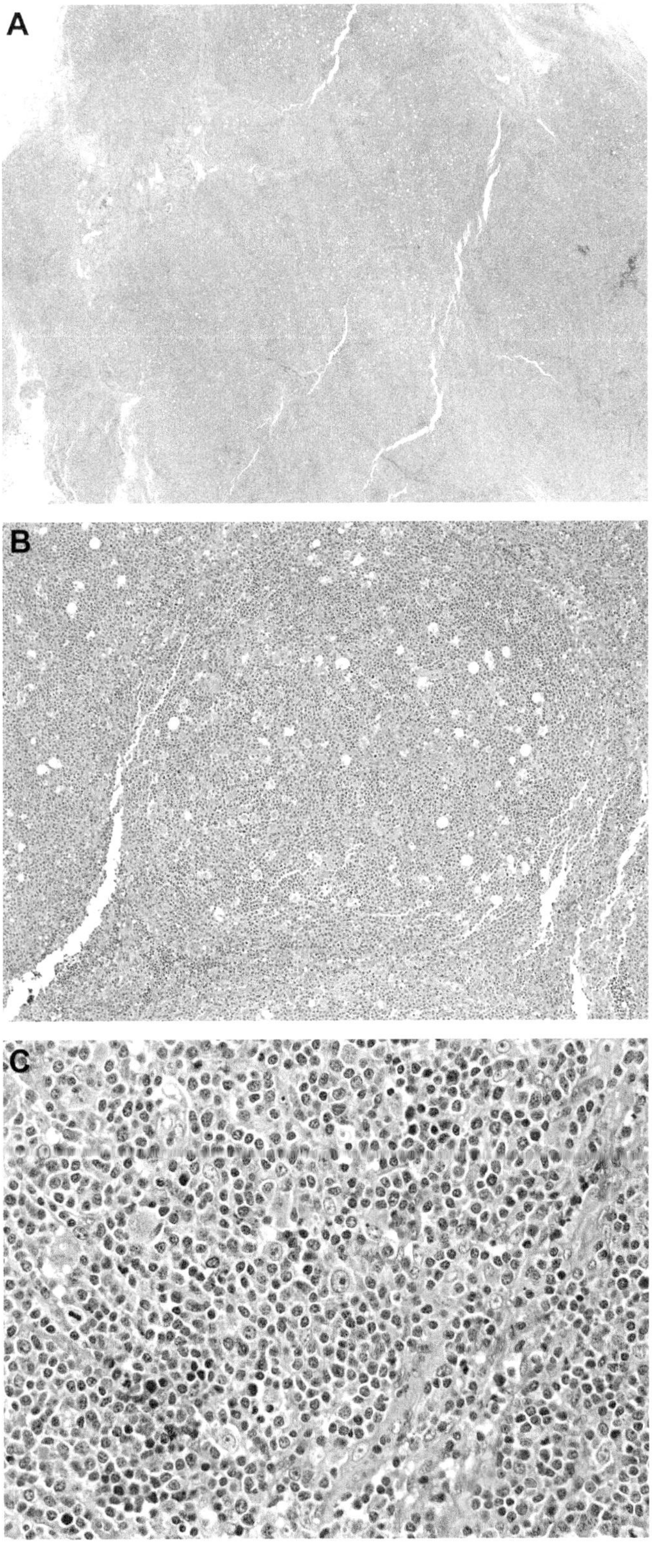

Fig. 10. Lymphocyte-rich CHL. (*A*) On low magnification, the lymph node architecture is effaced by a back-to-back nodular proliferation (H&E, 20x). (*B–D*) The nodules contain a predominance of mature-appearing small lymphocytes and scattered large atypical cells with prominent eosinophilic nuclei (*B*, H&E, 200x), including both mononuclear (*C*, 400x) and binucleate

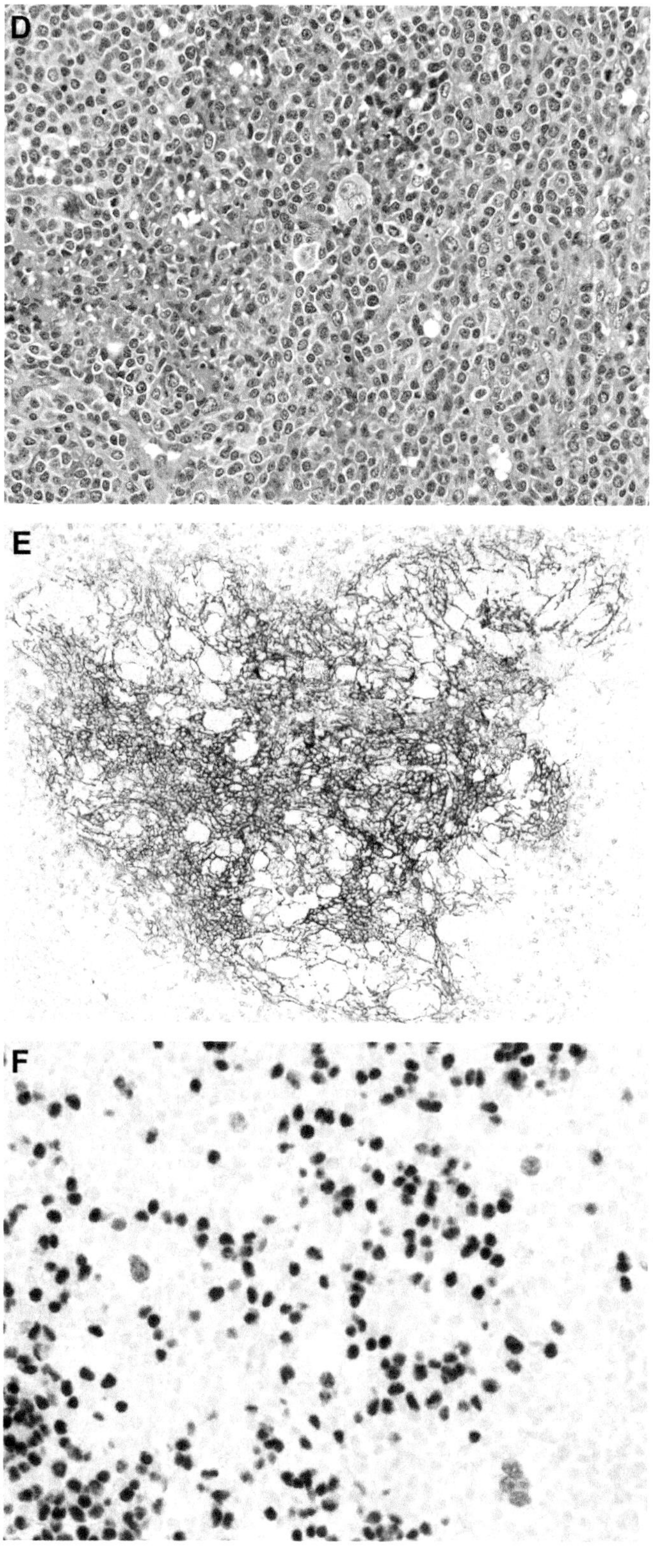

Fig. 10. (*D*) forms. (*E*) CD21 highlights expanded follicular dendritic cell meshworks, indicating that the atypical proliferation is centered on follicles. (*F*) The large, atypical cells are weakly positive for PAX5 and are present in a background containing loose clusters of small B cells with strong staining for PAX5, further supporting the presence of underlying B-cell follicles.

Fig. 10. (*G–H*) The large cells are positive for CD30 (*G*) and CD15 (*H*) and negative for CD20 (not shown), indicating a classic Hodgkin/Reed-Sternberg cell phenotype.

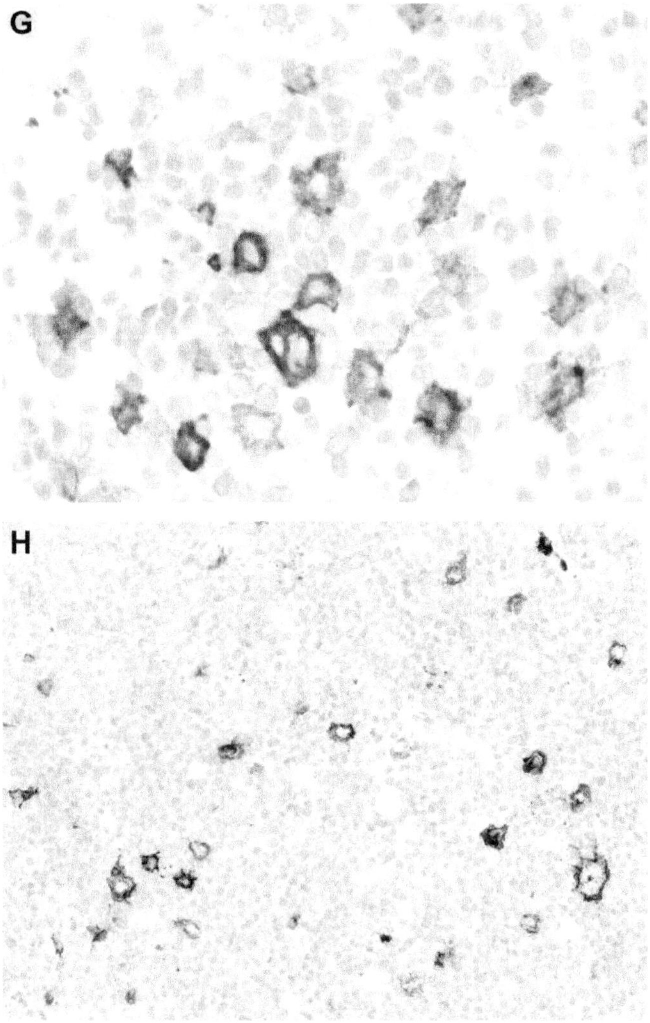

of germinal centers (PTGC). This pattern of reactive hyperplasia often coexists with reactive follicular hyperplasia; some cases of NLPHL may also contain areas of PTGC (Fig. 11A). The progressively transformed germinal centers are characterized by involution of mantle zone B cells with disruption of the germinal center and expansion of the B-cell follicle, which may be marked (Fig. 11B).

Given the overall nodular architecture and follicular expansion, PTGC may mimic NLPHL in cases in which this pattern of reactive hyperplasia predominates.[30] However, the expanded follicles of PTGC contain scattered centroblasts that lack the frank neoplastic appearance of lymphocyte-predominant cells, and T-follicular helper cell rosettes are less prominent (Fig. 11C, D). In addition, most cases of PTGC have at least a component of typical reactive follicles that are present in between the nodules of PTGC (see Fig. 11A). In contrast, NLPHL usually shows more overt nodal architectural effacement without admixed reactive follicles, which, if present, are located in a rim of normal lymph node outside of the area of NLPHL. In difficult cases of nodal architectural distortion with scattered centroblast-like cells demonstrating some cytologic atypia and without a reactive follicular component, it may be best to report

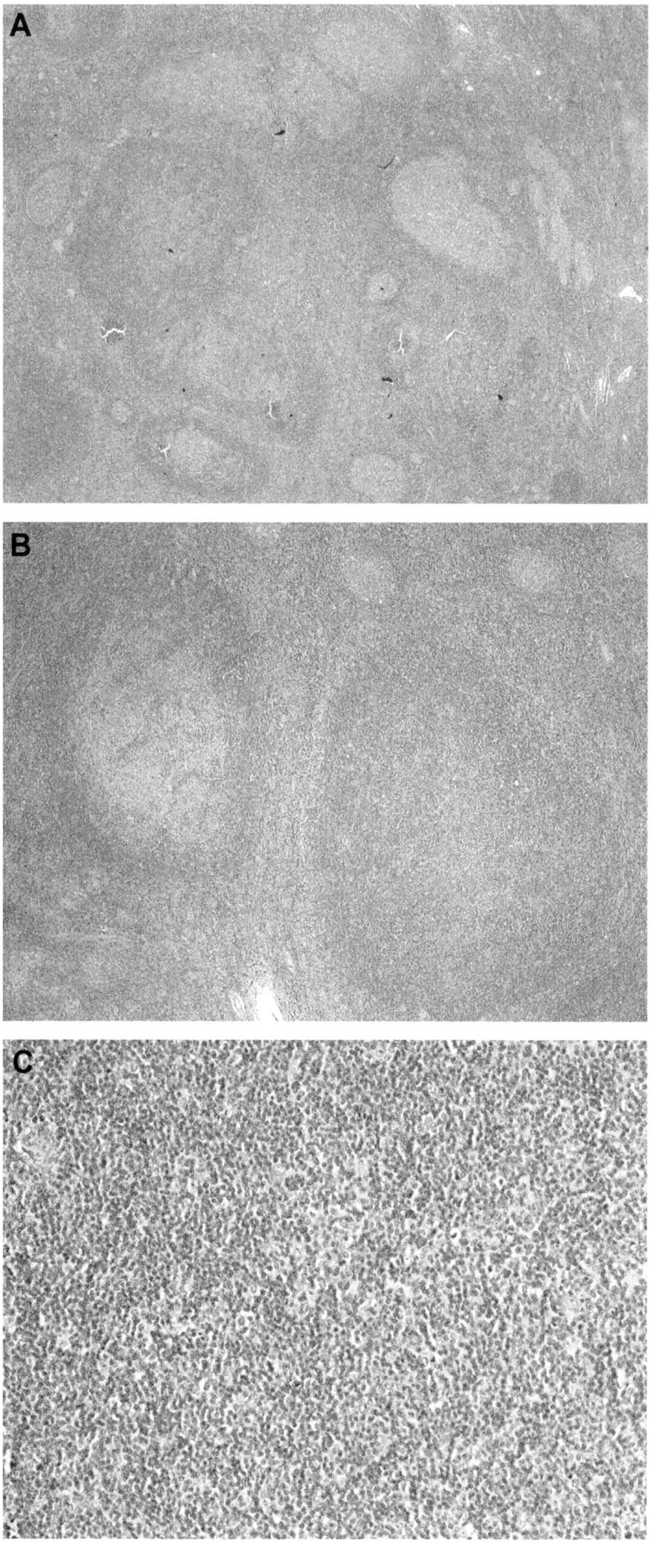

Fig. 11. PTGC. (*A*) On low magnification, the lymph node architecture is overall preserved but distorted by a proliferation of expanded reactive follicles consisting of intermingled typical hyperplastic germinal centers (*upper right*) and progressively transformed germinal centers (*lower left*) (H&E, 20x). (*B*) An intermediate magnification view shows 2 progressively transformed germinal centers at an earlier (*left*) and later (*right*) stage characterized by infiltration of the germinal center by mantle zone cells that disrupt and eventually replace the germinal center with resulting expansion of the follicle. Note the presence of adjacent small reactive follicles with typical hyperplastic germinal centers (H&E, 100x).

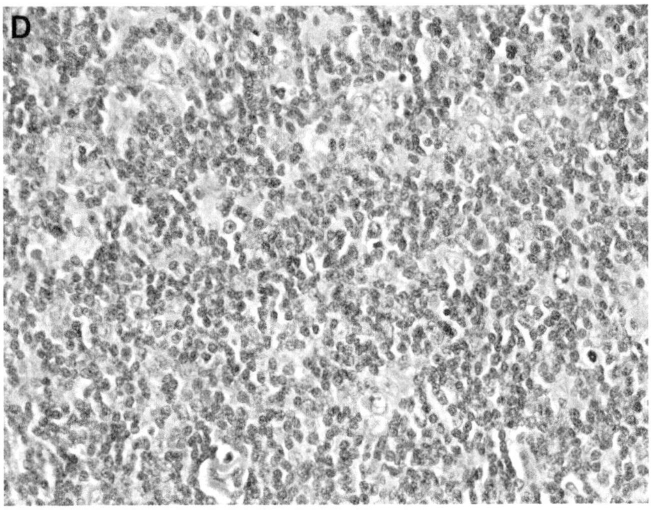

Fig. 11. (*C, D*) Higher magnification views show a predominance of small, mature-appearing lymphocytes, occasional histiocytic and follicular dendritic cells, and scattered centroblasts lacking cytologic atypia reminiscent of lymphocyte-predominant cells.

the issues of diagnostic uncertainty and state that early involvement by NLPHL cannot be entirely excluded. This will likely lead to complete excision of the area of atypical lymph node enlargement, which in certain patients with localized disease is considered adequate treatment for NLPHL, followed by close clinical follow-up for development of additional areas of nodal enlargement with subsequent biopsy.

Interestingly, some patients with NLPHL have metachronous nodal involvement by PTGC either preceding or following their diagnosis of NLPHL, and the $CD4^{+}$/CD8dim double-positive T-cell population detected by flow cytometry in NLPHL has also been reported, albeit less frequently, in PTGC but is rarely seen in CHL and other patterns of reactive lymphoid hyperplasia.[24,25] Although these findings may suggest a pathogenetic link between PTGC and NLPHL, not all patients with PTGC go on to develop NLPHL. Therefore, PTGC is not considered a precursor lesion to NLPHL but an unusual reactive hyperplasia that, if florid, is likely best managed by complete excision and close clinical follow-up, similar to other forms of atypical nodal hyperplasia.

NODULAR LYMPHOCYTE-PREDOMINANT HODGKIN LYMPHOMA WITH CYTOMORPHOLOGIC T-CELL ATYPIA

Another unusual finding in NLPHL with respect to T cells is that rare cases may show mild but conspicuous cytologic atypia of background T cells. This feature has been described mainly in cases with immunoarchitectural patterns showing increased numbers of extrafollicular lymphocyte-predominant cells (pattern C) or T-cell–rich backgrounds (patterns D and E), which are variably associated with more aggressive disease. The atypical T cells in these cases have slightly enlarged and/or irregular nuclei, more vesicular chromatin, and small nucleoli and exhibit increased mitotic activity (Fig. 12A–G). Despite these features, the T cells have preserved pan–T-cell antigen expression and lack clonal T-cell receptor gene rearrangements.[31] Affected patients are usually young men or boys, and in many of these cases, the lymphocyte-predominant cells express IgD, a feature also linked to younger age and male gender (Fig. 12H).[31,32] An emerging hypothesis is that NLPHL with IgD-positive lymphocyte-predominant cells may be precipitated by *Moraxella catarrhalis* bacterial infection followed by clonal transformation; this infectious trigger may explain the younger demographic and cytologic atypia in background T cells that presumably develops in the setting of an exuberant immune response in susceptible patients.[33,34]

NODAL T-FOLLICULAR HELPER CELL LYMPHOMA

Some cases of peripheral T-cell lymphoma may mimic NLPHL or lymphocyte-rich CHL. The T cells of such cases often harbor a T-follicular helper

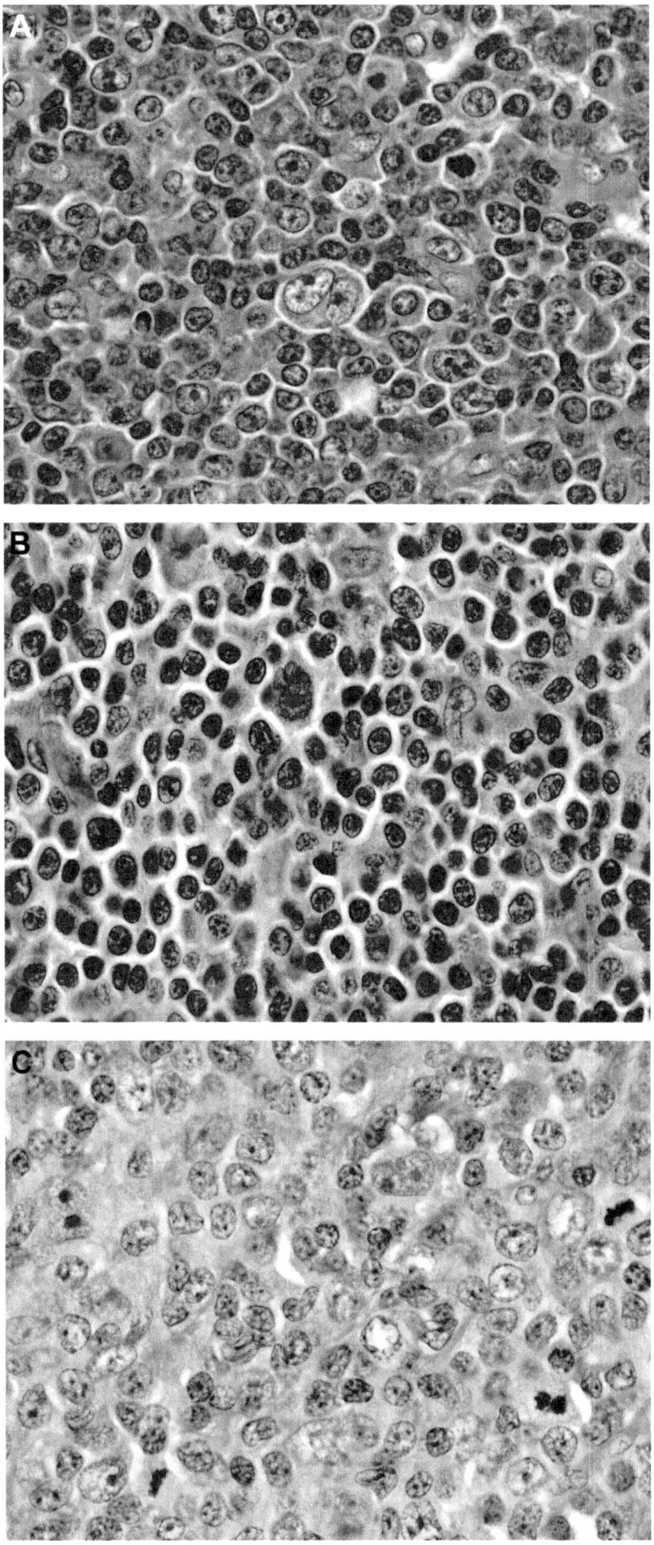

Fig. 12. NLPHL with cytomorphologic T-cell atypia. (*A–G*) Occasional cases of NLPHL show prominent cytologic atypia in T cells consisting of enlarged or irregular nuclei, vesicular or clumped chromatin, small prominent nucleoli, and increased mitotic activity (H&E, 1000x). Each image of this series is taken from a different case of NLPHL. These features are most conspicuous in T cells in the immediate vicinity of lymphocyte-predominant cells

Fig. 12. (*Continued*)

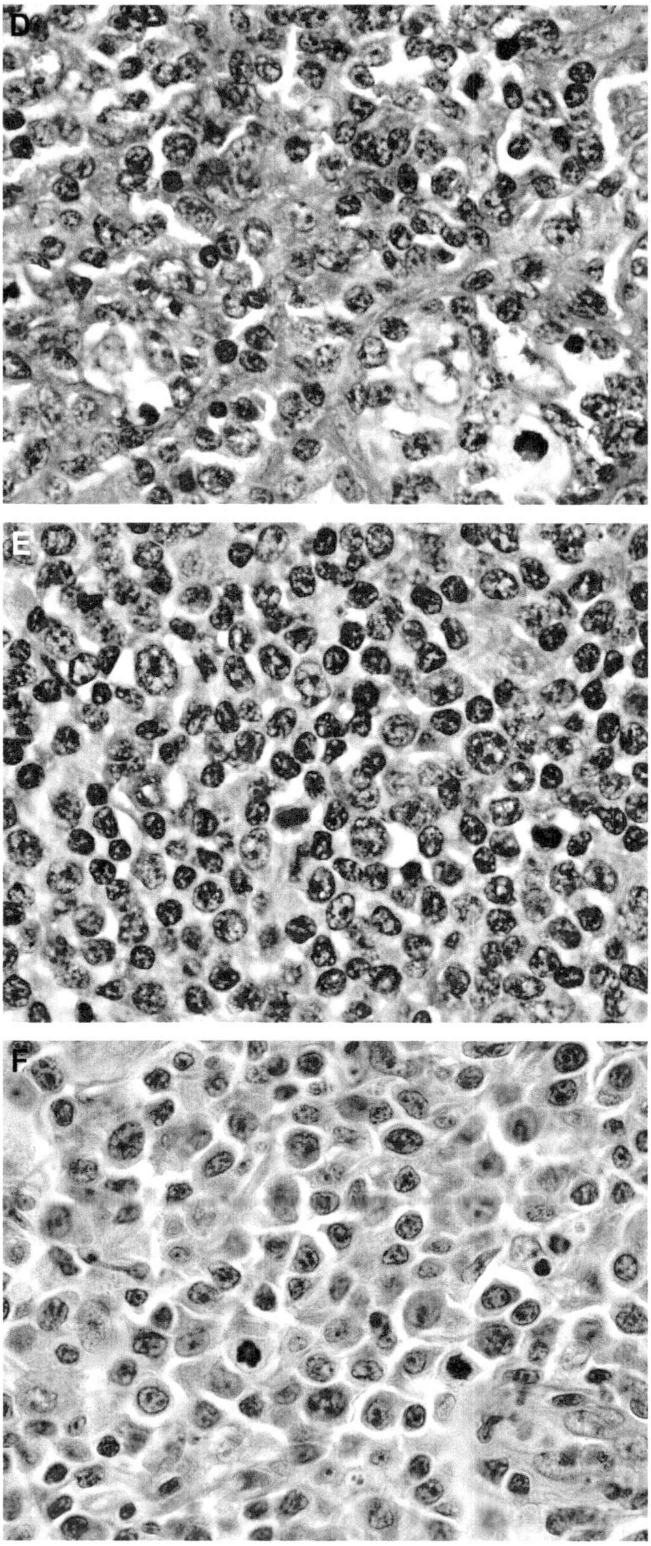

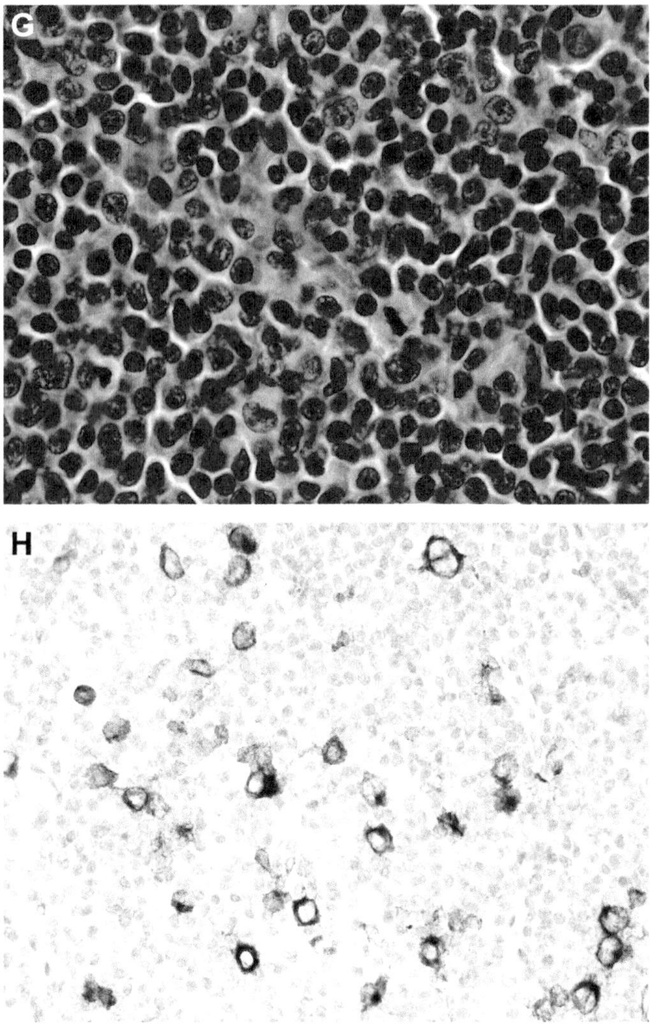

Fig. 12. (*A–E*) and are more often seen in younger male patients. (*H*) The lymphocyte-predominant cells in such cases frequently express IgD heavy chain.

phenotype, and the nomenclature of such cases has been updated in the 5th edition of the WHO Classification of Haematolymphoid Tumours to reflect this key feature. This newly named category of nodal T-follicular helper cell lymphoma includes cases of angioimmunoblastic type (formerly angioimmunoblastic T-cell lymphoma), follicular type (formerly follicular T-cell lymphoma), and NOS.[4] In these cases, the localized lack of T-cell immune surveillance leads to the proliferation of variable numbers of large atypical B cells with features of centroblasts or immunoblasts or with features resembling Hodgkin/Reed-Sternberg or lymphocyte-predominant cells (Fig. 13A–E). The large B cells are often positive for PAX5, CD30, and CD15, variably positive for CD20 and other pan–B-cell markers, and may be EBV-positive or EBV-negative with the former often meeting criteria for nodal T-follicular helper cell lymphoma, angioimmunoblastic type (Fig. 13F–J, M).[35] The predominant cellularity consists of small- to medium-sized, monomorphic T cells thereby mimicking the background cellularity of lymphocyte-rich CHL or NLPHL. The cytologic atypia of the T cells is often subtle, although some clues favoring a diagnosis of nodal T-follicular helper cell lymphoma over Hodgkin lymphoma include the presence of slight nuclear irregularities, clumped or dispersed chromatin, and moderate amounts of pale or clear cytoplasm (see Fig. 13B–E). In some cases, scattered eosinophils may be seen, a

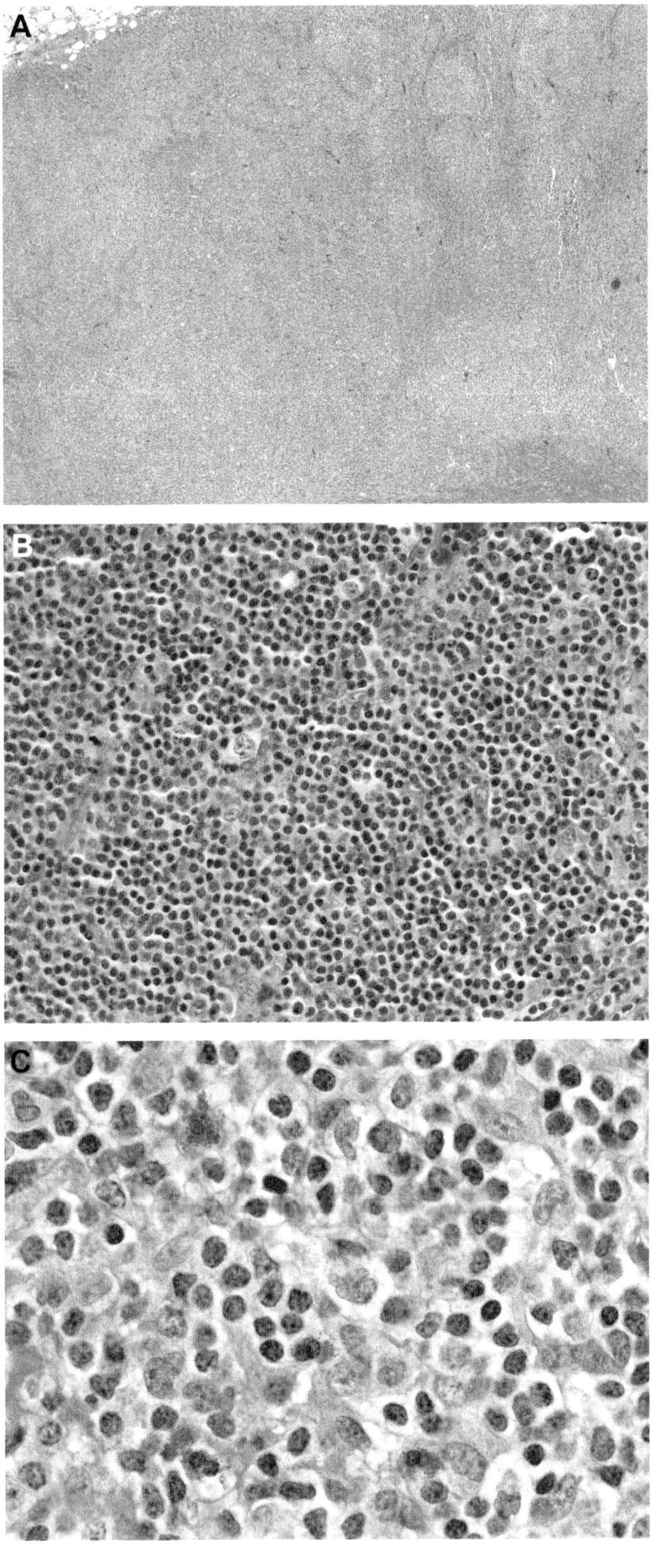

Fig. 13. Nodal T-follicular helper cell lymphoma. (*A–E*) This axillary lymph node excised from a 67-year-old woman with multifocal lymphadenopathy accompanied by a 30-pound weight loss shows complete architectural effacement by a vaguely nodular infiltrate (*A*, H&E, 20x) consisting of numerous small- to medium-sized monomorphic lymphocytes with slightly irregular nuclei, clumped chromatin, and moderate pale cytoplasm (*B*, H&E, 200x; *C–E*, H&E, 1000x), occasional eosinophils (*C*), and scattered large atypical cells with oval to irregular nuclei and prominent eosinophilic nucleoli with paranuclear chromatin clearing resembling lymphocyte-predominant cells or Hodgkin/Reed-Sternberg variants

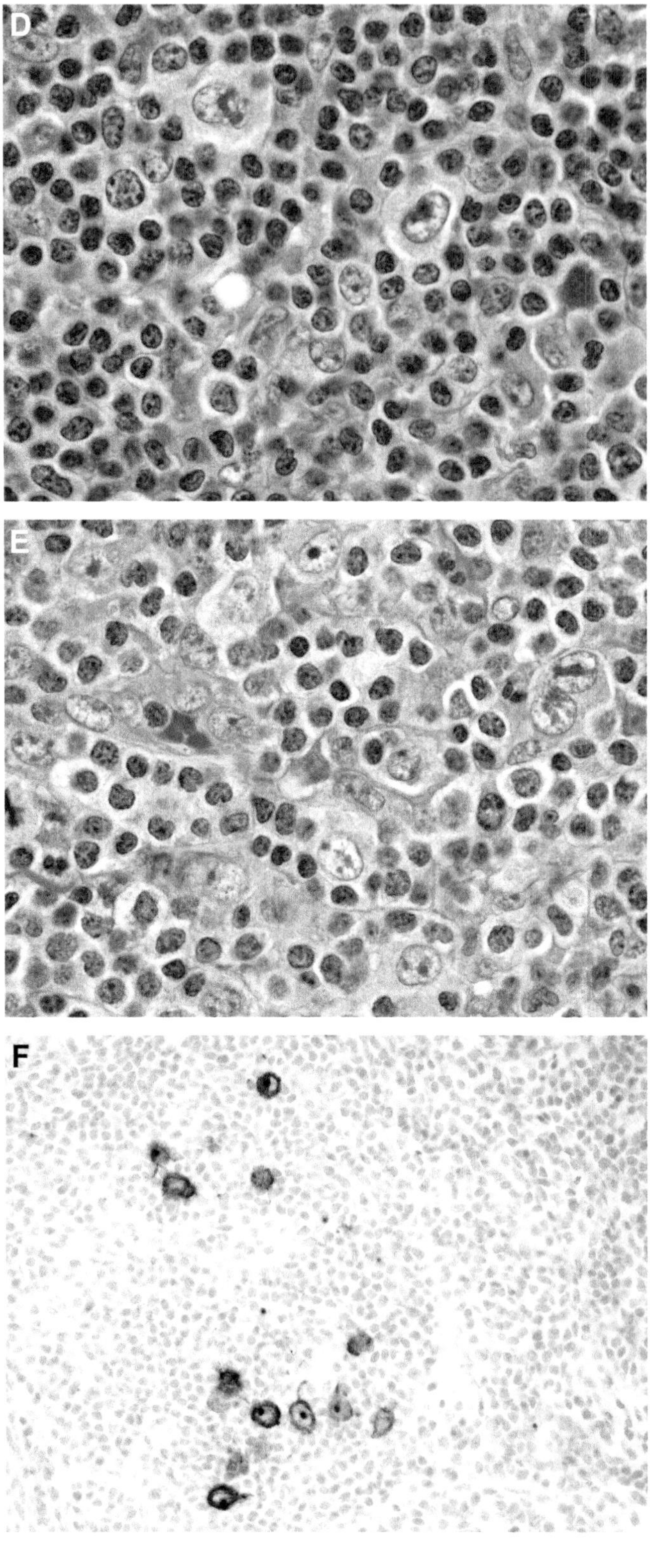

Fig. 13. (*D, E*), including occasional binucleate forms (*E*). (*F–J*) Immunohistochemical stains demonstrate that the large atypical cells are positive for CD30 (*F*)

Fig. 13. and CD15 (*G*), with weak, variable staining for PAX5 (*H*), and coexpression of OCT2 (*I*)

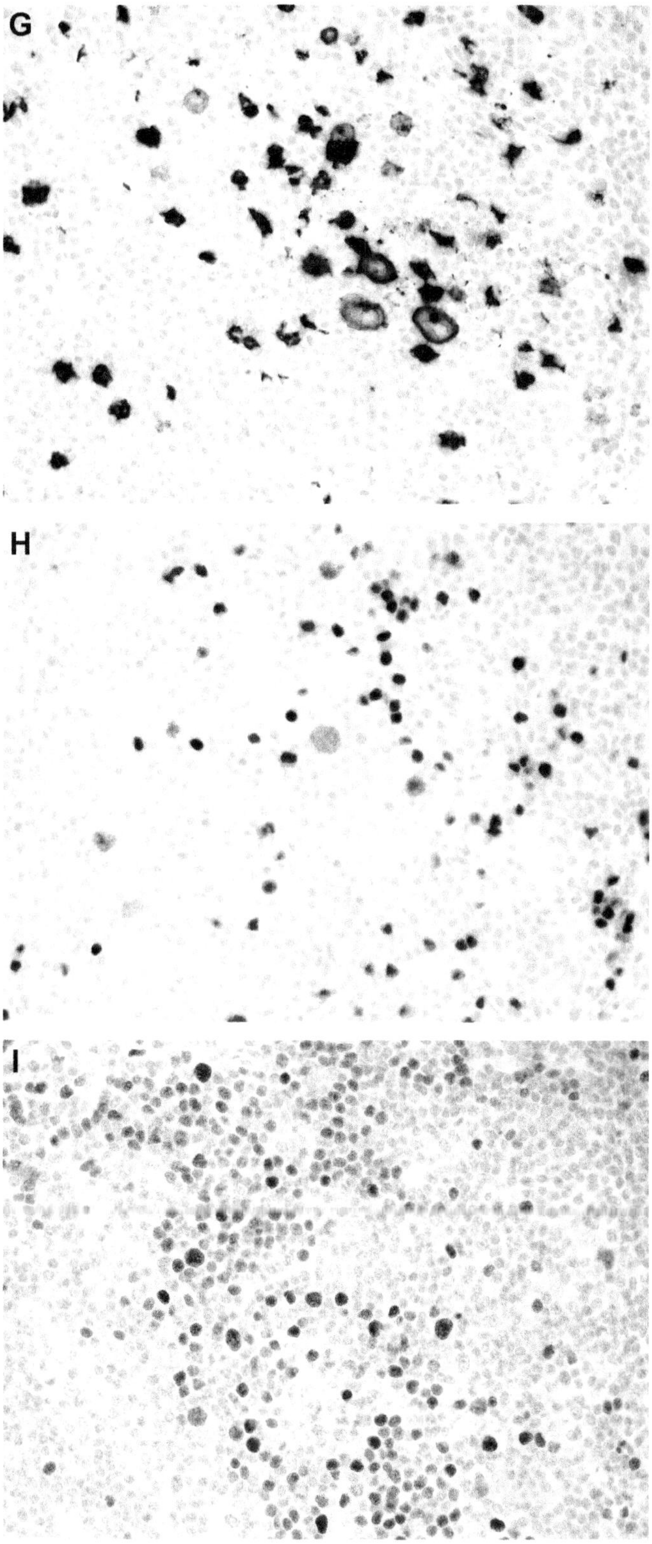

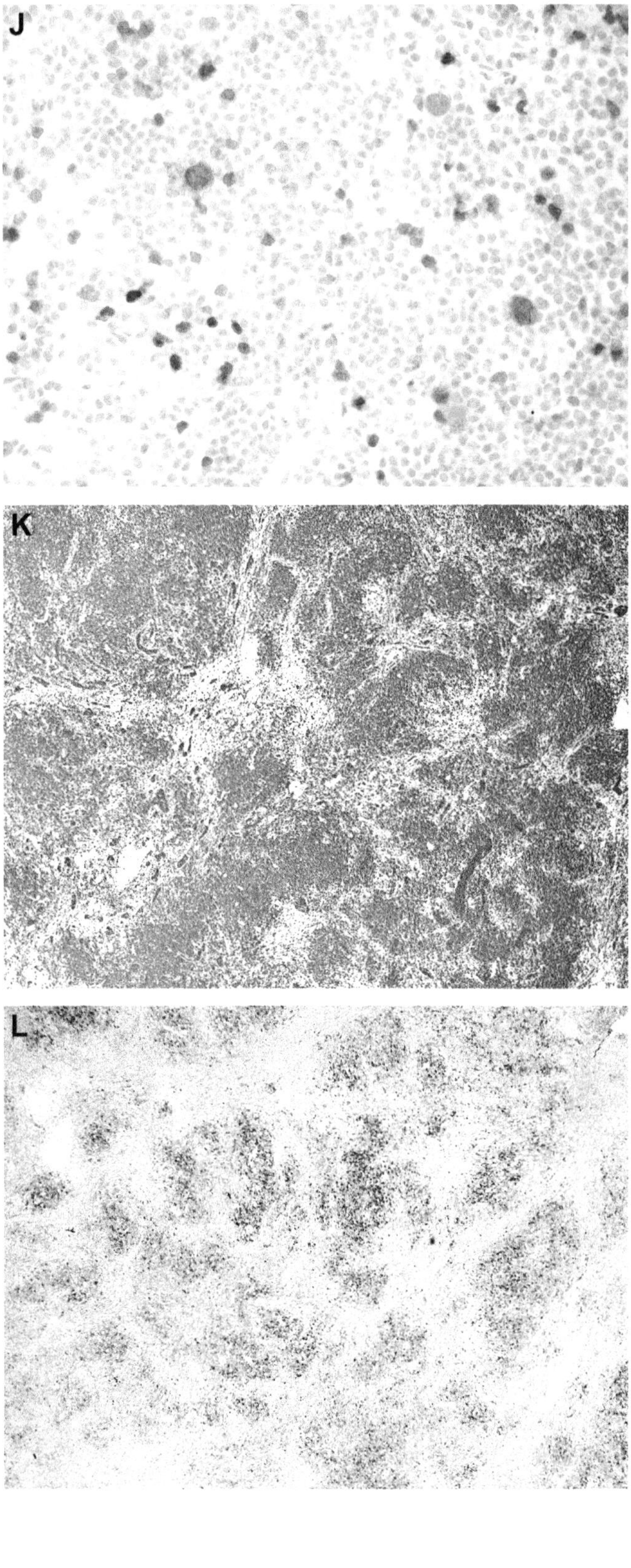

Fig. 13. and BOB1 (*J*). (*K–M*) Background small lymphocytes comprise an abundance of CD2-positive T cells (*K*) with co-expression of T-follicular helper antigens, ICOS (*L*), and PD1 (not shown), with many fewer CD20-positive small B cells present in focal clusters in the residual cortex; note that the large cells are negative for CD20 in this case

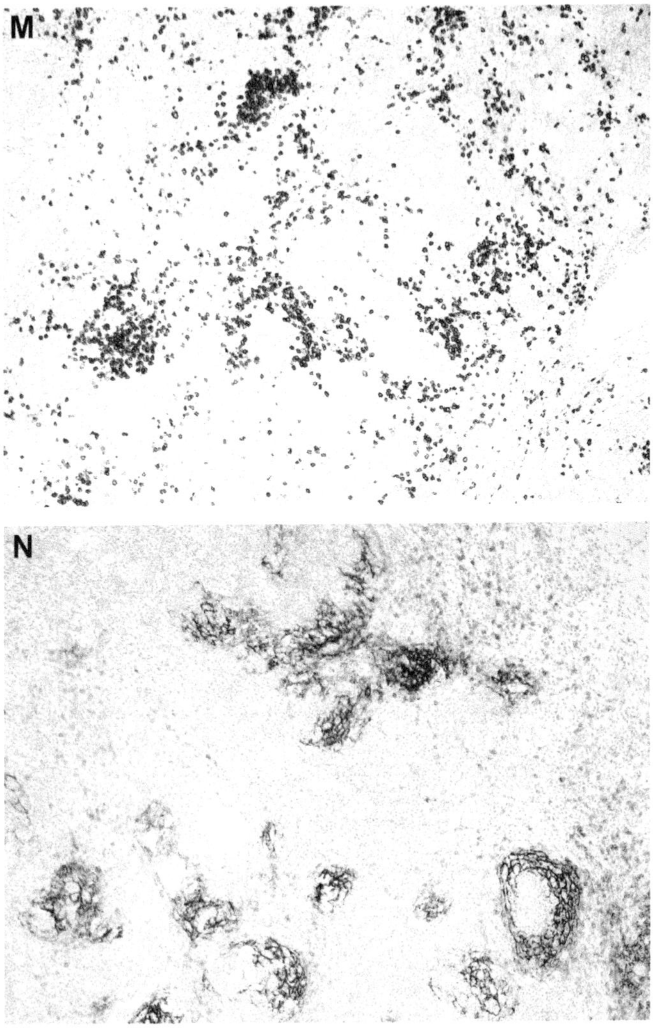

Fig. 13. (*M*), as well as EBER (not shown). (*N*) A stain for CD21 highlights focally expanded and distorted follicular dendritic cell meshworks that extend beyond residual B-cell follicles into areas occupied by atypical T cells.

background cell type often present in peripheral T-cell lymphoma but rare in lymphocyte-rich CHL or NLPHL (see Fig. 13C). The predominant atypical T-cell population is positive for CD4 with coexpression of at least 2 T-follicular-helper markers; CD21 may also be helpful in identifying expanded follicular dendritic cell aggregates associated with atypical T cells (Fig. 13K, L, N).[35] A helpful feature that has been reported in many cases of nodal T-follicular helper cell lymphoma is the detection of an abnormal CD4-positive T-cell population by flow cytometry that is typically dim or negative for surface CD3; this finding is more common than aberrant coexpression of CD10 by the neoplastic T cells and is not seen in lymphocyte-rich CHL or NLPHL (Fig. 14).[36] The utility of flow cytometry in these cases underscores the importance of sending tissue for this study at time of frozen section evaluation in cases with a cellular background rich in small lymphocytes, even if features are suspected to represent Hodgkin lymphoma. Cases found to have subtle morphologic abnormalities or diminished surface CD3 by flow cytometry should be evaluated further by performing an extended immunohistochemical panel to characterize the CD4:CD8 ratio, look for expression of T-follicular helper markers (CD10, BCL6, PD1, ICOS, CXCL13), and assess for T-cell antigen loss, as well as sending for T-cell

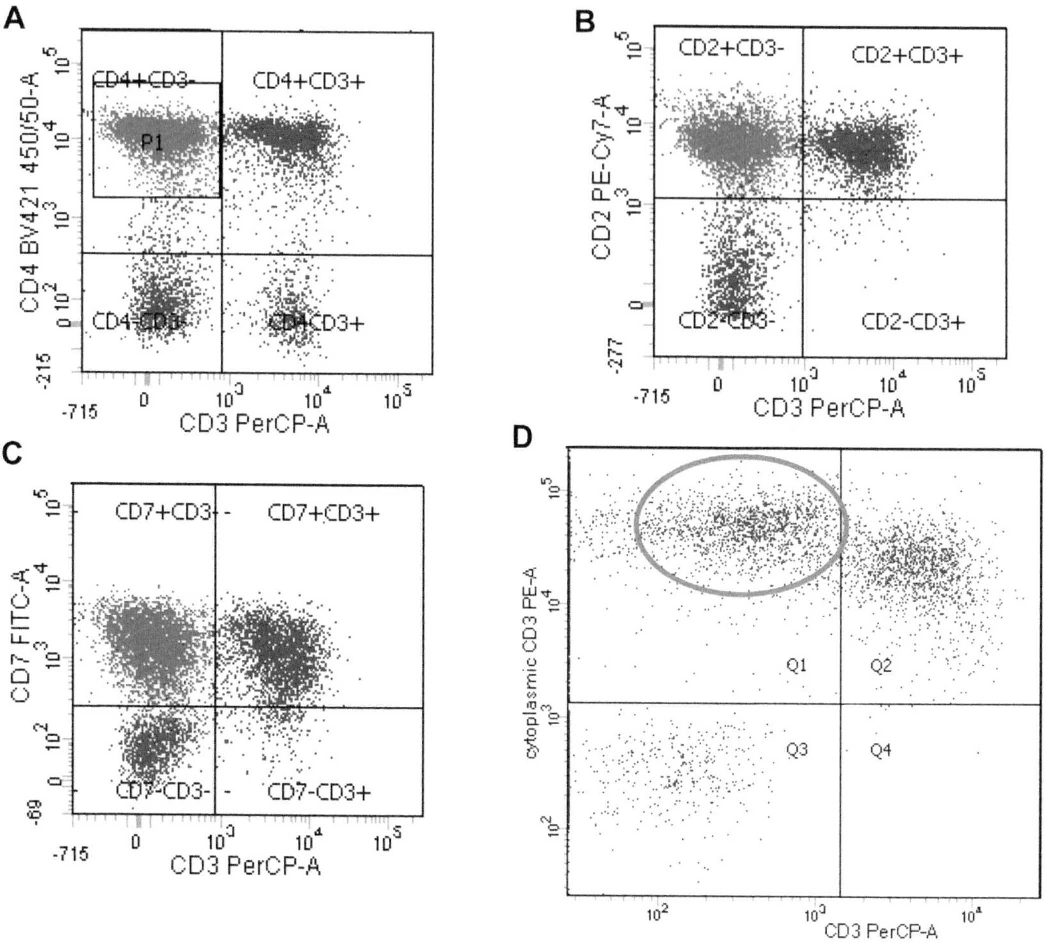

Fig. 14. Flow cytometric analysis of a case of nodal T-follicular helper cell lymphoma. (*A–D*) A portion of fresh tissue from the case illustrated in Fig. 13 was sent for flow cytometry, which showed an abnormal CD4-positive (*A*), CD2-positive (*B*), CD7-positive (*C*) T-cell population that was negative for surface CD3 (*A–C, green population*) but positive for cytoplasmic CD3 (*D, green circle*) present in a background of normal T cells (*A–C, red population*) and polytypic B cells (not shown). T-cell clonality PCR demonstrated a biclonal T-cell population with *TRG* Vgamma1-8 primers (not shown). The overall morphologic, immunophenotypic, and molecular genetic findings in this case support a diagnosis of nodal T-follicular helper cell lymphoma rather than Hodgkin lymphoma of any subtype. (BV421, brilliant violet 421; FITC, fluorescein isothyocyanate; PE, phycoerythrin; PE-Cy7, phycoerythrin-cyanine 7; PerCP, peridinin-chlorophyll protein complex.)

receptor gene rearrangement studies and NGS analysis, given the vast prognostic and therapeutic implications of establishing a diagnosis of peripheral T-cell lymphoma versus Hodgkin lymphoma.

SUMMARY

As described in this review and illustrated by historical precedent, the diagnosis of CHL and NLPHL may be challenging in some cases, and the differential diagnosis includes reactive conditions, lymphoproliferative diseases, and other lymphoid neoplasms. Being aware of this broad differential diagnosis, maintaining a low threshold for performing ancillary studies in cases with unusual morphologic or immunophenotypic features, and correlating with clinical features are all keys to establishing the correct diagnosis even in challenging cases of these fascinating lymphoid neoplasms and their related entities.

CLINICS CARE POINTS

- Reactive immunoblastic proliferations mimicking CHL generally show at least focal areas of nodal architectural preservation with an absence of fibrosis and retention of B-cell antigen expression on immunoblasts with polytypic expression of light chains by immunohistochemistry.
- Consider a diagnosis of EBV-positive MCU in cases with a localized, CHL-like infiltrate involving a mucosal or cutaneous site.
- The diagnosis of MGZL should be considered in cases with sheeting out of neoplastic cells that express of Hodgkin markers, such as CD30 and CD15, or in cases with scattered neoplastic cells that express multiple B-cell markers often absent in CHL, such as CD19 and CD79a.
- Awareness of variant patterns in NLPHL is important for disease prognostication and recognition of progression to large B-cell lymphoma.
- Some cases of NLPHL show reactive cytologic atypia in background T cells by histology or may contain reactive T cells with coexpression of CD4 and dim CD8 by flow cytometry.
- Because some cases of nodal T-follicular helper cell lymphoma with large B cells may closely resemble Hodgkin lymphoma, it is important to have a low threshold for performing additional T-cell markers, including T-follicular helper antigens, flow cytometry, and gene rearrangement studies, in cases of suspected Hodgkin lymphoma with a lymphocyte-rich background or unusual morphologic and immunophenotypic features.

DISCLOSURES

Consulting: Mersana Therapeutics Inc, AbbVie Inc; Scientific Advisory Board: AbbVie Inc; Expert Review: Levin Papantonio Rafferty PA, Seeger Devine LLP, Abbot Nicholson PC, Foley Baron Metzger & Juip PLLC.

REFERENCES

1. Lakhtakia R, Burney I. A historical tale of two lymphomas: part I: Hodgkin lymphoma. Sultan Qaboos Univ Med J 2015;15(2):e202–6.
2. Stein H, Pileri SA, Weiss LM, et al. Hodgkin lymphomas: Introduction. In: Swerdlow SH, Campo E, Harris NL, et al, editors. WHO Classification of Tumours of Haematopoietic and Lymphoid Tissues. revised 4th edition. Lyon: IARC; 2017. p. 424–30.
3. Campo E, Jaffe ES, Cook JR, et al. The International Consensus Classification of mature lymphoid neoplasms: a report from the Clinical Advisory Committee. Blood 2022;140(11):1229–53.
4. Alaggio R, Amador C, Anagnostopoulos I, et al. The 5th edition of the World Health Organization Classification of Haematolymphoid Tumours: lymphoid neoplasms. Leukemia 2022;36(7):1720–48.
5. Stein H, Pileri SA, Weiss LM, et al. Nodular sclerosis classic Hodgkin lymphoma. In: Swerdlow SH, Campo E, Harris NL, et al, editors. WHO Classification of Tumours of Haematopoietic and Lymphoid Tissues. revised 4th edition. Lyon: IARC; 2017. p. 435–7.
6. Weiss LM, Poppema S, Jaffe ES, et al. Mixed cellularity classic Hodgkin lymphoma. In: Swerdlow SH, Campo E, Harris NL, et al, editors. WHO Classification of Tumours of Haematopoietic and Lymphoid Tissues. revised 4th edition. Lyon: IARC; 2017. p. 440.
7. Huppmann AR, Nicolae A, Slack GW, et al. EBV may be expressed in the LP cells of nodular lymphocyte-predominant Hodgkin lymphoma (NLPHL) in both children and adults. Am J Surg Pathol 2014;38(3): 316–24.
8. Louissaint A Jr, Ferry JA, Soupir CP, et al. Infectious mononucleosis mimicking lymphoma: distinguishing morphological and immunophenotypic features. Mod Pathol 2012;25(8):1149–59.
9. Dojcinov SD, Venkataraman G, Raffeld M, et al. EBV positive mucocutaneous ulcer–a study of 26 cases associated with various sources of immunosuppression. Am J Surg Pathol 2010;34(3):405–17.
10. Gratzinger D, Jaffe ES. Mucocutaneous ulcer: a mimic of EBV + diffuse large B cell lymphoma in the immunodeficiency setting. Leuk Lymphoma 2016;57(8):1982–3.
11. Gaulard P, Harris NL, Pileri SA, et al. Primary mediastinal (thymic) large B-cell lymphoma. In: Swerdlow SH, Campo E, Harris NL, et al, editors. WHO Classification of Tumours of Haematopoietic and Lymphoid Tissues. revised 4th edition. Lyon: IARC; 2017. p. 314–6.
12. Dorfman DM, Shahsafaei A, Alonso MA. Utility of CD200 immunostaining in the diagnosis of primary mediastinal large B cell lymphoma: comparison with MAL, CD23, and other markers. Mod Pathol 2012;25(12):1637–43.
13. Gentry M, Bodo J, Durkin L, et al. Performance of a commercially available MAL antibody in the diagnosis of primary mediastinal large B-cell lymphoma. Am J Surg Pathol 2017;41(2):189–94.
14. Rodig SJ, Savage KJ, LaCasce AS, et al. Expression of TRAF1 and nuclear c-Rel distinguishes primary mediastinal large cell lymphoma from other types

of diffuse large B-cell lymphoma. Am J Surg Pathol 2007;31(1):106–12.
15. Bledsoe JR, Redd RA, Hasserjian RP, et al. The immunophenotypic spectrum of primary mediastinal large B-cell lymphoma reveals prognostic biomarkers associated with outcome. Am J Hematol 2016;91(10):E436–41.
16. Zhang ML, Sohani AR. Lymphomas of the mediastinum and their differential diagnosis. Semin Diagn Pathol 2020;37(4):156–65.
17. Harris NL. Shades of gray between large B-cell lymphomas and Hodgkin lymphomas: differential diagnosis and biological implications. Mod Pathol 2013;26(Suppl 1):S57–70.
18. Jaffe ES, Stein H, Swerdlow SH, et al. B-cell lymphoma, unclassifiable, with features intermediate between diffuse large B-cell lymphoma and classic Hodgkin lymphoma. In: Swerdlow SH, Campo E, Harris NL, et al, editors. WHO Classification of Tumours of Haematopoietic and Lymphoid Tissues. revised 4th edition. Lyon: IARC; 2017. p. 342–4.
19. Stein H, Swerdlow SH, Gascoyne RD, et al. Nodular lymphocyte predominant Hodgkin lymphoma. In: Swerdlow SH, Campo E, Harris NL, et al, editors. WHO Classification of Tumours of Haematopoietic and Lymphoid Tissues,. revised 4th edition. Lyon: IARC; 2017. p. 431–4.
20. Fan Z, Natkunam Y, Bair E, et al. Characterization of variant patterns of nodular lymphocyte predominant Hodgkin lymphoma with immunohistologic and clinical correlation. Am J Surg Pathol 2003;27(10):1346–56.
21. Menke JR, Spinner MA, Natkunam Y, et al. CD20-negative nodular lymphocyte-predominant Hodgkin lymphoma: a 20-year consecutive case series from a tertiary cancer center. Arch Pathol Lab Med 2021;145(6):753–8.
22. Seliem RM, Ferry JA, Hasserjian RP, et al. Nodular lymphocyte-predominant Hodgkin lymphoma (NLPHL) with CD30-positive lymphocyte-predominant (LP) cells. J Hematop 2011;4(3):175.
23. Venkataraman G, Raffeld M, Pittaluga S, et al. CD15-expressing nodular lymphocyte-predominant Hodgkin lymphoma. Histopathology 2011;58(5):803–5.
24. Rahemtullah A, Reichard KK, Preffer FI, et al. A double-positive CD4+CD8+ T-cell population is commonly found in nodular lymphocyte predominant Hodgkin lymphoma. Am J Clin Pathol 2006 Nov;126(5):805–14.
25. Rahemtullah A, Harris NL, Dorn ME, et al. Beyond the lymphocyte predominant cell: CD4+CD8+ T-cells in nodular lymphocyte predominant Hodgkin lymphoma. Leuk Lymphoma 2008 Oct;49(10):1870–8.
26. Anagnostopoulos I, Piris MA, Isaacson PG, et al. Lymphocyte-rich classic Hodgkin lymphoma. In: Swerdlow SH, Campo E, Harris NL, et al, editors. WHO Classification of Tumours of Haematopoietic and Lymphoid Tissues. revised 4th edition. Lyon: IARC; 2017. p. 438–40.
27. Xia D, Sayed S, Moloo Z, et al. Geographic variability of nodular lymphocyte-predominant Hodgkin lymphoma. Am J Clin Pathol 2022;157(2):231–43.
28. Gerhard-Hartmann E, Jöhrens K, Schinagl LM, et al. Epstein-Barr virus infection patterns in nodular lymphocyte-predominant Hodgkin lymphoma. Histopathology 2022;80(7):1071–80.
29. Fei F, Kiruthiga KG, Younes S, et al. EBV-positive nodular lymphocyte predominant Hodgkin lymphoma: a single institution experience. Hum Pathol 2022;129:32–9.
30. Younes S, Rojansky RB, Menke JR, et al. Pitfalls in the diagnosis of nodular lymphocyte predominant Hodgkin lymphoma: variant patterns, borderlines and mimics. Cancers 2021;13(12):3021.
31. Sohani AR, Jaffe ES, Harris NL, et al. Nodular lymphocyte-predominant Hodgkin lymphoma with atypical T cells: a morphologic variant mimicking peripheral T-cell lymphoma. Am J Surg Pathol 2011; 35(11):1666–78.
32. Prakash S, Fountaine T, Raffeld M, et al. IgD positive L&H cells identify a unique subset of nodular lymphocyte predominant Hodgkin lymphoma. Am J Surg Pathol 2006;30(5):585–92.
33. Thurner L, Hartmann S, Fadle N, et al. Lymphocyte predominant cells detect *Moraxella catarrhalis*-derived antigens in nodular lymphocyte-predominant Hodgkin lymphoma. Nat Commun 2020;11(1):2465.
34. Poppema S. Lymphocyte predominant Hodgkin lymphoma, antigen-driven after all? J Pathol 2021; 253(1):1–10.
35. Nicolae A, Pittaluga S, Venkataraman G, et al. Peripheral T-cell lymphomas of follicular T-helper cell derivation with Hodgkin/Reed-Sternberg cells of B-cell lineage: both EBV-positive and EBV-negative variants exist. Am J Surg Pathol 2013;37(6):816–26.
36. Alikhan M, Song JY, Sohani AR, et al. Peripheral T-cell lymphomas of follicular helper T-cell type frequently display an aberrant CD3(−/dim)CD4(+) population by flow cytometry: an important clue to the diagnosis of a Hodgkin lymphoma mimic. Mod Pathol 2016;29(10):1173–82.

Breast Implant-Associated Anaplastic Large Cell Lymphoma

Updates in Diagnosis and Specimen Handling

Mario L. Marques-Piubelli, MD[a], L. Jeffrey Medeiros, MD[b], John Stewart, MD[c], Roberto N. Miranda, MD[b,*]

KEYWORDS

- Breast implant-associated anaplastic large cell lymphoma • Breast implants • ALCL
- Breast capsule

Key points

- Pathologic staging including assessment of margins is essential for the proper diagnosis and management of patients with breast implant-associated anaplastic large-cell lymphoma (BIA-ALCL).
- Strategic sampling of capsules in the absence of grossly detected tumor mass is recommended.
- Concomitant or sequential cytologic, histologic, immunohistochemical, flow cytometric, and molecular testing may be necessary to achieve a diagnosis of BIA-ALCL.

ABSTRACT

Pathologic staging including assessment of margins is essential for the proper management of patients with breast implant-associated anaplastic large-cell lymphoma (BIA-ALCL). As most patients present with effusion, cytologic examination with immunohistochemistry and/or flow cytometry immunophenotyping are essential for diagnosis. Upon a diagnosis of BIA-ALCL, en bloc resection is recommended. When a tumor mass is not identified, a systematic approach to fixation and sampling of the capsule, followed by pathologic staging and assessment of margins, is essential. Cure is likely when lymphoma is contained within the en bloc resection and margins are negative. Incomplete resection or positive margins require a multidisciplinary team assessment for adjuvant therapy.

OVERVIEW

DEFINITION

Breast implant-associated anaplastic large cell lymphoma (BIA-ALCL) is an extranodal CD30-positive T-cell lymphoma that arises around textured breast implants. The first description of this disease is credited to Keech and Creech.[1] However, it seems likely that the first reported case was by Said and colleagues,[2] who reported the disease as a primary effusion lymphoma.[3] The disease has been considered as a distinct entity by the Word Health Organization Classification of Breast Tumors since 2019[4] and by the WHO Classification of Hematolymphoid Tumors since 2022, although it was highlighted by the latter as a provisional entity in 2017.[5] This lymphoma is morphologically and immunophenotypically similar to systemic or primary cutaneous ALCL;

[a] Department of Translational Molecular Pathology, The University of Texas MD Anderson Cancer Center; [b] Department of Hematopathology, The University of Texas MD Anderson Cancer Center; [c] Department of Pathology, The University of Texas MD Anderson Cancer Center
* Corresponding author. 1515 Holcombe Boulevard, Houston, TX 77030.
E-mail address: Roberto.miranda@mdanderson.org

Surgical Pathology 16 (2023) 347–360
https://doi.org/10.1016/j.path.2023.01.003

however, this disease has a distinctive pathogenesis and prognosis.[6]

In this review, we discuss the pathogenic and epidemiologic features of the disease, and we present an updated review of cytologic and histopathologic features. We also discuss handling protocols for specimens obtained from patients with a suspected diagnosis of BIA-ALCL.

EPIDEMIOLOGY

BIA-ALCL is an unusual lymphoma and represents less than 1% of all non-Hodgkin lymphomas and approximately 2% to 3% of all lymphomas involving the breast.[7–9] Almost all patients have been cisgender women, but there are reports of this neoplasm occurring in transgender women. The median age of patients is 50 years at diagnosis and there is no predilection for side of involvement.[10] In patients with BIA-ALCL, the most common reason for breast augmentation is aesthetic, followed by reconstruction after breast cancer surgery.[10–12]

Despite multinational efforts, there remain significant barriers to understanding the precise epidemiology of patients with breast implants and the number of patients affected by BIA-ALCL. The reasons for this deficiency in the literature include inaccurate records, lack of systematic follow-up of patients with implants, and misdiagnosis of the disease.[13] Based on worldwide health regulatory agencies, 949 cases were reported by the end of 2021 and more than 30 patients died from this disease.[14] Excerpts of the fourth World Consensus Conference on BIA-ALCL held in Houston, Texas, United States noted that approximately 1300 cases were recognized worldwide up to September 2022. There is a geographic variation in the reported incidence, which varies from 1:-350 to 1:30,000, and most cases have been reported in Europe, North America, and Australia.[15] The highest incidence may be related to the study population of patients with breast cancer, having received textured implants and followed systematically.[16] A recent study conducted by Kinslow and colleagues[8] reported an age-adjusted incidence of eight cases per 100 million women per year in the United States between 2000 and 2018. As also observed in other countries, this incidence rate is increasing and may be related to the increased use of textured breast implants and increased recognition of the disease.[8,17]

RISK FACTORS

During the past years, several factors have been implicated in the risk assessment of BIA-ALCL. The most important seems to be the quality of the implant shell. There is a substantial pathogenic relationship between a macro-textured (ISO 14607:2018) outer shell of saline and silicone-filled breast implants and the relative risk of developing BIA-ALCL.[11–13,15] No cases have been reported in patients who only underwent reconstruction with smooth outer shell implants.[18]

In a recent systematic review conducted by Lynch and colleagues,[19] the overall risk of BIA-ALCL in patients with textured breast implants in the United States varied from 0.002% to 0.2% according to patient age and time of implantation. When assessing patients in a single center cohort who underwent mastectomy due to breast cancer or contralateral prophylaxis, this risk was 0.311 cases per 1000 women-years or 0.3%.[16]

Other risk factors are less well established. An increased risk of BIA-ALCL in patients carrying *BRCA1* or *BRCA2* germline mutations has been reported, but this conclusion remains premature and larger cohorts are needed to establish a precise risk assessment for patients with these mutations.[12] Other rare cancer predisposition conditions, such as Li-Fraumeni syndrome, have also been suspected as an additional risk factor for the development of BIA-ALCL; however, only a few such cases have been reported.[20]

Bacterial biofilm of *Ralstonia* spp. was initially implicated in the etiology of BIA-ALCL, but no consistent differences between the microbiome of BIA-ALCL patients and normal controls have been found.[20] Importantly, with the recent removal of Allergan BIOCELL implants from the market due to the increased risk of BIA-ALCL development, there is an increased need for evaluation of other risk factors involved in the development of the disease.

PATHOGENESIS

The role of chronic inflammation associated with implants has been consistently noted as a factor triggering lymphocyte transformation and lymphomagenesis.[21–23] Chronic antigenic stimulation may lead to the recruitment, proliferation, and expansion of T cells. As a result, T-cell lifespan is prolonged making these cells more susceptible to genetic abnormalities that eventually lead to malignant transformation. Silicone has been known to be immunogenic since its original use as a liquid for breast expansion in the 1940s.[24–27] Silicone implants and silicone elastomeric capsules lining saline implants are plausible sources of a chronic immune-mediated inflammatory response. Presumably, the shell of the implant degrades over time resulting in leakage of antigens that elicit a host immune response.[28] The shedding of silicone particles is more pronounced with textured implants.[29] In a study by Meza-Britez and colleagues,[30] inflammation around breast implants, predominantly with a T-cell phenotype, was statistically more common in patients with textured breast implants as compared with smooth implants.

In vitro studies of BIA-ALCL cells by Xu and colleagues[31] and Wolfram and colleagues[32] revealed a genetic and cytokine profile consistent with interleukin (IL)-17-producing T-cells (Th17 cells) rather than Th1 or Th2 patterns. Th17 cells are thought to be important drivers of the inflammatory process in tissue-specific autoimmunity.[31,33] Th17 cells also have been implicated in stimulating the immune response to silicone implants.[32] Kadin and colleagues[34] reported that BIA-ALCL cell lines and anaplastic cells in clinical specimens produce IL-13, a signature cytokine of allergic inflammation, further supporting the role of inflammation in the pathogenesis of BIA-ALCL. Kadin and colleagues[35] also used gene expression array analysis, flow cytometry, and immunohistochemistry to study BIA-ALCL cell lines, reporting high expression of JunB, interferon-gamma, and IL-17F suggestive of a Th17/Th1 phenotype.

CLINICAL FEATURES

Breast swelling and asymmetry due to effusion (or seroma) around the affected implants is a very common presentation.[3,9,14,36] Breast pain, skin rash, pruritus, and capsule contracture with or without breast effusions are also commonly reported symptoms.[13,14] Around 70% of patients with BIA-ALCL present with only local symptoms, whereas a tumor mass with or without effusion occurs in approximately 30% of patients. Patients with a tumor mass are more likely to develop ipsilateral palpable axillary or infra/supraclavicular lymphadenopathy.[9,37] Systemic symptoms, such as fever and weight loss, are usually absent in patients with effusion only disease, but may be present in patients with invasive neoplasms.[3] Patients with BIA-ALCL usually have an indolent clinical course. The average interval from implantation to diagnosis varies from 8 to 10 years and more than 90% of patients are diagnosed in the early stage of disease (Ann Arbor Stage I/II).[10,14] Bilateral involvement is usually incidentally detected when the contralateral capsule and implant are removed and is reported in up to 5% of patients.[11,15,38–40] Imaging studies of breast involved by BIA-ALCL usually show an effusion around the breast implant, with or without a distinct mass (Fig. 1). Adrada and colleagues[41] found that the most sensitive procedure to detect this effusion is ultrasound, which in their hands achieved 84% sensitivity and 75% specificity. Mortality rate is low for BIA-ALCL, occurring in less than 5% of all patients.[14]

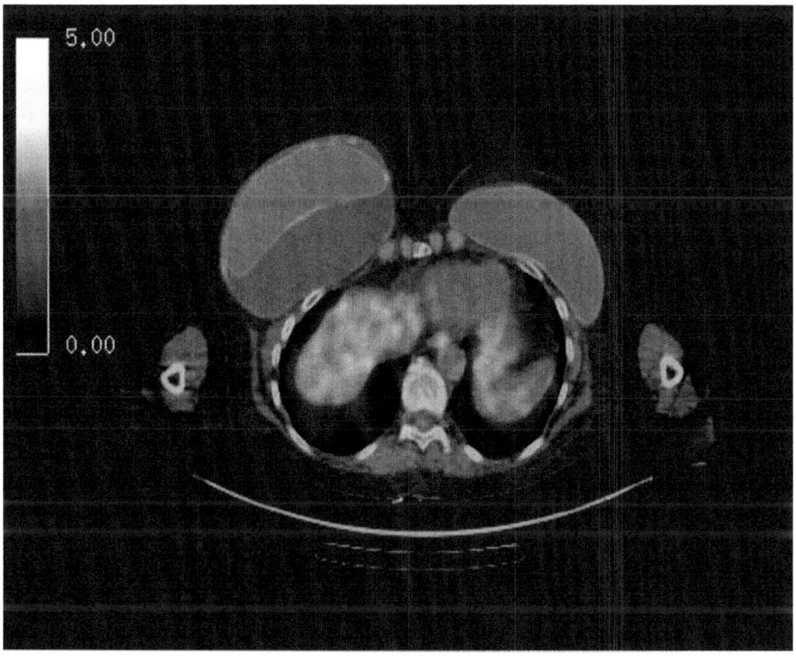

Fig. 1. Imaging of BIA-ALCL. PET-computed tomography (CT) scan showing right-sided effusion displacing the implant forward.

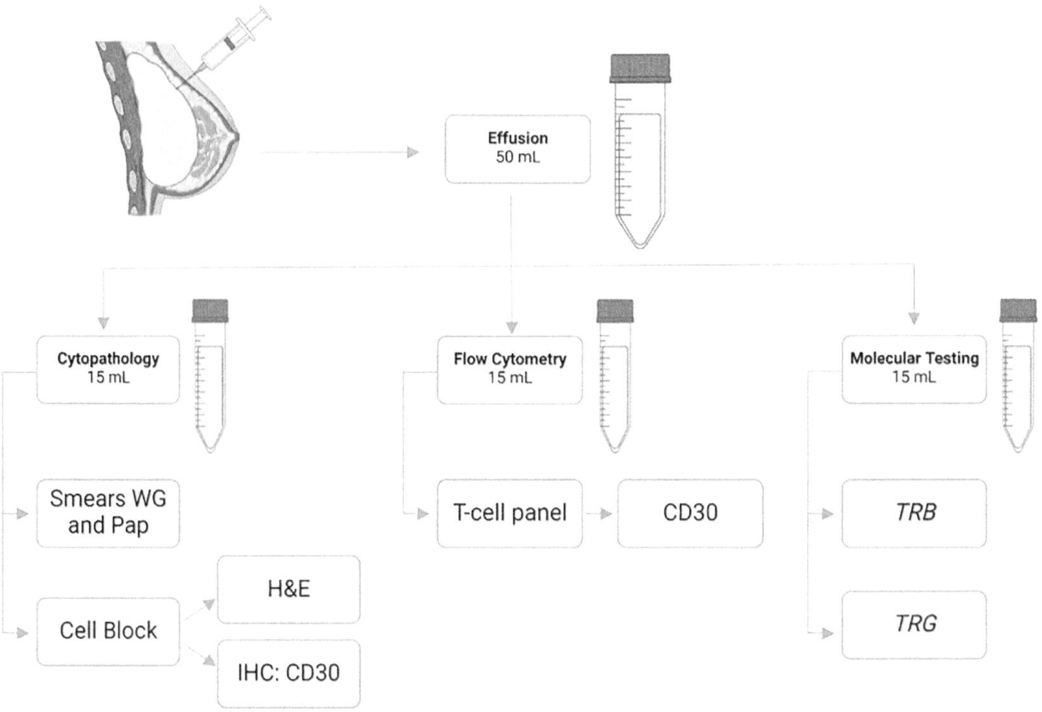

Fig. 2. Algorithm for screening of periprosthetic effusion. It is recommended to obtain between 20 and 50 mL of fluid for processing, and distribute in three Falcon tubes, between 5 and 15 mL each. The first tube is for cytopathology to perform Wright–Giemsa (WG) and Papanicolaou stain (Pap), as well as cell block for CD30 immunohistochemistry. The second tube is for flow-cytometry immunophenotyping for T-cell markers, including CD30 and TRBC1 restriction. The third tube is for molecular assessment of the *TRG* and *TRB* genes to determine clonality. (Created with BioRender.com.)

PROCESSING AND HANDLING OF PATHOLOGIC SPECIMENS

Here we discuss the standard protocol for handling breast implant capsules and peri-implant fluids and we summarize the main aspects of the pathologic staging and differential diagnosis. Our strategy to evaluate periprosthetic effusions is shown in **Fig. 2**. We recommend the aspiration of 20 to 50 mL of fluid that can be divided into three equal parts for cytopathology, flow cytometry immunophenotyping, and molecular genetic testing.

CYTOLOGY: SMEARS AND CELL BLOCK

Fluid collections shortly after the placement of breast implants are common and often represent a hematoma, an effusion related to the surgical procedure itself, or possibly infection. Unlike this scenario, effusions in the context of BIA-ALCL typically occur several years after implantation and are known as "late" seromas, defined as an effusion occurring $\geq$ 1 year after initial surgery.[42,43] In patients with effusion, the most remarkable feature is the presence of a turbid effusion accumulating in the space between the implant and fibrous capsule. Fine needle aspiration with cytologic evaluation provides a fast, safe, and effective method for evaluating the effusion in patients with BIA-ALCL. Fluid volume may range from minimal to more than 500 mL.[4,10] Morphologic evaluation of the aspirated fluid is aided by cytocentrifugation concentration. The quality of the resulting cytospin slides is greatly enhanced by the use of a ficoll-hypaque density gradient, which removes otherwise obscuring degenerated cells and debris. The lymphoma cells of BIA-ALCL resemble systemic ALCL at nodal or extranodal sites in cytologic preparations.[21,39,44–49] Wright-Giemsa or May-Grünwald-Giemsa-stained slides show highly cellular specimens composed of a homogeneous population of noncohesive large cells with irregularly lobated nuclei, prominent nucleoli, and abundant cytoplasm.[21,29,45,46,49–51] Cells are typically four to five times larger than a small mature lymphocyte. The cytoplasm is clear or light blue, usually containing scattered small vacuoles, and the cellular outlines show cytoplasmic fragmentation (Fig. 3A, B). Less frequently, the cytoplasmic vacuoles are abundant and confluent giving the neoplastic cells a signet ring appearance. The background is granular or fibrinoid, sometimes with karyorrhectic debris. Inflammatory cells in the background are variable and can range from few to abundant small lymphocytes, neutrophils, histiocytes, or eosinophils. Papanicolaou-stained slides show nuclei that are hyperchromatic with nuclear lobation and prominent nucleoli. The cytoplasm of these lymphoma cells appears opaque, basophilic, or cyanophilic.[45,47,49,52]

Preparation of a cell block is of great benefit for both morphologic and immunohistochemical evaluation (Fig. 3C, D).[45,46,50] Immunohistochemistry for CD30 is highly reliable for highlighting BIA-ALCL, and most viable and many ghost of necrotic cells are highlighted. Thus, CD30 usually reveals many more lymphoma cells than appreciated on routine hematoxylin and eosin (H&E) stains. Other markers frequently expressed in BIA-ALCL include CD43 (~80%), CD4 (~80%), TIA-1 (~70%), granzyme B (~70%), epithelial membrane antigen (~60%), CD3 (~33%), and CD8 (~10%).[9] Although most cases of BIA-ALCL do not express a T-cell receptor (TCR), TCR αβ (βF1) and TCR γδ have been reported in about 11% and 10% of cases, respectively. In our experience with over 200 cases of BIA-ALCL, all cases have been negative for anaplastic lymphoma kinase (ALK). Of interest, Taylor and colleagues[53] reported ALK1 expression in 8% of their cases. Cases of BIA-ALCL are negative for CD1a, TdT, and cyclin D1. In situ hybridization for Epstein-Barr virus (EBV) small encoded RNA (EBER) is negative in 100% of cases. Importantly, EBV(+) large B-cell lymphoma (LBCL) associated with breast implants has been recently recognized.[54]

The diagnosis of BIA-ALCL may be challenging if the patient recently (days to few weeks) underwent drainage or aspiration of the neoplastic effusion; the newly reaccumulated fluid may contain few tumor cells with a predominance of neutrophils or histiocytes.[55] Furthermore, there are patients who have recently undergone removal of an implant without capsulectomy or have had a drain placed to avoid fluid accumulation. In these circumstances, cytology samples may yield a false negative result for tumor cells even when using CD30 immunohistochemistry.

FLOW-CYTOMETRY IMMUNOPHENOTYPIC ANALYSIS

The availability of fluid in a patient with a suspicion for BIA-ALCL should lead to flow cytometry immunophenotyping to assess T cells for potential CD30 expression or an aberrant immunophenotype. Recently, clonality assessment by flow cytometry can be performed by assessing TRBC1 expression.[56]

ASSESSMENT OF CLONALITY USING POLYMERASE CHAIN REACTION-BASED METHODS

Both fluid specimens and fixed paraffin-embedded sections of cell blocks can be analyzed by polymerase chain reaction (PCR)-based methods to assess for T-cell receptor gene rearrangements. Cases of BIA-ALCL carry monoclonal *TRG* or *TRB* rearrangements. Based on our review of the literature, 5/12 (41.7%) had monoclonal *TRB* and 26/34 (76.5%) had monoclonal *TRG*. We suspect that the rate of monoclonality in BIA-ALCL cases is likely higher. The success rate of molecular testing may be limited by a paucity of tumor cells or the common presence of abundant necrosis.[10]

DETECTION OF INCIPIENT CD30(+) LYMPHOPROLIFERATION

An incontrovertible diagnosis of BIA-ALCL can be established in the presence of abundant large pleomorphic cells that react strongly with CD30 by immunohistochemistry or flow cytometry, as well as by showing aberrant loss of antigens and/or TRBC1 restriction by flow cytometry, and monoclonal T-cell receptor gene rearrangements. However, because of increased awareness of BIA-ALCL by patients and physicians, the disease is suspected more frequently, and it seems likely that early stages of the disease may become more prevalent. In effect, we have observed cases presenting with effusion where there are only scattered large atypical cells, usually CD30(+), admixed with variable numbers of inflammatory cells that make establishing the diagnosis of BIA-ALCL more difficult. Similarly, flow cytometry immunophenotyping may not show obvious aberrancies in T cells, and clonality studies may not be definitive for monoclonal T-cell receptor gene rearrangements. In an attempt to overcome these uncertainties, Kadin and colleagues[57] suggested that phosphorylated STAT3 (pSTAT3) is expressed in lymphoma cells of BIA-ALCL, but not in reactive processes. A similar finding was reported by Oishi and colleagues[58] who reported activating mutations of *JAK1* and *STAT3* in ~30% of cases of BIA-ALCL, whereas 100% of cases expressed pSTAT3 by immunohistochemistry. Furthermore, Oishi and colleagues[6] reported that carbonic

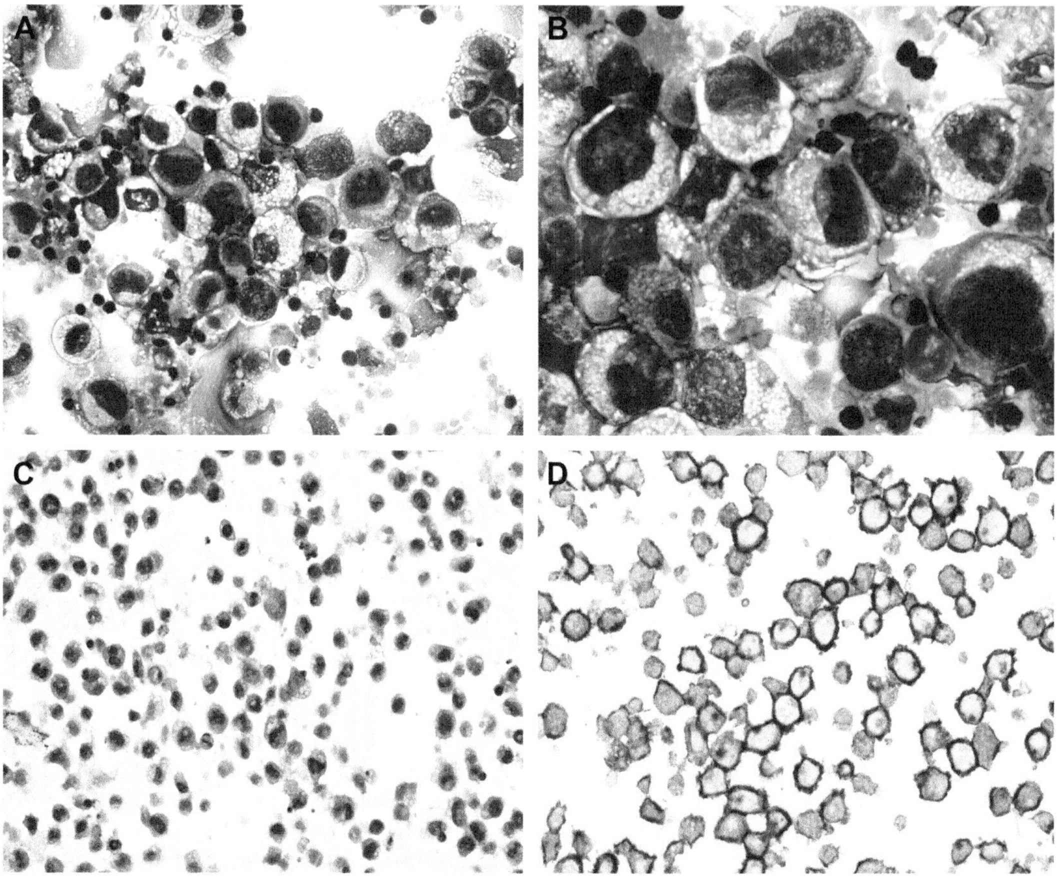

Fig. 3. Cytologic features of BIA-ALCL. (*A, B*) Cytospin slide after ficoll cytocentrifugation. Large anaplastic lymphoma cells with irregular nuclei, prominent nucleoli and abundant, occasionally vacuolated cytoplasm. Wright-Giemsa stain, 500X (*A*), 1000x (*B*). (*C*) Cell block preparation of effusion fluid showing scattered large lymphoma cells; H&E, 400x. (*D*) Immunohistochemistry for CD30 highlights most cells in the cell block. CD30 immunohistochemistry with hematoxylin counterstain.

anhydrase 9 (CA9) is inducible by BIA-ALCL cells in the hypoxic environment of the peri-implant space and showed overexpression of CA9 in all cases. We believe that pSTAT3 and CA9 are promising immunohistochemical markers, but further testing is necessary to establish their clinical utility in the diagnosis of BIA-ALCL.

PROCESSING CAPSULES

Because of the random distribution of lesions on the capsular surface of BIA-ALCL cases without a grossly identifiable lesion, we proposed a systematic approach for sampling capsules obtained from en bloc resections. The intact specimen with surgical orientation is handled by the pathologist, who will correlate with any clinically suspicious lesion, any suspicious feature detected by imaging studies, or track the margins provided by the surgeon. Based on the orientation of the specimen, the operative specimen is arbitrarily assigned sides like in a cube, and the specimen is opened sequentially from the posterior aspect. An intact specimen consists of a fibrous capsule, the implant in place, and non-disturbed effusion fluid. Opening the capsule reveals a yellowish turbid fluid, sometimes with fibrinoid strands; in some cases membranous material or a fibrous membrane is floating in the cavity, deemed a "second capsule" by radiologists. The implant is opaque and is covered by a thin layer of white or yellow material that may be misinterpreted as pus or fibrin. Routine microbiologic cultures are almost always negative, and if positive, most likely represent contamination from handling.[4,10] After a transverse and a longitudinal excision of the posterior surface of the capsule, the capsule becomes flat, ready to be pinned to a wax board for fixation overnight in buffered formalin. Full display of the capsule typically shows a pink luminal surface, occasionally with fibrinoid

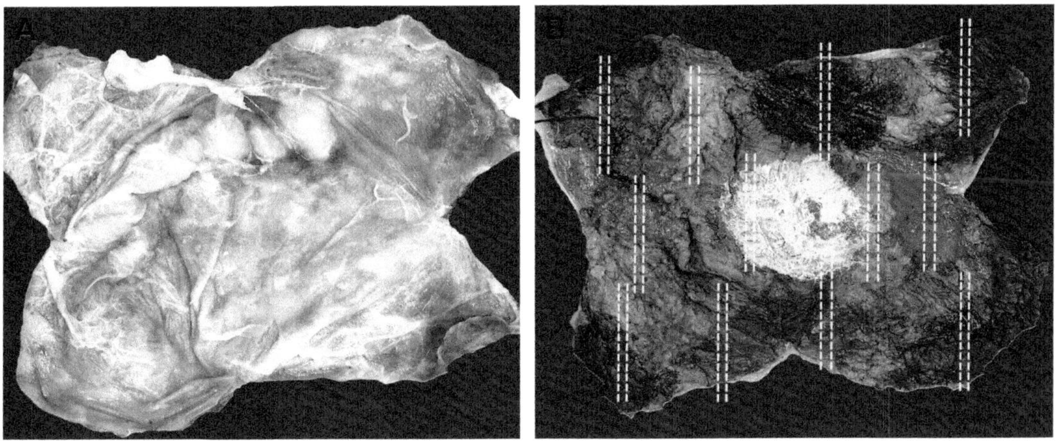

Fig. 4. Gross appearance of resected capsules of BIA-ALCL. (*A*) Fibrous capsule opened to show luminal surface displaying an irregular surface involved by lymphoma. (*B*) Breast implant capsule displaying the abluminal surface post fixation overnight. The surface has been inked with six colors that indicate the six "sides" of an imaginary cube. Each aspect is sampled and submitted for processing "on edge" to assess luminal side and margin. The dotted lines indicate 12 areas for random sampling of the capsule.

strands or detached fragments of pseudomembranous tissue, but without a distinct mass. The next day the specimen is reconstructed and the abluminal surface is carefully inked with six colors denoting the sides of an imaginary cube (Fig. 4). Two sections measuring 2 cm × 0.2 cm of each of all six "sides" are obtained and submitted for processing and histologic sectioning "on edge". A common routine may use six cassettes containing two sections each. However, when the capsule is pliable and thin, more sections can be placed in each cassette, with the benefit of saving some cassettes, and without detriment to section quality. This procedure was published by Lyapichev and colleagues[59] and subsequently endorsed in a US publication on best practice guidelines for processing BIA-ALCL specimens, the United Kingdom Guidelines on the diagnosis and treatment of BIA-ALCL, and by the National Comprehensive Cancer Network (NCCN).[60–62]

In capsules removed incidentally in asymptomatic patients, the luminal side of the capsule is typically smooth and the overall thickness of the capsule is < 1 mm. Histologic examination shows synovial-type cells lining the luminal side of the capsule but otherwise shows no or minimal inflammatory cells and no large or atypical cells.[45] A CD30 stain performed on the capsule is negative, but on occasion there are rare positive small to intermediate-size cells in the stroma, consistent with benign activated histiocytes or fibroblasts, but not clusters or aggregates of large cells on the luminal side.

In patients who present with effusion and no grossly identifiable capsule lesions, the most characteristic microscopic finding is a layer of tumor cells with extensive necrosis along the luminal side of the capsule. In most cases of BIA-ALCL, we estimate that more than 90% of the lymphoma cells are necrotic. Some areas of capsule lining are devoid of cells or necrotic material. In some cases, no viable cells are found attached to the capsule; however, cytologic preparations of the effusion are likely to reveal viable tumor cells. Lastly, scrapings of the implant surface submitted as cytologic smears or a cell block also may be helpful to detect lymphoma cells.[4]

If a tumor mass is detected preoperatively, we recommend en bloc resection with clear margins. The specimen should be intact when submitted to the pathologist. Orientation of the specimen should match the preoperative imaging studies or the areas of greatest concern should be clearly indicated by the surgeon. Areas of tumor are generally felt or readily visualized.[4,44] In some patients, tumor infiltrating the capsule may be firmly attached to the implant surface, causing distortion of the implant. The tumor may present as a localized mass that is highly necrotic, often leading to the mistaken impression of an abscess. Sometimes the tumor appears as a plaque, of variable size within or beyond the outer portion of the capsule. We recommend inking the resection margins and performing extensive sampling of any areas of suspected tumor.

PATHOLOGIC STAGING, PROGNOSIS, AND NATIONAL COMPREHENSIVE CANCER NETWORK GUIDELINES

Sections of capsules of BIA-ALCL without grossly identifiable lesions usually show lymphoma cells in

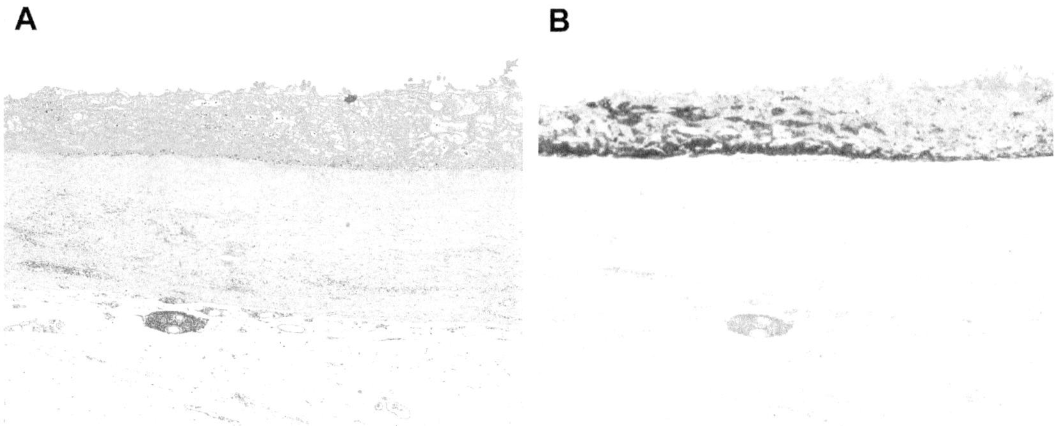

Fig. 5. Histologic staging of BIA-ALCL: (*A*) pT1, lymphoma cells are confined to the luminal space. H&E, 100x. (*B*). T1, CD30 immunohistochemistry with hematoxylin counterstain.

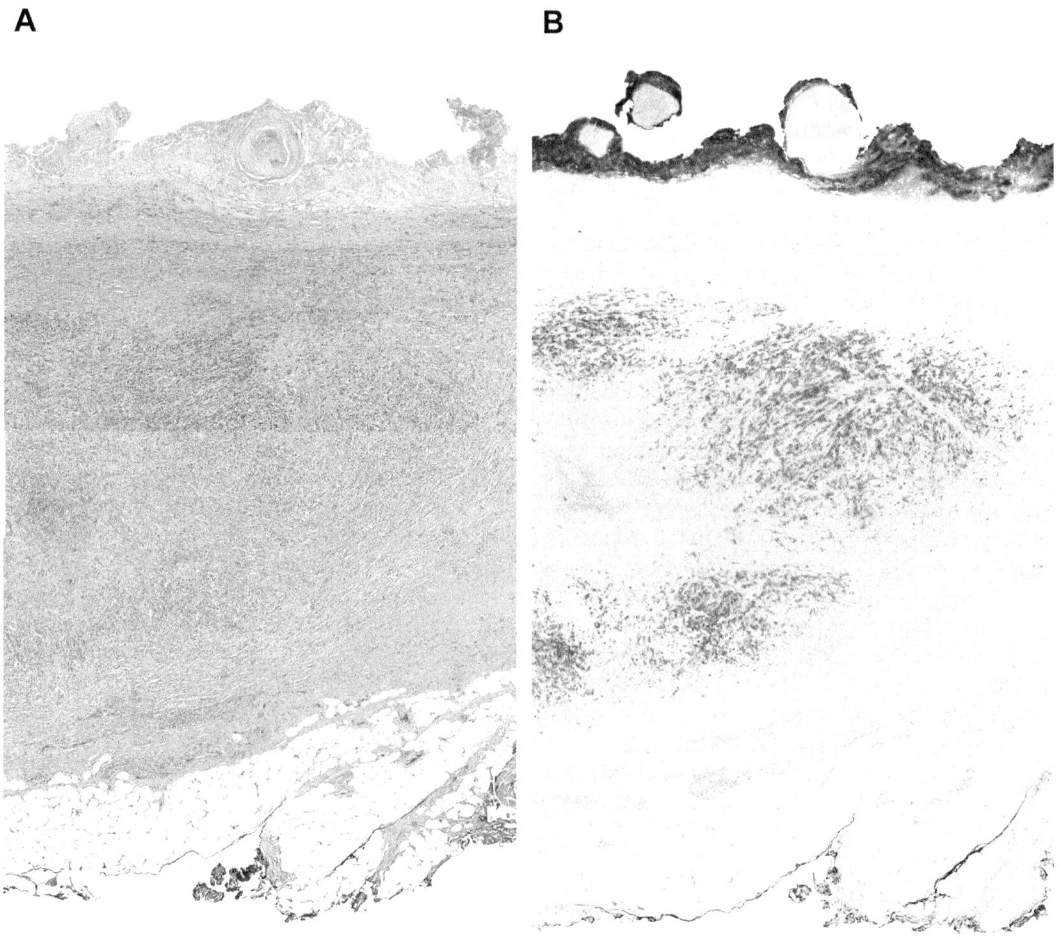

Fig. 6. Histologic staging of BIA-ALCL. (*A*) pT4, lymphoma cells are in the luminal space as well as deep through and beyond the capsule. H&E, 40x. (*B*). pT4, CD30 immunohistochemistry with hematoxylin counterstain displays reactivity both on the luminal side (*superior*) as well as through and beyond the capsule. 40x. Note that the inked margin (*bottom*) is away from CD30(+) cells, and is thus not involved by tumor.

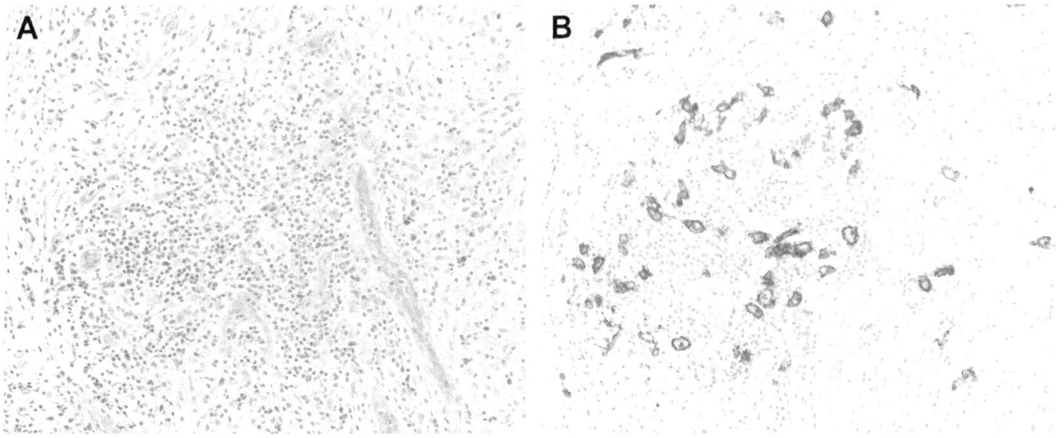

Fig. 7. Histologic staging of BIA-ALCL. (*A*) pT4, lymphoma cells are noted invading into breast parenchyma, denoting a highly aggressive behavior. H&E, 200x. (*B*). pT4, CD30 immunohistochemistry with hematoxylin counterstain displays reactivity of CD30(+) lymphoma cells amidst breast ducts. 200x.

small clusters within the effusion or as floating clots similar to the inner lining of the fibrous capsule. Although the background eosinophilic material has a low magnification resemblance to fibrin, this material is in fact composed of abundant necrotic "ghost" cells. Immunohistochemistry using CD30 highlights almost all the identified lymphoma cells on H&E stain, as well as the outlines of ghost cells or the distinctly granular necrotic debris. We have proposed a tumor staging system to assess the degree of tumor infiltration into the capsule.[4,63] T0 indicates that the tumor cells are confined to the fluid, and no tumor cells are detected in the capsule. T1 signifies that the lymphoma cells are attached to and confined to the luminal surface and are not admixed with inflammatory cells (Fig. 5). T2 occurs when there is minimal infiltration into the capsule and the tumor cells are minimally admixed with inflammatory cells. T3 indicates that tumor cells are invasive into the capsule and notably surrounded by many inflammatory cells. T4 designates the presence of tumor cells beyond the capsule (Fig. 6), where many viable tumor cells, usually in sheets, and areas of necrosis are commonly detected. T4 includes cases where the lymphoma is in the soft tissue around the implant, as well as when tumor infiltrates the breast parenchyma; we consider these latter cases a more aggressive stage of the disease (Fig. 7). T4 usually correlates with the clinical detection of a mass.[10,64] This pathologic T stage is included in a clinical tumor node metastasis (TNM) solid tumor staging system modeled after the American Joint Committee on Cancer TNM solid tumor staging, and is now advocated by the NCCN.[61,63] Using this TNM system, the distribution of stages in BIA-ALCL in our experience is as follows: IA, 36%; IB, 12%; IC, 14%; IIA, 25%; IIB, 5%; III, 9%; and IV, 0% to 9%.[64]

LYMPH NODE INVOLVEMENT

About 35% of patients with BIA-ALCL have clinical or radiologically enlarged regional lymph nodes.[10,41] It is well known that silicone can elicit regional lymphadenopathy in patients with breast implants, with or without BIA-ALCL, causing a reaction of foamy histiocytes or foreign body giant cell reaction to silicone. The frequency of these histiocytic reactions in patients with BIA-ALCL is unknown at this time. The frequency of lymphadenopathy as a result of dissemination of BIA-ALCL proven by biopsy or highly suspicious cases by imaging studies is 23% at diagnosis or during follow-up.[37] The incidence is 17% when the definition of lymph node involvement is limited only to patients with pathologic assessment of lymph nodes.[37] BIA-ALCL involves lymph nodes most often in a sinusoidal pattern, in over 90% of cases, but perifollicular (Fig. 8), interfollicular, and diffuse patterns of involvement may also occur and, in some cases, the neoplasm can mimic classic Hodgkin lymphoma.[37] The number and extent of lymph nodes involved by BIA-ALCL should be clearly stated, as it may reflect the aggressiveness of disease. These data also may be a factor in the decisions to use chemotherapy, immunotherapy, or radiation therapy by the multidisciplinary management team.

DIFFERENTIAL DIAGNOSIS

With increased attention to the pathology of periimplant capsules, a variety of benign, and malignant processes have been identified. Of most importance is the presence of lymphoma types other than BIA-ALCL, most of which appear to have a similar anatomic distribution when compared with BIA-ALCL. More experience is needed to better understand the natural history

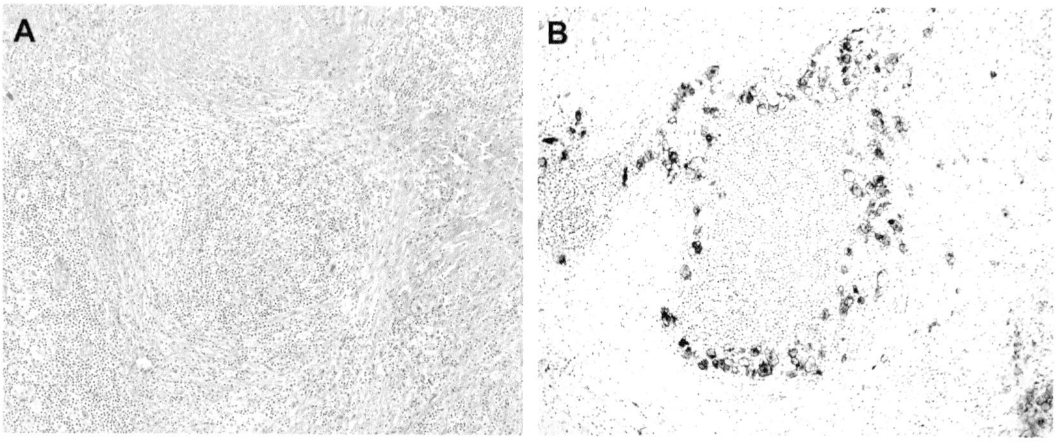

Fig. 8. Lymph node involvement by BIA-ALCL. (*A*). Effacement of the architecture of an axillary lymph node in a patient with BIA-ALCL, displaying a vaguely nodular distorted lymphoid follicle in this field. H&E, 200x. (*B*). CD30 immunohistochemistry highlights CD30(+) in a perifollicular pattern.

of the other lymphoma types that involve peri-implant capsules.

EPSTEIN–BARR VIRUS-POSITIVE LARGE B-CELL LYMPHOMA ASSOCIATED WITH BREAST IMPLANTS

EBV-positive LBCL associated with breast implants is a lymphoma associated with textured breast implants that are grossly and microscopically similar to BIA-ALCL. Unlike BIA-ALCL, however, the fibrous capsule is thicker, and the necrosis is more abundant and arranged in layers.[54,65] The neoplastic cells express pan B-cell antigens and have a nongerminal center immunophenotype. EBER is positive and shows a latency type III pattern of infection. CD30 is variably expressed, with some cases strongly and diffusely positive, whereas others are negative. EBV appears to be essential in the pathogenesis and diagnosis of this disease. The unifying hypothesis is centered on chronic inflammation and persistent antigenic stimulation. Some researchers have proposed that EBV(+) LBCL associated with breast implants has a pathogenesis similar to fibrin-associated EBV(+) LBCL.[6665]

SYSTEMIC ANAPLASTIC LARGE CELL LYMPHOMA, ANAPLASTIC LYMPHOMA KINASE-NEGATIVE, AND ANAPLASTIC LYMPHOMA KINASE-POSITIVE

Most patients with systemic ALCL do not have breast implants. The histopathologic and immunophenotypic features of systemic ALCL overlap with BIA-ALCL, but patients with systemic ALCL usually have systemic disease whereas BIA-ALCL involves the capsule around the implants.[4,67] In addition, ALK-positive ALCL cases are easily distinguished from BIA-ALCL based on ALK expression.[4]

DIFFUSE LARGE B-CELL LYMPHOMA, NOT OTHERWISE SPECIFIED

Rare cases of diffuse large B-cell lymphoma (DLBCL), not otherwise specified have been reported,[68] with an anatomic distribution very similar to BIA-ALCL, and these patients apparently have an excellent prognosis after complete resection and treatment with standard frontline DLBCL therapy. Most of the few cases of DLBCL associated with implants reported have had a non-germinal center B-cell immunophenotype.[69]

PLASMABLASTIC LYMPHOMA AND PRIMARY EFFUSION LYMPHOMA

Both of these lymphomas arise in the setting of immunodeficiency, most commonly HIV. Plasmablastic lymphoma is an aggressive type of lymphoma composed of cells that resemble large, immature plasma cells, and thus lack B-cell markers, but express plasma cell markers such as CD138 and/or MUM1/IRF4, and frequently express CD30. These cases commonly show kappa or lambda light chain restriction, and about 70% of cases are positive for EBER.[70] Primary effusion lymphoma typically involves body cavity sites without associated mass lesions and thus may enter the differential diagnosis of BIA-ALCL.[2] Its morphology and immunophenotype are similar to plasmablastic lymphoma and most cases show co-infection with EBV (EBER-positive) and human herpes virus-8 (HHV8).[5] Another rare LBCL with plasmablastic morphology, ALK(+) LBCL, may also enter this differential diagnosis, but positivity for ALK, typically in a cytoplasmic distribution, and absence of CD30 expression distinguish these neoplasms from BIA-ALCL.

EXTRANODAL MARGINAL ZONE LYMPHOMA

Extranodal marginal zone lymphoma has been noted rarely to occur in breast capsules around implants and patients with these neoplasms seem to have an indolent clinical course.[71] Grossly, extranodal marginal zone lymphoma shows thickening of the fibrous capsule. Microscopically there is a diffuse infiltrate of small, mature lymphocytes with a variable number of plasmacytic cells along the fibrous capsule. Regional lymph nodes may be involved.

EXTRANODAL NATURAL Killer/T-CELL LYMPHOMA

Extranodal NK/T-cell lymphoma involving the capsule surrounding an implant has been reported. These neoplasms are locally aggressive, pleomorphic and angiocentric, and exhibit a latency type III pattern of EBV infection. The tumor cells have a cytotoxic NK immunophenotype positive for TIA-1, granzyme B and CD56, and are partially CD30 positive. One reported patient was alive at last follow-up after removal of the neoplasm.[72]

SQUAMOUS CELL CARCINOMA

Of interest is the presence of squamous cell carcinoma arising in longstanding capsules around breast implants.[73] Most reported cases present with an invasive mass and exhibit an aggressive clinical behavior. The entirely different histology of squamous cell carcinoma, as compared with lymphomas, raises questions about its pathogenesis. These neoplasms are relatively easy to distinguish from BIA-ALCL based on their morphologic features and expression of keratin and other epithelial-associated markers such as p63 and CK5/6.

MESENCHYMAL TUMORS

Most mesenchymal tumors around breast implants have been classified as fibromatosis and tend to recur. Sarcomas appear to be extremely rare.[74]

TREATMENT AND PROGNOSIS

Following the 2019 NCCN consensus guidelines, the standard therapy for patients with disease confined to the capsule (T1 to T3) or to adjacent soft tissue or underlying breast parenchyma (T4) is en bloc complete capsulectomy with negative margins,[9,40,75] with a recommendation for resection of contralateral implant and capsule to address the possibility of asymptomatic contralateral tumor. After complete surgical excision, surveillance follow-up and imaging are recommended every 3 to 6 months in the first 2 years. A complete remission rate, more properly designated as a cure, is achievable in up to 90% of patients in this setting.[9,36,75] Importantly, if the diagnosis is initially missed, the evaluation of sequential specimens of patients with BIA-ALCL who did not undergo complete capsulectomy will show persistence or progression of disease.[76]

Patients with incomplete surgical resection or with successful complete capsulectomy but local lymph node involvement are usually treated with protocols similar to those used to treat systemic ALCL, such as cyclophosphamide, doxorubicin, vincristine, and prednisone (CHOP)-based regimens or anti-CD30 immunotherapy (brentuximab vedotin) with or without radiation therapy.[9] However, there are no prospective trials to evaluate the efficacy of these different types of regimens.[15,75] No standard of care is established in advanced clinical stage of disease and, in this scenario, neoadjuvant therapy followed by palliative resection with debulking and adjuvant chemotherapy could be a possible regimen.[40]

Finally, a prophylactic capsulectomy in patients with textured implants, who are otherwise asymptomatic, is not recommended to reduce the risk of BIA-ALCL.[15]

SUMMARY

BIA-ALCL is an uncommon type of non-Hodgkin lymphoma with an increasing incidence worldwide. Use of appropriate handling protocols for specimens obtained from patients with a suspected diagnosis of BIA-ALCL is important for precise pathologic staging and for determining the best treatment options in these patients. BIA-ALCL can be cured in most patients who present with effusion only; however, substantial morbidity and mortality can occur in patients who present with advanced disease.

DISCLOSURE

The authors have nothing to disclose.

REFERENCES

1. Keech JA Jr, Creech BJ. Anaplastic T-cell lymphoma in proximity to a saline-filled breast implant. Plast Reconstr Surg 1997;100(2):554–5.

2. Said JW, Tasaka T, Takeuchi S, et al. Primary effusion lymphoma in women: report of two cases of Kaposi's sarcoma herpes virus-associated effusion-based lymphoma in human immunodeficiency virus-negative women. Blood 1996;88(8):3124–8.
3. Lyapichev KA, Medeiros L, Clemens M, et al. Reconsideration of the first recognition of breast implant-associated anaplastic large cell lymphoma: A critical review of the literature. Ann Diagn Pathol 2020;45:151474.
4. Miranda RN, Feldman AL, Soares FA. Breast implant-associated anaplastic large cell lymphoma. In: Allison KH, Edi B, Ellis IO, et al, editors. World Health Organization Breast Tumours. 5th edition. Lyon: IARC; 2019. p. 245–8.
5. Alaggio R, Amador C, Anagnostopoulos I, et al. The 5th edition of the World Health Organization Classification of Haematolymphoid Tumours: Lymphoid Neoplasms. Leukemia 2022;36(7):1720–48.
6. Oishi N, Hundal T, Phillips JL, et al. Molecular profiling reveals a hypoxia signature in breast implant-associated anaplastic large cell lymphoma. Haematologica 2021;106(6):1714–24.
7. Talwalkar SS, Miranda RN, Valbuena JR, et al. Lymphomas involving the breast: a study of 106 cases comparing localized and disseminated neoplasms. Am J Surg Pathol 2008;32(9):1299–309.
8. Kinslow CJ, Kim A, Sanchez GI, et al. Incidence of anaplastic large cell lymphoma of the breast in the US, 2000 to 2018. JAMA Oncol 2022;8(9):1354–6.
9. Quesada AE, Medeiros LJ, Clemens MW, et al. Breast implant-associated anaplastic large cell lymphoma: a review. Mod Pathol 2019;32(2):166–88.
10. Miranda RN, Aladily TN, Prince HM, et al. Breast implant-associated anaplastic large-cell lymphoma: long-term follow-up of 60 patients. J Clin Oncol 2014;32(2):114–20.
11. Loch-Wilkinson A, Beath KJ, Magnusson MR, et al. Breast implant-associated anaplastic large cell lymphoma in Australia: a longitudinal study of implant and other related risk factors. Aesthet Surg J 2020;40(8):838–46.
12. de Boer M, Hauptmann M, Hijmering NJ, et al. Increased prevalence of BRCA1/2 mutations in women with macrotextured breast implants and anaplastic large cell lymphoma of the breast. Blood 2020;136(11):1368–72.
13. Collett DJ, Rakhorst H, Lennox P, et al. Current risk estimate of breast implant-associated anaplastic large cell lymphoma in textured breast implants. Plast Reconstr Surg 2019;143(3S):30s–40s.
14. Ionescu P, Vibert F, Amé S, et al. New data on the epidemiology of breast implant-associated anaplastic large cell lymphoma. Eur J Breast Health 2021;17(4):302–7.
15. Santanelli di Pompeo F, Clemens MW, Atlan M, et al. 2022 Practice recommendation updates from the World Consensus Conference on BIA-ALCL. Aesthet Surg J 2022;42(11):1262–78.
16. Cordeiro PG, Ghione P, Ni A, et al. Risk of breast implant associated anaplastic large cell lymphoma (BIA-ALCL) in a cohort of 3546 women prospectively followed long term after reconstruction with textured breast implants. J Plast Reconstr Aesthet Surg 2020;73(5):841–6.
17. Magnusson M, Beath K, Cooter R, et al. The Epidemiology of breast implant–associated anaplastic large cell lymphoma in Australia and New Zealand confirms the highest risk for grade 4 surface breast implants. Plast Reconstr Surg 2019;143(5):1285–92.
18. Doren EL, Miranda RN, Selber JC, et al, U.S. Epidemiology of breast implant-associated anaplastic large cell lymphoma. Plast Reconstr Surg 2017;139(5):1042–50.
19. Lynch EB, DeCoster RC, Vyas KS, et al. Current risk of breast implant-associated anaplastic large cell lymphoma: a systematic review of epidemiological studies. Ann Breast 2021;5:30.
20. Wang Y, Zhang Q, Tan Y, et al. Current progress in breast implant-associated anaplastic large cell lymphoma. Front Oncol 2021;11:785887.
21. Roden AC, Macon WR, Keeney GL, et al. Seroma-associated primary anaplastic large-cell lymphoma adjacent to breast implants: an indolent T-cell lymphoproliferative disorder. Mod Pathol 2008;21(4):455–63.
22. Story SK, Schowalter MK, Geskin LJ. Breast implant-associated ALCL: a unique entity in the spectrum of CD30+ lymphoproliferative disorders. Oncologist 2013;18(3):301–7.
23. Talmadge JE, Donkor M, Scholar E. Inflammatory cell infiltration of tumors: Jekyll or Hyde. Cancer Metastasis Rev 2007;26(3–4):373–400.
24. Malcolm TI, Hodson DJ, Macintyre EA, et al. Challenging perspectives on the cellular origins of lymphoma. Open Biol 2016;6(9):1–12.
25. Multhoff G, Molls M, Radons J. Chronic inflammation in cancer development. Front Immunol 2011;2:98.
26. Rauch D, Gross S, Harding J, et al. T-cell activation promotes tumorigenesis in inflammation-associated cancer. Retrovirology 2009;6:116.
27. Bondurant S, Ernster V, Herdman R. Safety of silicone breast implants. Washington, DC: National Academies Press; 2000.
28. Lazzeri D, Agostini T, Bocci G, et al. ALK-1-negative anaplastic large cell lymphoma associated with breast implants: a new clinical entity. Clin Breast Cancer 2011;11(5):283–96.
29. Lechner MG, Megiel C, Church CH, et al. Survival signals and targets for therapy in breast implant-associated ALK–anaplastic large cell lymphoma. Clin Cancer Res 2012;18(17):4549–59.
30. Meza Britez ME, Caballero Llano C, Chaux A. Periprosthetic breast capsules and immunophenotypes

of inflammatory cells. Eur J Plast Surg 2012;35(9): 647–51.
31. Xu S, Cao X. Interleukin-17 and its expanding biological functions. Cell Mol Immunol 2010;7(3):164–74.
32. Wolfram D, Rabensteiner E, Grundtman C, et al. T regulatory cells and TH17 cells in peri-silicone implant capsular fibrosis. Plast Reconstr Surg 2012;129(2):327e–37e.
33. Leung S, Liu X, Fang L, et al. The cytokine milieu in the interplay of pathogenic Th1/Th17 cells and regulatory T cells in autoimmune disease. Cell Mol Immunol 2010;7(3):182–9.
34. Kadin ME, Morgan J, Kouttab N, et al. Comparative analysis of cytokines of tumor cell lines, malignant and benign effusions around breast implants. Aesthet Surg J 2019;40(6):630–7.
35. Kadin ME, Deva A, Xu H, et al. Biomarkers provide clues to early events in the pathogenesis of breast implant-associated anaplastic large cell lymphoma. Aesthet Surg J 2016;36(7):773–81.
36. Yoo H, Park JU, Chang H. Comprehensive evaluation of the current knowledge on breast implant associated-anaplastic large cell lymphoma. Arch Plast Surg 2022;49(2):141–9.
37. Ferrufino-Schmidt MC, Medeiros LJ, Liu H, et al. Clinicopathologic features and prognostic impact of lymph node involvement in patients with breast implant-associated anaplastic large cell lymphoma. Am J Surg Pathol 2018;42(3):293–305.
38. Stuver R, Lewis NE, Ewalt MD, et al. First report of bilateral breast-implant associated anaplastic large cell lymphoma caused by identical T-cell clone. Leuk Lymphoma 2022;63(11):2747–50.
39. Bautista-Quach MA, Nademanee A, Weisenburger DD, et al. Implant-associated primary anaplastic large-cell lymphoma with simultaneous involvement of bilateral breast capsules. Clin Breast Cancer 2013;13(6):492–5.
40. Lillemoe HA, Miranda RN, Nastoupil LJ, et al. Clinical manifestations and surgical management of breast implant-associated anaplastic large cell lymphoma: Beyond the NCCN guidelines. Ann Surg Oncol 2022;29(9):5722–9.
41. Adrada BE, Miranda RN, Rauch GM, et al. Breast implant-associated anaplastic large cell lymphoma: sensitivity, specificity, and findings of imaging studies in 44 patients. Breast Cancer Res Treat 2014;147(1):1–14.
42. Chourmouzi DVT, Drevelegas A. New spontaneous breast seroma 5 years after augmentation: a case report. Cases J 2009;2:7126.
43. Mazzocchi MDL, Corrias F, Scuderi N. A clinical study of late seroma in breast implantation surgery. Aesthet Plast Surg 2012;36:97–104.
44. Carty MJ, Pribaz JJ, Antin JH, et al. A patient death attributable to implant-related primary anaplastic large cell lymphoma of the breast. Plast Reconstr Surg 2011;128(3):112e–8e.
45. Chai SM, Kavangh S, Ooi SS, et al. Anaplastic large-cell lymphoma associated with breast implants: A unique entity within the spectrum of peri-implant effusions. Diagn cytopathology 2014;42(11):929–38.
46. Farkash EA, Ferry JA, Harris NL, et al. Rare lymphoid malignancies of the breast: a report of two cases illustrating potential diagnostic pitfalls. J Hematop 2009;2(4):237–44.
47. Popplewell L, Thomas SH, Huang Q, et al. Primary anaplastic large-cell lymphoma associated with breast implants. Leuk Lymphoma 2011;52(8): 1481–7.
48. Smith TJ, Ramsaroop R. Breast implant related anaplastic large cell lymphoma presenting as late onset peri-implant effusion. Breast 2012;21(1): 102–4.
49. Talagas M, Uguen A, Charles-Petillon F, et al. Breast implant-associated anaplastic large-cell lymphoma can be a diagnostic challenge for pathologists. Acta Cytol 2014;58(1):103–7.
50. George EV, Pharm J, Houston C, et al. Breast implant-associated ALK-negative anaplastic large cell lymphoma: a case report and discussion of possible pathogenesis. Int J Clin Exp Pathol 2013; 6(8):1631–42.
51. Singh E, Frost E, Morris EJ, et al. Anaplastic lymphoma masquerading as breast abscess in a patient with silicone implants. Breast J 2013;19(5): 543–5.
52. Li S, Lee AK. Silicone implant and primary breast ALK1-negative anaplastic large cell lymphoma, fact or fiction? Int J Clin Exp Pathol 2009;3(1): 117–27.
53. Taylor CR, Siddiqi IN, Brody GS. Anaplastic large cell lymphoma occurring in association with breast implants: review of pathologic and immunohistochemical features in 103 cases. Appl Immunohistochem Mol Morphol : AIMM 2013;21(1):13–20.
54. Medeiros LJ, Marques-Piubelli ML, Sangiorgio VFI, et al. Epstein-Barr-virus-positive large B-cell lymphoma associated with breast implants: an analysis of eight patients suggesting a possible pathogenetic relationship. Mod Pathol 2021;34(12):2154–67.
55. Fleming D, Stone J, Tansley P. Spontaneous regression and resolution of breast implant-associated anaplastic large cell lymphoma: Implications for research, diagnosis and clinical management. Aesthet Plast Surg 2018;42(3):672–8.
56. Horna P, Wang SA, Wolniak KL, et al. Flow cytometric evaluation of peripheral blood for suspected Sézary syndrome or mycosis fungoides: International guidelines for assay characteristics. Cytometry B, Clin cytometry 2021;100(2):142–55.
57. Kadin ME, Xu H, Hunsicker LM, et al. Non-malignant CD30+ cells in contralateral peri-Implant capsule of patient with BIA-ALCL: A premalignant step? Aesthet Surg J 2021;42(2):NP125–9.

58. Oishi N, Brody G, Ketterling R, et al. Genetic subtyping of breast implant-associated anaplastic large cell lymphoma. Blood 2018;132(5):544–7.
59. Lyapichev KA, Pina-Oviedo S, Medeiros LJ, et al. A proposal for pathologic processing of breast implant capsules in patients with suspected breast implant anaplastic large cell lymphoma. Mod Pathol 2020;33(3):367–79.
60. Horwitz SM, Ansell S, Ai WZ, et al. T-Cell Lymphomas, Version 2.2022, NCCN Clinical Practice Guidelines in Oncology. J Natl Compr Canc Netw 2022;20(3):285–308.
61. Jaffe ES, Ashar BS, Clemens MW, et al. Best practices guideline for the pathologic diagnosis of breast implant-associated anaplastic large-cell lymphoma. J Clin Oncol 2020;38(10):1102–11.
62. Turton P, El-Sharkawi D, Lyburn I, et al. UK guidelines on the diagnosis and treatment of breast implant-associated anaplastic large cell lymphoma (BIA-ALCL) on behalf of the Medicines and Healthcare products Regulatory Agency (MHRA) Plastic, Reconstructive and Aesthetic Surgery Expert Advisory Group (PRASEAG). J Plast Reconstr Aesthet Surg 2021;74(1):13–29.
63. Clemens MW, Horwitz SM. NCCN Consensus guidelines for the diagnosis and management of breast implant-associated anaplastic large cell lymphoma. Aesthet Surg J 2017;37(3):285–9.
64. Clemens MW, Medeiros LJ, Butler CE, et al. Complete surgical excision Is essential for the management of patients with breast implant-associated anaplastic large cell lymphoma. J Clin Oncol 2016; 34(2):160–8.
65. Rodríguez-Pinilla SM, García FJS, Balagué O, et al. Breast implant-associated Epstein-Barr virus-positive large B-cell lymphomas: a report of three cases. Haematologica 2020;105(8):e412–4.
66. Boroumand N, Ly TL, Sonstein J, et al. Microscopic diffuse large B-cell lymphoma (DLBCL) occurring in pseudocysts: do these tumors belong to the category of DLBCL associated with chronic inflammation? Am J Surg Pathol 2012;36(7):1074–80.
67. Miranda RN. Anaplastic large cell lymphoma involving the breast: a clinicopathologic study of 6 cases and review of the literature. Arch Pathol Lab Med 2009;133:1383–90.
68. Smith BK, Gray SS. Large B-cell lymphoma occurring in a breast implant capsule. Plast Reconstr Surg 2014;134(4):670e–1e.
69. Larrimore C, Jaghab A. A rare case of breast implant-associated diffuse large B-cell lymphoma. Case Rep Oncological Med 2019;2019:1801942.
70. Geethakumari PR, Markantonis J, Shah JL, et al. Breast implant-associated plasmablastic lymphoma: a case report and discussion of the literature. Clin Lymphoma Myeloma Leuk 2019;19(10): e568–72.
71. Evans MG, Miranda RN, Young PA, et al. B-cell lymphomas associated with breast implants: Report of three cases and review of the literature. Ann Diagn Pathol 2020;46:151512.
72. Aladily TN, Nathwani BN, Miranda RN, et al. Extranodal NK/T-cell lymphoma, nasal type, arising in association with saline breast implant: expanding the spectrum of breast implant-associated lymphomas. Am J Surg Pathol 2012;36(11):1729–34.
73. Olsen DL, Keeney GL, Chen B, et al. Breast implant capsule-associated squamous cell carcinoma: a report of 2 cases. Hum Pathol 2017;67:94–100.
74. Balzer BL, Weiss SW. Do biomaterials cause implant-associated mesenchymal tumors of the breast? Analysis of 8 new cases and review of the literature. Hum Pathol 2009;40(11):1564–70.
75. Clemens MW, Jacobsen ED, Horwitz SM. 2019 NCCN Consensus guidelines on the diagnosis and treatment of breast implant-associated anaplastic large cell lymphoma (BIA-ALCL). Aesthet Surg J 2019;39(Supplement_1):S3–13.
76. Evans MG, Medeiros LJ, Marques-Piubelli ML, et al. Breast implant-associated anaplastic large cell lymphoma: clinical follow-up and analysis of sequential pathologic specimens of untreated patients shows persistent or progressive disease. Mod Pathol 2021;34(12):2148–53.

Aggressive Cutaneous Lymphomas and Their Mimics

Andrea P. Moy, MD*, Melissa P. Pulitzer, MD

KEYWORDS

• Cutaneous lymphoma • Cutaneous T-cell lymphoma • Cutaneous B-cell lymphoma • Diffuse large B-cell lymphoma, leg type • Primary cutaneous gamma-delta T-cell lymphoma • Primary cutaneous CD8+ aggressive epidermotropic cytotoxic T-cell lymphoma • Extranodal NK/T-cell lymphoma • Adult T-cell leukemia/lymphoma

Key points

- Histopathologic features of aggressive primary cutaneous lymphomas can overlap with those of indolent lymphomas/lymphoproliferative disorders (LPDs), systemic lymphomas, and reactive processes, making clinicopathologic correlation critical for diagnosis.
- Diffuse large B-cell lymphoma, leg type most commonly requires distinction from primary cutaneous follicle center lymphoma with a diffuse growth pattern; molecular studies, including the presence of *MYD88* mutation, may assist in this distinction.
- The diagnosis of aggressive cutaneous T-cell lymphomas, including primary cutaneous gamma/delta T-cell lymphoma and CD8+ aggressive epidermotropic cytotoxic T-cell lymphoma, requires correlation with clinical and immunophenotypic features; the presence of molecular alterations involving the JAK/STAT signaling pathway may also be helpful.
- EBV-associated cutaneous lymphomas/LPDs that may arise in the differential diagnosis of extranodal NK/T-cell lymphoma include hydroa vacciniforme lymphoproliferative disorder and some cases of lymphomatoid granulomatosis, mucocutaneous ulcer, and methotrexate-associated lymphoproliferative disorder.
- Adult T-cell leukemia/lymphoma is distinguished from its mimics (ie, mycosis fungoides and Sézary syndrome) by correlation with HTLV-1 serologic studies.

ABSTRACT

Cutaneous lymphomas encompass a heterogeneous group of neoplasms with a wide spectrum of clinical presentations, histopathologic features, and prognosis. Because there are overlapping pathologic features among indolent and aggressive forms and with systemic lymphomas that involve the skin, clinicopathologic correlation is essential. Herein, the clinical and histopathologic features of aggressive cutaneous B- and T-cell lymphomas are reviewed. Indolent cutaneous lymphomas/lymphoproliferative disorders, systemic lymphomas, and reactive processes that may mimic these entities are also discussed. This article highlights distinctive clinical and histopathologic features, increases awareness of rare entities, and presents new and evolving developments in the field.

OVERVIEW

The heterogeneous, complex, yet often subtle presentation of cutaneous lymphoma poses significant diagnostic and therapeutic challenge for pathologists, oncologists, and dermatologists alike. The

Department of Pathology and Laboratory Medicine, Memorial Sloan Kettering Cancer Center, 1275 York Avenue, New York, NY 10065, USA
* Corresponding author.
E-mail address: moya@mskcc.org

Surgical Pathology 16 (2023) 361–383
https://doi.org/10.1016/j.path.2023.01.009

most common B-cell and T-cell subtypes are typically associated with an indolent clinical course and good prognosis. However, some less common subtypes are characterized by aggressive behavior and poor outcomes, requiring intensive and multimodal therapeutic intervention. These aggressive subtypes can have clinical and pathologic features that mimic indolent lymphoma/lymphoproliferative disorders (LPDs) or secondary cutaneous involvement by a systemic lymphoma. Thus, careful integration of clinical characteristics, histopathologic data, and results of ancillary and molecular studies is required to make the most accurate diagnosis, thereby directing appropriate clinical management. Herein, we present key clinicopathologic markers and the constellations of findings most important for the recognition of aggressive cutaneous lymphomas. We discuss the differential diagnoses, highlighting distinguishing features and rare entities. We also review new developments regarding molecular attributes, which may facilitate more precise classification and identify prognostic markers and therapeutic targets.

CUTANEOUS DIFFUSE LARGE B-CELL LYMPHOMA, LEG TYPE

Diffuse large B-cell lymphoma, leg-type (DLBCL-LT) is a malignant lymphoma of postgerminal center/activated B-cell origin, which accounts for approximately 10% to 20% of primary cutaneous B-cell lymphomas.[1]

CLINICAL FEATURES

DLBCL-LT typically occurs on the legs of elderly patients with a mean age between 70 and 80 years, with a female predisposition. In about 10% to 20% of cases, other body sites are affected, including the trunk, arm, head, and neck. Patients often present with rapidly growing skin nodules/tumors, infiltrative plaques, large subcutaneous tumors, or leg ulceration.[2] Some present with a solitary lesion, although more commonly multifocal lesions develop. B-symptoms occur in a minority of patients. Early DLBCL-LT can occasionally present with mycosis fungoides (MF)-like patches or annular changes resembling erythema chronicum migrans or gyrate erythema.[3,4] Recurrent or advanced-stage DLBCL-LT demonstrates clinical features similar to primary lesions, with retained tropism for the leg.

MICROSCOPIC FEATURES

Skin biopsy shows a dense dermal infiltrate of predominantly large immunoblastic and centroblastic cells with round nuclei and variably prominent nucleoli, extending into the subcutis. Frequent mitotic figures are present and necrosis may be seen. Rare patterns include a starry-sky appearance, superficial to middermal bandlike infiltrate, angiocentricity, epidermal involvement, and spindle cells.[5,6] Early lesions may show few perivascular aggregates of large cells, foreshadowing a challenging diagnostic process. The neoplastic cells express traditional B-cell markers, including CD20, PAX5, and CD79a. BCL2, MUM1, and FOX-P1 are strongly positive in most cases. The significance of the lack of BCL2 and MUM1 expression in cases that otherwise meet clinicopathologic criteria for DLBCL-LT is unclear.[2,6–9] Typically, BCL6 is positive and CD10 is negative.[10] IgM is strongly expressed, sometimes with coexpression of IgD. MYC expression is present in about half of cases and CD30 expression may be seen.[11–13] Ki67 proliferative index is high. FOXP3 labeling of cells may indicate a better prognostic group.[14] Most cases show no follicular dendritic cell meshworks with CD21, CD23, or CD35. Sparse admixed, predominantly perivascular reactive T cells may be present.

GENETIC AND MOLECULAR FEATURES

Monoclonal rearrangement of the immunoglobulin genes is present. Mutations in *MYD88* and other genes involved in the nuclear factor-κB signaling pathway (including *CD79 B*, *TNFAIP3*, and *CARD11*) is found in most cases.[15–19] Studies have shown recurrent DNA amplifications of chromosome 18q21.31 to 33, which involves *BCL2* and *MALT1*, and inactivation of 9p21.3, containing *CDKN2A* and *CDKN2B*, by deletion or promoter hypermethylation.[20–22] Despite BCL2 expression, there is no t(14;18) translocation involving *BCL2* and *IGH* genes. Rearrangements involving *MUM1/IRF4* or *FOXP1* are also not present despite expression by immunohistochemistry (IHC).[23,24] *MYC* rearrangement may be identified and rarely a second "hit" occurs with *BCL2* or *BCL6* rearrangement; however, these cases are likely best classified separately.[22–27]

PROGNOSIS

The 5-year survival of patients with DLBCL-LT is poor compared with more common primary cutaneous B-cell lymphomas types and may be up to 50% to 70%.[28–31] Multifocal tumors, location on the leg, inactivation of *CDKN2A*/loss of 9p21, and the presence of *MYD88* L265 R mutation are associated with an unfavorable prognosis.[2,22] The prognostic significance of MYC expression or rearrangement in DLBCL-LT is unclear.[26,27] Also, data regarding the significance of CD30 expression are lacking.[11–13]

DIFFERENTIAL DIAGNOSIS

The differential diagnosis of DLBCL-LT is broad and includes cutaneous and systemic B-cell lymphomas. Perhaps most commonly in the differential diagnosis is primary cutaneous follicle center lymphoma (PCFCL). In contrast to DLBCL-LT, PCFCL is indolent and of germinal center origin. Although it typically presents as plaques, nodules, or tumors on the head, neck, or trunk, rare cases occur on the leg. It remains unclear if cases that present on the leg behave more aggressively than PCFCL at other sites and more similarly to DLBCL-LT.[2,8,31] PCFCL shows an infiltrate of centrocytes and variable numbers of centroblasts with a follicular, follicular and diffuse, or diffuse growth pattern; associated stromal fibrosis/sclerosis is common. PCFCL cases with a diffuse pattern and a predominance of large centrocytes and centroblasts is challenging to distinguish from DLBCL-LT. PCFCL is typically positive for BCL6, ± CD10 (less often seen in the diffuse pattern), and negative for MUM1 and FOXP1. Although PCFCL is typically BCL2 negative, approximately 20% of cases are BCL2-positive and rarely PCFCL can have a *BCL2* rearrangement[8,32,33]; therefore, BCL2 negativity cannot be used to distinguish PCFCL from DLBCL-LT. IgM ± IgD expression supports DLBCL-LT over PCFCL. Gene expression profiling studies have shown that there is overlap in patterns associated with cell of origin among some cases of DLBCL-LT and PCFCL and suggest a more integrated diagnostic approach incorporating mutational profile may be needed for precise classification.[34–37]

Systemic DLBCL involving the skin is difficult to distinguish from DLBCL-LT on histopathologic and immunophenotypic findings alone. A clinical history of systemic disease is most helpful. However, cutaneous involvement by systemic DLBCL can precede or appear concomitantly with the diagnosis of systemic disease, complicating precise clinicopathologic classification. Of note, although the presence of *MYD88* mutation supports a diagnosis of DLBCL-LT over systemic DLBCL or PCFCL with BCL2 positivity, clinical correlation is needed to exclude the possibility of secondary cutaneous involvement by a primary central nervous system (CNS) or testicular lymphoma, both of which may harbor the same mutation. The identification of rearrangement of *MYC* in addition to *BCL2* and/or *BCL6* within DLBCL characterizes "double-hit" or "triple-hit" lymphoma, which is now recognized as a specific category of high-grade B-cell lymphoma with aggressive behavior.

Epstein-Barr virus (EBV)-positive DLBCL, not otherwise specified (NOS), in patients older than 50 years and without evidence of immunosuppression, can arise in the skin with or without extracutaneous disease, and may precede systemic involvement. Because patients may present with solitary tumors on the leg, DLBCL-LT may be considered. Skin lesions show an infiltrate composed of centroblasts, immunoblasts, plasmablasts, and/or large cells resembling Hodgkin or Reed-Sternberg cells. Necrosis is commonly seen. In contrast to DLBCL-LT, the tumor cells may show loss of CD20 expression with retained expression of PAX5 and CD79a. EBV, MUM1, and often CD30 are positive; BCL6 is negative.

Cutaneous lesions of angioimmunoblastic T-cell lymphoma (AITL) contain variable numbers of EBV-positive or negative immunoblastic B cells and can mimic DLBCL when these cells are prominent.[38] Thus, recognition of the associated atypical clonal T-cell infiltrate is critical and may be facilitated by IHC for CD4, T-follicular helper antigens (eg, PD1, ICOS, BCL6), and T-cell receptor (TCR) gene rearrangement studies. Furthermore, EBV-positive immunoblastic B-cell proliferations in AITL can rarely progress to DLBCL.[39–41] In these cases, initial biopsies typically show AITL; B-cell lymphoma occurs on follow-up biopsy, with or without coexisting AITL.

Intravascular B-cell lymphoma is an exceedingly rare extranodal B-cell lymphoma that most often affects the skin; rarely, only the skin may be involved. Ill-defined indurated and erythematous plaques, telangiectatic macules or patches, and panniculitis-like lesions are seen.[42,43] Because clinically normal skin may be involved, random biopsy of unremarkable skin may be used for diagnosis.[44,45] Because neoplastic cells may colonize cutaneous hemangiomas, biopsy of a hemangioma may result in higher diagnostic yield.[46] Although DLBLC-LT can show intravascular tumor cells, the predominant localization of large, atypical lymphocytes within the lumens of dermal and subcutaneous small vessels is characteristic of intravascular B-cell lymphoma. The neoplastic cells express pan-B-cell markers, BCL2, and MUM1. MYC is often positive. Expression of CD5, CD10, and BCL6 is seen in a minority of cases. Molecular studies have detected *MYD88* and *CD79 B* mutations, such as other DLBCLs of nongerminal center origin.[47,48]

Other systemic B-cell lymphomas that rarely involve the skin may also be considered in the morphologic differential diagnosis of DLBCL-LT.

Cases with a "starry sky" pattern raise the possibility of Burkitt lymphoma. Although most common in young patients, Burkitt lymphoma involving the skin occurs in older patients as solitary, multiple, or generalized tumors. In contrast to DLBCL-LT, CD10 and BCL6 are positive and BCL2 is negative, consistent with a germinal center phenotype. Ki67 stains nearly all cells. MYC expression and the characteristic t(8;14) involving *MYC* are present. Cutaneous involvement of blastoid or pleomorphic variants of mantle cell lymphoma could mimic DLBCL-LT. However, mantle cell lymphoma is typically positive for cyclin D1 and SOX11 and t(11;14) involving *IGH::CCND1* is characteristic.

Primary effusion B-cell lymphoma (PEL) is Kaposi sarcoma herpesvirus/human herpes virus-8–associated and typically involves serous effusions in HIV-positive or other immunocompromised patients. When present as a solid mass, so-called "extracavitary" PEL, secondary cutaneous involvement may occur as nonspecific localized or generalized nodules. Plasmablastic lymphoma (PBL) also occurs in the setting of HIV infection or other immunodeficiency and can rarely involve the skin[49]; oral mucosal involvement is more common. Although histopathologic analysis of PEL and PBL may raise consideration of DLBCL given the presence of large cells with anaplastic, plasmablastic, or immunoblastic features, PEL and PBL are positive for plasmacytic markers (ie, CD38, CD138) and EBV and negative for B-cell markers (although PBL can express CD79a). PEL is also positive for human herpes virus-8.

Lymphomatoid granulomatosis (LYG) and mucocutaneous ulcer (MCU) are EBV-associated B-cell lymphoproliferative disorders that may mimic DLBCL-LT. LYG most commonly involves the lungs, followed by the skin and CNS. Cutaneous involvement can occur concurrently with or preceding pulmonary disease and is characterized by papules, plaques, or tumors on the trunk or extremities. Histopathologic features vary depending on grade; grade 2 and 3 lesions show an angiocentric and angiodestructive lymphoid infiltrate with frequent large EBV-positive B cells amid a polymorphous inflammatory background. MCU occurs in elderly patients and/or in the setting of immunosuppression, typically in oropharyngeal mucosa and less commonly the skin, as large, ulcerated tumors. Biopsies show a dense, diffuse infiltrate of enlarged atypical cells within a polymorphous background that includes numerous T-cells. Angiocentricity may be seen. Like DLBCL-LT, the tumor cells are positive for PAX5 and MUM1; however, expression of CD20 and CD79a is variable and CD30 and/or CD15 coexpression may be seen, sometimes mimicking Reed-Sternberg cells. EBV is positive. Monoclonal B- and T-cell gene rearrangements may be present. MCU may regress when immunosuppressive causes are removed.

Monomorphic posttransplant lymphoproliferative disorder (PTLD), considered under the nomenclature of lymphoid proliferations and lymphomas that arise in the setting of immune deficiency/dysregulation in the upcoming fifth edition World Health Organization classification,[50] has clinicopathologic features that parallel B-cell or NK/T-cell lymphomas in immunocompetent hosts.[51] B-cell PTLDs most often resemble DLBCL of nongerminal center B-cell type, although they may also be similar to PBL, plasmacytoma, or LYG.[52–55] A clinical history of solid organ or bone marrow transplantation is critical for accurate diagnosis. Cases presenting in the skin may respond to reduction of immunosuppression; however, occasionally more aggressive therapy is needed.

Methotrexate-associated LPDs (MTX-LPD) occur in the setting of chronic MTX therapy, typically for rheumatoid arthritis, and may be associated with EBV. Most cases present like B-cell lymphoma, most often DLBCL, manifesting clinically as multiple plaques or tumors on the lower legs. As with MCU and PTLD, MTX-LPD may regress on withdrawal of immunosuppression (in these cases, specifically MTX); therefore, distinction from DLBCL is critical. EBV-positive cases show expression of CD30 and MUM1 and may show loss of expression of CD20 and CD79a; in contrast, EBV-negative cases are positive for MYC and FOXP1.[56]

PRIMARY CUTANEOUS GAMMA/DELTA T-CELL LYMPHOMA

Primary cutaneous gamma/delta T-cell lymphoma (PCGDTL) is an aggressive cytotoxic cutaneous T-cell lymphoma (CTCL) characterized by cutaneous and/or subcutaneous infiltrates of atypical T cells expressing the $\gamma\delta$ TCR heterodimer. In the past, the ability to diagnose PCGDTL was limited because of the lack of a reliable marker on paraffin-embedded tissue and a $\gamma\delta$ immunophenotype was sometimes inferred based on lack of expression of $\alpha\beta$TCR using beta-F1 IHC. However, confirmation of the positive expression of $\gamma\delta$ TCR is now standard of care to avoid misdiagnosis of TCR-silent $\alpha\beta$ CTCLs.[57,58]

CLINICAL FEATURES

PCGDTL occurs in adults as rapidly progressive localized or generalized patches, plaques, or dermal or panniculitic tumors, frequently with associated ulceration or erosion. Lesions are most often on the lower extremities; the trunk, upper extremities, and head and neck can also be affected. Epidermal changes, such as scaling, is seen before erosion or ulceration develop, mimicking eczema, MF, or psoriasis. Disseminated disease can involve mucosal or other extranodal sites; involvement of lymph nodes, spleen, or bone marrow is rare. Patients may have constitutional symptoms, such as low-grade fever and fatigue, and hematophagocytic lymphohistiocytosis occurs in approximately half of cases, particularly those with subcutaneous involvement.[59,60] Most cases are sporadic; however, an association with autoimmune diseases, other LPDs, and malignancy have been reported, possibly suggesting a risk factor for clonal expansion of γδ T cells.[60–62]

MICROSCOPIC FEATURES

Biopsies show an infiltrate of atypical lymphocytes with variable involvement of the epidermis, dermis, and subcutis (Fig. 1). Histopathologic patterns may vary among biopsies taken from the same patient. Epidermotropism is subtle or marked and associated interface changes with dyskeratosis may be seen. Dermal involvement can show a perivascular, periadnexal, lichenoid, interstitial, nodular, or diffuse pattern. Subcutaneous involvement displays a lobular panniculitic-like pattern and may show rimming of adipocytes by neoplastic lymphocytes. Apoptosis, necrosis, and angioinvasion may be seen. The neoplastic cells range in size from small to large. They are CD3+, CD2+ CD5-, CD7+/−, CD56+/−, express TCRγ and TCRδ proteins, and are negative for TCRβ protein expression. Most cases are negative for CD4, CD8, and CD30; however, CD8 positivity can occur in up to 40% of cases[63] and CD30 is variably expressed.[50] Cytotoxic markers, including granzyme B, perforin, and TIA1, are strongly expressed. EBV is negative. The Ki67 proliferative index is typically high (>50%).

Apparent immunophenotypic switch of TCR or dual expression of αβ and γδ has been reported in rare cases of PCGDTL.[64–67] Some of these cases may represent disease progression through immune escape. More in-depth data and close clinicopathologic correlation are needed to confirm and appropriately classify such cases.

GENETIC AND MOLECULAR FEATURES

Clonal TCR gene rearrangement is present. Some tumors have activating mutations in *STAT5B* and, less often, *STAT3*.[68] A sequencing study has suggested that PCGDTL involving the epidermis or dermis is more likely to derive from Vδ1 cells, whereas panniculitic cases derive from Vδ2 cells, aligning with the respective predominant location of Vδ1 and Vδ2 cells in normal skin. Vδ2 lymphomas showed higher levels of cytotoxic and inflammatory genes by RNA-Seq analysis and were associated with adverse prognostic parameters, including lymph node involvement.[69] Frequent mutations in oncogenic pathways, such as MAPK signaling, JAK-STAT signaling, and chromatin modification, have been identified, including potentially targetable mutations in genes, such as *KRAS*, *NRAS*, *MAPK1*, and *JAK3*.[69]

PROGNOSIS

PCGDTL is associated with a poor prognosis, despite aggressive systemic therapy. The 5-year overall survival rate is approximately 30%.[60,70] Prognosis does not seem to correlate with extent of skin disease (ie, localized vs generalized).[60] There is controversy regarding the prognostic significance of the localization of tumors to the superficial versus deep skin compartments.[60,70–73]

DIFFERENTIAL DIAGNOSIS

Although documenting a γδ immunophenotype is needed to make the diagnosis of PCGDTL, the presence of slight increases in γδ T cells in the skin should be interpreted with caution because γδ T cells may be seen in other lymphoma subtypes, such as MF and lymphomatoid papulosis (LYP). Certain reactive conditions, including pityriasis lichenoides, may also harbor increased γδ T cells, although these typically represent a minority of lymphocytes that mostly express CD4 (or CD8 in younger patients).[74–76]

Subcutaneous panniculitis-like T-cell lymphoma (SPTCL), another mimic of PCGDTL, is a cytotoxic T-cell lymphoma that predominantly involves subcutaneous fat lobules, classically with rimming of medium-sized atypical lymphocytes around individual adipocytes; it typically spares the dermis (except for periadnexal aggregates) and epidermis. Florid involvement of the dermis and epidermis, and the presence of necrosis and angiocentricity/angiodestruction on histopathologic examination favor PCGDTL. Although PCGDTL is typically negative for CD4 and CD8, SPTCL is characteristically CD8+. However, because clinical and microscopic features are similar, documentation of an αβ or γδ phenotype is needed for differentiation and is critical because SPTCL has an indolent clinical course.

The presence of a lobular panniculitic lymphocytic infiltrate may raise the differential diagnosis

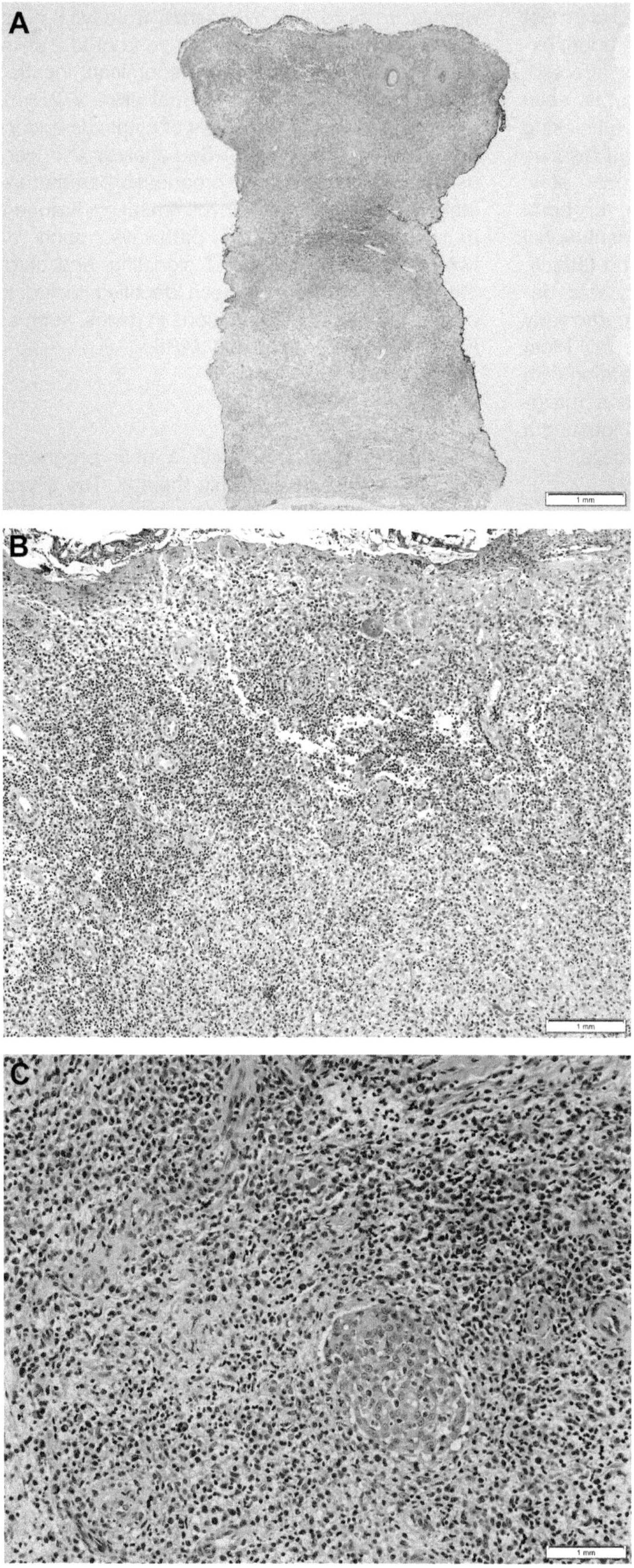

Fig. 1. Primary cutaneous gamma/delta T-cell lymphoma. There is a dense dermal atypical lymphocytic infiltrate with extension into the subcutis and overlying ulceration (*A–C*; hematoxylin-eosin [H&E], original magnification ×20, ×100, and ×200, respectively). The neoplastic cells are positive for CD3

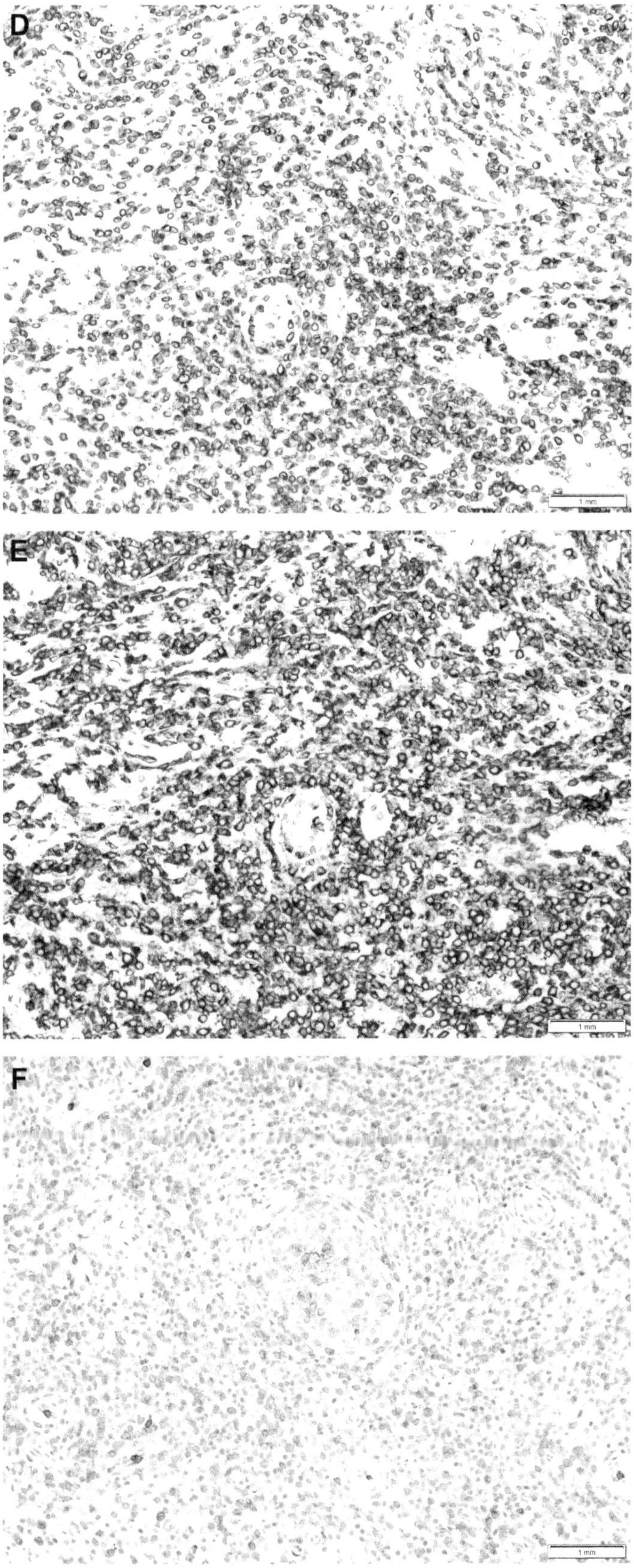

Fig. 1. (*continued*). (*D*; original magnification ×200), CD8 (*E*; original magnification ×200), and TCR-delta (*F*; original magnification ×200).

of inflammatory processes, such as lupus panniculitis/lupus profundus. Lupus panniculitis shows a lobular lymphoplasmacytic infiltrate; overlying interface changes and dermal mucin may also be present. The lack of cytologic atypia among the lymphoid infiltrate, and the presence of subcutaneous hyaline necrosis and germinal centers or B-cell aggregates, an admixture of CD4+ and CD8+ T cells, and clusters of CD123+ plasmacytoid dendritic cells support a diagnosis of lupus panniculitis. In a subset of cases, there are overlapping features of lupus panniculitis and SPTCL[77]; although these entities likely exist on a spectrum, they are distinguished from PCGDTL by demonstrating an αβ phenotype.

Cases of PCGDTL with epidermal involvement may mimic MF clinically and microscopically. However, in contrast to PCGDTL, MF patients tend to have an indolent, protracted course. Most MF cases demonstrate an αβ phenotype, although rare cases of classic MF with a γδ phenotype have been reported.[58,60,76,78] Thus, although cases with superficial skin involvement, a γδ phenotype, and an indolent clinical course may be best considered MF, precise clinicopathologic classification may be difficult. Patients should be followed and managed carefully because PCGDTL can initially have an indolent course and subsequently become aggressive.[76,79–81] Expression of CCR4, a chemokine receptor associated with Th2-like lymphocytes, may be useful in distinguishing MF from PCGCTL with an epidermotropic pattern; whereas most cases of MF, including CD8+ cases, are positive for CCR4, PCGDTL rarely expresses CCR4.[82,83]

Rare cases of CD30+ LPD/LYP can show expression of γδ TCR and be indistinguishable from PCGDTL on histopathologic analysis.[74,76] Clinically, LYP is characterized by recurrent and transient crops of papules and nodules; thus, clinicopathologic correlation is essential.

Distinction from primary aggressive epidermotropic CD8+ cytotoxic T-cell lymphoma (AECTCL), discussed next, may be difficult. Although PCGDTL tends to show more prominent subcutaneous involvement, CD8+ cases with prominent epidermotropism require staining for αβ and γδ TCR for distinction. CD8+ AECTCL can further be distinguished from PCGDTL by demonstration of *JAK2* rearrangement with fluorescence in situ hybridization or targeted next-generation sequencing.[84,85]

Hepatosplenic T-cell lymphoma is a rare systemic extranodal lymphoma of cytotoxic T cells of γδ TCR type characterized by infiltration of the liver, spleen, and bone marrow. Although hepatosplenic T-cell lymphoma can typically be distinguished from PCGDTL based on clinical characteristics, it can rarely involve the skin, potentially complicating diagnosis given overlapping immunophenotypes of neoplastic cells. A clue to the extracutaneous "leukemic" spread from a systemic origin that is seen in these cases is the presence of a grenz zone and a diffuse monomorphic T-cell infiltrate. Rare cases of presentation in the skin at initial diagnosis or preceding relapsed disease have been reported.[86–88]

PRIMARY CUTANEOUS CD8+ AGGRESSIVE EPIDERMOTROPIC CYTOTOXIC T-CELL LYMPHOMA

Primary cutaneous CD8+ AECTCL is characterized by, as its name implies, an aggressive clinical behavior and a proliferation of epidermotropic CD8+ cytotoxic T cells. In the past, these cases may have been classified as an aggressive MF or disseminated pagetoid reticulosis (Ketron-Goodman disease).

CLINICAL FEATURES

CD8+ AECTCL occurs in older adults with a male predominance and typically presents with the rapid development of generalized patches, plaques, and nodules/tumors, often associated with ulceration. Involvement of oral mucosa or perimucosal skin is common. Some patients may show early "prodromal" eczematous, psoriasiform, or erythema multiforme-like skin lesion clinically and microscopically, making diagnosis difficult. Dissemination to extracutaneous sites including the lungs, testes, and CNS may occur; bone marrow involvement is less common and lymph nodes are typically not involved.

MICROSCOPIC FEATURES

Biopsies show a dense band-like, nodular, or diffuse proliferation of lymphocytes within the dermis with epidermotropism. Although epidermotropism can be minimal, there is characteristically striking pagetoid epidermotropism (**Fig. 2**). The epidermis may be acanthotic or atrophic with associated spongiosis and vesiculation, epidermal necrosis, or ulceration. Adnexal involvement is often present, but angiocentricity is uncommon. The neoplastic cells are small, medium, or large and pleomorphic. Exclusive involvement of the subcutis is not common. The tumor cells are CD3+, CD8+, CD4-, and express αβ TCR and cytotoxic markers (granzyme B, perforin, and TIA1); expression of CD2 and CD5 is often negative and CD7 is variable although often retained.[89]

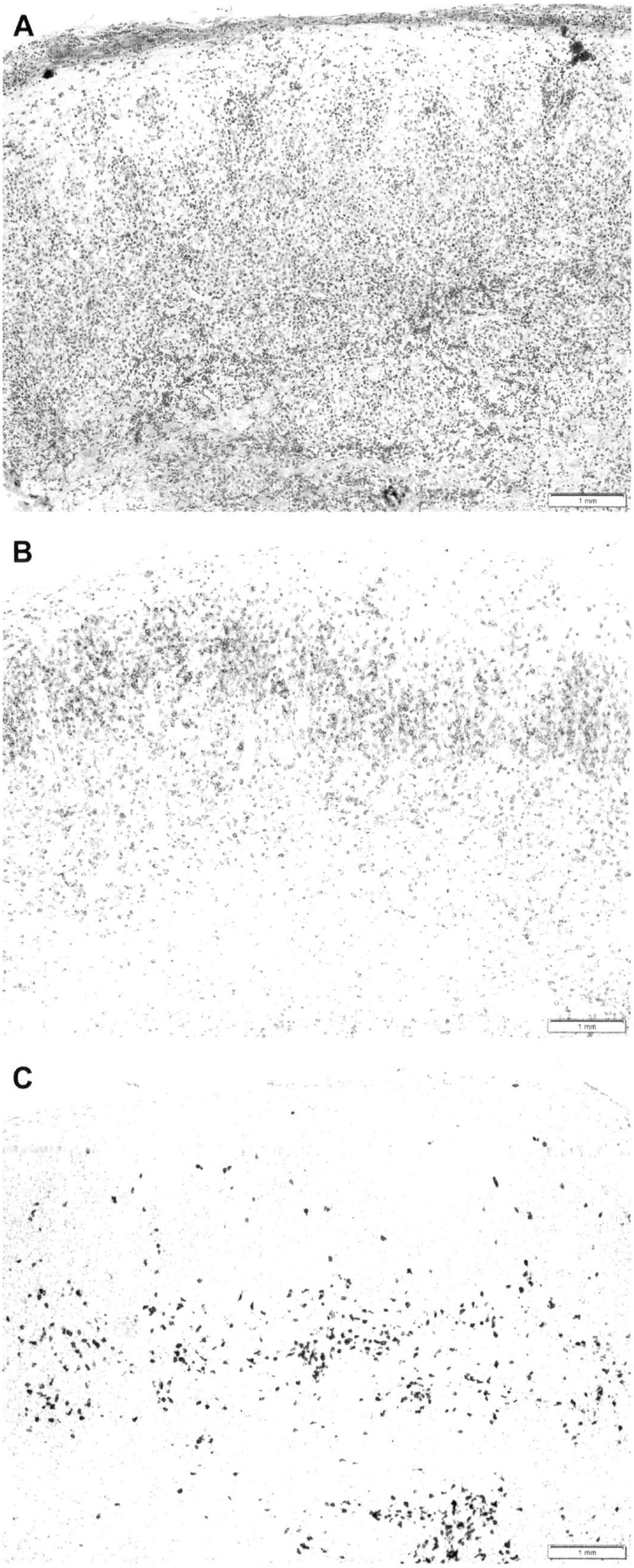

Fig. 2. Primary cutaneous CD8+ aggressive epidermotropic cytotoxic T-cell lymphoma. Biopsy shows a markedly epidermotropic atypical lymphoid infiltrate (*A*; H&E, original magnification ×100). The neoplastic cells are CD2+ (*B*; original magnification ×100), CD5- (*C*; original magnification ×100), CD8+ (weak)

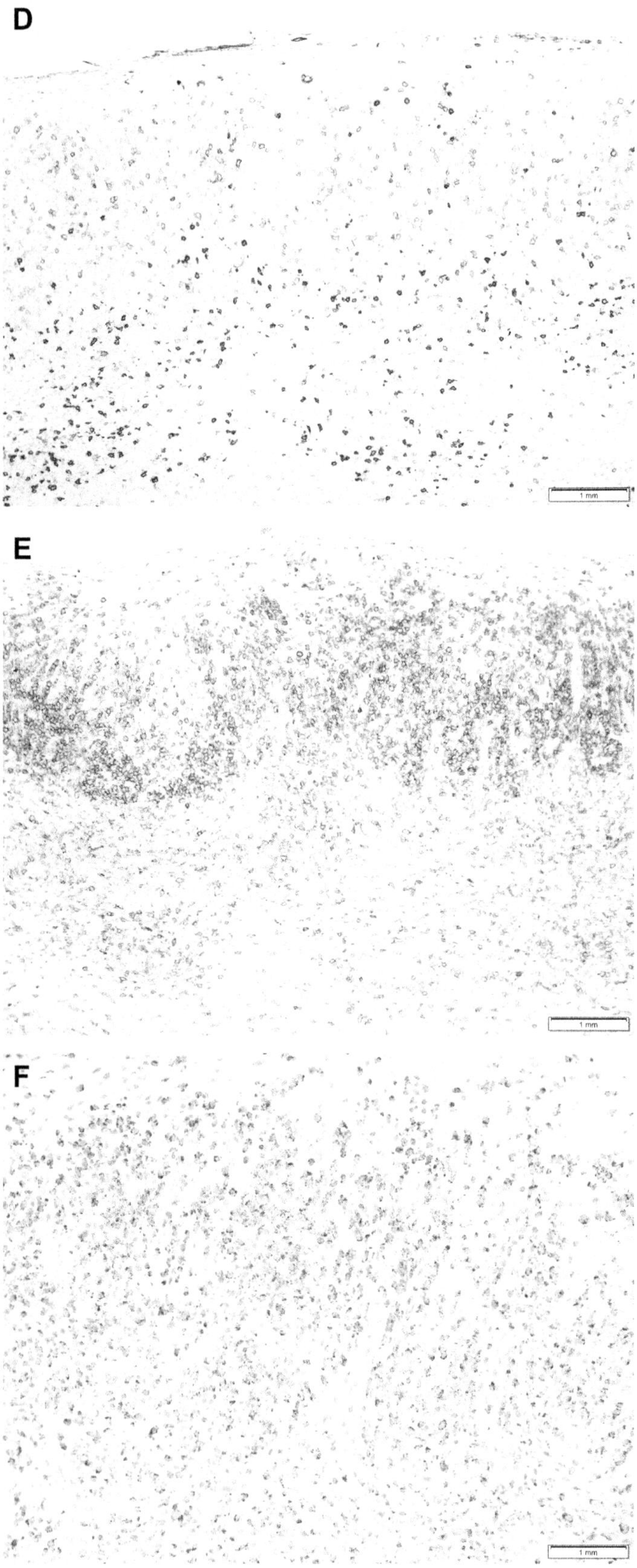

Fig. 2. (*continued*). (*D*; original magnification ×100), CD56+ (*E*; original magnification ×100), and TIA1+ (*F*; original magnification ×200).

Rarely, despite its name, CD8 expression may be weak or negative.[90] CD30 is generally negative. EBV in situ hybridization is negative. The Ki67 proliferative index is generally high (>75%).

GENETIC AND MOLECULAR FEATURES

Monoclonal rearrangement of TCR genes can be detected. Array-based comparative genomic hybridization studies have detected numerous genetic alterations affecting all chromosomes; however, no specific recurring chromosomal gains or losses have been found.[91] Subsequent whole-genome and RNA sequencing studies identified recurrent *JAK2* fusions in CD8+ AECTCL, and mutually exclusive fusions involving regulators of the JAK-STAT pathway, implicating a role of overactive JAK2 signaling in tumor pathogenesis and suggesting benefit from treatment with JAK2 inhibitors.[84,85] Although other cytotoxic CTCLs, including PCGDTL, showed somatic single-nucleotide variants that activate JAK-STAT signaling, *JAK2* fusions were not identified in these cases.[85]

PROGNOSIS

AECTCL has an aggressive clinical course with a median survival of 12 months.[92,93] Aggressive therapeutic intervention is used, including systemic chemotherapy and stem cell transplantation.

DIFFERENTIAL DIAGNOSIS

AECTCL may be histopathologically indistinguishable from type D LYP. Clinical correlation is also needed to distinguish CD8+ AECTCL from CD8+ MF; AECTCL, like PCGDTL, characteristically has a short duration of disease onset. Pagetoid roticulosis (also known as Woringer-Kolopp disease) is a rare unilesional variant of MF, which may be considered in the histopathologic differential diagnosis; this is clinically characterized by an indolent psoriasiform or verrucous plaque typically present on acral skin. Microscopic examination shows a prominent epidermotropic infiltrate of medium-sized T cells within an acanthotic epidermis. The lesional cells are typically CD8+, but CD4+ and CD4/CD8-double-negative cases have been described.[94,95]

Primary cutaneous CD8+ acral T-cell lymphoproliferative disorder encompasses a rare group of lymphoproliferative lesions characterized by a cutaneous infiltrate of cytotoxic T cells that may histopathologically mimic AECTCL. These lesions have an indolent clinical course and it remains controversial if these are true lymphomas, pseudolymphomas, or indeterminate lymphoproliferative disorders[96]; chronic local antigen stimulation has been suggested as a possible cause, but no definitive antigen has been identified. Patients typically present with a solitary slow-growing papule or nodule up to 5 cm in size, most commonly on the ear; involvement of other facial sites, including the nose and eyelid, and extrafacial sites, including the extremities and trunk, has been reported.[96–100] Microscopic evaluation shows a dense dermal infiltrate of atypical monomorphic small- to medium-sized lymphocytes, without epidermotropism or adnexotropism. The lesional cells are T-cell positive for CD3, CD8, betaF1, and TIA1+. They rarely express perforin or granzyme B. CD4, CD30, CD56, and EBV are negative. CD2, CD5, and CD7 are typically expressed but may show weak or loss of expression. Unlike AECTCL, the Ki67 proliferative index is generally low (generally <10%). These tumors are characterized by an excellent prognosis, typically with complete remission after excision or radiotherapy.

Other cytotoxic CTCLs, including PCGDTL, extranodal NK/T-cell lymphoma (ENKTCL), and peripheral T-cell lymphoma, NOS (PTCL-NOS), may also be considered in the differential diagnosis. PCGDTL is distinguished by documenting a $\gamma\delta$ T-cell phenotype. ENKTCL, discussed next, is associated with EBV, unlike CD8+ AECTCL. PTCL-NOS remains a heterogenous groups of tumors that do not meet diagnostic criteria for other T-cell lymphoma types. Although most primary cutaneous PTCL-NOS cases show a CD4+ immunophenotype, some cases are negative for CD4 and CD8, or rarely CD8 is positive. A subset of cases show expression of at least one cytotoxic marker.[101]

EXTRANODAL NK/T-CELL LYMPHOMA

ENKTCL, formerly extranodal NK/T-cell lymphoma, nasal type, is an aggressive cytotoxic lymphoma associated with EBV infection, most common in Asia and South and Central America.

CLINICAL FEATURES

Patients most commonly present with a mass involving the nasopharynx or upper aerodigestive tract, which can cause nasal obstruction or epistaxis. The skin and subcutis are also common sites of disease, characterized by erythematous to violaceous plaques or tumors with ulceration on the trunk and extremities. Primary cutaneous disease occurs in about 10% of cases.[102] Systemic symptoms, including fever, malaise, and weight loss, and hemophagocytic lymphohistiocytosis may occur.

MICROSCOPIC FEATURES

Biopsies show a diffuse, perivascular, and/or periadnexal dermal atypical lymphoid infiltrate, variably extending into the subcutis. Angiocentricity, angiodestruction, and necrosis are common (Fig. 3). Tumor cells may vary in size but are typically medium-sized and pleomorphic. Mitotic figures are present and a background reactive inflammatory infiltrate comprised of small lymphocytes, histiocytes, eosinophils, and plasma cells may be seen. Most commonly, the tumor cells are positive for CD2, CD56, and cytotoxic markers. In cases with an NK-cell phenotype, surface CD3, CD4, CD8, CD5, and CD7 are negative. About 10% of cases show a T-cell phenotype and usually express CD8 and TCRαβ or TCRγ.[103] Although surface CD3 expression is typically negative by flow cytometry, cytoplasmic CD3 expression is detected by this method or may be visualized by IHC as weak staining, supporting the diagnosis. EBV is detected in most tumor cells.

GENETIC AND MOLECULAR FEATURES

Monoclonal TCR gene rearrangements are not present in NK-cell derived tumors but may be identified in those of T-cell derivation. Cytogenetic abnormalities, including 6q21 deletion, 1q21 gain, and 17p11 deletion, and somatic mutations in several genes including *DDX3X*, members of the JAK/STAT signaling pathway, *TP53*, *RAS*, *MYC*, *KMT2D*, and *CDKN2A* have been identified.[104]

PROGNOSIS

ENKTCL has aggressive clinical behavior with a median survival of 12 to 15 months.[105,106] Primary and secondary cutaneous disease are aggressive; localized disease is associated with a better prognosis but the presence of extracutaneous involvement and generalized skin lesions has a particularly poor prognosis.[105,107,108] Extranasal tumors, stage, performance status, number of involved extranodal sites, and EBV viral load in tissue are also associated with poor prognosis.[109,110]

DIFFERENTIAL DIAGNOSIS

Because ENKTCL can show a range of histopathologic appearances, the diagnosis may be challenging. In cases with an NK-cell phenotype, lack of expression of T-cell markers, absences of T-cell clonality by molecular studies, and detection of EBV support the diagnosis of ENKTCL. However, cases with a T-cell immunophenotype require distinction from other CTCLs, including PCGDTL, SPTCL, and PTCL-NOS, all of which are negative for EBV.

Other EBV-positive lymphomas/LPDs may also be considered. LYG may also show angiocentricity and angiodestruction; although of B-cell origin, few B cells may be present, requiring clinical correlation and careful consideration. Additionally, in contrast to LYG, ENKTCL rarely involves the lungs and more commonly involves the upper aerodigestive tract. MCU may have overlapping clinical and histopathologic features; although MCU typically expresses B-cell markers, nonneoplastic T cells may predominate in some cases, complicating diagnosis. Rarely, MTX-LPD may manifest with features of ENKTCL, requiring clinical correlation.[111]

Hydroa vacciniforme lymphoproliferative disorder (HVLPD) is a cutaneous manifestation of chronic active EBV disease typically observed in children and young adults from Latin America or Asia. Chronic active EBV disease encompasses a broad spectrum of related lesions including HVLPD-classic form; severe mosquito bite allergy/hypersensitivity; and systemic disease characterized by fever, hepatosplenomegaly, and lymphadenopathy with or without skin involvement.[50] Clinically, HVLPD-classic form is characterized by recurrent papulovesicular skin lesions with necrotic areas present on sun-exposed sites that can develop into pitted scars. Cases are characterized by localized lesions in sun-exposed sites with no systemic symptoms and an indolent clinical course. In contrast, HVLPD cases with a more protracted course with systemic symptoms (fever, lymphadenopathy, and hepatosplenomegaly) and progression to severe disease are now considered HVLPD-systemic form.[50] Microscopic examination shows variable epidermal spongiosis, vesicle formation, and necrosis with a perivascular, periadnexal, or diffuse dermal lymphocytic infiltrate. HVLPD is typically a CD8+ T-cell process; expression of cytotoxic markers is usually present and variable loss of pan-T-cell markers may be seen. T cells may express αβ or γδ TCR. Less commonly, lesional cells are negative for CD4 and CD8, and show an NK-cell phenotype with CD56 expression, making it difficult to distinguish histopathologically from ENKTCL. CD30 may be expressed on a subset of cells. EBV expression is present in all cases.[104,112]

ADULT T-CELL LEUKEMIA/LYMPHOMA

Adult T-cell leukemia/lymphoma (ATLL) is a peripheral T-cell malignancy associated with human

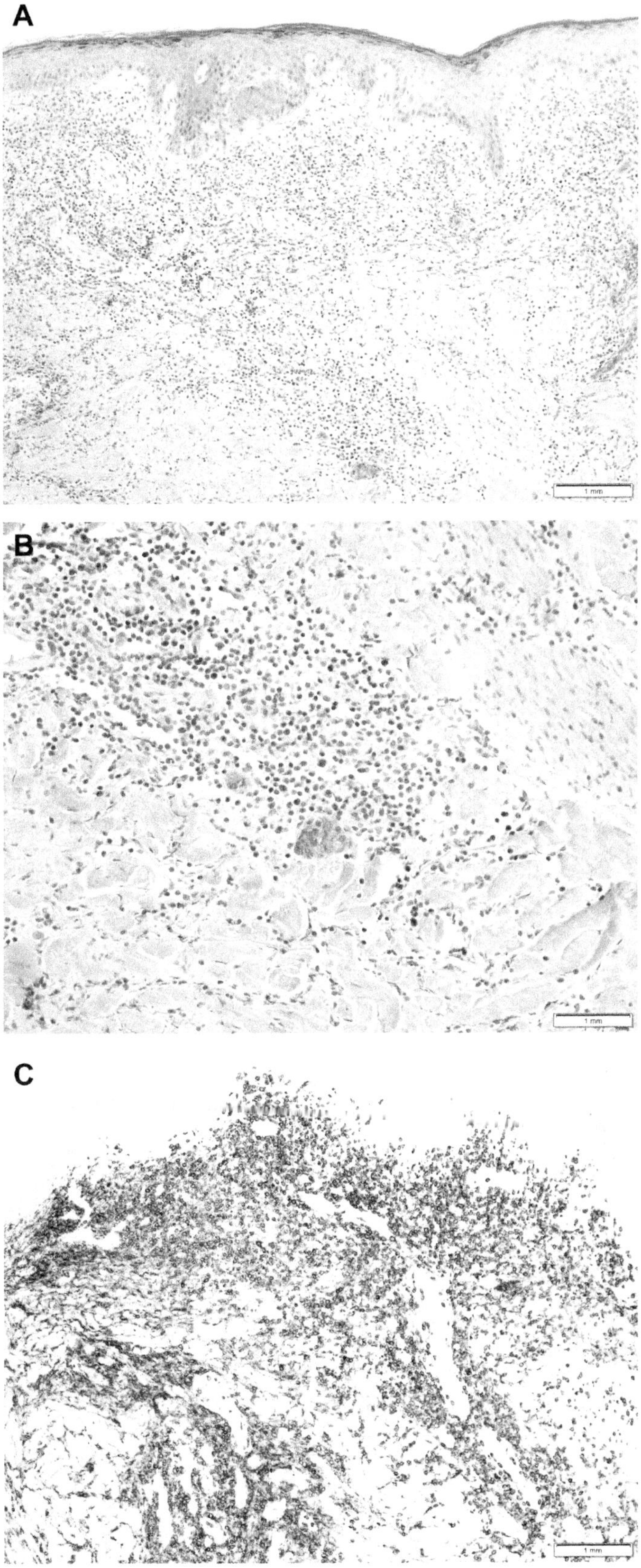

Fig. 3. Extranodal NK/T-cell lymphoma. There is an atypical dermal lymphoid infiltrate with angiocentricity (*A, B*; H&E, original magnification ×100 and ×200, respectively). The neoplastic cells are positive for CD3 (*C*; original magnification ×100), CD56, and granzyme B

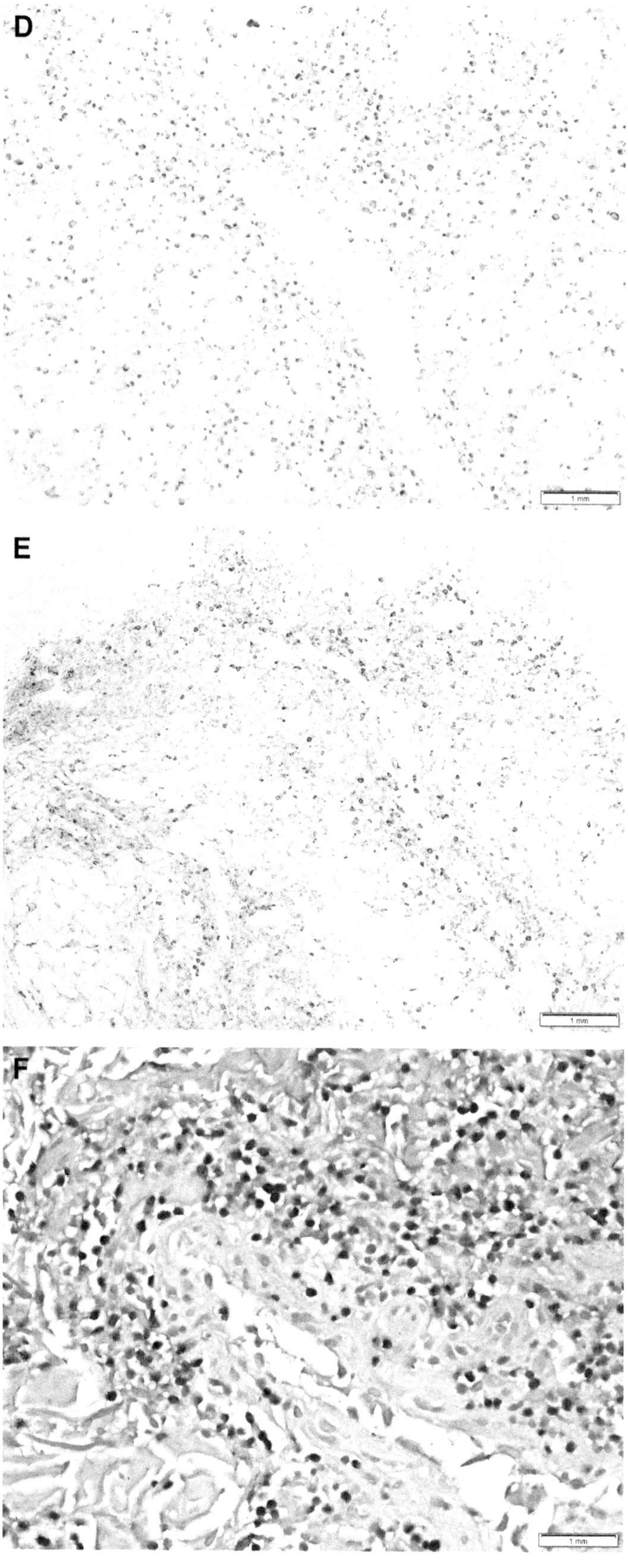

Fig. 3. (*continued*). (*D*; original magnification ×200), and showed weak expression for CD7 (*E*; original magnification ×100). EBER is positive (*F*; original magnification ×400).

T-lymphotropic virus-1 (HTLV-1) infection. It occurs most often in patients from endemic areas, including parts of Japan, the Caribbean, South and Central America, and Africa. Classification as a leukemia or lymphoma depends on clinical presentation resulting from infiltration of the blood or lymphoid organs.

CLINICAL FEATURES

ATLL typical presents in adults or elderly patients with a male predominance. About a third of patients present with disease limited to the skin; however, more often systemic disease is present at presentation.[113] Overall, cutaneous involvement is present in about half of patients, most often in chronic and smoldering subtypes (vs acute and lymphomatous types).[114] Cutaneous lesions may be localized or generalized and occur in the form of macules, papules, plaques, and tumors. Erythroderma and subcutaneous tumors may also be seen. Anti-HTVL-1 antibodies are present in the serum of affected individuals, which supports the diagnosis. Of note, patients with ATLL have an impaired immune response and are susceptible to infection, including cutaneous fungal infections.

MICROSCOPIC FEATURES

Cutaneous involvement most often occurs as an epidermotropic infiltrate of atypical pleomorphic lymphocytes. Pautrier-like microabscesses are common and generally prominent (Fig. 4). Perivascular, nodular, and diffuse infiltrates may be seen, as well as angiocentricity and/or angiodestruction, bullous lesions, perineural invasion, adnexotropism, and follicular mucinosis.[113,115] Microscopic features may vary in different skin biopsies from the same patient. The neoplastic cells are positive for CD3 (although expression may be decreased), CD2, CD4, and CD5. CD25 is characteristically strongly positive. CD30 and FOXP3 may also be positive, typically in the Caribbean population.[113,116] CD7 and CD8 are usually negative.

GENETIC AND MOLECULAR FEATURES

Monoclonal rearrangement of TCR genes and monoclonal integration of HTLV-1 DNA can be detected, although the latter assay is not performed in routine clinical practice. The HTLV-1 oncoviral proteins TAX and HBZ are associated with tumorigenesis; although TAX mRNA is only identified in a subset of cases, HBZ mRNA is present in almost all cases.[117–119] A recent study has suggested that differential expression of HBZ and TAX mRNA are associated with distinct clinicopathologic features and could potentially help guide therapy in the future.[120] Mutations in several genes have been identified in ATLL, including *PLCG1*, *PRKCB*, *IRF4*, *CARD11*, *STAT3*, and *CCR4*.[121,122] ATLL cases with an indolent behavior more commonly have mutations in *STAT3*, whereas aggressive cases have a greater number of alterations, more commonly mutations in *TP53* and *IRF4* and deletions in *CDKN2A*.[123]

PROGNOSIS

The prognosis of ATLL is typically poor. Disease limited to the skin or presenting first in the skin, most often seen in chronic and smoldering types, has a better prognosis as compared with acute and lymphomatous types.[113,124,125] Controversy exists as to whether cutaneous involvement in patients with systemic disease portends a poor prognosis.[126] It has been suggested that cutaneous patch/plaque disease has a better prognosis than patients with erythroderma, multipapular, nodular-tumoral, or purpuric lesions.[127] Additionally, deep skin involvement may be associated with a worse prognosis in comparison with superficial skin involvement.[126]

DIFFERENTIAL DIAGNOSIS

ATLL is histopathologically indistinguishable from other CTCLs, including MF and Sézary syndrome (SS). MF typically shows an indolent clinical course and good prognosis, although advanced disease is associated with a more dismal prognosis. MF typically shows progression through patch, plaque, and tumor stages. In contrast, ATLL often shows a more rapid onset with evidence of systemic involvement. Unlike MF, the atypical lymphocytes are large and pleomorphic, typically without cerebriform morphology. ATLL frequently shows strong CD25 expression, although CD25 may also be seen in MF/SS. Thus, distinction of ATLL from MF/SS relies on documentation of HTLV-1 positivity and viral DNA integration when available.[128] Although not currently used in routine clinical practice, GEP studies have shown differential patterns in MF and ATLL.[129]

Primary cutaneous PTCL-NOS is also within the differential diagnosis. This diagnosis is made when clinicopathologic features do not fit into other defined cutaneous lymphoma subtypes and is typically characterized by widespread tumors. Like MF/SS, there is no association with HTLV-1. In one study, GEP allowed four PTCL-NOS to be reclassified as ATLL; of note, these cases were associated with poor clinical outcome and HTLV-1 seropositivity.[130]

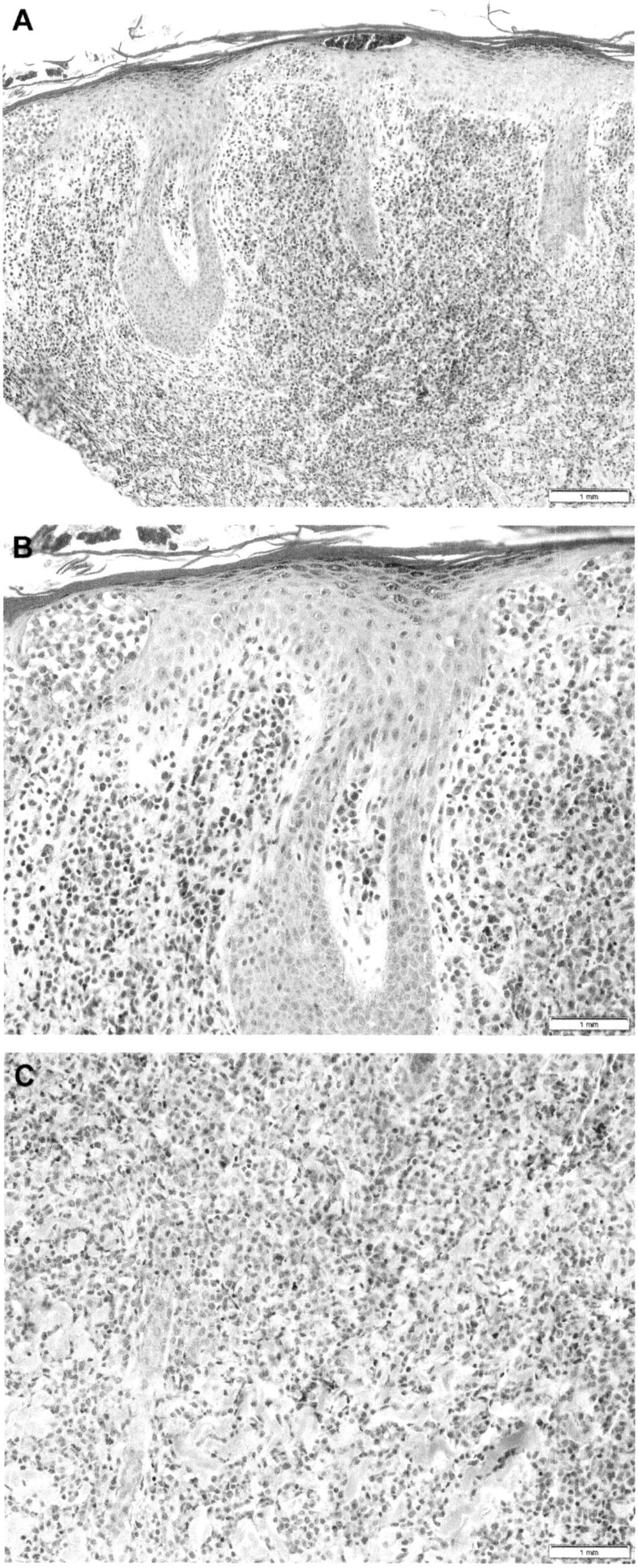

Fig. 4. Adult T-cell leukemia/lymphoma. Cutaneous involvement is characterized by a dense infiltrate of atypical lymphoid cells with epidermotropism and Pautrier-like microabscesses (*A, B*; H&E, original magnification ×100 and ×200, respectively). The tumor cells are large and pleomorphic with scattered mitotic figures (*C*; H&E, original magnification ×200). The tumor cells are positive for CD3

Fig. 4. (*continued*). (*D*; original magnification ×100), CD4 (*E*; original magnification ×100), and CD25 (*F*; original magnification ×100).

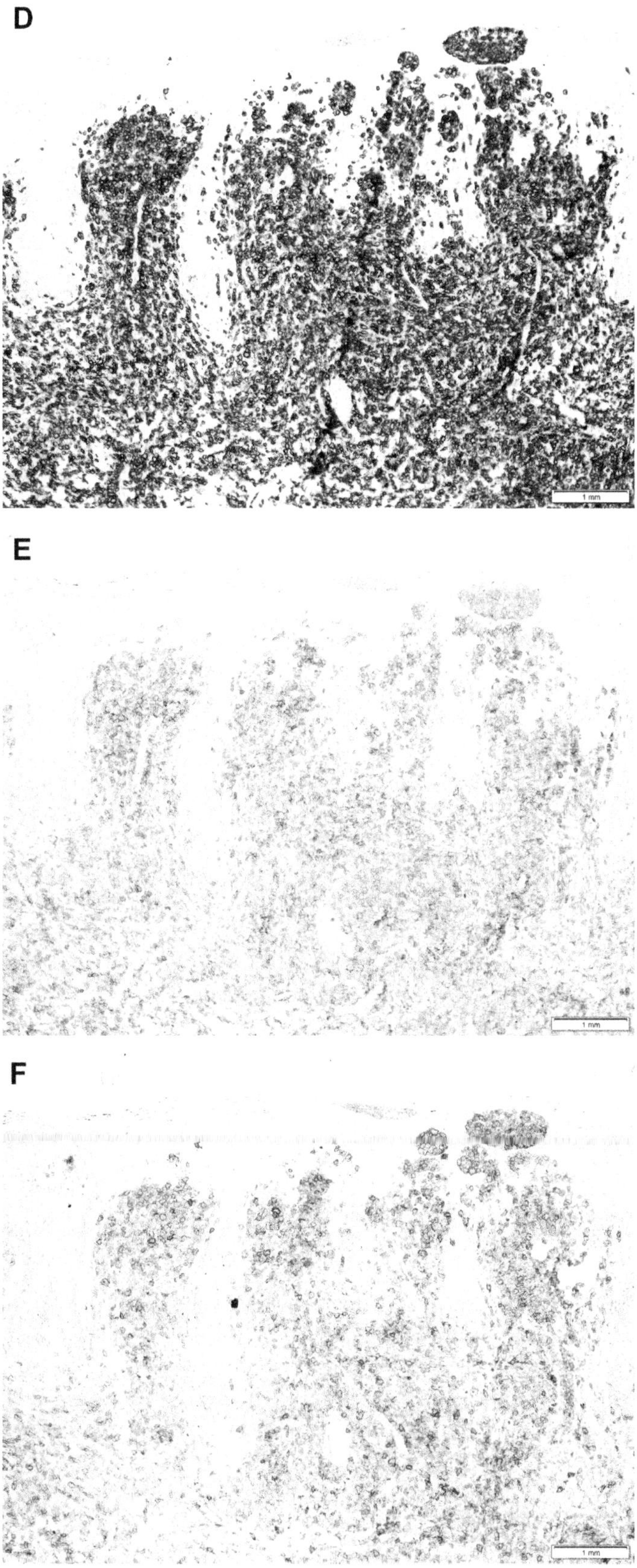

SUMMARY

Accurate diagnosis of cutaneous lymphomas requires careful consideration and integration of clinical characteristics, histopathologic and immunophenotypic features, and increasingly, molecular findings. Distinguishing aggressive forms of cutaneous lymphoma from more indolent processes and systemic lymphomas is critical and has important clinical and therapeutic implications. As more is learned about lymphomagenesis, clinicians will continue to refine the ability to classify tumors with overlapping features, predict biologic behavior, and better guide therapeutic interventions.

CLINICS CARE POINTS

- Aggressive cutaneous lymphomas, including B-cell and T-cell neoplasms, can show a wide spectrum of overlapping clinical and histopathologic features and must be differentiated from indolent lymphomas/LPDs and systemic lymphomas.
- Differentiating DLBCL-LT and PCFCL with a diffuse growth pattern and a predominance of large centroblasts is difficult. Although not currently used routinely, molecular insights may prove to be helpful. Clinical correlation is required to exclude secondary cutaneous involvement by a systemic DLBCL.
- Primary cutaneous gamma/delta T-cell lymphoma should be distinguished from other lymphoid proliferations, which may show a $\gamma\delta$ phenotype, including MF and LYP.
- Primary cutaneous CD8+ aggressive epidermotropic cytotoxic T-cell lymphoma has been associated with *JAK2* fusions, which can assist in diagnosis because the histopathologic differential diagnosis includes indolent processes, including type D LYP and primary cutaneous CD8+ acral T-cell LPD.
- Extranodal NK/T-cell lymphoma is an EBV-associated aggressive cytotoxic lymphoma that may show an NK- or T-cell phenotype; cases with a T-cell phenotype must be distinguished from HV-LPD, LYG, MCU, and MTX-LPD.
- Adult T-cell leukemia/lymphoma is an HTLV-1-associated peripheral T-cell neoplasm that often involves or presents in the skin and can mimic MF, SS, and PTCL-NOS.

DISCLOSURE

A.P. Moy is a collaborator/coinvestigator on a National Institute of Arthritis and Musculoskeletal and Skin Diseases, United States/National Institutes of Health funded grant (1U01AR077511–01) and has no commercial or financial conflicts of interest. M.P. Pulitzer declares no conflicts of interest.

REFERENCES

1. Willemze R, Vergier B, Duncan LM. Primary cutaneous diffuse large B-cell lymphoma. In: Swerdlow SH, Campo E, Harris NL, et al, editors. WHO classification of tumours of haematopoietic and lymphoid tissue. 4th edition. Lyon: IARC Press; 2017. p. 202–4. Revised.
2. Grange F, Beylot-Barry M, Courville P, et al. Primary cutaneous diffuse large B-cell lymphoma, leg type: clinicopathologic features and prognostic analysis in 60 cases. Arch Dermatol 2007;143(9):1144–50.
3. Ekmekci TR, Koslu A, Sakiz D, et al. Primary cutaneous large B-cell lymphoma, leg type, presented with a migratory lesion. J Eur Acad Dermatol Venereol 2007;21:1000–1.
4. Massone C, Fink-Puches R, Wolf I, et al. Atypical clinicopathologic presentation of primary cutaneous diffuse large B-cell lymphoma, leg type. J Am Acad Dermatol 2015;72:1016–20.
5. Hu S, Xi-Monette ZY, Tzankov A, et al. MYC/BCL2 protein coexpression contributes to the inferior survival of activated B-cell subtype of diffuse large B-cell lymphoma and demonstrates high-risk gene expression signatures: a report from The International DLBCL Rituximab-SHOP Consortium Program. Blood 2013;121:4021–31.
6. Plaza JA, Kacerovska D, Stockman DL, et al. The histomorphologic spectrum of primary cutaneous diffuse large B-cell lymphoma: a study of 79 cases. Am J Dermatopathol 2011;33(7):649–955, [quiz; 656-658].
7. Gronbaeck K, Moller PH, Nedergaard, et al. Primary cutaneous B-cell lymphoma: a clinical, histopathological, phenotypic and genotypic study of 21 cases. Br J Dermatol 2000;142:913–23.
8. Kodama K, Massone C, Chott A, et al. Primary cutaneous large B-cell lymphomas: clinicopathologic features, classification, and prognostic factors in a large series of patients. Blood 2005;106(7):2491–7.
9. Senff NJ, Hoefnagel JJ, Jansen PM, et al. Reclassification of 300 primary cutaneous B-cell lymphomas according to the new WHO-EORTC classification for cutaneous lymphomas: comparison with previous classifications and identification of prognostic markers. J Clin Oncol 2007;25(12):1581–7.

10. Hoefnagel JJ, Vermeer MH, Jansen PM, et al. Bcl-2, Bcl-6 and CD10 expression in cutaneous B-cell lymphoma: further support for a follicle centre cell origin and differential diagnostic significance. Br J Dermatol 2003;149:1183–91.
11. Herrera E, Gallardo M, Bosch R, et al. Primary cutaneous CD30 (Ki-1)-positive non-anaplastic B-cell lymphoma. J Cutan Pathol 2002;29:181–4.
12. Magro CM, Nash JW, Werling RW, et al. Primary cutaneous CD30+ large cell B-cell lymphoma: a series of 10 cases. Appl Immunohistochem Mol Morphol 2006;14(1):7–11.
13. Hu S, Xu-Monette ZY, Balasubramanyam A, et al. CD30 expression defines a novel subgroup of diffuse large B-cell lymphoma with favorable prognosis and distinct gene expression signature: a report from the International DLBCL Rituximab-CHOP Consortium Program Study. Blood 2013;121:2715.
14. Felcht M, Heck M, Weiss C, et al. Expression of the T-cell regulatory marker FOXP3 in primary cutaneous large B-cell lymphoma tumour cells. Br J Dermatol 2012;167(2):348–58.
15. Pham-Ledard A, Cappellen D, Martinez F, et al. MYD88 somatic mutation is a genetic feature of primary cutaneous diffuse large B-cell lymphoma, leg type. J Invest Dermatol 2012;132(8):2118–20.
16. Menguy S, Gros A, Pham-Ledard A, et al. MYD88 somatic mutation is a diagnostic criterion in primary cutaneous large B-cell lymphoma. J Invest Dermatol 2016;136:1741–4.
17. Koens L, Zoutman WH, Ngarmlertsirichai P, et al. Nuclear factor-κB pathway-activating gene aberrancies in primary cutaneous large B-cell lymphoma, leg type. J Invest Dermatol 2014;134(1):290–2.
18. Mareschal S, Pham-Ledard A, Viailly PJ, et al. Identification of somatic mutations in primary cutaneous diffuse large B-cell lymphoma, leg type by massive parallel sequencing. J Invest Dermatol 2017;137(9):1984–94.
19. Zhou XA, Louissaint A Jr, Wenzel A, et al. Genomic analyses identify recurrent alterations in immune evasion genes in diffuse large B-cell lymphoma, leg type. J Invest Dermatol 2018;138:2365–76.
20. Gimenez S, Costa C, Espinet B, et al. Comparative genomic hybridization analysis of cutaneous large B-cell lymphomas. Exp Dermatol 2005;14(12):883–90.
21. Dijkman R, Tensen CP, Jordanova ES, et al. Array-based comparative genomic hybridization analysis reveals recurrent chromosomal alterations and prognostic parameters in primary cutaneous large B-cell lymphoma. J Clin Oncol 2006;24(2):296–305.
22. Senff NJ, Zoutman WH, Vermeer MH, et al. Fine-mapping chromosomal loss at 9p21: correlation with prognosis in primary cutaneous diffuse large B-cell lymphoma, leg type. J Invest Dermatol 2009;129(5):1149–55.
23. Pham-Ledard A, Prochazkova-Carlotti M, Vergier B, et al. IRF4 expression without IRF4 rearrangement is a general feature of primary cutaneous diffuse large B-cell lymphoma, leg type. J Invest Dermatol 2010;130(5):1470–2.
24. Espinet B, García-Herrera A, Gallardo F, et al. FOXP1 molecular cytogenetics and protein expression analyses in primary cutaneous large B cell lymphoma, leg-type. Histol Histopathol 2011;26(2):213–21.
25. Pham-Ledard A, Prochazkova-Carlotti M, Andrique L, et al. Multiple genetic alterations in primary cutaneous large B-cell lymphoma, leg type support a common lymphomagenesis with activated B-cell-like diffuse large B-cell lymphoma. Mod Pathol 2014;27:402–11.
26. Schrader AMR, Jansen PM, Vermeer MH, et al. High incidence and clinical significance of MYC rearrangements in primary cutaneous diffuse large B-cell lymphoma, leg type. Am J Surg Pathol 2018;42:1488–94.
27. Menguy S, Frison E, Prochazkova-Carlotti M, et al. Double-hit or dual expression of MYC and BCL2 in primary cutaneous large B-cell lymphomas. Mod Pathol 2018;31:1332–42.
28. Senff NJ, Willemze R. The applicability and prognostic value of the new TNM classification system for primary cutaneous lymphomas other than mycosis fungoides and Sézary syndrome: results on a large cohort of primary cutaneous B-cell lymphomas and comparison with the system used by the Dutch Cutaneous Lymphoma Group. Br J Dermatol 2007;157(6):1205–11.
29. Hallermann C, Niermann C, Fischer RJ, et al. Survival data for 299 patients with primary cutaneous lymphomas: a monocentre study. Acta Derm Venereol 2011;91(5):521–5.
30. Bessell EM, Humber CE, O'Connor S, et al. Primary cutaneous B-cell lymphoma in Nottinghamshire U.K.: prognosis of subtypes defined in the WHO-EORTC classification. Br J Dermatol 2012;167(5):1118–23.
31. Grange F, Joly P, Barbe C, et al. Improvement of survival in patients with primary cutaneous diffuse large B-cell lymphoma, leg type, in France. JAMA Dermatol 2014;150(5):535–41.
32. Child FJ, Russell-Jones R, Woolford AJ, et al. Absence of the t(14;18) chromosomal translocation in primary cutaneous B-cell lymphoma. Br J Dermatol 2001;144(4):735–44.
33. Zhou XA, Yang J, Ringbloom KG, et al. Genomic landscape of cutaneous follicular lymphomas reveals 2 subgroups with clinically predictive molecular features. Blood Adv 2021;5(3):649–61.

34. Hoefnagel JJ, Dijkman R, Basso K, et al. Distinct types of primary cutaneous large B-cell lymphoma identified by gene expression profiling. Blood 2005;105(9):3671–8.
35. Cretella P, Peluso AL, Picariello C, et al. Immunohistochemical algorithms and gene expression profiling in primary cutaneous B-cell lymphoma. Pathol Res Pract 2022;231:153804.
36. Schrader AMR, de Groen RAL, Willemze R, et al. Cell-of-origin classification using the Hans and Lymph2Cx algorithms in primary cutaneous large B-cell lymphomas. Virchows Arch 2022;480(3): 667–75.
37. Gros A, Menguy S, Bobée V, et al. Integrative diagnosis of primary cutaneous large B-cell lymphomas supports the relevance of cell of origin profiling. PLoS One 2022;17(4):e0266978.
38. Szablewski V, Dereure O, René C, et al. Cutaneous localization of angioimmunoblastic T-cell lymphoma may masquerade as B-cell lymphoma or classical Hodgkin lymphoma: a histologic diagnostic pitfall. J Cutan Pathol 2019;46:102–10.
39. Lee MH, Moon IJ, Lee WJ, et al. A case of cutaneous Epstein-Barr virus-associated diffuse large B-cell lymphoma in an angioimmunoblastic T-cell lymphoma. Ann Dermatol 2016;28(6): 789–91.
40. Yang QX, Pei XJ, Tian XY, et al. Secondary cutaneous Epstein-Barr virus-associated diffuse large B-cell lymphoma in a patient with angioimmunoblastic T-cell lymphoma: a case report and review of the literature. Diagn Pathol 2012;7:7.
41. Poon F, Ieremia E, Collins G, et al. Epstein–Barr virus–induced cutaneous diffuse large B-cell lymphoma in a patient with angioimmunoblastic T-cell lymphoma. Am J Dermatopathol 2019;41(12): 927–30.
42. Wahie S, Dayala S, Husain A, et al. Cutaneous features of intravascular lymphoma. Clin Exp Dermatol 2011;36(3):288–91.
43. Feldmann R, Schierl M, Sittenthaler M, et al. Intravascular large B-cell lymphoma of the skin: typical clinical manifestations and a favourable response to rituximab-containing therapy. Dermatology 2009;219(4):344–6.
44. Matsue K, Abe Y, Narita K, et al. Diagnosis of intravascular large B-cell lymphoma: novel insights into clinicopathologic features from 42 patients at a single institution over 20 years. Br J Haematol 2019; 187:328–66.
45. Rozenbaum D, Tung J, Xue Y, et al. Skin biopsy in the diagnosis of intravascular lymphoma: a retrospective diagnostic accuracy study. J *Am Acad Dermatol* 2021;85(3):665–70.
46. Cerroni L, Zalaudek I, Kerl H. Intravascular large B-cell lymphoma colonizing cutaneous hemangiomas. Dermatology 2004;209:132–4.
47. Schrader AMR, Jansen PN, Willemze R, et al. High prevalence of MYD88 and CD79B mutations in intravascular large B-cell lymphoma. Blood 2018; 131:2086–9.
48. Bauer WM, Aichelburg MC, Griss J, et al. Molecular classification of tumour cells in a patient with intravascular large B-cell lymphoma. Br J Dermatol 2018;178:215–21.
49. Jordan LB, Lessells AM, Goodlad JR. Plasmablastic lymphoma arising at a cutaneous site. Histopathology 2005;46:113–5.
50. Alaggio R, Amador C, Anagnostopoulos I, et al. The 5th edition of the World Health Organization Classification of Haematolymphoid Tumours: Lymphoid Neoplasms. Leukemia 2022;36(7): 1720–48.
51. Campo E, Jaffe ES, Cook JR, et al. The international consensus classification of mature lymphoid neoplasms: a report from the Clinical Advisory Committee. Blood 2022;140(11):1229–53.
52. Nicol I, Boye T, CarsuzaaF, et al. Post-transplant plasmablastic lymphoma of the skin. Br J Dermatol 2003;149:889–91.
53. Samolitis J, Bharadwaj JS, Weis JR, et al. Post-transplant lymphoproliferative disorder limited to the skin. J Cutan Pathol 2004;31:453–7.
54. Salama S, Todd S, Cina DP, et al. Cutaneous presentation of post-renal transplant lymphoproliferative disorder: a series of four cases. J Cutan Pathol 2010;37(6):641–53.
55. Seçkin D, Barete S, Euvrard S, et al. Primary cutaneous posttransplant lymphoproliferative disorders in solid organ transplant recipients: a multicenter European case series. Am J Transplant 2013; 13(8):2146–53.
56. Koens L, Senff NJ, Vermeer MH, et al. Methotrexate-associated B-cell lymphoproliferative disorders presenting in the skin: a clinicopathologic and immunophenotypical study of 10 cases. Am J Surg Pathol 2014;38(7):999–1006.
57. Garcia-Herrera A, Song JY, Chuang SS, et al. Nonhepatosplenic γ/δ T-cell lymphomas represent a spectrum of aggressive cytotoxic T-cell lymphomas with a mainly extranodal presentation. Am J Surg Pathol 2011;35:1214–25.
58. Rodriguez-Pinilla SM, Ortiz-Romero PL, Monsalvez V, et al. TCR-γ expression in primary cutaneous T-cell lymphomas. Am J Surg Pathol 2013;37(3):375–84.
59. Lee DE, Martinez-Escala ME, Serrano LM, et al. Hematophagocytic lymphohistiocytosis in cutaneous T-cell lymphoma. JAMA Dermatology 2018; 154:828–31.
60. Guitart J, Weisenburger DD, Subtil A, et al. Cutaneous gamma/delta T-cell lymphomas. A spectrum of presentations with overlap with other cytotoxic lymphomas. Am J Surg Pathol 2012;36:1656–65.

61. Swerdlow SH, Jaffee ES, Brousset P, et al. Cytotoxic T-cell and NK-cell lymphomas: current questions and controversies. Am J Surg Pathol 2014;38:e60–71.
62. Tripodo C, Iannitto E, Florena AM, et al. Gamma-delta T-cell lymphomas. Nat Rev Clin Oncol 2009;6(12):707–17.
63. Guitart J, Martinez-Escala ME. Gamma/delta T-cell in cutaneous and subcutaneous lymphoid infiltrates: malignant or not? J Cutan Pathol 2016;43:1242–4.
64. Omland SH, Gjerdrum LM, Walter L, et al. Primary cutaneous gamma-delta T-cell lymphoma positive for both T-cell receptor gamma and T-cell receptor beta. Pathol Case Rev 2014;19:216–20.
65. Patsatsi A, Kolesta T, Sotiriadis D, et al. Silent T-cell lymphoma of gamma/delta T-cell origin initially presented as panniculitis. J Eur Acad Dermatol Venereol 2015;29:1244–5.
66. Agbay RLMC, Torres-Cabala CA, Patel KP, et al. Immunophenotypic shifts in primary cutaneous gamma/delta T-cell lymphoma suggest antigentic modulation: a study of sequential biopsy specimens. Am J Surg Pathol 2017;41:431–45.
67. Tomasini D, Croci GA, Hotz A, et al. Gamma/delta T-cell lymphoma with mycosis fungoides-like clinical course transforming to "T-cell-receptor-silent" aggressive lymphoma: description of one case. J Cutan Pathol 2021;48(9):1197–203.
68. Kucuk C, Jiang B, Hu X, et al. Activating mutations of STAT5B and STAT3 in lymphomas derived from γδ-T or NK cells. Nat Commun 2015;6:6025.
69. Daniels J, Doukas PG, Escala MEM, et al. Cellular origins and genetic landscape of cutaneous gamma delta T cell lymphomas. Nat Commun 2020;11:1806.
70. Toro JR, Liewehr DJ, Pabby N, et al. Gamma-delta T-cell phenotype is associated with significantly decreased survival in cutaneous T-cell lymphoma. Blood 2003;101(9):3407–12.
71. Merrill ED, Agbay R, Miranda RN, et al. Primary cutaneous T-cell lymphomas showing gamma-delta phenotype and predominnalty epidermotropic pattern are clinicopathologically distinct from classic primary cutaneous gamma/delta T-cell lymphomas. Am J Surg Pathol 2017;41:204–15.
72. Kempf W, Kazakov DV, Scheidegger PE, et al. Two cases of primary cutaneous lymphoma with a γ/δ+ phenotype and an indolent course. Am J Dermatopathol 2014;36(7):570–7.
73. Goyal A, O'Leary D, Duncan LM. The significance of epidermal involvement in primary cutaneous gamma/delta (γδ) T-cell lymphoma: a systematic review and meta-analysis. J Cutan Pathol 2021;48(12):1449–54.
74. Martinez-Escala ME, Sidiropoulos M, Deonizio J, et al. γδ T-cell-rich variants of pityriasis lichenoides and lymphomatoid papulosis: benign cutaneous disorders to be distinguished from aggressive cutaneous γδ T-cell lymphomas. Br J Dermatol 2015;172(2):372–9.
75. Martin SM, Fowers R, Saavedra AP, et al. A reactive peripheral gamma-detla T-cell lymphoid proliferation after a tick bite. Am J Dermatopathol 2019;41:e73–5.
76. Pulitzer M, Geller S, Kumar E, et al. T-cell receptor-δ expression and γ/δ+ T-cell infiltrates in primary cutaneous γδ T-cell lymphoma and other cutaneous T-cell lymphoproliferative disorders. Histopathology 2018;73:653–62.
77. Bosisio F, Boi S, Caputo V, et al. Lobular panniculitic infiltrates with overlapping histopathologic features of lupus panniculitis (lupus profundus) and subcutaneous T-cell lymphoma: a conceptual and practical dilemma. Am J Surg Pathol 2015;39(2):206–11.
78. Massone C, Crisman G, Kerl H, et al. The prognosis of early mycosis fungoides is not influenced by phenotype and T-cell clonality. Br J Dermatol 2008;159(4):881–6.
79. Hosler GA, Liegeois N, Anhalt GJ, et al. Transformation of cutaneous gamma/delta T-cell lymphoma following 15 years of indolent behavior. J Cutan Pathol 2008;35(11):1063–7.
80. Alexander RE, Webb AR, Abuel-Haija M, et al. Rapid progression of primary cutaneous gamma-delta T-cell lymphoma with an initial indolent clinical presentation. Am J Dermatopathol 2014;36(10):839–42.
81. Ferrier A, Soong L, Alabdulsalam A, et al. Diagnosis of gamma/delta mycosis fungoides requires longitudinal clinical observation. J Am Acad Dermatol 2021;85(5):1352–3.
82. Jour G, Aung PP, Merrill ED, et al. Differential expression of CCR4 in primary cutaneous gamma/delta (γ/δ) T cell lymphomas and mycosis fungoides: significance for diagnosis and therapy. J Dermatol Sci 2018;89(1):88–91.
83. Geller S, Hollmann TJ, Horwitz SM, et al. C-C chemokine receptor 4 expression in CD8+ cutaneous T-cell lymphomas and lymphoproliferative disorders, and its implications for diagnosis and treatment. Histopathology 2020;76(2):222–32.
84. Bastidas Torres AN, Cats D, Out-Luiting JJ, et al. Deregulation of JAK2 signaling underlies primary cutaneous CD8+ aggressive epidermotropic cytotoxic T-cell lymphoma. Haematologica 2022;107(3):702–14.
85. Lee K, Evans MG, Yang L, et al. Primary cytotoxic T-cell lymphomas harbor recurrent targetable alterations in the JAK-STAT pathway. Blood 2021;138(23):2435–40.
86. Hocker TL, Wada DA, McPhail ED, et al. Relapsed hepatosplenic T-cell lymphoma heralded by a

solitary skin nodule. J Cutan Pathol 2011;38(11): 899–904.
87. Santonja C, Carrasco L, Pérez-Sáenz MLÁ, et al. A skin plaque preceding systemic relapse of gamma-delta hepatosplenic T-cell lymphoma. Am J Dermatopathol 2020;42(5):364–7.
88. Karpate A, Barcena C, Hohl D, et al. Cutaneous presentation of hepatosplenic T-cell lymphoma: a potential mimicker of primary cutaneous gamma-delta T-cell lymphoma. Virchows Arch 2016;469: 591–6.
89. Geller S, Myskowski PL, Pulitzer M. NK/T-cell lymphoma, nasal type, γδ T-cell lymphoma, and CD8-positive epidermotropic T-cell lymphoma-clinical and histopathologic features, differential diagnosis, and treatment. Semin Cutan Med Surg 2018;37(1):30–8.
90. Guitart J, Martinez-Escala ME, Subtil A, et al. Primary cutaneous aggressive epidermotropic cytotoxic T-cell lymphomas: reappraisal of a provisional entity in the 2016 WHO classification of cutaneous lymphomas. Mod Pathol 2017;30: 761–72.
91. Fanoni D, Corti L, Alberti-Violetti S, et al. Array-based CGH of primary cutaneous CD8+ aggressive EPIDERMO-tropic cytotoxic T-cell lymphoma. Genes Chromosomes Cancer 2018;57(12):622–9.
92. Robson A, Assaf C, Bagot M, et al. Aggressive epidermotropic cutaneous CD8+ lymphoma: a cutaneous lymphoma with distinct clinical and pathological features. Report of an EORTC Cutaneous Lymphoma Task Force Workshop. Histopathology 2015;67(4):425–41.
93. Berti E, Tomasini D, Vermeer MH, et al. Primary cutaneous CD8-positive epidermotropic cytotoxic T cell lymphomas. A distinct clinicopathological entity with an aggressive clinical behaviour. Am J Pathol 1999;155:483–92.
94. Haghighi B, Smoller BR, LeBoit PE, et al. Pagetoid reticulosis (Woringer-Kolopp disease): an immunophenotypic, molecular, and clinicopathologic study. Mod Pathol 2000;13(5):502–10.
95. Mourtzinos N, Puri PK, Wang G, et al. CD4/CD8 double negative pagetoid reticulosis: a case report and literature review. J Cutan Pathol 2010;37(4): 491–6.
96. Hagen JW, Magro CM. Indolent CD8+ lymphoid proliferation of the face with eyelid involvement. Am J Dermatopathol 2014;36(2):137–41.
97. Suchak R, O'Connor S, McNamara C, et al. Indolent CD8-positive lymphoid proliferation on the face: part of the spectrum of primary cutaneous small-/medium-sized pleomorphic T-cell lymphoma or a distinct entity? J Cutan Pathol 2010;37(9): 977–81.
98. Kempf W, Kazakov DV, Cozzio A, et al. Primary cutaneous CD8(+) small- to medium-sized lymphoproliferative disorder in extrafacial sites: clinicopathologic features and concept on their classification. Am J Dermatopathol 2013;35(2): 159–66.
99. Greenblatt D, Ally M, Child F, et al. Indolent CD8(+) lymphoid proliferation of acral sites: a clinicopathologic study of six patients with some atypical features. J Cutan Pathol 2013;40(2):248–58.
100. Li JY, Guitart J, Pulitzer MP, et al. Multicenter case series of indolent small/medium-sized CD8+ lymphoid proliferations with predilection for the ear and face. Am J Dermatopathol 2014;36(4): 402–8.
101. Weaver J, Mahindra AK, Pohlman B, et al. Non-mycosis fungoides cutaneous T-cell lymphoma: reclassification according to the WHO-EORTC classification. J Cutan Pathol 2010;37(5):516–24.
102. Takata K, Hong ME, Sitthinamsuwan P, et al. Primary cutaneous NK/T-cell lymphoma, nasal type and CD56-positive peripheral T-cell lymphoma: a cellular lineage and clinicopathologic study of 60 patients from Asia. Am J Surg Pathol 2015;39(1): 1–12.
103. Pongpruttipan T, Sukpanichnant S, Assanasen T, et al. Extranodal NK/T-cell lymphoma, nasal type, includes cases of natural killer cell and αβ, γδ, and αβ/γδ T-cell origin: a comprehensive clinicopathologic and phenotypic study. Am J Surg Pathol 2012;36(4):481–99.
104. Montes-Mojarro IA, Kim WY, Fend F, et al. Epstein-Barr virus positive T and NK-cell lymphoproliferations: morphological features and differential diagnosis. Semin Diagn Pathol 2020;37(1):32–46.
105. Mraz-Gernhard S, Natkunam Y, Hoppe RT, et al. Natural killer/natural killer-like T-cell lymphoma, CD56+, presenting in the skin: an increasingly recognized entity with an aggressive course. J Clin Oncol 2001;19(8):2179–88.
106. Ahn HK, Suh C, Chuang SS, et al. Extranodal natural killer/T-cell lymphoma from skin or soft tissue: suggestion of treatment from multinational retrospective analysis. Ann Oncol 2012;23(10):2703–7.
107. Yu JB, Zuo Z, Tang Y, et al. Extranodal nasal-type natural killer/T-cell lymphoma of the skin: a clinicopathologic study of 16 cases in China. Hum Pathol 2009;40(6):807–16.
108. Bekkenk MW, Jansen PM, Meijer CJ, et al. CD56+ hematological neoplasms presenting in the skin: a retrospective analysis of 23 new cases and 130 cases from the literature. Ann Oncol 2004;15(7): 1097–108.
109. Suzuki R, Suzumiya J, Yamaguchi M, et al. NK-cell Tumor Study Group. Prognostic factors for mature natural killer (NK) cell neoplasms: aggressive NK cell leukemia and extranodal NK cell lymphoma, nasal type. Ann Oncol 2010;21(5):1032–40.

110. Hsieh PP, Tung CL, Chan AB, et al. EBV viral load in tumor tissue is an important prognostic indicator for nasal NK/T-cell lymphoma. Am J Clin Pathol 2007;128(4):579–84.
111. Tajima S, Takanashi Y, Koda K, et al. Methotrexate-associated lymphoproliferative disorder presenting as extranodal NK/T-cell lymphoma arising in the lungs. Pathol Int 2015;65(12):661–5.
112. Barrionuevo C, Anderson VM, Zevallos-Giampietri E, et al. Hydroa-like cutaneous T-cell lymphoma: a clinicopathologic and molecular genetic study of 16 pediatric cases from Peru. Appl Immunohistochem Mol Morphol 2002;10(1):7–14.
113. Marchetti MA, Pulitzer MP, Myskowski PL, et al. Cutaneous manifestations of human T-cell lymphotrophic virus type-1-associated adult T-cell leukemia/lymphoma: a single-center, retrospective study. J Am Acad Dermatol 2015;72(2):293–301.
114. Qayyum S, Choi JK. Adult T-cell leukemia/lymphoma. Arch Pathol Lab Med 2014;138(2):282–6.
115. Wada T, Yoshinaga E, Oiso N, et al. Adult T-cell leukemia/lymphoma associated with follicular mucinosis. J Dermatol 2009;36(12):638–42.
116. Yao J, Gottesman SR, Ayalew G, et al. Loss of Foxp3 is associated with CD30 expression in the anaplastic large cell subtype of adult T-cell leukemia/lymphoma (ATLL) in US/Caribbean patients: potential therapeutic implications for CD30 antibody-mediated therapy. Am J Surg Pathol 2013;37(9):1407–12.
117. Takeda S, Maeda M, Morikawa S, et al. Genetic and epigenetic inactivation of tax gene in adult T-cell leukemia cells. Inr J Cancer 2004;109(4):559–67.
118. Satou Y, Yasunaga J, Yoshida M, et al. HTLV-I basic leucine zipper factor gene mRNA supports proliferation of adult T cell leukemia cells. Proc Natl Acad Sci USA 2006;103:720–5.
119. Wang w, Zhou J, Shi J, et al. Human T-cell leukemia virus type I Tax-deregulated autophagy pathway and c-FLIP expression contribute to resistance against death receptor-mediated apoptosis. J Virol 2014;88(5):2786–98.
120. Yamada K, Miyoshi H, Yoshida N, et al. Human T-cell lymphotropic virus HBZ and tax mRNA expression are associated with specific clinicopathological features in adult T-cell leukemia/lymphoma. Mod Pathol 2021;34(2):314–26.
121. Kataoka K, Nagata Y, Kitanaka A, et al. Integrated molecular analysis of adult T cell leukemia/lymphoma. Nat Genet 2015;47(11):1304–15.
122. Vicente C, Cools J. The genomic landscape of adult T cell leukemia/lymphoma. Nat Genet 2015;47(11):1226–7.
123. Kataoka K, Iwanaga M, Yasunaga JI, et al. Prognostic relevance of integrated genetic profiling in adult T-cell leukemia/lymphoma. Blood 2018;131:215–25.
124. Amano M, Setoyama M, Grant A, et al. Human T-lymphotropic virus 1 (HTLV-1) infection: dermatological implications. Int J Dermatol 2011;50(8):915–20.
125. Hurabielle C, Battistella M, Ram-Wolff C, et al. Cutaneous presentation of adult T-cell leukemia/lymphoma (ATLL). Single-center study on 37 patients in metropolitan France between 1996 and 2016. Ann Dermatol Venereol 2018;145:405–12.
126. Setoyama M, Katahira Y, Kanzaki T. Clinicopathologic analysis of 124 cases of adult T-cell leukemia/lymphoma with cutaneous manifestations: the smouldering type with skin manifestations has a poorer prognosis than previously thought. J Dermatol 1999;26(12):785–90.
127. Sawada Y, Hino R, Hama K, et al. Type of skin eruption is an independent prognostic indicator for adult T-cell leukemia/lymphoma. Blood 2011;117(15):3961–7.
128. Yamaguchi T, Ohshima K, Karube K, et al. Clinicopathological features of cutaneous lesions of adult T-cell leukaemia/lymphoma. Br J Dermatol 2005;152(1):76–81.
129. Hashikawa K, Yasumoto S, Nakashima K, et al. Microarray analysis of gene expression by microdissected epidermis and dermis in mycosis fungoides and adult T-cell leukemia/lymphoma. Int J Oncol 2014;45(3):1200–8.
130. Iqbal J, Wright G, Wang C, et al. Lymphoma Leukemia Molecular Profiling Project and the International Peripheral T-cell Lymphoma Project. Gene expression signatures delineate biological and prognostic subgroups in peripheral T-cell lymphoma. Blood 2014;123(19):2915–23.

Controversies in the Spleen

Histiocytic, Dendritic, and Stromal Cell Lesions

Aaron Auerbach, MD, MPH[a], Mark Girton, MD[b], Nadine Aguilera, MD[b,*]

KEYWORDS

• Spleen • Mesothelial cyst • Sclerosing angiomatoid nodular transformation
• Inflammatory pseudotumor • EBV-positive inflammatory follicular dendritic cell sarcoma
• Histiocytic sarcoma

Key points

- To describe mesenchymal/stromal and histiocytic entities that occur as primary entities in the spleen.
- To describe the differential diagnoses of each histiocytic and stromal lesion.
- To describe the important workup of these lesions.
- To summarize the important new findings and possible further future study of these entities.

ABSTRACT

Histiocytic, dendritic, and stromal cell lesions that occur in the spleen are challenging diagnostically, not well studied due to their rarity, and therefore somewhat controversial. New techniques for obtaining tissue samples also create challenges as splenectomy is no longer common and needle biopsy does not afford the same opportunity for examination of tissue. Characteristic primary splenic histiocytic, dendritic, and stromal cell lesions are presented in this paper with new molecular genetic findings in some entities that help differentiate these lesions from those occurring in non-splenic sites, such as soft tissue, and identify possible molecular markers for diagnosis.

OVERVIEW

Histiocytic and mesenchymal neoplasms presenting primarily in the soft tissue and skin are very rare. Primary splenic histiocytic and mesenchymal neoplasms are even rarer and less well characterized. Histiocytoses are true proliferations of cells characterized by macrophage, dendritic cell, or monocytic lineage; stromal lesions are somewhat harder to define but include those lesions derived from the splenic stromal or framework cells. Histiocytic and dendritic neoplasms are classified together in the World Health Organization (WHO) Classification of Haematolymphoid Tumours (5th edition) in recognition of their derivation from common myeloid progenitors giving rise to monocytic, histiocytic and dendritic cell neoplasms, whereas tumors derived from stromal or mesenchymal cells are classified together in a separate category.[1]

The true incidence of histiocytic/dendritic and mesenchymal tumors in the spleen is unclear. Of histiocytic sarcoma (HS) cases reported in a single population-based study, approximately 5% occur in the spleen.[2] Of dendritic cell neoplasms reported in one large study, 7.2% of follicular dendritic cell sarcoma (FDCS) occur in the spleen and 10.5% of the fibroblastic reticular cell tumors

The authors have nothing to disclose. The views expressed by Dr A. Auerbach are his and do not reflect the official policy of the Department of Army/Navy/Air Force, Department of Defense, or US Government.
[a] Joint Pathology Center, Silver Spring, MD, USA; [b] University of Virginia Health System, Charlottesville, VA, USA
* Corresponding author.
E-mail address: na2d@virginia.edu

Surgical Pathology 16 (2023) 385–400
https://doi.org/10.1016/j.path.2023.01.004

(FRCTs) occur in the spleen.[3] These lesions are challenging in the spleen due to their rarity and the manner in which many of these lesions are biopsied for evaluation. Splenectomy now is uncommon and needle biopsies limit the evaluation of the tissue. Newer studies using next-generation sequencing (NGS) have found mutations in some of these tumors and these studies may aid in diagnosis in the future. This article presents some of the more enigmatic histiocytic and stromal lesions in the spleen and provides clarification regarding their diagnosis and differential diagnosis.

PELIOSIS

INTRODUCTION

Splenic peliosis is a rare, non-neoplastic condition of unknown etiology associated with endogenous and exogenous steroid use, oral contraceptives, alcoholism, intravenous drugs, cirrhosis, renal failure, and chronic infections including tuberculosis, human immunodeficiency virus, and *Bartonella henselae*.[4] Neoplastic hematologic conditions such as Hodgkin lymphoma[5] and myeloid neoplasms have also been documented in association with peliosis cases.[6,7] Grossly, peliosis shows numerous blood-filled cystic spaces of varying size and shape with demarcation from adjacent normal splenic parenchyma.[4,8] Classically described in reticuloendothelial (mononuclear phagocytic system) organs such as the liver, spleen, bone marrow, and lymph nodes, peliosis has also presumptively been identified at various other diverse sites including kidney, lung, pituitary, gastrointestinal tract, adrenal gland, pancreas, and parathyroid.[9–12]

PATHOLOGIC FEATURES

The first description of splenic peliosis is attributed to Cohnheim in 1866.[8,13] Spontaneous splenic rupture has been described in several case reports,[14,15] but most cases have been incidentally reported at autopsy. Peliosis shows variably sized and shaped blood-filled cystic spaces within the red pulp. The lesion is demarcated from normal splenic parenchyma and localized to parafollicular areas and may be found adjacent to periarteriolar lymphoid sheaths.[4,16] Microscopic examination shows the cyst walls generally lack a lining, with occasional CD34-positive endothelial cells present (**Fig. 1**). Attenuation of the white pulp may be seen. Peliosis is often described as involving red pulp only; the absence of white pulp in the lesion raises the possibility of an association with splenic hamartoma.

DIFFERENTIAL DIAGNOSIS

Other lesions of consideration include those in the vascular and cystic categories. Hemangioma and lymphangiectasia both may have cyst-like space formation but with a cellular lining. This is confirmed by immunohistochemical staining with vascular and lymphatic epithelial markers, respectively. Hairy cell leukemia may lead to the formation of blood lakes with red pulp involvement by neoplastic cells.[17] Chronic passive congestion may also result in blood-filled cystic spaces, but without localization to the parafollicular compartment.

SUMMARY

Peliosis is a lesion of cyst-like and blood-filled cavities in the spleen of unknown etiology. Hepatic peliosis and a variety of other diseases are associated with this idiopathic entity. Though peliosis is a benign lesion, splenic rupture and hemorrhage have been reported.

> **Key Features–Peliosis**
>
> - Asymptomatic cyst-like process that involves the red pulp primarily in a parafollicular distribution.
> - Cystic structures are unlined but may have sinusoidal-type cells.
> - Associated with various underlying illnesses, infection, pharmaceuticals, and intravenous drug use.
> - Unknown etiology.

MEOTHELIAL CYST–SOLID VARIANT

INTRODUCTION

Cystic lesions in the spleen are rare with an incidence rate of 0.07% as reported by autopsy review,[18] and occur in 0.5% of splenectomies.[19] Cysts are usually asymptomatic and found incidentally by radiologic studies or at autopsy. They are categorized as primary "true" cysts (epidermoid) and secondary "false" cysts, depending on the presence or absence of a cyst lining. Secondary cysts can further be divided as parasitic and non-parasitic.

Primary epidermoid cysts include epithelial and mesothelial cysts (MCSVs), which can occur in

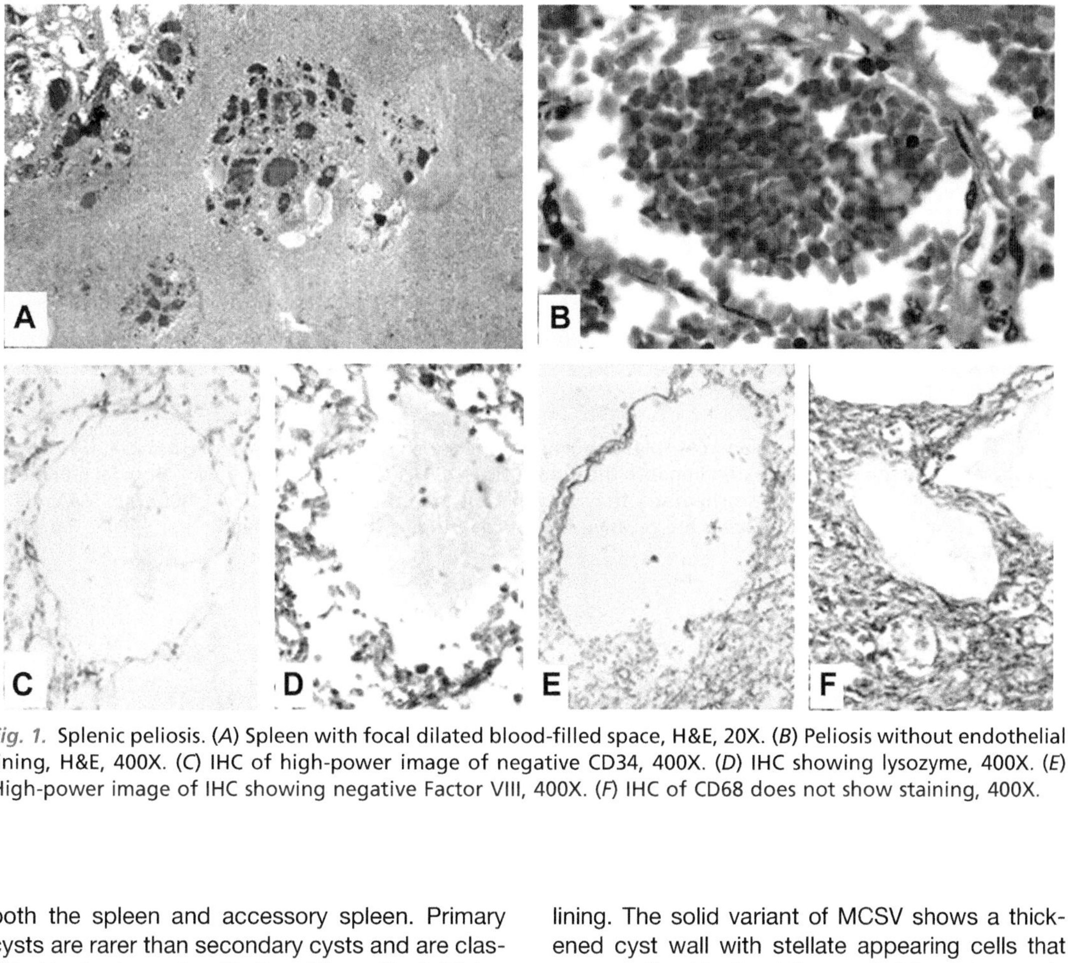

Fig. 1. Splenic peliosis. (*A*) Spleen with focal dilated blood-filled space, H&E, 20X. (*B*) Peliosis without endothelial lining, H&E, 400X. (*C*) IHC of high-power image of negative CD34, 400X. (*D*) IHC showing lysozyme, 400X. (*E*) High-power image of IHC showing negative Factor VIII, 400X. (*F*) IHC of CD68 does not show staining, 400X.

both the spleen and accessory spleen. Primary cysts are rarer than secondary cysts and are classified by the type of epithelium. The epithelial lining cells may be denuded; therefore, a thorough examination of the wall surface is necessary to find intact epithelium.

MCSVs are thought to be congenital, and it has been proposed that they derive from capsular mesothelium invaginating into the tissue of developing spleen during embryogenesis. This may also explain the occurrence of rare intrasplenic mesotheliomas.[20,21] There is a wide age range for splenic MCSVs, but primarily they present in pediatric and young adult patients. Clinical presentation is generally asymptomatic; however, thrombocytopenia has been reported and complications can occur with rupture and hemorrhage. Treatment is splenectomy but conservative treatment of small cysts includes percutaneous drainage, partial splenectomy, marsupialization, or cyst unroofing.

PATHOLOGIC FEATURES

Grossly, cysts may be unilocular or multilocular. Microscopically, MCSVs show a cuboidal to flat lining. The solid variant of MCSV shows a thickened cyst wall with stellate appearing cells that appear fibroblastic. The underlying stroma is thickened and shows ectatic vessels and fibrous tissue. The uninvolved spleen often shows red pulp congestion.

Immunohistochemistry shows the overlying lining is characteristically positive for cytokeratin, WT-1, and calretinin. The stellate cells in the wall are positive for smooth muscle actin (SMA), WT-1, and keratin Click or tap here to enter text.; calretinin is equivocal.[19,22] These cells have features of FRCT cells, but there is no mass lesion and they appear to be a benign proliferation (Fig. 2). The underlying stroma is thickened and shows ectatic vessels and fibrous tissue. The cyst fluid can show CD68- and CD163-positive histiocytes. Epstein–Barr virus (EBV), carcinoembryonic atigen (CEA), and CA19-9 are negative.[22,23]

There are no known genetic abnormalities in MCSVs; however, genetic evaluation of these lesions is rare. Guney and colleagues[22] evaluated MCSV nodules using an NGS panel of 479 genes, and no mutations, structural variants, or copy number alterations were identified. There have been reports of familial cases of mesothelial/

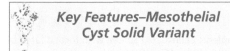

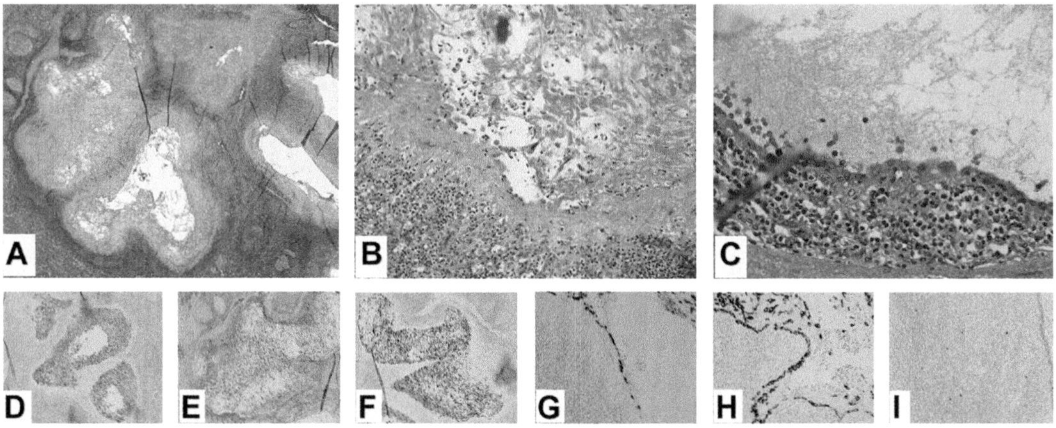

Fig. 2. Mesothelial cyst, solid variant. (*A*) Spleen showing cystic areas with thickened walls, H&E, 20X. (*B*) The cyst wall shows dense spindled cells extending into the lumen, H&E, 100X. (*C*) The cyst wall shows cuboidal lining cells focally, H&E 400X. By immunohistochemistry the cyst wall cells are positive for (*D*) D2-40, 400X, (*E*) SMA, 400X, and (*F*) keratin, 400X. The lining cells are positive for (*G*) calretinin, 400X and (*H*) cytokeratin, 400X. Rare cells are (*I*) EBV RNA (EBER)-positive.

epidermal cysts that have germline variants in genes associated with cyst development, including *HMCN1, CNTN2*, and *DDHD1*.[24,25]

DIFFERENTIAL DIAGNOSIS

Epithelial cysts must be differentiated from MCSV. Epithelial cysts show keratin positivity but lack calretinin expression.[23,26] Squamous differentiation may be present.

Fibroblastic reticular cell tumor (FBRCT) is also in the differential diagnosis, as they may have a stellate appearance and a similar immunophenotype with positivity for SMA, keratin, and WT1. FBRCT is an obscure lesion that is accepted by the 2017 WHO Classification of Haematopoietic Neoplasms that expresses SMA, desmin, cytokeratin (in a dendritic pattern), and CD68[27]; there are often interspersed collagen fibers. Rare FBRCT may show follicular dendritic cell features.[28]

Mesenchymal smooth muscle, vascular and inflammatory tumors including lipomas, angiomyolipoma, fibroma, fibrosarcoma, leiomyosarcoma, and benign spindle cell lesions are included in the differential diagnosis, but their morphology and immunophenotype should differentiate these neoplasms from MCSV.[22,29]

SUMMARY

MCSV of the spleen is rare and the cyst wall shows stellate cells that have characteristics of fibroblastic reticular cells.

Key Features–Mesothelial Cyst Solid Variant

- Cystic and solid areas on radiographic imaging.
- Flattened cuboidal mesothelial lining expresses keratin, WT1, and calretinin.
- Thickened wall with stellate-appearing cells expressing SMA, WT1, and keratin.

SCLEROSING ANGIOMATOID NODULAR TRANSFORMATION

INTRODUCTION

Sclerosing angiomatoid nodular transformation (SANT) is an unusual lesion that is not infrequently detected in spleens but continues to have many open questions related to its pathogenesis. It is included in the most recent WHO Classification of Haematolymphoid Tumours (5th edition) in a section on splenic vascular-stromal tumors, along with Littoral cell angioma and splenic hamartoma.[30] SANT typically is found in adults, usually incidentally, who usually present with vague abdominal symptoms.[31] It is sometimes considered a vascular lesion, although the fibrosclerosing component often makes up the majority of the lesion, so is it questionable whether it is truly a vascular lesion or rather more of a fibrosing process with entrapped vascular elements. It is also associated with increased immunoglobulin G4 (IgG4)-positive stromal plasma cells which, in the context of marked fibrosis, indicates that it could be an entity linked to IgG4-related disease. Recent demonstration of a gene alteration in SANT suggests that it may represent a preneoplastic or neoplastic process. Like sclerosing hemangioma, SANT has both a vascular and stromal sclerosis component, although the former is considered a neoplasm and the latter is typically considered a benign vascular lesion. The pathogenesis of SANT is controversial and remains in question.

PATHOLOGIC FEATURES

The term SANT was first coined as a distinct entity in 2004 by Martel and colleagues[32] to describe a vascular lesion of the spleen with distinctive angiomatoid nodules and associated bands of fibrosis. The medical literature was previously peppered with other terms such as cord capillary angioma, splenic hemangioendothelioma, nodular transformation of red pulp, and multinodular hemangioma to describe cases that are now considered to be SANT, and these other terms are considered obsolete and are no longer used.[33] However, this diversity of names describing SANT helps to show the lack of full understanding of the disease and its pathogenesis.

On gross examination and by imaging studies, SANT is typically a single large central mass that is well demarcated from the surrounded normal spleen and has a striking multinodular appearance.[34] This multinodular appearance can be appreciated at low magnification with multiple angiomatoid nodules, which sometimes coalesce and are variable in size with some nodules being large and others being small. The blood vessels in the angiomatoid nodules are thought to be composed of a mixture of capillaries, veins, and sinusoids recapitulating the normal red pulp of the spleen and it is distinctive that each of these three vessel types is found in this lesion. The vessels are small, round, to slit-like, or mildly irregular in shape, with plump endothelial cells lining the blood vessels, but without marked atypia or dysplasia (Fig. 3). The three different types of blood vessels can be teased out by using three immunohistochemical stains, CD8, CD31, and CD34: capillaries are highlighted by CD34 and CD31 but lack CD8, and small veins and sinusoids are highlighted by CD31 but lack CD8 and CD34.[35] The Ki-67 proliferation index by immunohistochemistry is low in the angiomatoid nodules. Red blood cells are seen within the vessels and may show extravasation, and fresh and old hemorrhage is often seen.

The angiomatoid nodules are typically surrounded by stroma which is variably sclerotic to myxoid to fibrotic with scattered mixed inflammatory cells. These stromal elements are important because they may be part of the pathogenesis, although the stroma may be sparse or loose within the angiomatoid areas. Thick bands of fibrosclerosis are often present and the center-most nodules may be entirely fibrotic. The variable numbers of inflammatory cells in the vasculature and fibrosclerosis mostly consist of small lymphocytes, IgG4-positive plasma cells, and histiocytes. Hemosiderin-laden macrophages are often conspicuous and may be focused around the angiomatoid nodules. Scattered bland spindle cells are also present that are immunoreactive for SMA, but negative for other dendritic cell markers such as CD21, CD23, CD35, and D2-40, consistent with myofibroblasts.[36] The lymphocytes within the angiomatoid nodules and the surrounding fibrosclerosis are mostly T cells and a subset are cytotoxic T cells expressing CD8, TIA1, granzyme B, perforin, and CD8. Fewer B cells expressing CD20 are also identified. The plasma cells usually lack atypia and are polytypic by kappa and lambda. No necrosis, granulomas, or microabscesses are present to consider an infectious process. The spleen surrounding the SANT is often unremarkable.

Although SANT is favored to be a benign process, there is some recent evidence to question whether it could be a neoplastic lesion. Multiple authors have noted that SANT is associated with other mass-like lesions including malignancies.[37] Although benign lesions, such as sarcoidosis, have been reported in patients with SANT, SANT has also been associated with metastatic colon cancer, lung cancer, and gastric cancer, as well as primary myelofibrosis and abdominal calcifying fibrous tumors. Most of the time, these have been considered incidental associations, but it is noteworthy that SANT has been associated with multiple different neoplasms.[38] Furthermore, SANT has recently shown loss of exon 3 of the β-catenin gene, *CTNNB1*. Other *CTNNB1* exon 3 mutations have been found in some rare fibrovascular lesions, such as juvenile nasopharyngeal angiofibroma, sclerosing hemangioma of the lung, and sinonasal hemangiopericytoma, suggesting that alterations in this gene may be related to different neoplasms with a component of fibrosclerosis. β-catenin immunohistochemical stain corresponding to the *CTNNB1* gene is negative in the angiomatoid nodules and stromal cells of SANT, although it is expressed in endothelial cells in the adjacent normal spleen. This begs the question as to whether *CTNNB1* exon 3 loss is an indication

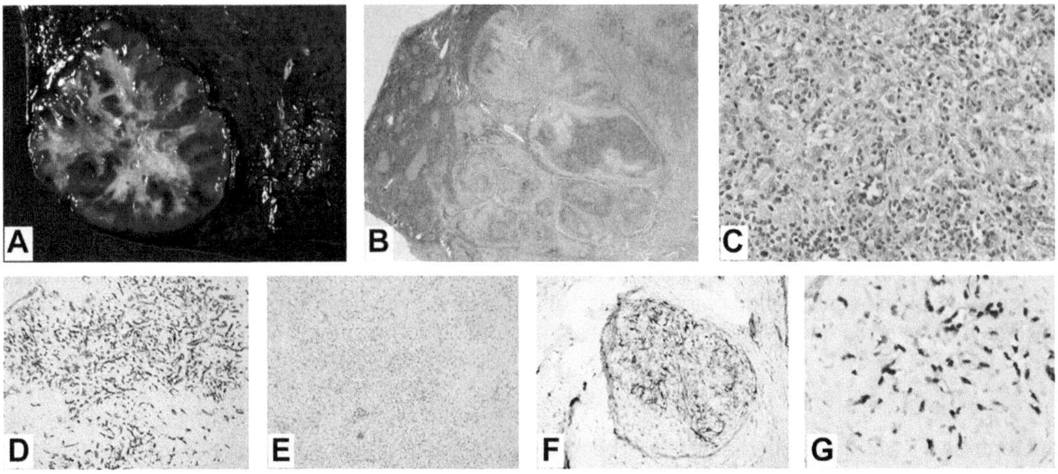

Fig. 3. SANT. (*A*) Gross image of spleen showing a well-demarcated mass composed of multiple smaller nodules. (*B*) Low-power view of spleen showing a multinodular mass, H&E,20X. (*C*) Image showing vessels with sclerosis and intervening inflammatory cells, H&E, 200X. (*D*) CD34 showing scattered capillaries, 200X (*E*) CD8 shows no residual sinuses within the lesion, X200. (*F*) WT1 highlights the vessels, 200X. (*G*) ERG stains the endothelial cells, 400X.

that SANT could represent a preneoplastic/neoplastic process or whether this is a gene alteration associated with a reactive process. β-catenin is a central component of the Wnt signaling pathway, which is altered in many other neoplasms. *CTNNB1* gene alteration with activation of the Wnt signaling pathway may play a role in the pathogenesis of SANT.[39] Cord capillary hemangioma is a dated term for lesions akin to SANT and one study showed that cord capillary hemangioma was clonal by performing clonality analysis for X-chromosome activation at the human androgen receptor locus (HUMARA).[40] However, another study using HUMARA shows conflicting results and favors SANT to be reactive in nature.[41] SANT is typically treated with splenectomy that is curative with no known recurrences or metastases.

DIFFERENTIAL DIAGNOSIS

The differential diagnosis of SANT includes several vascular lesions such as a sclerosing hemangioma, Littoral cell angioma, angiosarcoma, and even splenic hamartoma, but also includes stromal lesions including inflammatory pseudotumor (IPT) and IgG4-related disease.[42] The diversity of this differential diagnosis is indicative of the uncertainty of the pathogenesis of SANT.

Hemangiomas are the most common vascular tumor of the spleen that express vascular markers, factor VIII, CD8, CD31, and CD34. It is usually a single lesion but may be multifocal and is benign. Sclerosing hemangiomas consist of a vasculature with intermixed sclerosis that can be similar to, if not indistinguishable, from the fibrosclerosis and angiomatoid nodules of SANT. The vessels in sclerosing hemangioma do not show marked atypia, necrosis, sheets of endothelial cells, or atypical mitotic figures differentiating it from angiosarcoma, but hemangiomas can undergo infarction or cystic degeneration. Some question whether a sclerosing hemangioma is even a distinct lesion from SANT.

Angiosarcoma is a malignant vascular neoplasm, which often presents with multiple hemorrhagic nodules in the spleen. Microscopically, there are anastomosing vessels that consist of highly atypical endothelial cells with frequent atypical mitotic figures and necrosis. The endothelial cells are typically positive for CD31 and CD34, but negative for CD8. SANT does not show the atypia or necrosis of angiosarcoma and is often easy to distinguish. Littoral cell angioma is a multinodular cystic lesion in the spleen consisting of variably sized vascular structures often with plump, tall endothelial cells, sometimes showing papillary projections or desquamating into the cystic lumens. The lining cells in Littoral cell angioma are positive for factor VIII, CD31, CD68, and langerin, but lack CD8 and CD34. SANT differs from Littoral cell angioma in that it does not present as a cystic neoplasm with endothelial cells sloughing into the vascular lumina. Splenic hamartoma is a single, nodular lesion that consists of disorganized red pulp elements consisting of sinusoids and cords of Billroth. The large fibrosclerotic bands and angiomatoid nodules of SANT are not seen in splenic hamartoma.

IPT consists of small lymphocytes, plasma cells, myofibroblasts and histiocytes forming a mass-like lesion. These stromal elements are similar to the stroma of a SANT, but there is less fibrosclerosis.[43] It is possible that SANT and IPT are a spectrum of the same disease process in which SANT has angiomatoid nodules, prominent fibrosclerosis, and scant stromal inflammatory elements, whereas IPT has more inflammatory elements creating a mass-like lesion and less fibrosclerosis. An association between SANT and IPT has been noted in the literature, as rare cases of spleens with IPT and coexisting SANT have been described.[44] SANT may represent an end-stage mass-like lesion with a fibrotic component that started as IPT.

IgG4-related disease lies within the differential diagnosis and SANT may be one of the many entities that comprise IgG4-related disease. Multiple studies have shown that the stromal plasma cells in SANT are IgG4+.[45,46] There may be numerous plasma cells and the IgG4:IgG ratio may be elevated; however, elevated serum IgG4 is only infrequently detected in patients with SANT.[47]

SUMMARY

SANT is a not uncommon lesion of the spleen that has a very controversial and unclear pathogenesis. Although it typically shows the natural history of a benign lesion treated by splenectomy without recurrence or metastasis, it has been associated with different neoplasms and shows deletions of exon 3 of the *CTNNB1* gene.[48] It is generally thought to be a benign vascular lesion rather than a true neoplasm, but it also has distinctive stromal elements which in some cases cannot be distinguished from IPT or sclerosing hemangioma. Are SANTs, IPTs, and sclerosing hemangiomas different entities or are they all different presentations of the same process? Could SANT be a proliferating stromal lesion with entrapped red pulp elements that look like angiomatoid nodules? Trauma to the spleen frequently leads to hemorrhage, which can eventually lead to fibrosclerosis similar to that seen in SANT. This fibrosclerosis can then entrap normal splenic red pulp elements to look like the angiomatoid nodules of SANT. Thus, SANT may represent a splenic sclerotic and vascular reaction that evolves as part of the healing process following different insults and injuries, such as trauma, hemorrhage, infarction, neoplasm, or other inflammatory processes. Alternatively, SANT may be part of the spectrum of IgG4-related disease as it has IgG4+ polytypic plasma cells and distinctive fibrosis. The pathogenesis of SANT remains controversial and uncertain but the exon 3 *CTNNB1* deletions and downstream activation of the Wnt pathology are novel findings that may play a role in its pathogenesis.

Key Features–Sclerosing Angiomatoid Nodular Transformation

- SANT is generally considered a benign vascular lesion.
- SANT has been associated with other lesions including other tumors.
- May be healing/repair process in spleens with hemorrhage, inflammatory conditions, or neoplasms.
- Presence of IgG4+ plasma cells and fibrosis suggest overlap with IgG4-related disease in some cases.
- Presence of molecular alterations argues that SANT could be preneoplastic or neoplastic.

INFLAMMATORY PSUEDOTUMOR

INTRODUCTION

IPT of the spleen is a fascinating lesion that has an uncertain pathogenesis and a particularly challenging differential diagnosis.[49] In the past, it has been questioned as to whether it has any properties of a neoplastic process, although it is currently considered to be a reactive condition. Other entities, such as EBV-positive inflammatory FDCS, inflammatory myofibroblastic tumor (IMT), and post-chemotherapy histiocyte-rich pseudotumor, can have some overlapping morphologic features and are within the differential diagnosis of IPT, but these are different entities and are not considered to be part of IPT. The pathogenesis of IPT is equally unclear. An infectious etiology has been considered: specifically, *Legionella, Streptococcus*, and EBV have all been implicated and have been detected in patients with IPT.[50] However, no specific infectious agent has ever been consistently detected in patients with splenic IPT. IPT could also be a specific splenic reaction to trauma, as fresh or old hemorrhage may be identified in spleens with IPT. Vascular and autoimmune etiologies have also been proposed, but no definitive etiology is identified for IPT at this time.

PATHOLOGIC FEATURES

First described by Cotelingam and colleagues[51] in 1984, splenic IPT is a reactive condition in the spleen that presents as a mass-like lesion and is composed of inflammatory cells, spindle cells, and sometimes sclerosis. There is usually a single discrete hypodense mass, although it can rarely be multicentric, often with central calcification by CT scan.[52] Patients are either asymptomatic or have vague abdominal complaints and splenectomy is curative with an excellent prognosis and no evidence of recurrence.[53] The lesions tend to be well-circumscribed with normal adjacent white and red pulp. IPT has an abundant mixed inflammatory cell infiltrate that contains conspicuous numbers of plasma cells, as well as histiocytes and lymphocytes with fewer numbers of neutrophils and eosinophils.[54] The degree of inflammation is variable from case to case but also within a particular spleen with some areas showing larger aggregates of inflammatory cells. Plasma cells are seen dispersed or in clusters and look mature with occasional Russell bodies. Lymphocytes are usually small with coarse chromatin and indistinct nucleoli, although scattered larger immunoblasts are also seen. The lymphocytes are a mix of CD20+ B cells and CD3+ T cells, of which the latter usually predominate. IPT also has a component of bland spindle cells with oval/vesicular nuclei and small nucleoli lacking cytologic atypia. The spindle cell component can be hyper- or hypocellular and associated with vascular changes similar to granulation tissue. The spindle cells can form short fascicles and be focally storiform but do not show the marked atypia of a high-grade sarcoma. The spindle cells represent myofibroblasts that are often positive for SMA and CD68, although these can be focal, CD21, CD23, CD35, and CD30 are uniformly negative. These lesions can show some sclerosis or fibrosis, but they can also have focal necrosis often associated with neutrophils. New or old hemorrhage is also often present, as well as scattered hemosiderin-laden macrophages. The spleen outside of the IPT is usually morphologically unremarkable and CD8 negativity within the IPT supports the loss of the normal splenic architecture. No clonal genetic alterations have yet been detected in IPT, although genetic alterations are sometimes detected in reactive clinical entities. EBV has been detected by EBV-encoded small RNA (EBER) in situ hybridization (**Fig. 4**).

IPT has also been diagnosed in other anatomic sites including the lungs, gastrointestinal tract, lymph nodes, and spine. In general, splenic IPT looks similar if not identical to nodal IPT.[55] Some cases of IPT in these other sites have shown increased IgG4+ plasma cells and may be part of the spectrum of IgG4-related disease. EBER has been found to be positive in approximately 20% of lymph node IPT.[56,57]

DIFFERENTIAL DIAGNOSIS

The differential diagnosis of IPT may be particularly challenging and includes some more obscure entities such as EBV-positive inflammatory FDCS, post-chemotherapy histiocyte-rich pseudotumor, and IMT.

EBV-positive inflammatory FDCS, previously known as IPT-like FDCS, differs from IPT because it is a malignant neoplasm that can metastasize and has frequent recurrences.[58] In the 5th edition of the WHO Classification of Haematolymphoid Tumours, it has been moved from the category of histiocytic and dendritic cell neoplasms to the category of stroma-derived neoplasms of lymphoid tissues, because follicular dendritic cells are of mesenchymal origin and are not derived from hematopoietic stem cells. The tumor cells of EBV-positive inflammatory FDCS are spindle to epithelioid in shape, have a range of morphology from bland to more pleomorphic, and are usually more atypical than in IPT. They often form a whorled growth pattern and can rarely be seen with granulomas.[59] FDCS often has scattered inflammatory cells, but the inflammatory component is usually less than in IPT (**Fig. 5**). Furthermore, EBV-positive inflammatory FDCS involves both the spleen and liver, is positive for CD21, CD23, and CD35, and is EBV positive unlike IPT.[60] Many cases that were previously considered IPT in the spleen or the liver are now reclassified as EBV-positive inflammatory FDCS.[61]

IMT is a lesion that most often involves the soft tissue of children and young adults. Myofibroblasts are positive for SMA, and sometimes for cytokeratins, but are negative for CD21, CD23, and CD35. Along with the more spindle-shaped cells there can be scattered larger atypical cells, sometimes with a ganglion cell-like appearance and prominent nucleoli. ALK protein is not present by immunohistochemistry in splenic IPT, although it is detected in about half of cases of soft tissue IMT.[62] Molecular testing will show translocations involving the *ALK* gene found at 3p23 and this is commonly detected by a FISH *ALK* break-apart probe. It is controversial whether IMT can involve the spleen: there have been rare reports in the spleen, although these cases are ALK negative.

Post-chemotherapy histiocyte-rich pseudotumor is a benign histiocytic proliferation, often with xanthomatous histiocytes presenting as a mass after chemotherapy. It consists of non-neoplastic inflammatory cells, as well as necrotic neoplastic ghost cells. After chemotherapy, it is believed that circulating monocytes travel to the site of necrosis and become histiocytes creating a mass-like lesion. The histiocytes are often lipid-laden foamy cells

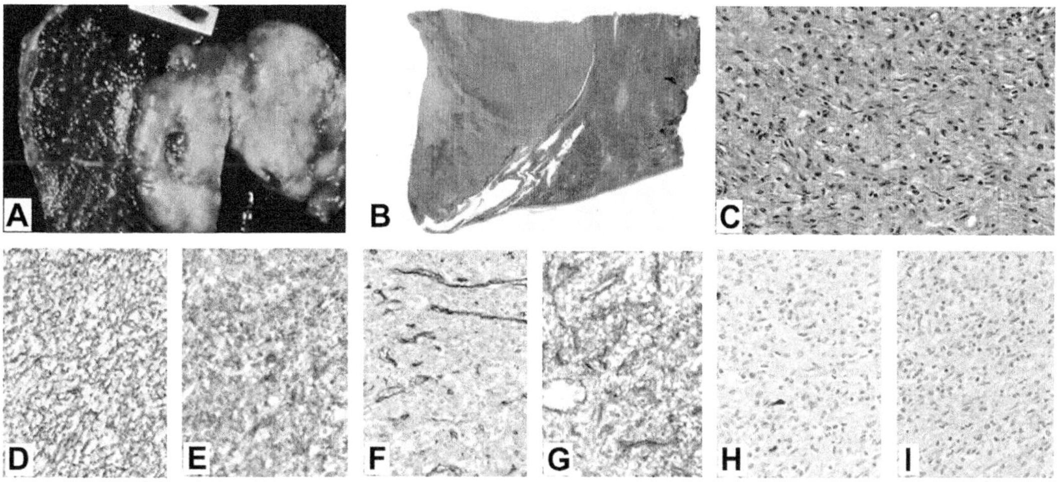

Fig. 4. IPT. (*A*) Gross image of a solitary mass in the spleen. (*B*) Low-power image showing normal spleen next to the IPT, H&E, 10X. (*C*) This image shows a relatively acellular area with scattered spindle cells, H&E, 20X. The spindle cells are positive for (*D*) SMA, 200X. (*E*) Lysozyme, 200X. (*F*) CD31, 200X. (*G*) CD34, 200X. The IPT was negative for (*H*) CD8, 200X, and (*I*) CD21; 200X.

and can have cytoplasmic vacuolization. There can also be scattered giant cells, cholesterol clefts, granulomas, and dystrophic calcification. Sclerosis can also develop in more chronic lesions. Post-chemotherapy histiocyte-rich pseudotumor should be considered in the differential diagnosis of IPT in patients with a known history of chemotherapy.

SUMMARY

Splenic IPT is a reactive condition with inflammatory cells, spindle cells, and sometimes sclerosis that has unclear pathogenesis and a complicated differential diagnosis. Infection, trauma, vascular and autoimmune diseases have all been

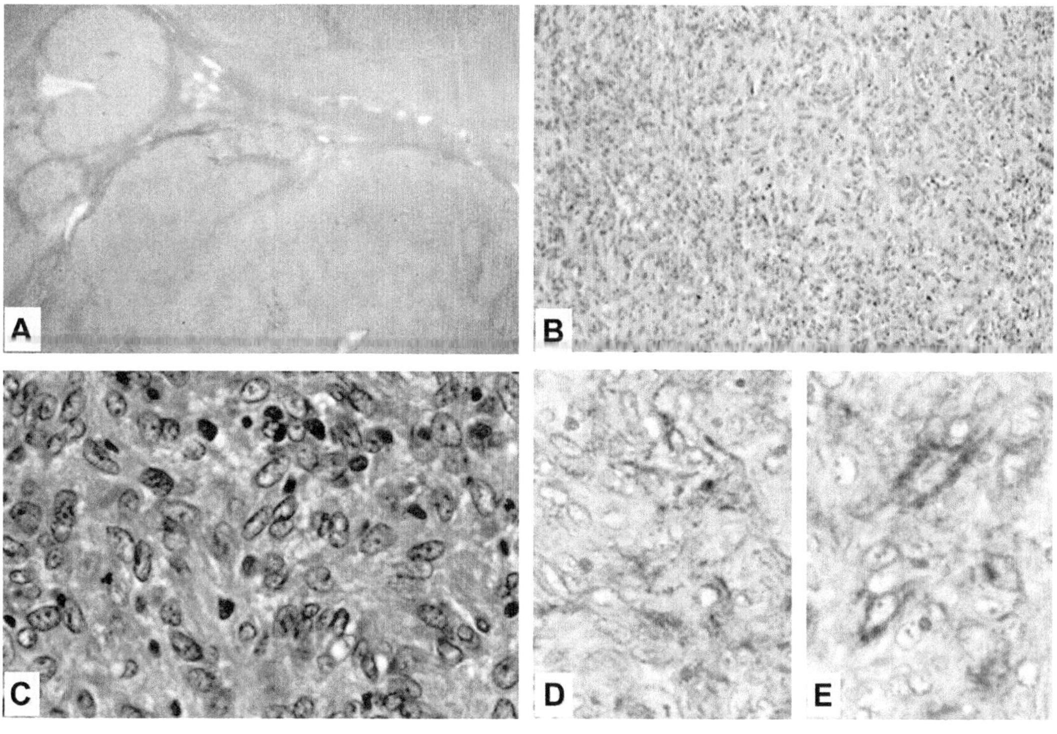

Fig. 5. FDCS. (*A*) Low power showing nodules, H&E, 10X. (*B*) Intermediate-power showing spindled cells, H&E, 200X. (*C*) High-power showing dendritic cells with intervening small lymphocytes, H&E, 400X. FDCS is positive for (*D*) CD21, 400X and (*E*) CD35, 400X.

associated with IPT and it is most likely that several conditions can result in splenic IPT. Regardless of the initiating event, IPT always has mixed inflammation forming a mass-like lesion.

> **Key Features–Inflammatory Pseudotumor**
>
> - Benign stromal tumor of uncertain etiology
> - Well-circumscribed mass comprised of mixed inflammatory cells.
> - SMA and vimentin expression; EBV may be positive.
> - No known genetic abnormalities.

EPSTEIN–BARR VIRUS-POSITIVE INFLAMMATORY FOLLICULAR DENDRITIC CELL SARCOMA

INTRODUCTION

EBV-positive inflammatory FDCS is a tumor with overlapping histomorphologic and immunophenotypic features with conventional FDCS. EBV-positive inflammatory FDCS has historically been considered a variant of FDCS, though compelling differences in site of occurrence, sex predilection, and EBV association call this subclassification into question. EBV-positive inflammatory FDCS shows primary splenic or liver involvement, whereas FDCS occurs most commonly in the head and neck region lymph nodes and at various soft tissue sites. Reported primary occurrence of FDCS in the spleen is very uncommon, and case reports may represent secondary involvement[63] or misclassification.[64] Furthermore, EBV-positivity, a female predilection, and a more indolent clinical course[65] in splenic EBV-positive inflammatory FDCS separate this diagnosis from FDCS. Limited molecular evidence also separates the two entities, with FDCS showing a complex karyotype,[66] whereas EBV-positive inflammatory FDCS lacks common genetic abnormalities.[67]

PATHOLOGIC FEATURES

EBV-positive inflammatory FDCS is comprised of a spindle cell neoplastic component with a prominent lymphoplasmacytic infiltrate. The spindle cells have nucleoli with vesicular chromatin and small, distinct nucleoli. Although the majority of cells usually have bland features, occasional cells with nuclear enlargement, folding, and hyperchromasia may be present with some cells resembling Reed–Sternberg cells. Hemorrhage and necrosis are common, and may be associated with granulomatous or histiocytic proliferation. Fibrinoid deposits may be seen in small vessel walls. The tumor cells may be hidden by eosinophils or epithelioid granulomatous inflammation (**Fig. 6**).[59] A follicular dendritic cell immunophenotype includes CD35, CD21, clusterin, CAN.42, D2-40, and CD23 with variable positivity and staining within the tumor. SMA may be expressed in areas of tumor without follicular dendritic cell markers, raising the possibility of fibroblastic reticular cell differentiation. Like FDCS, histiocytic markers CD68 and CD163 are occasionally expressed with a variable distribution.[60,68–70]

EBV is present in monoclonal episomal form.[36,71] The percentage of splenic cases with EBV positivity may approach 100% when consideration is given to cases that have likely been misclassified. Liver EBV-positive inflammatory FDCS has only rarely been reported to be negative for EBV.[72]

DIFFERENTIAL DIAGNOSIS

Although the histomorphologic differential diagnosis is broad for EBV-positive inflammatory FDCS, only FDCS shares a follicular dendritic cell phenotype. FDCS, as previously discussed, lacks EBV and does not typically have primary splenic involvement.

Splenic inflammatory pseudotumor is non-neoplastic, EBV negative, and lacks a population with follicular dendritic cell immunophenotype.

Classic Hodgkin lymphoma, especially the lymphocyte-depleted subtype, is a B cell lymphoma lacking follicular dendritic cell immunophenotype and may be positive for EBV by IHC. Neoplastic Hodgkin Reed-Sternberg cells are consistently positive for CD30, and PAX5 (weak), with or without expression of CD15. Similar large cells in EBV-positive inflammatory FDCS will not have these staining characteristics. Diffuse large B-cell lymphoma is a B-cell malignancy that expresses B-cell markers and lacks a follicular dendritic cell immunophenotype. EBV is occasionally positive, especially in the activated B-cell type.

SANT is EBV negative and lacks a follicular dendritic cell immunophenotype.

IMT is discussed in the IPT section above. This entity lacks EBV positivity and does not have a follicular dendritic cell immunophenotype. ALK is positive in a subset of cases.

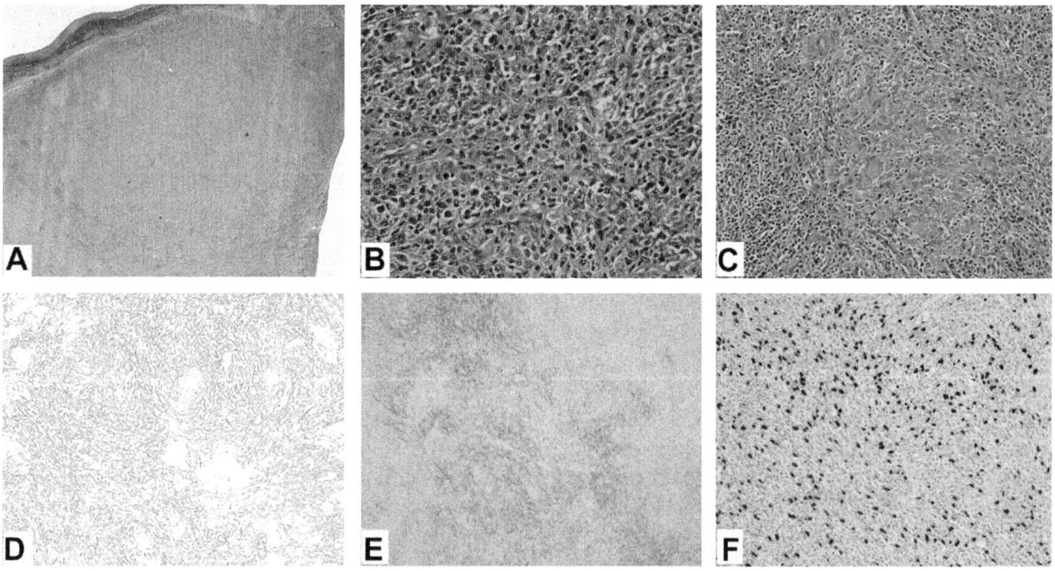

Fig. 6. EBV-positive inflammatory FDCS. (*A*) Low-power image; H&E, 20X. (*B*) High power showing a mixed inflammatory infiltrate, H&E, 400X. (*C*) Intermediate power of a granuloma, H&E, 200X. (*D*) SMA is positive, 200X. (*E*) CD35 is focally positive, 200X. (*F*) EBER is positive in the spindle cell areas, EBER ISH, 200X.

SUMMARY

EBV-positive inflammatory FDCS is a low-grade malignancy of the spleen and liver with follicular dendritic differentiation and an inflammatory background. It has histomorphologic and immunophenotypic overlap with FDCS, but with distinct clinicopathologic features.

Key Features–EBV-positive Inflammatory Follicular Dendritic Cell Sarcoma

- Low-grade malignant neoplasm of spleen and/or liver with indolent clinical course.
- Follicular dendritic cell immunophenotype with a prominent inflammatory component.
- Epstein-Barr Virus association.
- Female predilection.

HISTIOCYTIC SARCOMA

INTRODUCTION

HS is a rare malignant non-Langerhans cell histiocytosis; the incidence is 0.17 per million in adults.[2] Most commonly, HS occurs as a primary neoplasm in soft tissue but only rarely in the spleen. Approximately 25% of the cases occur in association with a preexisting hematolymphoid neoplasm and are presumed to occur by "transdifferentiation"[1,73–76]; however, this has raised speculation that HS and low-grade B-cell lymphoma derive from a common early precursor.[77] In adults, HS has been associated with germ cell tumor as a secondary malignancy, and in pediatric patients, HS is associated with the autoimmune lymphoproliferative disorder. The diagnosis is largely one of exclusion.

The clinical presentation is variable. There is a wide age distribution and HS is predominantly an adult disease, but pediatric cases occur. There is a bimodal age distribution with a peak from 0-29 years and a larger peak from 50-69 years of age. Approximately 5% of HS occur in the spleen.[2] HS may present as a solitary lesion or disseminated disease, with involvement of the gastrointestinal tract, skin, soft tissue, and hematopoietic system, including spleen. The clinical course in aggressive and median overall survival is six months.[2,73] Treatment is a combination of surgical resection and chemotherapy.[75] Patients with HS can be cured with aggressive surgical management in localized cases.

PATHOLOGIC FEATURES

Grossly, HS can present as a fleshy mass that is well circumscribed or infiltrative with variable necrosis. Histomorphologically, the architecture is diffuse. The neoplastic cells, which are large and discohesive, have abundant cytoplasm and ovoid to irregularly shaped nuclei. The neoplastic cells resemble histiocytes and macrophages but can be spindled or bizarre with morphologic features of frank malignancy. Giant cells may be present. Mitotic activity and necrosis may be present. Focally there can be a xanthomatous appearance or vacuoles. Hemophagocytosis may be present. A mixed inflammatory background including lymphocytes and neutrophils may also be present (**Fig. 7**).

Immunohistochemistry must show expression of at least one and preferably two histiocytic markers, including CD163, CD68, CD11c, or lysozyme.[74,75] PU1, CD4, S100 and CD45 are often positive. HS variably expresses CD15, HLA-DR, CD31, CD30, and factor VIII. Pertinent negative markers include CD13, CD33, myeloperoxidase, HMB45, and follicular dendritic cell markers, including CD21, CD23, CD35, and CD1a (although rare cases can show weak positivity). HS derived from low-grade B-cell lymphoma may have some retention of B-cell markers.

Molecular studies show a subset of de novo HS has clonal *IGH* rearrangement, and rarely *TCR* rearrangement has been identified. Mutations of RAS/RAF/MAPK signaling pathway *(NF1, MAP2K1, PTPPN11, KRAS, BRAF, NRAS, LZTR1)*, alterations of PI3K signaling pathway *(PTEN, MTOR, PIK3)*, and alterations of tumor suppressor gene *CDKN2A* are described in HS.[78,79] Mutations of *BRAF* V600E are seen in 63% of cases.[80] Tumors derived from low-grade B-cell lymphomas retain similar alterations as the prior B-cell lymphoma. HS associated with germ cell tumors have similar genetic findings to the germ cell tumor, including isochromosome 12p.[81]

DIFFERENTIAL DIAGNOSIS

HS must be differentiated from acute monocytic or monoblastic leukemia, which can present in the spleen as myeloid sarcoma resembling a mass of histiocytic cells. The morphology and Immunophenotype of myeloid sarcoma may be similar to HS. However, the common presentation with bone marrow and peripheral blood involvement and genetic findings more characteristic of acute monocytic/monoblastic leukemia, including lack of *BRAF* mutations, would favor acute leukemia.

Anaplastic large cell lymphoma (ALCL) is unusual in the spleen and should be excluded by immunohistochemistry. ALCL should be strongly positive for CD30 and at least one T-cell marker is typically expressed. CD68, CD163, lysozyme, and other histiocytic markers are negative.

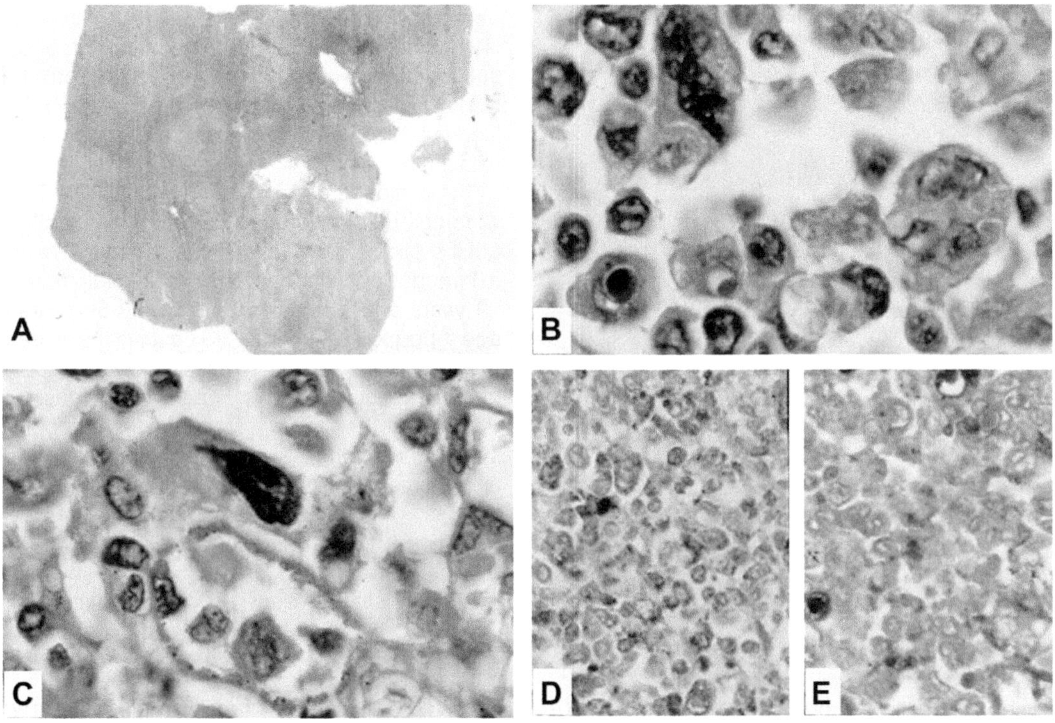

Fig. 7. Histiocytic sarcoma. (*A*) Spleen low power showing extensive involvement with histiocytic sarcoma showing vague nodularity, H&E, 10X. (*B*) High power showing pleomorphic histiocytes with erythrophagocytosis, H&E, 400X. (*C*) High power showing bizarre nuclei, H&E, 400X. (*D*) IHC for CD68 is positive, 200X. (*E*) IHC is positive for lysozyme; 200X.

Diffuse large B-cell lymphoma is a neoplasm of malignant large B cells with vesicular chromatin that can be excluded by immunohistochemistry. The neoplastic lymphocytes express B-cell markers such as CD20, PAX5, CD79a, CD22, and CD19 and lack histiocytic markers.

Malignant melanoma can resemble HS and should be excluded by expression of melanoma markers including HMB45, SOX10, and MelanA. Histiocytic markers are negative.

Metastatic carcinoma should be excluded by expression of keratin markers and lack of histiocytic markers.

Histiocytic processes, including Langerhans cell histiocytosis (LCH) and non-Langerhans cell histiocytoses such as Rosai–Dorfman disease (RDD), should be excluded by morphology and immunohistochemistry. LCH has a variety of presentations, shows ovoid histiocytic cells with longitudinal nuclear grooves, and has a spectrum of morphology from benign-appearing to frankly malignant. Eosinophils are usually present. LCH expresses S100 and CD1a, with variable expression of langerin (CD207). *BRAF* mutation is present in 50% to 60% of the cases. RDD morphologically shows large histiocytic cells with emperipolesis. Plasma cells are frequent and eosinophils are rare. The histiocytic cells are positive for S100, CD68, CD163, and lysozyme. They are negative for CD1a and langerin.

Reactive histiocytic processes in the spleen can include storage diseases, infection, and sarcoid. These lesions express histiocytic markers including CD68, CD163, CD4, and lysozyme, but lack cytologic atypia. *BRAF* mutation is absent.

Key Features–Histiocytic Sarcoma

- Malignant histiocytic neoplasm with pleomorphism and mitoses.
- Positive for histiocytc markers including CD68, CD163, lysozyme, CD4, MAC387.
- Most cases are de novo, but some are derived from low-grade B-cell lymphomas by presumed transdifferentiation.
- *IGH* may show clonal rearrangement and does not exclude the diagnosis even if de novo and not associated with a B-cell lymphoma.
- Mutations of RAS/RAF/MAPK signaling pathway *(NF1, MAP2K1, PTPPN11, KRAS, BRAF, NRAS, LZTR1)*, alterations of PI3K signaling pathway *(PTEN, MTOR, PIK3)*, and alterations of tumor suppressor gene *CDKN2A* have been described.

SUMMARY

HS is a true histiocytic malignant neoplasm that rarely occurs in the spleen. It is clinically aggressive, but potentially curable with aggressive management if discovered early.

SUMMARY

The histiocytic, dendritic, and stromal cell lesions that occur in the spleen are diagnostically challenging, not well studied due to their rarity, and therefore may be controversial. Newer techniques for obtaining tissue samples also create challenges, as splenectomy is no longer common and needle biopsy does not afford the same opportunity for morphologic examination of tissue. However, molecular genetic characterization, including NGS analysis, of primary splenic histiocytic, dendritic, and stromal cell lesions may offer potential molecular markers for diagnosis and further clarity with regard to their pathogenesis. Further study is needed to differentiate these lesions from those occurring in non-splenic sites, such as lymph nodes and soft tissues.

REFERENCES

1. Khoury JD, Solary E, Abla O, et al. The 5th edition of the World Health Organization Classification of Haematolymphoid Tumours: Myeloid and Histiocytic/Dendritic Neoplasms. Leukemia 2022;36(7). https://doi.org/10.1038/S41375-022-01613-1.
2. Kommalapati A, Tella SH, Durkin M, et al. Histiocytic sarcoma: a population-based analysis of incidence, demographic disparities, and long-term outcomes. Blood 2018;131(2):265–8.
3. Saygin C, Uzunaslan D, Ozguroglu M, et al. Dendritic cell sarcoma: a pooled analysis including 462 cases with presentation of our case series. Crit Rev Oncol Hematol 2013;88(2):253–71.
4. Auerbach A, Aguilera N. Diagnostic pathology: spleen. 2nd edition. Philadelphia, PA: Elsevier; 2022.
5. Taxy JB. Peliosis: A morphologic curiosity becomes an iatrogenic problem. Hum Pathol 1978;9(3):331–40.
6. Tada T, Wakabayashi T, Kishimoto H. Peliosis of the spleen. Am J Clin Pathol 1983;79(6):708–13.
7. Diebold J, Audouin J. Peliosis of the spleen. Report of a case associated with chronic myelomonocytic leukemia, presenting with spontaneous splenic rupture. Am J Surg Pathol 1983;7(2):197–204.
8. Tsokos M, Erbersdobler A. Pathology of peliosis. Forensic Sci Int 2005;149(1):25–33.

9. Ichijima K, Kobashi Y, Yamabe H, et al. PELIOSIS HEPATIS. An unusual case involving multiple organs. Pathol Int 1980;30(1):109–20.
10. Castelli MJ, Armin AR, Orfei E. Parathyroid peliosis: Report of a case and review of the literature. Fetal Pediatr Pathol 1986;6(2–3):127–30.
11. Lie JT. Pulmonary peliosis. Arch Pathol Lab Med 1985;109(9):878–9.
12. Kovacs K, Horvath E, Asa SL, et al. Microscopic peliosis of pancreatic islets in a woman with MEN-1 syndrome. Arch Pathol Lab Med 1986;110(7): 607–10.
13. Cohnheim J. Tod durch Berstung von Varicen der Milz. Arch für Pathol Anat Physiol für Klin Med 1866;37(3):413–5.
14. Gómez-Ramos JJ, Marín-Medina A, Lisjuan-Bracamontes J, et al. Adolescent with spontaneous splenic rupture as a cause of hemoperitoneum in the emergency department: case report and literature review. Pediatr Emerg Care 2020;36(12):E737–41.
15. Podduturi V, Blessing MM. Fatal Hemoperitoneum Due to Isolated Splenic Peliosis. Am J Forensic Med Pathol 2021;42(1):85–7.
16. Jaffe E, Arber D, Campo E, et al. Hematopathology. 2nd edition. Philadelphia, PA: Elsevier; 2017.
17. Nanba K, Soban EJ, Bowling MC, et al. Splenic pseudosinuses and hepatic angiomatous lesions. Distinctive features of hairy cell leukemia. Am J Clin Pathol 1977;67(5):415–26.
18. Ingle SB, Hinge CR, Patrike S. Epithelial cysts of the spleen: a minireview. World J Gastroenterol 2014; 20(38):13899–903.
19. Lucandri G, Felicioni F, Monsellato I, et al. Robotic splenectomy for mesothelial cyst: a case report. Surg Laparosc Endosc Percutan Tech 2011;21(2). https://doi.org/10.1097/SLE.0B013E31820B8A7C.
20. Giansanti M, Bellezza G, Guerriero A, et al. Localized intrasplenic mesothelioma: a case report. Int J Surg Pathol 2014;22(5):451–5.
21. D'Antonio A, Baldi C, Addesso M, et al. The first case of benign multicystic mesothelioma presenting as a splenic mass. Ecancermedicalscience 2016; 10. https://doi.org/10.3332/ECANCER.2016.678.
22. Guney E, Wah Wen K, Ruiz-Cordero R, et al. A solid variant of splenic mesothelial cyst, a case report with molecular analysis. Hum Pathol: Case Reports 2021;24:200509.
23. Palmieri I, Natale E, Crafa F, et al. Epithelial splenic cysts. Anticancer Res 2005;25(1B):515–21.
24. Omer WH, Narita A, Hosomichi K, et al. Genome-wide linkage and exome analyses identify variants of HMCN1 for splenic epidermoid cyst. BMC Med Genet 2014;15(1). https://doi.org/10.1186/S12881-014-0115-4.
25. Iwanaka T, Nakanishi H, Tsuchida Y, et al. Familial multiple mesothelial cysts of the spleen. J Pediatr Surg 1995;30(12):1743–5.
26. Bürrig KF. Epithelial (true) splenic cysts. Pathogenesis of the mesothelial and so-called epidermoid cyst of the spleen. Am J Surg Pathol 1988;12(4): 275–81.
27. Weiss LM, Chan JKC, Fletcher CDM. In: WHO Classification of tumours of haematopoietic and lymphoid tissues. Revised. 4th edition. Lyon: International Agency for Research on Cancer (IARC; 2017. p. 479.
28. Goto N, Tsurumi H, Takami T, et al. Cytokeratin-positive fibroblastic reticular cell tumor with follicular dendritic cell features: a case report and review of the literature. Am J Surg Pathol 2015;39(4):573–80.
29. Magro G. Differential diagnosis of benign spindle cell lesions. Surg Pathol Clin 2018;11(1):91–121.
30. Alaggio R, Amador C, Anagnostopoulos I, et al. The 5th edition of the World Health Organization Classification of Haematolymphoid Tumours: Lymphoid Neoplasms. Leukemia 2022;36(7):1720–48.
31. Sangiorgio VFI, Arber DA. Non-hematopoietic neoplastic and pseudoneoplastic lesions of the spleen. Semin Diagn Pathol 2021;38(2):159–64.
32. Martel M, Cheuk W, Lombardi L, et al. Sclerosing angiomatoid nodular transformation (SANT): report of 25 cases of a distinctive benign splenic lesion. Am J Surg Pathol 2004;28(10):1268–79.
33. Kato M, Lubitz C, Finley D, et al. Splenic cord capillary hemangioma and anemia: resolution after splenectomy. Am J Hematol 2006;81(7):538–42.
34. Wang H, Hu B, Chen W, et al. Clinicopathological features of sclerosing angiomatoid nodular transformation of the spleen. Pathol Res Pract 2021;224. https://doi.org/10.1016/J.PRP.2021.153490.
35. Pradhan D, Mohanty SK. Sclerosing angiomatoid nodular transformation of the spleen. Arch Pathol Lab Med 2013;137(9):1309–12.
36. Cao P, Wang K, Wang C, et al. Sclerosing angiomatoid nodular transformation in the spleen: a case series study and literature review. Medicine 2019;98(17). https://doi.org/10.1097/MD.0000000000015154.
37. Zhang Z bin, Li L. Splenic sclerosing angiomatoid nodular transformation in a patient with right renal carcinoma: a case report. Asian J Surg 2021;44(1): 396–7.
38. Efared B, Sidibé IS, Erregad F, et al. Sclerosing angiomatoid nodular transformation of the spleen (SANT) in a patient with clear cell carcinoma of the uterus: a case report. J Med Case Rep 2018;12(1). https://doi.org/10.1186/S13256-018-1907-5.
39. Uzun S, Özcan Ö, Işık A, et al. Loss of CTNNB1 exon 3 in sclerosing angiomatoid nodular transformation of the spleen. Virchows Arch 2021;479(4):747–54.
40. Chiu A, Czader M, Cheng L, et al. Clonal X-chromosome inactivation suggests that splenic cord capillary hemangioma is a true neoplasm and not a subtype of splenic hamartoma. Mod Pathol 2011; 24(1):108–16.

41. Chang KC, Lee JC, Wang YC, et al. Polyclonality in sclerosing angiomatoid nodular transformation of the spleen. Am J Surg Pathol 2016;40(10):1343–51.
42. Awamleh AA, Perez-Ordoñez B. Sclerosing angiomatoid nodular transformation of the spleen. Arch Pathol Lab Med 2007;131(6):974–8.
43. Rosai J. Is sclerosing angiomatoid nodular transformation (SANT) of the splenic red pulp identical to inflammatory pseudotumor? Report of 16 cases. Histopathology 2009;54(4):494.
44. Diebold J, le Tourneau A, Marmey B, et al. Is sclerosing angiomatoid nodular transformation (SANT) of the splenic red pulp identical to inflammatory pseudotumour? Report of 16 cases. Histopathology 2008;53(3):299–310.
45. Kim HH, Hur YH, Koh YS, et al. Sclerosing angiomatoid nodular transformation of the spleen related to IgG4-associated disease: report of a case. Surg Today 2013;43(8):930–6.
46. Kashiwagi S, Kumasaka T, Bunsei N, et al. Detection of Epstein-Barr virus-encoded small RNA-expressed myofibroblasts and IgG4-producing plasma cells in sclerosing angiomatoid nodular transformation of the spleen. Virchows Arch 2008;453(3):275–82.
47. Kuo TT, Chen TC, Lee LY. Sclerosing angiomatoid nodular transformation of the spleen (SANT): clinicopathological study of 10 cases with or without abdominal disseminated calcifying fibrous tumors, and the presence of a significant number of IgG4+ plasma cells. Pathol Int 2009;59(12):844–50.
48. Jin Y, Hu H, Regmi P, et al. Treatment options for sclerosing angiomatoid nodular transformation of spleen. HPB 2020;22(11):1577–82.
49. Ugalde P, García Bernardo C, Granero P, et al. Inflammatory pseudotumor of spleen: a case report. Int J Surg Case Rep 2015;7C:145–8.
50. Wiernik PH, Rader M, Becker NH, et al. Inflammatory pseudotumor of spleen. Cancer 1990;66(3): 597–600.
51. Cotelingam JD, Jaffe ES. Inflammatory pseudotumor of the spleen. Am J Surg Pathol 1984;8(5):375–80.
52. Monforte-Munoz H, Ro JY, Manning JT, et al. Inflammatory pseudotumor of the spleen. Report of two cases with a review of the literature. Am J Clin Pathol 1991;96(4):491–5.
53. Sheahan K, Wolf BC, Neiman RS. Inflammatory pseudotumor of the spleen: a clinicopathology study of three cases. Hum Pathol 1988;19(9):1024–9.
54. Kim N, Auerbach A, Manning MA. Algorithmic approach to the splenic lesion based on radiologic-pathologic correlation. Radiographics 2022;42(3):683–701.
55. Moran CA, Suster S, Abbondanzo SL. Inflammatory pseudotumor of lymph nodes: a study of 25 cases with emphasis on morphological heterogeneity. Hum Pathol 1997;28(3):332–8.
56. Puyan FO, Bilgi S, Unlu E, et al. Inflammatory pseudotumor of the spleen with EBV positivity: report of a case. Eur J Haematol 2004;72(4):285–91.
57. Neuhauser TS, Derringer GA, Thompson LDR, et al. Splenic inflammatory myofibroblastic tumor (inflammatory pseudotumor): a clinicopathologic and immunophenotypic study of 12 cases. Arch Pathol Lab Med 2001;125(3):379–85.
58. Krishnan J, Frizzera G. Two splenic lesions in need of clarification: hamartoma and inflammatory pseudotumor. Semin Diagn Pathol 2003;20(2):94–104.
59. Li XQ, Cheuk W, Lam PWY, et al. Inflammatory pseudotumor-like follicular dendritic cell tumor of liver and spleen: Granulomatous and eosinophil-rich variants mimicking inflammatory or infective lesions. Am J Surg Pathol 2014; 38(5):646–53.
60. Arber DA, Weiss LM, Chang KL. Detection of Epstein-Barr Virus in inflammatory pseudotumor. Semin Diagn Pathol 1998;15(2):155–60.
61. Lewis JT, Gaffney RL, Casey MB, et al. Inflammatory pseudotumor of the spleen associated with a clonal Epstein-Barr virus genome. Case report and review of the literature. Am J Clin Pathol 2003;120(1):56–61.
62. Kutok JL, Pinkus GS, Dorfman DM, et al. Inflammatory pseudotumor of lymph node and spleen: an entity biologically distinct from inflammatory myofibroblastic tumor. Hum Pathol 2001;32(12): 1382–7.
63. Sander B, Middel P, Gunawan B, et al. Follicular dendritic cell sarcoma of the spleen. Hum Pathol 2007;38(4):668–72.
64. Wang L, Xu D, Qiao Z, et al. Follicular dendritic cell sarcoma of the spleen: A case report and review of the literature. Oncol Lett 2016;12(3):2062–4.
65. Chen Y, Shi H, Li H, et al. Clinicopathological features of inflammatory pseudotumour-like follicular dendritic cell tumour of the abdomen. Histopathology 2016;68(6):858–65.
66. Perry AM, Nelson M, Sanger WG, et al. Cytogenetic abnormalities in follicular dendritic cell sarcoma: Report of two cases and literature review. Vivo (Brooklyn) 2013;27(2):211–4.
67. Bruehl FK, Azzato E, Durkin L, et al. Inflammatory Pseudotumor-Like Follicular/Fibroblastic Dendritic Cell Sarcomas of the Spleen Are EBV-Associated and Lack Other Commonly Identifiable Molecular Alterations. Int J Surg Pathol 2021;29(4):443–6.
68. Facchetti F, Simbeni M, Lorenzi L. Follicular dendritic cell sarcoma. Pathologica 2021;113(5):316–29.
69. Bui PL, Vicens RA, Westin JR, et al. Multimodality imaging of Epstein-Barr virus-associated inflammatory pseudotumor-like follicular dendritic cell tumor of the spleen: Case report and literature review. Clin Imaging 2015;39(3):525–8.

70. Horiguchi H, Matsui-Horiguchi M, Sakata H, et al. Inflammatory pseudotumor-like follicular dendritic cell tumor of the spleen. Pathol Int 2004;54(2):124–31.
71. Arber DA, Kamel OW, van de Rijn M, et al. Frequent presence of the epstein-barr virus in inflammatory pseudotumor. Hum Pathol 1995;26(10):1093–8.
72. Liu X, Cao L, Chin W, et al. Epstein-Barr virus-negative inflammatory pseudotumor-like variant of follicular dendritic cell sarcoma of the liver: A case report and literature review. Clin Res Hepatol Gastroenterol 2021;45(1):101457.
73. Andersen KF, Sjö LD, Kampmann P, et al. Histiocytic sarcoma: challenging course, dismal outcome. Diagnostics 2021;11(2). https://doi.org/10.3390/DIAGNOSTICS11020310.
74. Skala SL, Lucas DR, Dewar R. Histiocytic Sarcoma: Review, Discussion of Transformation From B-Cell Lymphoma, and Differential Diagnosis. Arch Pathol Lab Med 2018;142(11):1322–9.
75. Hung YP, Qian X. Histiocytic Sarcoma. Arch Pathol Lab Med 2020;144(5):650–4.
76. Feldman AL, Arber DA, Pittaluga S, et al. Clonally related follicular lymphomas and histiocytic/dendritic cell sarcomas: evidence for transdifferentiation of the follicular lymphoma clone. Blood 2008;111(12):5433–9.
77. Waanders E, Hebeda KM, Kamping EJ, et al. Independent development of lymphoid and histiocytic malignancies from a shared early precursor. Leukemia 2016;30(4):955–8.
78. Said J. Genomic profiling of histiocytic sarcoma: new insights into pathogenesis and subclassification. Haematologica 2020;105(4):854–5.
79. Egan C, Nicolae A, Lack J, et al. Genomic profiling of primary histiocytic sarcoma reveals two molecular subgroups. Haematologica 2020;105(4):951–60.
80. Go H, Jeon YK, Huh J, et al. Frequent detection of BRAF(V600E) mutations in histiocytic and dendritic cell neoplasms. Histopathology 2014;65(2):261–72.
81. Tashkandi H, Dogan A. Histiocytic sarcoma arising in patient with history of clonally-related germ cell tumour and myelodysplastic syndrome. Br J Haematol 2020;188(4). https://doi.org/10.1111/BJH.16372.

Molecular Diagnostics of Plasma Cell Neoplasms

Megan J. Fitzpatrick, MD[a], Mandakolathur R. Murali, MD[b,c], Valentina Nardi, MD[d,*]

KEYWORDS

• Plasma cell • Myeloma • Next-generation sequencing • Flow cytometry • Cell-free DNA • Circulating tumor cells • Mass spectrometry

Key points

- Plasma cell neoplasms are typically initiated by a primary genetic insult, predominately hyperdiploidy, or an immunoglobulin heavy chain translocation. Secondary genetic insults are subsequently acquired over time, including copy number alterations, structural variants, single-nucleotide variants, and small insertion/deletions, resulting in disease progression from monoclonal gammopathy of undetermined significance to myeloma.
- Genomic characterization of myeloma by interphase fluorescence in situ hybridization and next-generation sequencing (NGS) has helped elucidate disease pathogenesis and predict prognosis.
- Evaluation of measurable residual disease (MRD) is one of the most important prognostic indicators in myeloma. Current assessment of MRD involves bone marrow evaluation by next-generation flow cytometry or NGS; however, less-invasive techniques such as peripheral blood cell-free DNA assessment and mass spectrometry for M-protein have recently been evaluated as potential alternatives.

ABSTRACT

Genetic characterization of myeloma at diagnosis by interphase fluorescence in situ hybridization and next-generation sequencing (NGS) can assist with risk stratification and treatment planning. Measurable residual disease (MRD) status after treatment, as evaluated by next-generation flow cytometry or NGS on bone marrow aspirate material, is one of the most important predictors of prognosis. Less-invasive tools for MRD assessment such as liquid biopsy approaches have also recently emerged as potential alternatives.

OVERVIEW

Plasma cell myeloma is a common lymphoproliferative disorder, arising from the clonal expansion of malignant plasma cells. In recent years, myeloma has emerged as one of the most complex and heterogenous hematologic neoplasms. Foundational events in myeloma can broadly be divided into hyperdiploid and non-hyperdiploid groups, the latter being predominately characterized by recurrent translocations involving the immunoglobulin heavy chain (*IGH*) gene.[1–3] These initiating events are thought to result in an asymptomatic pre-malignant state termed monoclonal gammopathy of undetermined significance (MGUS), which can progress to myeloma through the acquisition of additional genetic insults including structural variants (SVs), copy number alterations (CNAs), single-nucleotide variants (SNVs), and small insertion/deletions (indels) (Fig. 1). Characterization of these genetic abnormalities is important for risk stratification and treatment planning. In addition, assessment for measurable residual disease (MRD) in response to treatment has also emerged as one of the best predictors of

The authors have no relevant conflicts of interest to disclose.

[a] Hospital Pathology Associates, 2800 10th Avenue South, Suite 2200, Minneapolis, MN 55407, USA; [b] Department of Pathology, Massachusetts General Hospital, Harvard Medical School, 55 Fruit Street, Boston, MA 02114, USA; [c] Division of Rheumatology, Allergy and Immunology, Department of Medicine, Massachusetts General Hospital, Boston, MA, USA; [d] Department of Pathology, Massachusetts General Hospital, Harvard Medical School, 55 Fruit Street, Warren 820A, Boston, MA 02114, USA
* Corresponding author.
E-mail address: vnardi@partners.org

Surgical Pathology 16 (2023) 401–410
https://doi.org/10.1016/j.path.2023.01.005
1875-9181/23/

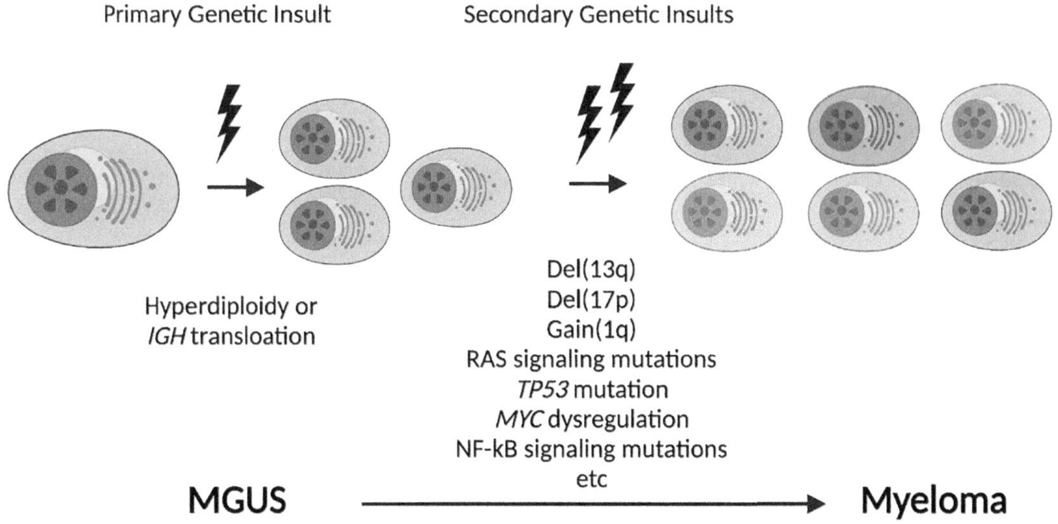

Fig. 1. Myeloma pathogenesis. A plasma cell clone is generated by an initiating genetic insult, generally either hyperdiploidy or an *IGH* gene rearrangement. This leads to the development of MGUS. Over time, the initial clone can acquire various secondary genetic insults, leading to the development of a complex genomic landscape including numerous subclones competing for dominance and subsequent disease progression to myeloma. (Created with BioRender.com.)

prognosis.[4] In this review, we outline the current and emerging molecular diagnostic methods used to characterize the genomic landscape of myeloma and assess treatment response.

MOLECULAR DIAGNOSTIC ASSAYS FOR RISK STRATIFICATION

KARYOTYPE AND INTERPHASE FLUORESCENCE IN SITU HYBRIDIZATION

Traditional karyotyping with G-banding is an insensitive method for detecting clonal abnormalities in myeloma, as only 30% of myeloma cases and essentially no MGUS cases show an abnormal karyotype, likely due to the low proliferative activity of malignant plasma cells and the often low number of plasma cells in bone marrow specimens.[5,6] More sensitive techniques, including comparative genomic hybridization (CGH) and interphase fluorescence in situ hybridization (iFISH) following plasma cell enrichment, have enabled the identification of recurrent chromosomal aberrations in >90% of myeloma cases, many of which are associated with prognostic implications.[7] The International Myeloma Working Group (IMWG) recommends performing iFISH at myeloma diagnosis to assist in risk stratification and has included certain high-risk abnormalities in the revised international staging system (R-ISS) for myeloma.[8]

Based on these techniques, plasma cell neoplasms can broadly be divided into two cytogenetic groups based on the founding clone: hyperdiploid and non-hyperdiploid.[6] Hyperdiploidy is defined as the detection of between 48 and 72 chromosomes, usually due to trisomies of the odd-numbered chromosomes 5, 7, 9, 11, 15, 19, and 21.[2,9,10] The non-hyperdiploid group is largely characterized by translocations involving the 14q32 *IGH* locus. These translocations result in the placement of oncogenes under the control of the constitutively active *IGH* gene.[2,11] Both the hyperdiploid and non-hyperdiploid pathways result in upregulation of cyclin D genes, which form complexes with cyclin-dependent kinases, leading to dysregulation of the cell cycle and accelerated progression through the G1/S checkpoint.[12]

Although co-occurrence of multiple primary aberrations has been reported in 5% to 10% of plasma cell neoplasms,[13] this finding is overall rare and primary abnormalities are generally thought to be mutually exclusive.[14] Primary genetic insults are thought to occur at the MGUS or smoldering myeloma stage and as a result, are present in nearly the whole plasma cell population.[15–17] Subclonal, secondary genetic insults are then acquired over time leading to the development of multiple subclones and subsequent disease progression. Common primary and secondary genetic abnormalities are summarized in **Table 1**.

NEXT-GENERATION SEQUENCING

Whole-genome sequencing (WGS) and whole-exome sequencing (WES) of myeloma have led to the discovery of recurrent SNVs and indels, with at least one SNV and/or indel driver present

Table 1
Common primary and secondary cytogenetic aberrations in plasma cell myeloma detectable by interphase fluorescence in situ hybridization

Alteration	Frequency (%)	Candidate Genes/ Chromosomes Involved	Associations	Risk	References
Primary Events					
Hyperdiploidy	45% to 50%	Trisomy 3, 5, 7, 9, 11, 15, 19, and 21	RAS signaling mutations, *MYC* dysregulation	Standard[a]	2,11,18
Non-hyperdiploid[c]					
t(11;14)	15% to 20%	*CCND1*	Mutations of *CCND1* and *IRF4*	Standard[b]	2,11,19
t(6;14)	1% to 2%	*CCND3*		Standard	2,11
t(4;14)	10% to 15%	*WHSC1* and *FGFR3*		High	8,20
t(14;16)	2% to 4%	*MAF*	*APOBEC* signature, gain 1q, del 17p	High	21,22
t(14;20)	1%	*MAFB*	*APOBEC* signature, gain 1q, del 17p	High	21,22
Secondary Events					
MYC (8q) Dysregulation					23–26
Translocations	18%	*IGH, IGL, IGK, FAM46C, FOXO3,* and *BMP6*[c]	Hyperdiploidy	Controversial	
Gain	19%		Hyperdiploidy	Standard	
Common Chromosomal Abnormalities					
Monosomy 13 Del 13q	50% 6% to 10%	*RB1, EBPL, RNASEH2B, RCBTB2, mir-16–1,* and *mir-15a*	Non-hyperdiploid	Standard	27–29
Gain 1q	20% to 30%	*CKS1B*	"Double-hit" high risk cohort	High[d]	30
Del 1p	30%	*FAM46C, CDKN2C,* and *MTF2*		High	27,31,32
Del 17p[e]	8% to 10%	*TP53*	"Double-hit" high risk cohort	High risk if *TP53* inactivated[e]	11,27,30

Abbreviation: Del, deletion.
[a] Recent studies have found <5 trisomies, >2 concurrent FISH abnormalities, and/or co-occurrence of *IGH* rearrangement is associated with a worse prognosis among hyperdiploid myeloma.[18]
[b] Adverse prognosis if associated with concurrent *CCND1* mutation.
[c] Five most common partners.
[d] High risk only if > 4 copy gain of 1q and R-ISS Stage III ("double hit"), present in approximately 6% of myeloma cases.
[e] High risk only if associated with *TP53* inactivation. Worse prognosis if biallelic inactivation ("double hit").
Fitzpatrick, M.J., Nardi, V. & Sohani, A.R. Plasma cell myeloma: role of histopathology, immunophenotyping, and genetic testing. Skeletal Radiol 51, 17–30 (2022). https://doi.org/10.1007/s00256-021-03754-3.

in 84% to 87% of myeloma.[11,33] An increased number of SNV and/or indel drivers is associated with an adverse prognosis, possibly due to increased genomic instability.[33–35] SNVs and indels can be clonal or subclonal events and there is marked variability across patients, with mutations occurring as clonal events in some patients and subclonal events in others.[34] Interestingly, despite the complex genomic landscape of myeloma, relatively few genes are recurrently mutated. Approximately 40% of myeloma will show mutations involving either genes in the MAPK signaling pathway including *NRAS*, *KRAS*, or the potentially targetable *BRAF* (**Table 2**).[11,33–36] Other recurrently mutated genes include the tumor suppressor *TP53*, as well as *DIS3* and *FAM46C*, involved in RNA processing and protein translation, and which are also thought to function as

Table 2
Most common somatic mutations in newly diagnosed myeloma

Gene	Frequency	Gene Function	Risk	References
NRAS	20% to 23%	MAPK signaling	Standard	11,33–36
KRAS	19% to 20%	MAPK signaling	Standard	11,33–36
FAM46C	6% to 11%	RNA processing and protein translation	Standard	11,33–36
BRAF	6% to 12%	MAPK signaling	Standard	11,33–36
TP53	3% to 12%	Cell cycle regulation	High	11,30,33–36
DIS3	1% to 11%	RNA processing and protein translation	High	11,33–36
EGR1	4% to 6%	Transcription regulation	Unknown	11,33–35
TRAF3	2% to 5%	NF-kB signaling	High	11,33–35
CYLD		NF-kB and WNT signaling	High	11,33–35
IRF4	2% to 3%	B-cell lineage differentiation	Standard	11,33,35
MAX	1% to 2%	*MYC* dysregulation	Unknown	11,33,35
PRDM1	0% to 5%	B-cell lineage differentiation	Unknown	11,34,35
SP140	0% to 6%	B-cell lineage differentiation	Unknown	11,34,35

tumor suppressors.[11,35] Mutations in genes involved in NF-κB signaling and *MYC* regulation have also been identified as drivers in a subset of myeloma, though no individual gene mutation appears to be significantly recurrent.[33,34]

MOLECULAR DIAGNOSTIC ASSAYS FOR DISEASE MONITORING

MEASURABLE RESIDUAL DISEASE

The prognosis of patients with myeloma has markedly improved in recent years largely due to the development of novel agents such as proteasome inhibitors, immunomodulatory agents, histone deacetylase inhibitors, monoclonal antibodies, and selective inhibitors of nuclear export.[37] This has resulted in >50% of patients achieving complete remission (CR), defined as undetectable M-protein by serum and urine immunofixation (IFE), disappearance of any soft-tissue plasmacytomas, and <5% plasma cells in bone marrow aspirates.[4] A further refinement of this definition, termed "stringent CR," is defined as CR in addition to a normal free light chain ratio and the absence of clonal plasma cells detected by immunohistochemistry on bone marrow core biopsies.[4]

Despite these apparent deep treatment responses most patients continue to relapse, suggesting frequent disease persistence below the level of CR or stringent CR, termed MRD. The IMWG has defined MRD-negative status in myeloma as an absence of clonal plasma cells by NGS or next-generation flow cytometry (NGF) performed on bone marrow aspirate material using a platform reaching a minimum sensitivity of 1 in 10^5 nucleated cells (**Table 3**).[4] In addition, PET and computed tomography (CT) is recommended in conjunction with MRD assessment to assess the extent of residual extramedullary disease, which would be missed by bone marrow-based MRD assays.[4] Patients achieving undetectable MRD show longer overall survival (OS) and progression-free survival (PFS) regardless of cytogenetic risk group and disease stage when compared with patients in CR with detectable

Table 3
Myeloma response criteria as defined by the International Myeloma Working Group

Complete response (CR)	1. Negative serum and urine immunofixation 2. Disappearance of soft-tissue plasmacytomas 3. <5% plasma cells in bone marrow aspirate
Stringent complete response (sCR)	1. Complete response criteria as defined above 2. Normal free light chain ratio 3. Absence of clonal plasma cells in bone marrow biopsy by immunohistochemistry
Negative measurable residual disease (MRD)	Absence of clonal plasma cells by NGF or NGS on bone marrow aspirate with assays reaching a minimum sensitivity of 1 in 10^5 nucleated cells

MRD. In addition, in multivariable analysis, when a sensitivity of 10^{-6} is achieved, MRD-negativity is one of the best predictors of prolonged PFS.[38–43] A recent study using an NGS-based MRD assay with a sensitivity of 10^{-6} found that nearly 60% of patients in CR were MRD-positive and this MRD-positive group showed worse OS compared with those in CR who were MRD-negative, suggesting that the survival benefit observed for patients in CR is largely attributable to MRD status.[44] There are multiple methods of evaluating MRD, all with advantages and disadvantages, including NGF (reviewed elsewhere[4,40]), allele-specific oligonucleotide quantitative polymerase chain reaction (ASO-qPCR), NGS-based assays, and most recently, liquid biopsy approaches (Table 4).

ALLELE-SPECIFIC OLIGONUCLEOTIDE QUANTITATIVE POLYMERASE CHAIN REACTION

ASO-qPCR identifies residual clonal plasma cells by detecting and quantifying plasma cell-specific *IGH* gene rearrangements using primers complementary to the junctional region.[4] This method can reach sensitivities of 10^{-4} and has been shown to have high correlation with flow cytometric methods; however, applicability is lower compared with NGF, with only 70% to 75% of patients harboring trackable clonal targets for amplification with consensus primers, usually due to somatic hypermutation within *IGH* resulting in reduced primer annealing.[4,39,45] If patient-specific primers to the V and J genes are used, applicability increases to 90% and sensitivity increases to 10^{-5}; however, this technique is laborious and standardized protocols for NGS-based approaches for MRD assessment show higher sensitivities of up to 10^{-6} with similar applicability.[38,44,46]

NEXT-GENERATION SEQUENCING

Several commercial NGS-based assays, including a US Food and Drug Administration (FDA)-approved assay (clonoSEQ, Adaptive Biotechnologies, Seattle, WA, United States), are available. These assays use consensus primers to amplify and sequence rearranged *IGH* and immunoglobulin kappa (*IGK*) and lambda (*IGL*) gene segments present in ≥90% of myeloma patients.[38,44] Multiple studies have shown that MRD-negative patients by NGS show significantly improved time to tumor progression and OS.[38,44] Importantly, low-level MRD at levels of $\geq 10^{-3}$ and $\geq 10^{-3}$ to 10^{-5} show worse survival outcomes relative to those found to be MRD-negative at levels of $<10^{-5}$, suggesting that assays reaching sensitivities of 10^{-6} may be important to ensure appropriate risk stratification.[44] In comparison to NGF, NGS can be performed on frozen specimens, increasing the flexibility of sample collection. In addition, results are reproducible with a digital readout, avoiding the need for expert review as well as the subjectivity inherent in flow cytometry data interpretation. Despite high sensitivity and applicability, NGS assays generally take days to weeks for results to become available and still suffer from pre-analytic variables related to bone marrow aspirate quality and concentration as well as sampling error related to patchy bone marrow involvement or isolated extramedullary disease.[44] To overcome some of these disadvantages, it has been proposed that MRD-negative status be confirmed by at least one additional bone marrow biopsy.[47]

LIQUID BIOPSY APPROACHES

The use of noninvasive liquid biopsy approaches, including the measurement and evaluation of cell-free DNA (cfDNA) and circulating tumor cells (CTCs) for the assessment of disease burden and development of therapy-resistant clones, have emerged as powerful techniques that can potentially overcome some of the limitations of methods reliant on bone marrow material, including spatial heterogeneity and poor aspirate quality, as well as avoid invasive procedures. cfDNA includes circulating tumor DNA that is shed through apoptosis and necrosis of tumor cells, whereas CTCs are malignant plasma cells hypothesized to egress from the bone marrow to the peripheral blood to escape hypoxic bone marrow niches and a pro-inflammatory tumor microenvironment.[48,49] Strategies to evaluate and characterize cfDNA vary and include WES and low-pass WGS for genomic characterization of disease, as well as NGS-based MRD assays designed to detect clonal rearrangements in immunoglobulin genes, similar to those currently used for MRD assessment on bone marrow aspirate material.[49–53] Analysis of CTCs has generally been restricted to enumeration tracking throughout disease progression and genomic characterization rather than MRD evaluation. Although in theory cfDNA and CTCs are derived from the same disease process, the relationship between the two is largely unknown.

CELL-FREE DNA

Assessment of cfDNA allows for real-time assessment of disease burden due to a short half-life of

Table 4
Laboratory methods for the measurement of measurable residual disease

Disease Evaluation Technique	Highest Sensitivity	Applicability	Specimen Requirements	Assay Speed	Assay Complexity
Bone Marrow Assays					
Immunohisto chemistry	10^{-2}	Nearly 100%, but insufficiently sensitive for MRD	Bone marrow core biopsy	Hours	• Low complexity • Subjective interpretation
Standard flow cytometry	10^{-4}	Nearly 100%, but insufficiently sensitive for MRD	Any fresh bone marrow aspirate	Hours	• Complex data with subjective interpretation • Difficult to standardize
Next-generation flow cytometry	10^{-6}	Approximately 100%	Any fresh bone marrow aspirate	Hours	• Complex data with subjective interpretation • Difficult to standardize, but standardized assays have been developed by EuroFlow
ASO-qPCR	10^{-5}	60% to 70% (higher with more laborious methods)	Baseline fresh or stored bone marrow aspirate	Days to weeks	• Complex and laborious • Can be standardized
Next-generation sequencing	10^{-6}	≥90%	Baseline fresh or stored bone marrow aspirate	Days to weeks	• Complex, but less laborious than ASO-qPCR and higher throughput • Can be standardized, but only one FDA-approved platform currently available.
Peripheral Blood Assays					
cfDNA	Varies	Unknown	Peripheral blood	Days to weeks	• Highly complex assays • Currently no standardized platform
MALD-TOF-MS	10^{-6}	~97%	Peripheral blood	Hours	• Complex assays • Objective measurement
LC-MS	$<10^{-6}$	~97%	Peripheral blood	Hours	• Complex assays • Objective measurement

approximately 1.5 hours.[50] Multiple small studies evaluating the use of cfDNA for the assessment of myeloma disease burden and genomic characterization have reported promising results, showing a high degree of correlation between mutations detected in bone marrow and those in cfDNA from peripheral blood.[49] A recent meta-analysis found that among two studies comprising 97 patients, high cfDNA levels were significantly associated with poor PFS, and among four studies comprising 164 patients, high cfDNA levels were significantly associated with worse OS.[51] Another recent study using low-pass WGS of cfDNA showed that in a cohort of 45 previously diagnosed patients undergoing identical treatment, a cfDNA tumor fraction ≥10% was associated with shorter PFS at both diagnosis and during treatment and was found to be an independent prognostic marker of poor outcome in multivariable analysis.[50] In addition, among patients with clinically stable disease and patients with partial response, higher levels of cfDNA portended a significantly shorter PFS.

Several studies have also evaluated the use of cfDNA for MRD assessment; however, results have been variable when compared with currently used NGS and NGF strategies. One study, which compared NGS for *IGH* rearrangements on bone marrow aspirate material to cfDNA in peripheral blood, found no correlation for quantitative MRD burden and reported that 69% of patients determined to be MRD-negative by cfDNA were MRD-positive by bone marrow NGS assessment.[52] Another small study of 12 patients comparing MRD assessment by NGF on bone marrow aspirate material to ASO-qPCR on cfDNA also found discordant results among 25% of patients.[53] In contrast, another study comparing NGF on aspirate material to NGS for *IGH* rearrangements in cfDNA found a complete correlation among 25 patients.[54] A recent meta-analysis reported that among five studies comprising 186 myeloma patients and including the three described above, overall sensitivity for MRD detection by cfDNA was 0.58 and specificity was 0.91.[51] Further studies with larger cohorts are needed to elucidate the reasons for the variable correlation between cfDNA and bone marrow MRD assessment and to better establish the applicability of cfDNA for MRD detection.

CIRCULATING TUMOR CELLS

CTCs are detectable in nearly all myeloma patients and increased numbers have been shown to be associated with an increased risk of progression from MGUS or smoldering myeloma to overt myeloma.[55,56] The genomic landscape of CTCs appears to show overall high correlation with both bone marrow clonal plasma cells and extramedullary plasmacytomas with the important exception of translocations.[55,57] One study found that only 39% of translocations present in bone marrow specimens were detectable in CTCs.[55] Additional important biological differences have also been noted including CTC overexpression of genes involved in hypoxia, cellular migration and adhesion, and inflammation, as well as downregulation of genes involved in cell cycle progression, suggesting that malignant plasma cells may egress to the peripheral blood due to a hypoxic and pro-inflammatory bone marrow microenvironment.[57] These findings suggest that CTCs can capture at least part of the bone marrow and extramedullary genomic landscape of myeloma; however, important limitations especially regarding risk stratification are present.

A recent study using a WES-based approach compared the mutational profiles of cfDNA and CTCs and found that although tumor fractions between the two liquid biopsy types did not correlate, both showed an overall correlation with disease stage and serum free light chain ratio.[49] Interestingly, although cfDNA and CTC sequencing found similar mutational profiles among paired samples, sequencing both was required to detect all clonal mutations identified in matched bone marrow specimens as several patients were found to harbor subclones present in only cfDNA or CTCs. These findings suggest that simultaneous sequencing may be necessary to capture the full mutational landscape of myeloma.

MASS SPECTROMETRY

Detection and quantification of serum and urine monoclonal immunoglobulin and/or monoclonal free light chains (M-proteins) secreted by malignant plasma cells have long been used as biomarkers to track disease course and treatment response through electrophoresis and immunofixation (IFE).[58] With improved treatments, an increased proportion of patients show undetectable M-protein by IFE during and after treatment, suggesting that more sensitive methods may be needed to determine treatment efficacy, especially in an evolving therapeutic era when MRD assessment has profound importance in predicting OS and PFS.

Recently, the use of matrix-assisted laser desorption/ionization-time of flight mass spectrometry (MALDI-TOF-MS) and liquid chromatography quadrupole time-of-flight mass spectrometry

(LC-MS) have been described as highly sensitive methods to detect and quantify M-proteins that can potentially be used in the MRD setting.[58–60] IFE has a lower limit of detection (LLoD) of 0.1 to 0.2 g/dL and as low as 0.04 g/dL if the M-protein is within the gamma-region. In comparison, MALDI-TOF-MS consistently shows an LLoD of 0.05 g/dL, whereas LC-MS shows an LLoD as low as 0.005 g/dL.[60] A recent study comparing MALD-TOF-MS to IFE found that among initial diagnostic samples in 223 newly diagnosed myeloma patients, there was >80% concordance at diagnosis, post-induction, post-autologous stem cell transplant, and post-consolidation.[58] Interestingly, among cases negative for M-protein by IFE, those positive by MALD-TOF-MS showed significantly shorter PFS compared with those negative by both methods, suggesting that MALDI-TOF-MS evaluation may result in a clinically meaningful increase in sensitivity. Another small study comparing MALDI-TOF-MS, LC-MS, and NGS for the assessment of MRD found that among 36 patients undergoing identical treatment for myeloma, peripheral blood assessment for M-protein by LC-MS was more sensitive ($<10^{-6}$) than either peripheral blood MALDI-TOF-MS and bone marrow NGS, both of which showed comparable sensitivities of 10^{-5} to 10^{-6}, and was a better predictor of PFS.[60] This study suggested that a multimodal MRD approach may be most efficacious, in which patients negative by IFE undergo LC-MS and if also found to be negative, MRD status should be confirmed by subsequent bone marrow evaluation whereas those positive by LC-MS could avoid invasive procedures.

SUMMARY

The molecular landscape of myeloma is markedly complex and heterogenous. An ancestral clone likely initiates disease, and the acquisition of secondary genetic insults then results in the development of numerous subclones that compete for dominance, resulting in both temporal and spatial heterogeneity. Molecular and immunophenotypic bone marrow assessment remains essential for initial disease characterization and prognostication. In addition, MRD assessment after treatment by NGS or NGF on bone marrow aspirate material has emerged as a powerful predictor of prognosis. Newer, less-invasive liquid biopsy approaches have also recently emerged as sensitive tools that can potentially be used for molecular characterization and to track disease progression and response to treatment.

CLINICS CARE POINTS

- Molecular characterization of myeloma at diagnosis with interphase fluorescence in situ hybridization is essential for appropriate risk stratification. Next-generation sequencing (NGS) performed at initial diagnosis can also supplement risk stratification, though is not currently included in the revised international staging system for myeloma.
- Measurable residual disease (MRD) evaluation is critical for risk stratification during and after treatment. Current best strategies include NGS-based assays or next-generation flow cytometry performed on bone marrow aspirate material.
- Liquid biopsy strategies for molecular characterization and MRD detection including cell-free DNA, circulating tumor cell evaluation, and M-protein detection by mass spectrometry are emerging technologies that show promising results; however, larger studies are needed to determine optimal applicability and appropriate use in clinical practice.

REFERENCES

1. Swerdlow SH, Campo E, Harris NL, et al. WHO classification of tumours of haematopoietic and lymphoid tissues. 4th edition. Lyon: IARC; 2017.
2. Manier S, Salem KZ, Park J, et al. Genomic complexity of multiple myeloma and its clinical implications. Nat Rev Clin Oncol 2017;14(2):100–13.
3. Fitzpatrick MJ, Nardi V, Sohani AR. Plasma cell myeloma: role of histopathology, immunophenotyping, and genetic testing. Skeletal Radiol 2022;51(1):17–30.
4. Kumar S, Paiva B, Anderson KC, et al. International Myeloma Working Group consensus criteria for response and minimal residual disease assessment in multiple myeloma. Lancet Oncol 2016;17(8):e328–46.
5. Saxe D, Seo EJ, Bergeron MB, et al. Recent advances in cytogenetic characterization of multiple myeloma. Int J Lab Hematol 2019;41(1):5–14.
6. Debes-Marun CS, Dewald GW, Bryant S, et al. Chromosome abnormalities clustering and its implications for pathogenesis and prognosis in myeloma. Leukemia 2003;17(2):427–36.
7. Hebraud B, Magrangeas F, Cleynen A, et al. Role of additional chromosomal changes in the prognostic value of t(4;14) and del(17p) in multiple myeloma: The IFM experience. Blood 2015;125(13):2095–100.

8. Palumbo A, Avet-Loiseau H, Oliva S, et al. Revised international staging system for multiple myeloma: A report from international myeloma working group. J Clin Oncol 2015;33(26):2863–9.
9. Vu T, Gonsalves W, Kumar S, et al. Characteristics of exceptional responders to lenalidomide- based therapy in multiple myeloma. Blood Cancer J 2015;(September):e363.
10. Maura F, Rustad EH, Boyle EM, et al. Reconstructing the evolutionary history of multiple myeloma. Best Pract Res Clin Haematol 2020;33(1):101145.
11. Maura F, Bolli N, Angelopoulos N, et al. Genomic landscape and chronological reconstruction of driver events in multiple myeloma. Nat Commun 2019;10(1):1–12.
12. Jannes Neuse C, Lomas O, Schliemann C, et al. Genome instability in multiple myeloma. Leukemia 2020;34:2887–97.
13. Pawlyn C, Melchor L, Murison A, et al. Coexistent hyperdiploidy does not abrogate poor prognosis in myeloma with adverse cytogenetics and may precede IGH translocations. Blood 2015;125(5):831–40.
14. Kumar SK, Rajkumar SV. The multiple myelomas - Current concepts in cytogenetic classification and therapy. Nat Rev Clin Oncol 2018;15(7):409–21.
15. López-Corral L, Mateos MV, Corchete LA, et al. Genomic analysis of high-risk smoldering multiple myeloma. Haematologica 2012;97(9):1439–43.
16. Fonseca R, Bailey RJ, Ahmann GJ, et al. Genomic abnormalities in monoclonal gammopathy of undetermined significance. Blood 2002;100(4):1417–24.
17. Rajkumar SV, Gupta V, Fonseca R, et al. Impact of primary molecular cytogenetic abnormalities and risk of progression in smoldering multiple myeloma. Leukemia 2013;27(8):1738–44.
18. Barilà G, Bonaldi L, Grassi A, et al. Identification of the true hyperdiploid multiple myeloma subset by combining conventional karyotyping and FISH analysis. Blood Cancer J 2020;10(2):1–5
19. Gasparetto C, Jagannath S, Rifkin RM, et al. Effect of t (11;14) Abnormality on outcomes of patients with newly diagnosed multiple myeloma in the connect MM registry. Clin Lymphoma, Myeloma Leuk 2022;22(3):149–57.
20. Foltz SM, Gao Q, Yoon CJ, et al. Evolution and structure of clinically relevant gene fusions in multiple myeloma. Nat Commun 2020;11(1):1–12.
21. Zhan F, Huang Y, Colla S, et al. The molecular classification of multiple myeloma. Blood 2006;108(6):2020–8.
22. Pawlyn C, Davies FE. Toward personalized treatment in multiple myeloma based on molecular characteristics. Blood 2019;133(7):660–75.
23. Misund K, Keane N, Stein CK, et al. MYC dysregulation in the progression of multiple myeloma. Leukemia 2020;34(1):322–6.
24. Walker B.A., Wardell C.P., Murison A., et al., APOBEC family mutational signatures are associated with poor prognosis translocations in multiple myeloma, *Nat Commun*, 6, 2015, 1-15.
25. Walker BA, Wardell CP, Brioli A, et al. Translocations at 8q24 juxtapose MYC with genes that harbor superenhancers resulting in overexpression and poor prognosis in myeloma patients. Blood Cancer J 2014;4(3):e191–7.
26. Sharma N, Smadbeck JB, Abdallah N, et al. The prognostic role of MYC structural variants identified by NGS and FISH in multiple myeloma. Clin Cancer Res 2021;27(19):5430–9.
27. Walker BA, Leone PE, Chiecchio L, et al. A compendium of myeloma-associated chromosomal copy number abnormalities and their prognostic value. Blood 2010;116(15):56–65.
28. Avet-Loiseau H, Daviet A, Saunier S, et al. Chromosome 13 abnormalities in multiple myeloma are mostly monosomy 13. Br J Haematol 2000;111(4):1116–7.
29. Avet-Loiseau H, Attal M, Moreau P, et al. Genetic abnormalities and survival in multiple myeloma: The experience of the Intergroupe Francophone du Myélome. Blood 2007;109(8):3489–95.
30. Walker BA, Mavrommatis K, Wardell CP, et al. A high-risk, Double-Hit, group of newly diagnosed myeloma identified by genomic analysis. Leukemia 2019;33(1):159–70.
31. Bustoros M, Sklavenitis-Pistofidis R, Park J, et al. Genomic profiling of smoldering multiple myeloma identifies patients at a high risk of disease progression. J Clin Oncol 2020;38(21):2380–9.
32. Maganti HB, Jrade H, Cafariello C, et al. Targeting the MTF2–MDM2 axis sensitizes refractory acute myeloid leukemia to chemotherapy. Cancer Discov 2018;8(11):1376–89.
33. Walker BA, Mavrommatis K, Wardell CP, et al. Identification of novel mutational drivers reveals oncogene dependencies in multiple myeloma. Blood 2018;132(6):687–97.
34. Bolli N., Avet-Loiseau H., Wedge D.C., et al., Heterogeneity of genomic evolution and mutational profiles in multiple myeloma, *Nat Commun*, 5, 2014, 1–16.
35. Lohr JG, Stojanov P, Carter SL, et al. Widespread genetic heterogeneity in multiple myeloma: Implications for targeted therapy. Cancer Cell 2014;25(1):91–101.
36. Chapman MA, Lawrence MS, Keats JJ, et al. Initial genome sequencing and analysis of multiple myeloma. Nature 2011;471(7339):467–72.
37. Moreau P, Kumar S, San Miguel J, et al. Treatment of relapsed and refractory multiple myeloma: recommendations from the International Myeloma Working Group. Lancet Oncol 2021;22(3):E105–18.
38. Perrot A, Lauwers-Cances V, Corre J, et al. Minimal residual disease negativity using deep sequencing

is a major prognostic factor in multiple myeloma. Blood 2018;132(23):2456–64.
39. Sarasquete ME, Garcia-Sanz R, Gonzalez D, et al. Minimal residual disease monitoring in multiple myeloma: a comparison between allelic-specific oligonucleotide real-time quantitative polymerase chain reaction and flow cytometry. Haematologica 2005;90(10):1365–72.
40. Flores-Montero J, Sanoja-Flores L, Paiva B, et al. Next Generation Flow for highly sensitive and standardized detection of minimal residual disease in multiple myeloma. Leukemia 2017;31(10):2094–103.
41. Lahuerta JJ, Paiva B, Vidriales MB, et al. Depth of response in multiple myeloma: a pooled analysis of three PETHEMA/GEM clinical trials. J Clin Oncol 2017;35(25):2900–10.
42. Paiva B, Vidriales MB, Cerveró J, et al. Multiparameter flow cytometric remission is the most relevant prognostic factor for multiple myeloma patients who undergo autologous stem cell transplantation. Blood 2008;112(10):4017–23.
43. Paiva B, Martinez-Lopez J, Vidriales MB, et al. Comparison of immunofixation, serum free light chain, and immunophenotyping for response evaluation and prognostication in multiple myeloma. J Clin Oncol 2011;29(12):1627–33.
44. Martinez-Lopez J, Lahuerta JJ, Pepin F, et al. Prognostic value of deep sequencing method for minimal residual disease detection in multiple myeloma. Blood 2014;123(20):3073–9.
45. Puig N, Sarasquete ME, Balanzategui A, et al. Critical evaluation of ASO RQ-PCR for minimal residual disease evaluation in multiple myeloma. A comparative analysis with flow cytometry. Leukemia 2014; 28(2):391–7.
46. Yao Q, Bai Y, Kumar S, et al. Minimal residual disease detection by next-generation sequencing in multiple myeloma: a comparison with real-time quantitative PCR. Front Oncol 2021;10(January):1–5.
47. Burgos L, Puig N, Cedena MT, et al. Measurable residual disease in multiple myeloma: ready for clinical practice? J Hematol Oncol 2020;13(1):1–8.
48. Pugh TJ. Circulating tumour DNA for detecting minimal residual disease in multiple myeloma. Semin Hematol 2018;55(1):38–40.
49. Manier S, Park J, Capelletti M, et al. Whole-exome sequencing of cell-free DNA and circulating tumor cells in multiple myeloma. Nat Commun 2018;9(1): 1–11.
50. Waldschmidt JM, Yee AJ, Vijaykumar T, et al. Cell-free DNA for the detection of emerging treatment failure in relapsed/refractory multiple myeloma. Leuk 2022;36(4):1078–87, 2021 364.
51. Ye X, Li W, Zhang L, et al. Clinical significance of circulating cell-free DNA detection in multiple myeloma: a meta-analysis. Front Oncol 2022; 12(February):1–8.
52. Mazzotti Ć, Buisson L, Maheo S, et al. Myeloma MRD by deep sequencing from circulating tumor DNA does not correlate with results obtained in the bone marrow. Blood Adv 2018;2(21):2811–3.
53. Vrabel D, Sedlarikova L, Besse L, et al. Dynamics of tumor-specific cfDNA in response to therapy in multiple myeloma patients. Eur J Haematol 2020;104(3): 190–7.
54. Biancon G, Gimondi S, Vendramin A, et al. Noninvasive molecular monitoring in multiple myeloma patients using cell-free tumor DNA: a pilot study. J Mol Diagnostics 2018;20(6):859–70.
55. Garcés JJ, Bretones G, Burgos L, et al. Circulating tumor cells for comprehensive and multiregional non-invasive genetic characterization of multiple myeloma. Leukemia 2020;34(11):3007–18.
56. Sanoja-Flores L, Flores-Montero J, Garcés JJ, et al. Next generation flow for minimally-invasive blood characterization of MGUS and multiple myeloma at diagnosis based on circulating tumor plasma cells (CTPC). Blood Cancer J 2018;8(12). https://doi.org/10.1038/s41408-018-0153-9.
57. Garcés JJ, Simicek M, Vicari M, et al. Transcriptional profiling of circulating tumor cells in multiple myeloma: a new model to understand disease dissemination. Leukemia 2020;34(2):589–603.
58. Puig N, Contreras M-T, Agulló C, et al. Mass spectrometry vs immunofixation for treatment monitoring in multiple myeloma. Blood Adv 2022;6(11): 3234–9.
59. Langerhorst P, Noori S, Zajec M, et al. Multiple myeloma minimal residual disease detection: targeted mass spectrometry in blood vs next-generation sequencing in bone marrow. Clin Chem 2021;67(12):1689–98.
60. Derman BA, Stefka AT, Jiang K, et al. Measurable residual disease assessed by mass spectrometry in peripheral blood in multiple myeloma in a phase II trial of carfilzomib, lenalidomide, dexamethasone and autologous stem cell transplantation. Blood Cancer J 2021;11(2):2–5.

Current Landscape of Ancillary Diagnostic Testing in Chronic Lymphocytic Leukemia

Julia T. Geyer, MD[a], Michael J. Kluk, MD, PhD[b,*]

KEYWORDS

• CLL • Chronic lymphocytic leukemia • MBL • Monoclonal B-cell lymphocytosis • Flow cytometry • Immunohistochemistry • Molecular • Cytogenetic

Key points

- Chronic lymphocytic leukemia (CLL) is a heterogeneous disease with variable patient outcomes, and a multidisciplinary evaluation (ie, flow cytometry, immunohistochemistry, molecular and cytogenetic analyses) is important in diagnostic and prognostic assessment and permits tracking of measurable residual disease during follow-up, thereby influencing therapeutic management.
- By flow cytometry, CLL typically expresses CD19, CD20 (dim), CD5, CD23, CD43, CD200 (bright), ROR1 (bright), and monotypic light chain (dim) and is negative for FMC7, CD10, CD25, CD22, CD79b, CD81, CD103, and SOX11. In tissue sections, immunohistochemistry for B-cell markers, CD5, LEF1, cyclin D1, SOX11, Ki67, and p53 is useful in the workup.
- Molecular studies evaluating mutational status of *TP53* and *IGHV*, as well as *IGHV3-21/IGLV3-21* and *IGHV4-39* gene usage, are increasingly helpful to guide therapy decisions. In addition, *BTK*, *PLCG2*, and *BCL2* mutational status may be helpful in the context of resistance to targeted therapies.
- In the context of Richter transformation, the clonal relatedness (by molecular methods) of the Richter transformation to the underlying/prior CLL has been shown to have prognostic significance.
- Cytogenetic/fluorescence in situ hybridization testing for *CCND1* translocation, del(17p), del(11q), trisomy 12, del(13q), and karyotype complexity is helpful in the diagnostic and/or prognostic workup of CLL.

ABSTRACT

Chronic lymphocytic leukemia (CLL) is the most common adult leukemia and is a heterogeneous disease with variable patient outcomes. A multidisciplinary technical evaluation, including flow cytometry, immunohistochemistry, molecular and cytogenetic analyses, can comprehensively characterize a patient's leukemia at diagnosis, identify important prognostic biomarkers, and track measurable residual disease; all of which can impact patient management. This review highlights the key concepts, clinical significance, and main biomarkers detectable with each of these technical approaches; the contents are a helpful resource for medical practitioners involved in the workup and management of patients with CLL.

OVERVIEW

Chronic lymphocytic leukemia (CLL) is the most common chronic leukemia in adults in Western countries.[1] It has a strong inherited genetic

[a] Department of Pathology and Laboratory Medicine, Weill Cornell Medicine, New York Presbyterian Hospital, Immunopathology, Starr 715, 525 East 68th Street, New York, NY 10065, USA; [b] Department of Pathology and Laboratory Medicine, Weill Cornell Medicine, Molecular Hematopathology Laboratory, Box 69, 1300 York Avenue, K509, New York, NY 10065, USA
* Corresponding author.
E-mail address: mik9095@med.cornell.edu

Surgical Pathology 16 (2023) 411–421
https://doi.org/10.1016/j.path.2023.01.012

component. Small lymphocytic lymphoma (SLL) represents overt tissue involvement by clonal B cells with the morphology and immunophenotype of CLL. Monoclonal B-cell lymphocytosis (MBL) is an asymptomatic precursor to CLL/SLL. The diagnostic criteria for MBL and CLL/SLL are well established and are similar in the updated 5th edition World Health Organization (WHO) Classification (WHO-HAEM5) and in the International Consensus Classification of mature lymphoid neoplasms (**Table 1**).[2–4] CLL/SLL demonstrates great heterogeneity in morphology, immunophenotypes, chromosomal abnormalities, and genetic mutations. As a result, the natural history of CLL/SLL is extremely variable. Median survival is approximately 10 years with a wide range from approximately 2 to 20 years. Some patients experience a long and indolent course, which may not require treatment. Other patients have a long-term benign course followed by rapid disease progression. The most unfavorable disease course is that of a rapid deterioration and death within 2 to 3 years from diagnosis.

The diagnostic approach to CLL/SLL is a paradigm of multidisciplinary specimen evaluation in hematopathology. Demonstration of classic immunophenotype by flow cytometry and immunohistology is part of the essential criteria, as highlighted by the updated WHO-HAEM5.[3] Cytogenetic and molecular genetic characterization of the samples is not necessarily required for diagnosis, but is the recommended investigation for prognostic purposes and may play an important role in selection of a personalized therapeutic approach.[3,5] At the authors' institution, every new patient diagnosed with CLL undergoes a peripheral blood sample evaluation by flow cytometry, CLL interphase fluorescence in situ hybridization (FISH) analysis, a targeted next-generation sequencing (NGS) panel, and an assessment of immunoglobulin heavy chain gene variable region (*IGHV*), as recommended by the consensus guidelines of the International Workshop on CLL.[4] Patients with relapsed disease have repeat evaluation with flow cytometry, FISH, and NGS. If the diagnostic evaluation is performed on a lymph node biopsy, the authors perform confirmatory immunohistochemistry, flow cytometry, and a full cytogenetic analysis to include karyotyping and interphase CLL FISH.

DISCUSSION

FLOW CYTOMETRY

CLL cells have a characteristic immunophenotype; therefore, flow cytometry analysis is routinely used for diagnosis and clinical follow-up of these patients (**Fig. 1**). The neoplastic cells typically express monotypic surface immunoglobulin M (IgM; dim), IgD (partial), CD5, CD19, CD20 (dim), CD23, CD43, CD200 (bright), and ROR1 (bright).[6–9] Classic cases are expected to be negative with FMC7, CD10, CD25, CD22/CD79b (weak or absent expression compared with normal B cells), CD81, CD103, or SOX11.[10,11] Dim monotypic light chain expression by flow cytometry is another characteristic feature. Atypical immunophenotypes, including negativity for CD5 or CD23, positivity for FMC7 or CD79b, or strong

Table 1
Diagnostic criteria of chronic lymphocytic leukemia/small lymphocytic lymphoma based on the updated 5th edition World Health Organization classification

	Category	Positive	Negative
Essential diagnostic criteria	PB	Classic morphology of CLL cells Absolute B-cell count $\geq 5 \times 10^9$/L	
	Tissue	Lymphadenopathy/organomegaly or altered architecture Classic morphology of SLL	
	Flow cytometry	CD19, CD5, CD20, CD23 (variable), monotypic light chain (dim)	
	IHC	CD20 (weak), CD5 (weak)	Cyclin D1[a]
Desirable criteria	Flow cytometry	CD200, ROR1, CD43	FMC7, CD10, CD79b, CD81
	IHC	CD23, LEF1, CD43, MUM1 (proliferation centers)	CD10, SOX11

Abbreviations: IHC, immunohistochemistry; PB, peripheral blood.
[a] For cyclin D1 IHC, weak positivity in subset of cells in proliferation centers is allowed.

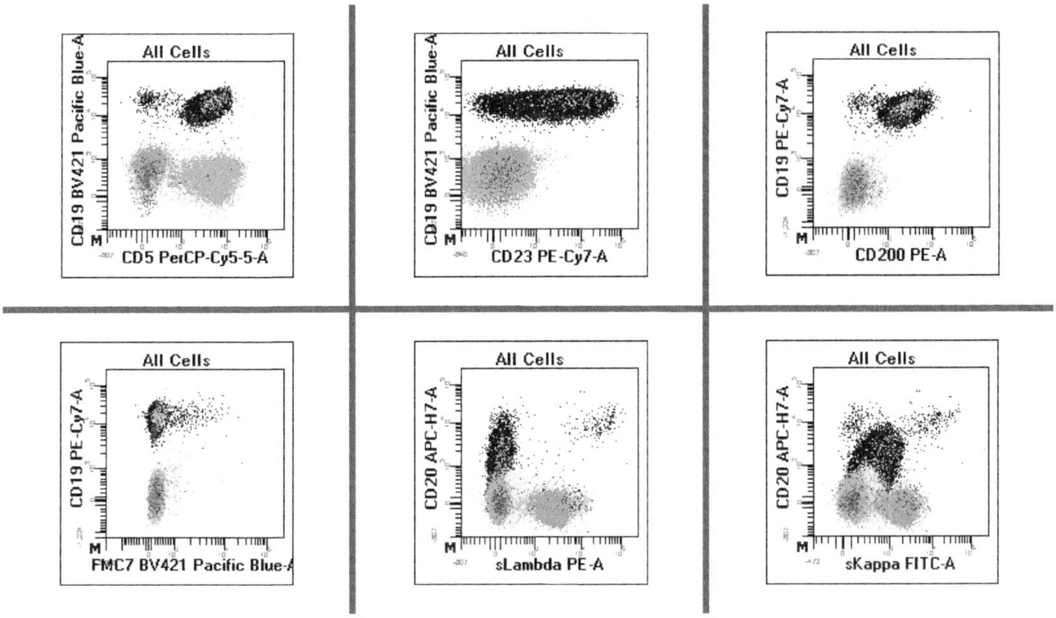

Fig. 1. Flow cytometric representation diagnostic of CLL with classic immunophenotype. The neoplastic B cells (*blue*) express CD19, dim CD20, CD5, CD23, bright CD200, and show dim surface immunoglobulin kappa light chain restriction. Tumor cells are negative for FMC7. Note a small population of residual benign CD20-brightly positive, FMC7-positive, CD5-negative, CD200-negative polytypic B cells.

expression of CD20 or surface immunoglobulin, may be present. In 2018, a large European consensus harmonization effort identified CD19, CD20, CD5, CD23, kappa, and lambda as "required" markers to be tested for a diagnosis of CLL. Additional "recommended" markers (CD43, CD79b, CD81, CD200, CD10, and ROR1) were suggested to refine the differential diagnosis from other small B-cell lymphomas/leukemias in borderline CLL cases with atypical immunophenotype.[12]

The characteristic immunophenotypic features of CLL are very useful in designing flow cytometry techniques to assess for measurable residual disease (MRD). MRD in CLL is considered positive if there is ≥1 leukemic cell per 10,000 normal leukocytes (≥0.01%).[4] Prospective clinical trials have provided a large body of evidence that therapies that eradicate MRD lead to an improved clinical outcome.[13–15] In both peripheral blood and bone marrow, MRD status is strongly prognostic for progression-free survival and overall survival in patients with CLL; along these lines, undetectable MRD (<1 cell per 10,000, $<10^{-4}$) in blood or bone marrow at the end of therapy has been associated with improved survival.[1,16,17] Concordance between peripheral blood and bone marrow MRD status is approximately 85% at the 10^{-4} threshold, but can be affected by treatment type (for example, it is lower in patients treated with rituximab and alemtuzumab).[18–20] MRD assessment in peripheral blood is useful for screening and for informing bone marrow aspiration decisions.[13] For example, if MRD is detected in blood, then usually bone marrow aspiration is not needed.

Multicolor flow cytometry remains the most widely applied method for MRD assessment owing to extensive availability, rapid turnaround time, reliable detection of currently applied MRD limits ($<10^{-4}$), and relatively low costs. In 2021, an international, multidisciplinary, 174-member panel published their consensus recommendations for MRD in CLL.[13] The panel recommends using the following nomenclature: MRD instead of minimal residual disease and "undetectable MRD" instead of "MRD negative." The gold standard for flow cytometric MRD testing is considered to be the 8-color panel designed by European Research Initiative on CLL (ERIC) group in 2016.[21] In the United States and many other countries outside of Europe, numerous institutions use "home-brew" panels developed in-house and based on the technology and antibodies that are available (**Fig. 2**). Recently, a 10-color panel modified from the EuroFlow LST screening tube was published by the McGill University group.[22] Most in-house validations are for internal use only and are not publicly disseminated. Examples of the MRD multicolor flow cytometry panels are summarized in **Table 2**.

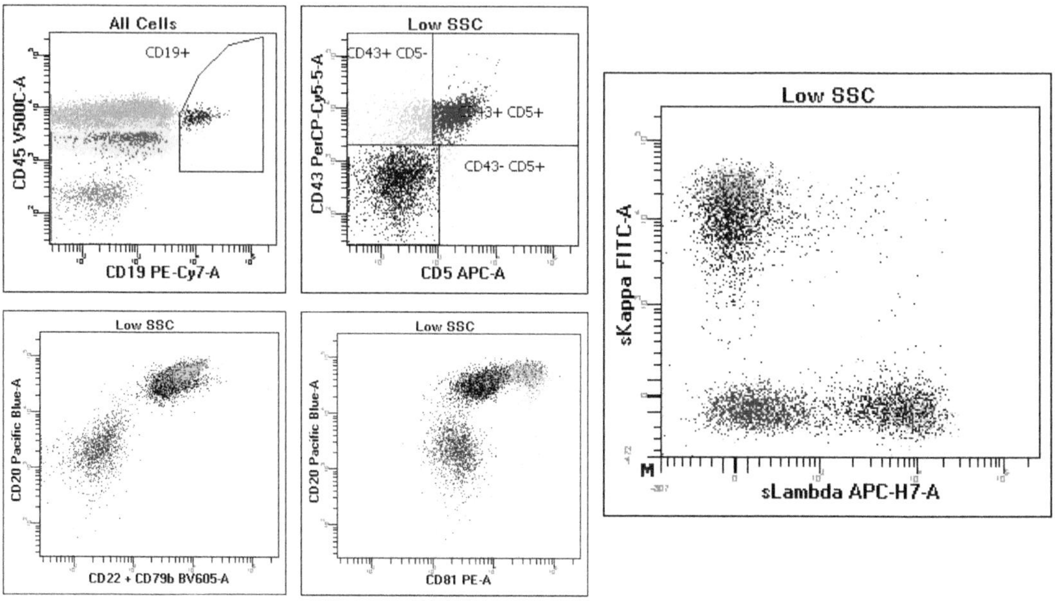

Fig. 2. Flow cytometric evaluation of CLL MRD assessment internally validated at Weill Cornell Medicine. CD19-positive B lymphocytes are selected for initial gating (*blue*). Subsequently, these cells are separated into 4 distinct populations based on expression of CD5 and CD43 (the neoplastic population of CD5-positive, CD43-positive B cells is highlighted in *purple*). The neoplastic B cells aberrantly express dim CD20, dim CD22/CD79b, and dim CD81 and show dim surface immunoglobulin lambda light chain restriction. Compare this expression pattern with that of residual normal CD5-negative B lymphocytes in blue and green.

Flow cytometry is also routinely used to evaluate prognostic markers in CLL. Expression of ZAP-70, CD38, and CD49d reflects activation and proliferation of CLL cells and tends to correlate with genetic markers, such as unmutated *IGHV* genes (Zap-70, CD38) and trisomy 12/*NOTCH* mutations (CD49d).[23,24] The presence of these markers is typically associated with an aggressive clinical course. ZAP-70 is expressed by T cells and a subset of normal B cells and may be assessed by either flow cytometry or immunohistochemistry. Flow cytometry is a preferred method, as it allows for a more straightforward and precise quantification of ZAP-70 expression on the neoplastic B lymphocytes. ZAP-70 evaluation has been a subject of some debate because of the lack of standardization of technical procedures. Currently, the most common approach is based on methods relying on evaluation of mean fluorescence intensity (MFI) values, as measured in the context of

Table 2
Selected multiparameter flow cytometry panels for detection of measurable residual disease in chronic lymphocytic leukemia

Panel, Year	No. of Markers	Sensitivity	Antibody Panel
ERIC,[21] 2016	8-color	10^{-5}	CD3, CD5, CD19, CD20, CD22, CD43, CD79b, CD81
DuraClone,[59] 2020	8-color	10^{-4}	CD5, CD19, CD20, CD43, CD45, CD79b, CD81, ROR1
McGill (Montreal),[22] 2021	10-color	10^{-4}	CD3, CD5, CD19, CD20, CD23, CD43, CD45, CD200, kappa, lambda
Weill Cornell (New York), 2022[a]	9-color	10^{-4}	CD5, CD19, CD20, CD43, CD45, CD22^{+}CD79b, CD81, kappa, lambda

Abbreviation: DuraClone, dry antibody reagents by Beckman Coulter.
[a] See Fig. 2.

both CLL cells and residual normal B or T cells. Various cutoffs have been proposed in the literature.[25–28] The authors' laboratory at Weill Cornell Medicine has determined the optimal cutoff of 0.4 B-cell/T-cell ZAP-70 ratio (ie, ZAP-70-positive cases have ≥0.4 MFI; ZAP-70-negative cases are <0.4 MFI) after extensive internal validation studies (Fig. 3). CD38 expression in ≥30% of CLL cells was found to be associated with aggressive clinical course and to correlate with *IGHV* mutational status.[29–32] However, the 30% cutoff represents a general consensus, as some studies have suggested a lower cutoff. CD49d expression by ≥30% of the CLL cells is an independent indicator of poor prognosis and may be superior to CD38 and ZAP-70 in predicting clinical progression in patients with CLL.[33] CD49d expression is stable over time, and determination of a positive or negative status appears straightforward.[34–36]

IMMUNOHISTOCHEMISTRY

Immunohistochemical staining of CLL/SLL shows the same characteristic immunophenotype as described above for flow cytometry. Typically, expression of CD20 is dim and partial, whereas other B-cell markers, such as CD19, PAX5, and CD79a, are strongly expressed by the neoplastic lymphocytes. Therefore, performing 2 B-cell markers is recommended when working up either de novo or posttreatment cases of CLL/SLL. LEF1 is a useful diagnostic marker because it is strongly diffusely expressed in up to 95% of CLL and is typically negative in other small B-cell lymphomas.[37,38] Like CD5, LEF1 is a T-cell marker, but is expressed by both B and T cells in CLL/SLL. Last, cyclin D1 and SOX11 immunostaining are also useful tools to help rule out mantle cell lymphoma, which is a distinct CD5$^+$ B-cell lymphoma separate from CLL.

WHO-HAEM5 designates a new category of "histologically aggressive CLL/SLL" defined as tissue cases with either very large, prominent/confluent proliferation centers (>20× field) or with high proliferation indices (>2.4 mitoses per proliferation center or >40% Ki67-positive cells in proliferation centers; Fig. 4).[3] This category now represents one of 2 subsets of cases under the umbrella term of "accelerated CLL/SLL."[39,40] MYC and MUM1 can be helpful immunohistochemical stains to highlight the proliferation centers, and Ki67 is routinely performed to assess for increased proliferation.

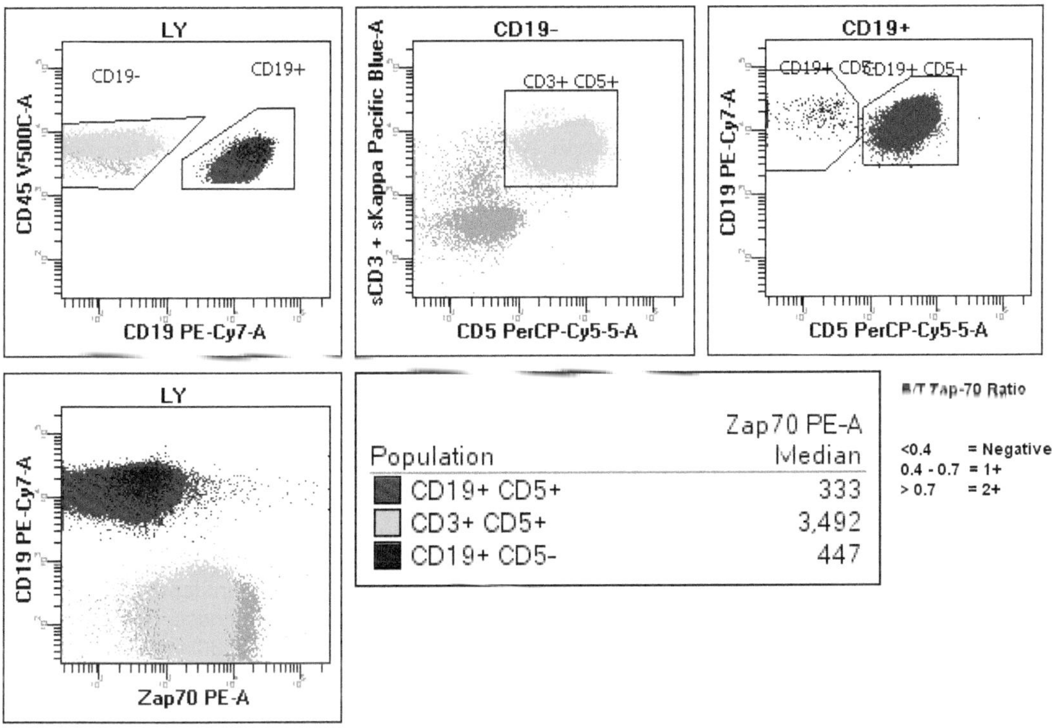

Fig. 3. Flow cytometric evaluation of ZAP-70 on CLL cells. CD19-positive B lymphocytes (*blue*) are separated from CD19-negative, CD3-positive, CD5-positive T cells (*green*). Subsequently, the neoplastic CD19-positive, CD5-positive B cells are gated and highlighted in purple. MFI values for ZAP-70 are tabulated for each population. The ratio of neoplastic B to T cells is calculated and compared with the cutoff value of 0.4. The CLL is this example is negative for ZAP-70.

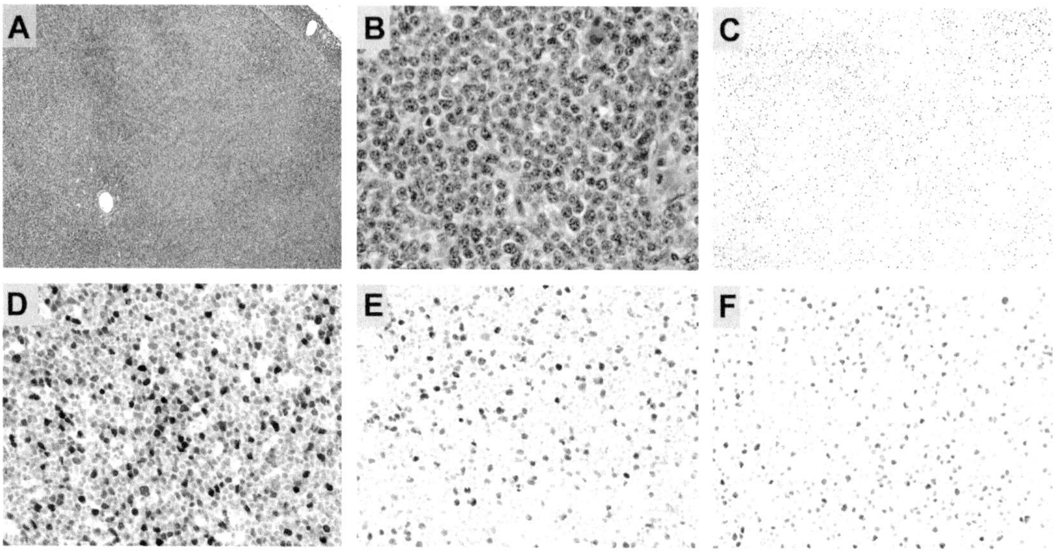

Fig. 4. Morphology and immunophenotype of a histologically aggressive case of CLL/SLL with 17p deletion by FISH. (*A*) The lymph node architecture is effaced by markedly enlarged, confluent proliferation centers. (*B*) High-power view of an abnormal proliferation center with sheets of medium-sized cells with variably open chromatin and small nucleoli (formerly called paraimmunoblastic transformation). (*C*) Ki67 immunohistochemical stain highlights increased proliferation within the atypically large proliferation centers. (*D*) MUM1 and (*E*) MYC immunohistochemical stains are positive in many cells within proliferation centers. (*F*) p53 is strongly expressed in a subset of tumor cells. Hematoxylin and eosin stain (*A,B*). Diaminobenzidine stain (*C-F*). Original magnification: (A) 40x, (B) 400x, (C) 40X, (D-F) 200X.

Patients with *TP53* alterations frequently show atypical morphologic features, including lymphocytes with cleaved/irregularly shaped nuclei or increased prolymphocytoid/prolymphocytic cells (prolymphocytes) in peripheral blood; lymph nodes with prominent proliferation centers corresponding to histologically aggressive cases described above; or cases with increased number of medium- to large-sized cells without expanded proliferation centers ("paraimmunoblastic variant") in bone marrow and lymph nodes.[40,41] Cases of prolymphocytic progression are defined as having greater than 15% circulating prolymphocytes with enlarged nuclei, basophilic cytoplasm, and a prominent nucleolus, and represent the second subset of accelerated CLL/SLL cases outlined by WHO-HAEM5. In a large study of 95 patients with CLL with *TP53* alterations, 91% of the patients demonstrated 17p deletion by FISH studies, whereas 84% had *TP53* mutations identified through Sanger sequencing. Only about half of these patients (49%) demonstrated positive staining for p53 by immunohistochemistry, defined as strong staining in greater than 5% of total cells (see **Fig. 4**).[40] Importantly, among the 49 patients evaluated by all 3 methods (FISH, Sanger sequencing, and p53 immunohistochemistry), 26% had a *TP53* alteration identifiable by only FISH or sequencing; however, no patient with *TP53* alteration was identified by immunohistochemistry alone.[40] Therefore, p53 immunohistochemistry is specific, but not sensitive, for *TP53* alterations, and this study provides support for the need for both molecular and cytogenetic analyses of patient samples.

MOLECULAR TESTING

According to the National Comprehensive Cancer Network guidelines,[1] a variety of molecular tests may be performed during the workup of CLL. Currently, there are no so-called CLL-specific mutations or genetic alterations that definitively establish a diagnosis of CLL. Nevertheless, once the diagnosis of CLL is established, molecular testing is playing an increasing role in the prognostication and therapeutic decision-making process.[16,42] This includes testing for *TP53* mutation status (by sequencing) and assessment for del(17p) (by cytogenetic analysis/FISH), because *TP53* mutation is present in approximately 80% of patients with del(17p)[16] and both are associated with the unfavorable risk category.[1,42] *TP53* mutation/del(17p) status influences the decision to use chemoimmunotherapy, given that CLL with del(17p)/*TP53* mutation has been associated with low response rates to conventional chemoimmunotherapy. Thus, in CLL with del17p/*TP53* mutation, regimens that include various combinations of first- and second-generation Bruton tyrosine kinase (BTK) inhibitor compounds, anti-CD20 therapies, and BCL2 inhibitors are typically preferred.[1] Of note, these same targeted regimens are also typically preferred in CLL without del(17p)/*TP53* mutation.[1]

In addition, molecular testing for *IGHV* mutation status can be done at diagnosis of CLL, given the prognostic significance and potential role in therapeutic planning of *IGHV* status.[16] *IGHV* mutations are the result of the physiologic process of somatic hypermutation that occurs during B-cell maturation.[42] It is thought that *IGHV* mutational status remains constant over time during the patient's disease course.[16,42] Molecular analysis to determine *IGHV* mutation status is recommended, especially when considering chemoimmunotherapy. Molecular methods are preferred over immunohistochemistry or flow cytometry, given the challenges in interpreting the results of these techniques, although they may be used to assess *IGHV* mutation status if molecular testing for *IGHV* is not available.[1] *IGHV* mutation status showing ≤2% mutation (or ≥98% homology with germline gene sequence, ie, "unmutated IGHV" or "unmutated CLL") is associated with unfavorable risk category and poor prognosis.[1,16] *IGHV*-mutated CLL (defined as *IGHV* sequence that varies by >2% from the germline sequence due to somatic hypermutation[16]) is associated with longer survival than unmutated CLL[1,16] and appears to influence response to chemoimmunotherapy, with long-term disease-free survival noted for *IGHV*-mutated CLL in the context of fludarabine, cyclophosphamide, and rituximab (FCR) treatment.[1,16,43] Conversely, unmutated CLL appears to respond better to the BTK inhibitor, ibrutinib, than mutated CLL.[16,44,45] Continued study in this area has shown that unmutated CLL had superior outcomes with ibrutinib-rituximab versus FCR, suggesting that BTK-inhibitor–based therapy may be an appropriate upfront strategy for unmutated CLL.[16,46] Optimal therapeutic strategies for the different subtypes of CLL continue to be studied.

Another molecular prognostic marker of disease, which is somewhat related to *IGHV* mutational status, is the identification of the exact subset of *IGHV* alleles used[16]; for example, *IGHV* gene usage involving *IGHV3-21/IGLV3-21* may be associated with a poor prognosis even when mutated (ie, independent of *IGHV* mutational status),[1,16,47,48] and usage of *IGHV4-39* has been reported to have an aggressive course and increased risk of Richter transformation.[16,49] Testing of *IGHV* subtypes in the clinical setting is not yet performed at many institutions, but its availability continues to expand.

During therapy, if the patient shows no response or disease progression, *TP53* mutational status and del(17p) FISH may be reevaluated. Also, testing for *BTK* and *PLCG2* mutations[42] may be useful in patients with lack of response or progressive disease during therapy with a BTK inhibitor; nevertheless, it has been suggested that *BTK* or *PLCG2* mutation status alone is not an indication to alter therapy.[1] This may be due, in part, to the observation that the reported variant allele frequencies (VAF) of *BTK* or *PLCG2* mutations may be low (ie, <10% VAF) at the time of progression on ibrutinib and may occur up to 15 months before clinical progression; therefore, these mutations may not entirely explain resistance to BTK-targeted therapy.[50,51] In the context of venetoclax therapy, the presence of *BCL2* mutations has been associated with treatment resistance; similar to mutations in *BTK* or *PLCG2* during ibrutinib therapy, *BCL2* mutation during venetoclax therapy may show a low VAF (<10%) and may be seen many months before clinical evidence of progression.[52,53] Currently, routine screening for *BTK* and *BCL2* mutations to assess for ibrutinib or venetoclax resistance is not recommended.[1]

During the course of disease, CLL may transform to diffuse large B-cell lymphoma (DLBCL) (so-called Richter transformation). The pathogenic evolution of this process is influenced by several variables, including the extent and types of prior therapies as well as certain molecular (eg, unmutated *IGHV*, *NOTCH1* mutation, *TP53* mutation) and cytogenetic (eg, del(17p) and complex karyotype) characteristics.[1] The transformed DLBCL may be either clonally related or clonally unrelated to the CLL. Clonally unrelated DLBCL has a lower prevalence of *TP53* abnormalities and a longer survival than clonally related DLBCL.[1,54]

As described above, assessment for MRD is increasingly being incorporated into the follow-up protocols for patients with CLL. The presence of del(17p), complex karyotype, and unmutated *IGHV* has been associated with increased risk of MRD conversion among those patients who had previously undetectable MRD at the end of therapy.[55] In addition, the presence of *TP53*, *NOTCH1*, and *BIRC3* mutations has been associated with lower rates of undetectable MRD.[14] The molecular-based methods of MRD assessment include allele-specific oligonucleotide (ASO)-polymerase chain reaction (PCR) and DNA-based NGS assays.[21,56] NGS-based approaches and 6-color flow cytometry have been observed to show appropriate concordance at the 10^{-4} threshold.[16] Currently, flow cytometry–based approaches are the most widely available method. Regardless of the test method used, an MRD assay with a sensitivity of at least 10^{-4} is recommended.[1] Among the molecular methods, NGS-based approaches are increasingly being implemented over ASO-PCR given the workflow efficiency and sensitivity of the NGS-based approach. Of note, MRD by NGS of bone marrow samples has been observed to show a lower rate of MRD negativity than peripheral blood, suggesting the potential importance of performing MRD analysis on marrow samples.[16,57]

In addition to the molecular findings described above, the presence of mutations in *NOTCH1*, *SF3B1*, *ATM*, and *BIRC3* has been reported in a subset of patients with CLL (ranging from 4% to 25%); among these, *BIRC3* and *ATM* have been associated with higher-risk disease and *NOTCH1* and/or *SF3B1* mutations with intermediate-risk disease.[1,16] Several other genes are recurrently mutated at lower frequency in CLL and tend to coalesce around select signaling pathways (eg, NOTCH1 signaling, B-cell receptor and Toll-like receptor signaling, MAPK/ERK pathway, NF-κB signaling, cell cycle, DNA damage response pathway, RNA splicing, and chromatin modifiers).[48] Testing for somatic mutations in CLL is expanding, most often in the context of clinical trials.[16]

CYTOGENETIC ANALYSIS BY FLUORESCENCE IN SITU HYBRIDIZATION AND CONVENTIONAL KARYOTYPE

Cytogenetic testing by FISH may be required initially to help establish the diagnosis of CLL and differentiate it from mantle cell lymphoma; in this context, FISH for *CCND1* translocation status may be helpful if cyclin D1 immunostaining is not available. Once the diagnosis of CLL is established, the following cytogenetic analysis is recommended in order to acquire prognostic information and guide therapy: FISH for del(17p), del(11q), trisomy 12, and del(13q), as well as CpG-stimulated metaphase karyotype.[58] Cytogenetic abnormalities have been reported in approximately 80% of untreated CLL, with del(13q) being the most frequent finding. Isolated del(13q) is reported to be associated with a favorable prognosis.[1,16,42] The presence of del(17p), del(11q), or complex karyotype (≥3 unrelated chromosomal abnormalities in more than 1 cell), is typically associated with unfavorable risk category,[1,42] although the prognostic significance of del(11q) may be evolving in the context of BTK-directed therapy.[16] Del(17p) is often associated with mutations in the remaining *TP53* allele, which may be detected by sequencing studies. During therapy, if the patient shows no response to treatment and/or demonstrates disease progression (including progression to DLBCL), then FISH for del(17p), in addition to TP53 sequencing, trisomy 12, del(11q), del(13q), and CpG-stimulated metaphase karyotype (to assess for a complex karyotype), may be reevaluated.[1] Given that the results of cytogenetic analysis continue to be clinically relevant, it is often included in the work-up of patients with CLL, in the appropriate clinical context.

SUMMARY

CLL is the most common adult leukemia and is a heterogeneous disease with variable patient outcomes that are due in part to a range of alterations in protein, molecular, and cytogenetic biomarkers that contribute to the underlying pathogenesis. A multidisciplinary technical evaluation, including flow cytometry, immunohistochemistry, molecular and cytogenetic analyses, can comprehensively characterize a patient's leukemia at diagnosis and identify important prognostic and therapeutic biomarkers. Much remains to be learned as technical advances improve the ability of these methods to evaluate CLL. Alongside discovering novel biomarkers and therapeutic targets, interesting emerging concepts to consider in the future, which have been raised by some investigators, include that CLL is clonally diverse, being composed of a heterogeneous tumor cell population, even in an individual patient; therefore, technological advances that permit learning more about the potential clinical importance of the subclonal populations in a patient may become increasingly relevant.[16,42,48] Likewise, studying the significance of specific compartments of disease (eg, lymph node vs peripheral blood vs bone marrow) may also become increasingly relevant in the future, given the evolving role of the microenvironment in CLL.[16,42,48]

CLINICS CARE POINTS

- Chronic lymphocytic leukemia/small lymphocytic lymphoma is the most common chronic leukemia in adults. It demonstrates heterogeneity in morphology, immunophenotype, chromosomal abnormalities, and genetic mutations. As a result, the natural history of chronic lymphocytic leukemia is extremely variable.
- Chronic lymphocytic leukemia typically expresses CD19, CD20 (dim), CD5, CD23, CD43, CD200 (bright), LEF1, ROR1 (bright), and monotypic light chain (dim) and is negative for cyclin D1, SOX11, FMC7, CD10, CD25, CD22/CD79b, CD81, and CD103.

- Measurable residual disease in chronic lymphocytic leukemia is considered positive if there is ≥1 leukemic cell per 10,000 normal leukocytes (≥0.01%). Published evidence has shown that therapies that eradicate measurable residual disease lead to an improved clinical outcome. Flow cytometric approaches for measurable residual disease measurement are the most widely available method. Next-generation sequencing–based molecular techniques to detect measurable residual disease are increasingly being adopted and used.
- Molecular studies evaluating mutational status of *TP53* and *IGHV*, as well as *IGHV3-21/IGLV3-21* and *IGHV4-39* gene usage, are increasingly used to guide therapy. In addition, *BTK*, *PLCG2*, and *BCL2* mutational status may be helpful in the context of resistance to targeted therapies.
- Cytogenetic analysis, including fluorescence in situ hybridization for *CCND1* rearrangement, del(17p), del(11q), trisomy 12, del(13q), and karyotype to assess for complexity, is helpful in the diagnostic and/or prognostic workup of chronic lymphocytic leukemia.

DISCLOSURES

The authors have no conflicts of interest to disclose.

REFERENCES

1. NCCN Clinical Practice Guidelines in Oncology. Chronic Lymphocytic Leukemia/Small Lymphocytic Lymphoma. Clinical Practice Guideline. www.NCCN.org Version 2.2022. 2022.
2. Marti GE, Rawstron AC, Ghia P, et al. Diagnostic criteria for monoclonal B-cell lymphocytosis. Br J Haematol 2005;130(3):325–32.
3. Alaggio R, Amador C, Anagnostopoulos I, et al. The 5th edition of the World Health Organization Classification of Haematolymphoid Tumours: Lymphoid Neoplasms. Leukemia 2022;36(7):1720–48.
4. Hallek M, Cheson BD, Catovsky D, et al. iwCLL guidelines for diagnosis, indications for treatment, response assessment, and supportive management of CLL. Blood 2018;131(25):2745–60.
5. Campo E, Jaffe ES, Cook JR, et al. The International Consensus Classification of Mature Lymphoid Neoplasms: A Report from the Clinical Advisory Committee. Blood 2022;140(11):1229–53.
6. Uhrmacher S, Schmidt C, Erdfelder F, et al. Use of the receptor tyrosine kinase-like orphan receptor 1 (ROR1) as a diagnostic tool in chronic lymphocytic leukemia (CLL). Leuk Res 2011;35(10):1360–6.
7. Hoffmann J, Rother M, Kaiser U, et al. Determination of CD43 and CD200 surface expression improves accuracy of B-cell lymphoma immunophenotyping. Cytometry B Clin Cytom 2020;98(6):476–82.
8. Challagundla P, Medeiros LJ, Kanagal-Shamanna R, et al. Differential expression of CD200 in B-cell neoplasms by flow cytometry can assist in diagnosis, subclassification, and bone marrow staging. Am J Clin Pathol 2014;142(6):837–44.
9. Sandes AF, de Lourdes Chauffaille M, Oliveira CR, et al. CD200 has an important role in the differential diagnosis of mature B-cell neoplasms by multiparameter flow cytometry. Cytometry B Clin Cytom 2014;86(2):98–105.
10. Wasik AM, Priebe V, Lord M, Jeppsson-Ahlberg Å, Christensson B, Sander B. Flow cytometric analysis of SOX11: a new diagnostic method for distinguishing B-cell chronic lymphocytic leukemia/small lymphocytic lymphoma from mantle cell lymphoma. Leuk Lymphoma 2015;56(5):1425–31.
11. Afacan-Öztürk HB, Falay M, Albayrak M, et al. CD81 Expression in the Differential Diagnosis of Chronic Lymphocytic Leukemia. Clin Lab 2019;65(3). https://doi.org/10.7754/Clin.Lab.2018.180802.
12. Rawstron AC, Kreuzer KA, Soosapilla A, et al. Reproducible diagnosis of chronic lymphocytic leukemia by flow cytometry: An European Research Initiative on CLL (ERIC) & European Society for Clinical Cell Analysis (ESCCA) Harmonisation project. Cytometry B Clin Cytom 2018;94(1):121–8.
13. Wierda WG, Rawstron A, Cymbalista F, et al. Measurable residual disease in chronic lymphocytic leukemia: expert review and consensus recommendations. Leukemia 2021;35(11):3059–72.
14. Kater AP, Wu JQ, Kipps T, et al. Venetoclax Plus Rituximab in Relapsed Chronic Lymphocytic Leukemia: 4-Year Results and Evaluation of Impact of Genomic Complexity and Gene Mutations From the MURANO Phase III Study. J Clin Oncol 2020;38(34):4042–54.
15. Kovacs G, Robrecht S, Fink AM, et al. Minimal Residual Disease Assessment Improves Prediction of Outcome in Patients With Chronic Lymphocytic Leukemia (CLL) Who Achieve Partial Response: Comprehensive Analysis of Two Phase III Studies of the German CLL Study Group. J Clin Oncol 2016;34(31):3758–65.
16. Hotinski AK, Best OG, Kuss BJ. The future of laboratory testing in chronic lymphocytic leukaemia. Pathology 2021;53(3):377–84.
17. Molica S, Giannarelli D, Montserrat E. Minimal Residual Disease and Survival Outcomes in Patients With Chronic Lymphocytic Leukemia: A Systematic Review and Meta-analysis. Clin Lymphoma Myeloma Leuk 2019;19(7):423–30.

18. Rawstron AC, Villamor N, Ritgen M, et al. International standardized approach for flow cytometric residual disease monitoring in chronic lymphocytic leukaemia. Leukemia 2007;21(5):956–64.
19. Abrisqueta P, Villamor N, Terol MJ, et al. Rituximab maintenance after first-line therapy with rituximab, fludarabine, cyclophosphamide, and mitoxantrone (R-FCM) for chronic lymphocytic leukemia. Blood 2013;122(24):3951–9.
20. Böttcher S, Ritgen M, Fischer K, et al. Minimal residual disease quantification is an independent predictor of progression-free and overall survival in chronic lymphocytic leukemia: a multivariate analysis from the randomized GCLLSG CLL8 trial. J Clin Oncol 2012;30(9):980–8.
21. Rawstron AC, Fazi C, Agathangelidis A, et al. A complementary role of multiparameter flow cytometry and high-throughput sequencing for minimal residual disease detection in chronic lymphocytic leukemia: an European Research Initiative on CLL study. Leukemia 2016;30(4):929–36.
22. Bazinet A, Rys RN, Barry A, et al. A 10-color flow cytometry panel for diagnosis and minimal residual disease in chronic lymphocytic leukemia. Leuk Lymphoma 2021;62(10):2352–9.
23. Malavasi F, Deaglio S, Damle R, et al. CD38 and chronic lymphocytic leukemia: a decade later. Blood 2011;118(13):3470–8.
24. Benedetti D, Tissino E, Pozzo F, et al. NOTCH1 mutations are associated with high CD49d expression in chronic lymphocytic leukemia: link between the NOTCH1 and the NF-κB pathways. Leukemia 2018;32(3):654–62.
25. Rossi FM, Del Principe MI, Rossi D, et al. Prognostic impact of ZAP-70 expression in chronic lymphocytic leukemia: mean fluorescence intensity T/B ratio versus percentage of positive cells. J Transl Med 2010;8:23.
26. Gachard N, Salviat A, Boutet C, et al. Multicenter study of ZAP-70 expression in patients with B-cell chronic lymphocytic leukemia using an optimized flow cytometry method. Haematologica 2008;93(2):215–23.
27. Degheidy HA, Venzon DJ, Farooqui MZ, et al. Combined normal donor and CLL: Single tube ZAP-70 analysis. Cytometry B Clin Cytom 2012;82(2):67–77.
28. Marquez ME, Deglesne PA, Suarez G, et al. MFI ratio estimation of ZAP-70 in B-CLL by flow cytometry can be improved by considering the isotype-matched antibody signal. Int J Lab Hematol 2011;33(2):194–200.
29. Hamblin TJ, Orchard JA, Ibbotson RE, et al. CD38 expression and immunoglobulin variable region mutations are independent prognostic variables in chronic lymphocytic leukemia, but CD38 expression may vary during the course of the disease. Blood 2002;99(3):1023–9.
30. Jelinek DF, Tschumper RC, Geyer SM, et al. Analysis of clonal B-cell CD38 and immunoglobulin variable region sequence status in relation to clinical outcome for B-chronic lymphocytic leukaemia. Br J Haematol 2001;115(4):854–61.
31. Dürig J, Naschar M, Schmücker U, et al. CD38 expression is an important prognostic marker in chronic lymphocytic leukaemia. Leukemia 2002;16(1):30–5.
32. Damle RN, Wasil T, Fais F, et al. Ig V gene mutation status and CD38 expression as novel prognostic indicators in chronic lymphocytic leukemia. Blood 1999;94(6):1840–7.
33. Bulian P, Shanafelt TD, Fegan C, et al. CD49d is the strongest flow cytometry-based predictor of overall survival in chronic lymphocytic leukemia. J Clin Oncol 2014;32(9):897–904.
34. Gattei V, Bulian P, Del Principe MI, et al. Relevance of CD49d protein expression as overall survival and progressive disease prognosticator in chronic lymphocytic leukemia. Blood 2008;111(2):865–73.
35. Gooden CE, Jones P, Bates R, et al. CD49d shows superior performance characteristics for flow cytometric prognostic testing in chronic lymphocytic leukemia/small lymphocytic lymphoma. Cytometry B Clin Cytom 2018;94(1):129–35.
36. Salem DA, Stetler-Stevenson M. Clinical Flow-Cytometric Testing in Chronic Lymphocytic Leukemia. Methods Mol Biol 2019;2032:311–21.
37. Menter T, Trivedi P, Ahmad R, et al. Diagnostic Utility of Lymphoid Enhancer Binding Factor 1 Immunohistochemistry in Small B-Cell Lymphomas. Am J Clin Pathol 2017;147(3):292–300.
38. Tandon B, Peterson L, Gao J, et al. Nuclear overexpression of lymphoid-enhancer-binding factor 1 identifies chronic lymphocytic leukemia/small lymphocytic lymphoma in small B-cell lymphomas. Mod Pathol 2011;24(11):1433–43.
39. Giné E, Martinez A, Villamor N, et al. Expanded and highly active proliferation centers identify a histological subtype of chronic lymphocytic leukemia ("accelerated" chronic lymphocytic leukemia) with aggressive clinical behavior. Haematologica 2010;95(9):1526–33.
40. Liu YC, Margolskee E, Allan JN, et al. Chronic lymphocytic leukemia with TP53 gene alterations: a detailed clinicopathologic analysis. Mod Pathol 2020;33(3):344–53.
41. Garces S, Khoury JD, Kanagal-Shamanna R, et al. Chronic lymphocytic leukemia with proliferation centers in bone marrow is associated with younger age at initial presentation, complex karyotype, and TP53 disruption. Hum Pathol 2018;82:215–31.
42. Lee J, Wang YL. Prognostic and Predictive Molecular Biomarkers in Chronic Lymphocytic Leukemia. J Mol Diagn 2020;22(9):1114–25.

43. Thompson PA, Tam CS, O'Brien SM, et al. Fludarabine, cyclophosphamide, and rituximab treatment achieves long-term disease-free survival in IGHV-mutated chronic lymphocytic leukemia. Blood 2016;127(3):303–9.
44. Byrd JC, Furman RR, Coutre SE, et al. Three-year follow-up of treatment-naive and previously treated patients with CLL and SLL receiving single-agent ibrutinib. Blood 2015;125(16):2497–506.
45. Byrd JC, Furman RR, Coutre SE, et al. Targeting BTK with ibrutinib in relapsed chronic lymphocytic leukemia. N Engl J Med 2013;369(1):32–42.
46. Shanafelt TD, Wang XV, Kay NE, et al. Ibrutinib-Rituximab or Chemoimmunotherapy for Chronic Lymphocytic Leukemia. N Engl J Med 2019;381(5): 432–43.
47. Baliakas P, Agathangelidis A, Hadzidimitriou A, et al. Not all IGHV3-21 chronic lymphocytic leukemias are equal: prognostic considerations. Blood 2015; 125(5):856–9.
48. Delgado J, Nadeu F, Colomer D, et al. Chronic lymphocytic leukemia: from molecular pathogenesis to novel therapeutic strategies. Haematologica 2020; 105(9):2205–17.
49. Rossi D, Spina V, Cerri M, et al. Stereotyped B-cell receptor is an independent risk factor of chronic lymphocytic leukemia transformation to Richter syndrome. Clin Cancer Res 2009;15(13):4415–22.
50. Ahn IE, Underbayev C, Albitar A, et al. Clonal evolution leading to ibrutinib resistance in chronic lymphocytic leukemia. Blood 2017;129(11):1469–79.
51. Woyach JA, Ruppert AS, Guinn D, et al. BTKC481S-Mediated Resistance to Ibrutinib in Chronic Lymphocytic Leukemia. J Clin Oncol 2017;35(13): 1437–43.
52. Blombery P, Anderson MA, Gong J-n, et al. Acquisition of the Recurrent Gly101Val Mutation in BCL2 Confers Resistance to Venetoclax in Patients with Progressive Chronic Lymphocytic Leukemia. Cancer Discov 2019;9(3):342–53.
53. Eugen T, William C, Anna D, et al. Venetoclax resistance and acquired BCL2 mutations in chronic lymphocytic leukemia. Haematologica 2019;104(9): e434–7.
54. Rossi D, Spina V, Deambrogi C, et al. The genetics of Richter syndrome reveals disease heterogeneity and predicts survival after transformation. Blood 2011;117(12):3391–401.
55. Kater AP, Kipps TJ, Eichhorst B, et al. Five-Year Analysis of Murano Study Demonstrates Enduring Undetectable Minimal Residual Disease (uMRD) in a Subset of Relapsed/Refractory Chronic Lymphocytic Leukemia (R/R CLL) Patients (Pts) Following Fixed-Duration Venetoclax-Rituximab (VenR) Therapy (Tx). Blood 2020;136(Supplement 1):19–21.
56. Aw A, Kim HT, Fernandes SM, et al. Minimal residual disease detected by immunoglobulin sequencing predicts CLL relapse more effectively than flow cytometry. Leuk Lymphoma 2018;59(8):1986–9.
57. Thompson PA, Srivastava J, Peterson C, et al. Minimal residual disease undetectable by next-generation sequencing predicts improved outcome in CLL after chemoimmunotherapy. Blood 2019; 134(22):1951–9.
58. Miller CR, Heerema NA. Culture and Harvest of CpG-Stimulated Peripheral Blood or Bone Marrow in Chronic Lymphocytic Leukemia. In: Malek SN, editor. Chronic lymphocytic leukemia: methods and protocols. New York, NY: Springer New York; 2019. p. 27–34.
59. Bento L, Correia R, de Sousa F, et al. Performance of eight-color dry antibody reagent in the detection of minimal residual disease in chronic lymphocytic leukemia samples. Cytometry B Clin Cytom 2020;98(6): 529–35.

Diagnostic Flow Cytometry in the Era of Targeted Therapies

Lessons from Therapeutic Monoclonal Antibodies and Chimeric Antigen Receptor T-cell Adoptive Immunotherapy

Ifeyinwa Obiorah, MD, PhD, Elizabeth L. Courville, MD*

KEYWORDS

• Immunotherapy • CAR-T • Flow cytometry • Therapeutic monoclonal antibodies • Leukemia • Lymphoma • Daratumumab • Rituximab

Key points

- Use of targeted therapy with therapeutic monoclonal antibodies or adoptive immunotherapy for leukemia/lymphoma is growing, and this has important implications for diagnostic flow cytometry.
- Populations of interest may be difficult to identify in patients who have received therapeutic monoclonal antibodies or adoptive immunotherapy.
- Therapeutic monoclonal antibody therapy can cause test interference in flow cytometry resulting in pseudo-light chain restriction.
- Established guidelines do not exist for the evaluation of antigen expression by flow cytometry for therapeutic purposes, introducing variation in such evaluation.
- Awareness of the practical implications of targeted therapy in diagnostic flow cytometry can help the practitioner avoid diagnostic errors.

ABSTRACT

Therapeutic monoclonal antibodies (therapeutic mAb) and adoptive immunotherapy have become increasingly more common in the treatment of hematolymphoid neoplasms, with practical implications for diagnostic flow cytometry. Their use can reduce the sensitivity of flow cytometry for populations of interest owing to downregulation/loss of the target antigen, competition for the target antigen, or lineage switch. Expanded flow panels, marker redundancy, and exhaustive gating strategies can overcome this limitation. Therapeutic mAb have been reported to cause pseudo-light chain restriction, and awareness of this potential artifact is key. Established guidelines do not yet exist for antigen expression by flow cytometry for therapeutic purposes.

OVERVIEW

Targeted therapies use drugs or other substances to identify and attack specific types of cancer cells with less harm to normal cells. Targeted therapies relevant to diagnostic flow cytometry include therapeutic monoclonal antibodies (therapeutic mAb;

Department of Pathology, University of Virginia Health, PO Box 800214, Charlottesville, VA 22908, USA
* Corresponding author.
E-mail address: Ec8kk@hscmail.mcc.virginia.edu

Surgical Pathology 16 (2023) 423–431
https://doi.org/10.1016/j.path.2023.01.006

a type of protein therapeutics) and chimeric antigen receptor T-cell (CAR-T) adoptive immunotherapy.

THERAPEUTIC MONOCLONAL ANTIBODIES

The field of monoclonal antibody therapeutics has shown remarkable growth over the past 30 years owing to a variety of scientific and technological advances that have facilitated their discovery and development.[1] Recombinant DNA technology has allowed for the production of therapeutic mAb by a single clone of B cells, making them monospecific and homogenous. As of 2022, more than 100 mAb therapeutic products have been approved in the United States, with most being treatment for cancer (45%) or immune-mediated disorders (27%).[2] **Table 1** shows selected examples of therapeutic mAb relevant to hematolymphoid cells and processes.[3]

Many therapeutic mAb guide the patient's own immune system to destroy targeted cells or molecules via a variety of mechanisms.[4] A full discussion of the pharmacodynamics and pharmacokinetics of mAb therapeutics is beyond the scope of this article; however, it is worth noting that they are varied and not entirely understood for all mAb therapeutics.[5] Rituximab, a widely used therapeutic mAb, is thought to eliminate CD20-positive cells by at least 4 mechanistic pathways: antibody-dependent cellular cytotoxicity, antibody-dependent cellular phagocytosis, complement-dependent cytotoxicity, and direct antitumor effects via either apoptosis or other cell death pathways.[6]

Other types of therapeutic mAb include bispecific T-cell–engaging small molecules (BiTEs). These are genetically engineered proteins designed to bind to a tumor antigen as well as an effector cell antigen (often a T-cell antigen). Blinatumomab is a BiTE with a high affinity for target CD19-positive cells as well as T cells, thus driving T-cell–mediated cytotoxicity.[7,8] Antibody-drug conjugates use monoclonal antibodies to deliver other compounds or proteins; for example, gemtuzumab ozogamicin links the binding region of an anti-CD33 monoclonal antibody with calicheamicin, a small molecule chemotherapeutic agent. Monoclonal antibodies have also been used for selective delivery of radioisotopes to cancer cells.[3]

CHIMERIC ANTIGEN RECEPTOR T-CELL ADOPTIVE IMMUNOTHERAPY

Adoptive immunotherapy involves using T cells that are genetically engineered ex vivo to express CAR that mediate the lysis of cancer cells. The CAR is an artificial immunoreceptor consisting of an extracellular single-chain antibody fragment (scFv), intracellular signaling domains, and a costimulatory domain.[9,10] In response to the scFv-induced recognition of the tumor-expressing antigens, the CAR directs the T cells to proliferate and eliminate the neoplastic cells.[11]

CAR-T cells are used in the treatment of B-cell malignancies, using CD19 as a target (**Table 2**).

Table 1
Select examples of therapeutic monoclonal antibodies

Antibody	Type	Target	Select Medical Uses[a]
Alemtuzumab	Monoclonal antibody	CD52	Multiple sclerosis, chronic lymphocytic leukemia
Blinatumomab	BiTE	CD19	B-lymphoblastic leukemia
Brentuximab vedotin	Antibody-drug conjugate	CD30	Hodgkin lymphoma, $CD30^+$ T-cell neoplasms
Daratumumab	Monoclonal antibody	CD38	Multiple myeloma
Gemtuzumab ozogamicin	Antibody-drug conjugate	CD33	Acute myeloid leukemia
Inotuzumab ozogamicin	Antibody-drug conjugate	CD22	B-lymphoblastic leukemia
Obinutuzumab	Monoclonal antibody	CD20	Chronic lymphocytic leukemia
Ofatumumab	Monoclonal antibody	CD20	Refractory chronic lymphocytic leukemia
Rituximab	Monoclonal antibody	CD20	Rheumatoid arthritis, $CD20^+$ B-cell non-Hodgkin lymphoma and chronic lymphocytic leukemia

[a] There may be other uses of these therapies, including off-label uses.

Modified from Castelli MS, McGonigle P, Hornby PJ. The pharmacology and therapeutic applications of monoclonal antibodies. *Pharmacol Res Perspect.* 2019;7(6):e00535.

Table 2
Examples of chimeric antigen receptor T-cell therapy

CAR T-Cell Therapy	Target	Medical Uses
Tisagenlecleucel	CD19	B-lymphoblastic leukemia/lymphoma, non-Hodgkin B-cell lymphoma
Axicabtagene ciloleucel	CD19	Non-Hodgkin B-cell lymphoma, follicular lymphoma
Brexucabtagene autoleucel	CD19	B-lymphoblastic leukemia/lymphoma, mantle cell lymphoma
Lisocabtagene maraleucel	CD19	Non-Hodgkin B-cell lymphoma
Idecabtagene vicleucel	BCMA	Multiple myeloma
Ciltacabtagene autoleucel	BCMA	Multiple myeloma

Several factors make CD19 an ideal target for therapy: it is highly expressed on essentially all B-cell neoplasms, is required for normal B-cell development, and is rarely expressed in non–B-lineage cells.[11] CAR-T therapy has been used most effectively in the treatment of B-lymphoblastic leukemia/lymphoma (B-ALL)[12,13] and mature B-cell neoplasms,[14,15] even in patients resistant to multiple lines of therapy.[16,17] CAR-T therapy has moved beyond the CD19 target with anti-CD22 CAR-T cells shown to induce remission in B-ALL that is naive or resistant to CD19-targeted CAR immunotherapy.[18] In addition, Ali and colleagues[19] conducted the first in-human clinical trial of CAR-T cells targeting B-cell maturation antigen (BCMA) in patients with multiple myeloma, with 2 patients showing excellent response. Despite promising results of CAR-T therapy, relapse has been described, attributed to a number of factors, including lack of persistence of CAR-T cells, antigen loss, and product manufacturing failures.[20–23]

PRACTICAL IMPLICATIONS

TARGETED THERAPIES CAN REDUCE THE SENSITIVITY FOR POPULATIONS OF INTEREST

It may be more difficult to identify the population of interest in patients who have received therapeutic mAb or adoptive immunotherapy (Fig. 1). Neoplastic cells escape targeted therapies by a variety of mechanisms, including mutation or alternative splicing of the target antigen, resulting in downregulation or loss of target antigen expression. In some cases, competition for the target antigen may be the mechanism for antigen loss by flow cytometric immunophenotyping.[24]

Awareness of the issue and a thoughtful approach by the clinical flow cytometry laboratory can help overcome the potential difficulty introduced by antigen loss. Flow cytometry panels can be designed to contain multiple identifying markers for the population of interest. Incorporation of new markers may be needed in the setting of new targeted therapies, necessitating vigilance on the part of the flow cytometry laboratory. When multiple markers are used to identify the population of interest, gating strategies to screen for populations in multiple ways are needed.

From a workflow perspective, the approach to samples from patients treated with therapeutic mAb or CAR-T therapy may vary among clinical flow cytometry laboratories. Some laboratories will have access to patient medication history and may choose to tailor their panels to the specific targeted therapy. This approach is limited by uncertainty as to how long the phenotypic effects of therapeutic mAb last, and in some laboratories may be limited by a paucity of available clinical information.

Evaluating for Plasma Cells in the Setting of Daratumumab

Daratumumab is an anti-CD38 therapeutic mAb used in the treatment of multiple myeloma. There is evidence that there is long-term persistence of daratumumab on the cell surface of CD38-positive cells, lasting up to several months after the last dose.[24,25] As standard monoclonal diagnostic CD38 antibodies bind to epitopes overlapping with the daratumumab binding site, alternative strategies (other than CD38 expression) are needed to identify residual plasma cell myeloma in the setting of such therapy.

CD138 may be a helpful alternative marker but is not always reliable, as its expression can deteriorate over time[26] or may show aberrant dim to negative expression by neoplastic plasma cells. A multiepitope CD38 antibody was included in the EuroFlow multiple myeloma minimal residual disease (MRD) panel to overcome interference by daratumumab.[27] Alternatively, studies have shown that the monoclonal antibody VS38, recognizing a

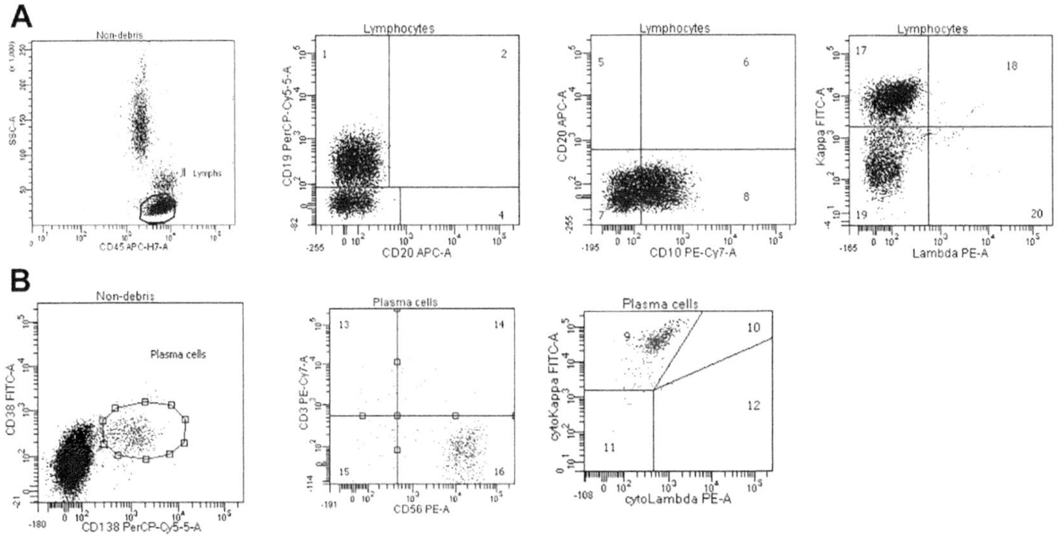

Fig. 1. (*A*) Peripheral blood specimen from a patient with a history of follicular lymphoma on rituximab (anti-CD20) maintenance therapy with evidence of disease progression on imaging. Within the mature lymphocyte gate from a side scatter versus CD45 plot, there is a population of neoplastic $CD19^+$, $CD20^-$ B cells with expression of CD10 and monotypic kappa surface light chains. (*B*) Bone marrow specimen from a patient with a history of plasma cell myeloma on treatment with a regimen including daratumumab (anti-CD38). As shown, a $CD138^+$, $CD38^-$ plasma cell population (*magenta*) is identified with aberrant coexpression of CD56 and cytoplasmic kappa light chain restriction. The corresponding morphologic evaluation of the bone marrow specimen showed scattered abnormal clusters and aggregates of plasma cells showing kappa immunoglobulin light chain restriction by in situ hybridization stains for kappa and lambda.

nonglycated type II transmembrane protein (p63) residing in the rough endoplasmic reticulum, is a reliable marker for plasma cell identification.[25,28] Broijl and colleagues[29] recently compared the VS38 and CD38 multiepitope antibodies and found that both provided similar MRD data in patients with multiple myeloma. Other markers to replace CD38 in plasma cell identification have been investigated, including CD272, CD319, CD229, and CD48.[30]

Evaluating for Minimal Residual Disease After Chimeric Antigen Receptor T-Cell for B-Lymphoblastic Leukemia/Lymphoma

CD19 is generally the gating reagent of choice used in the identification of neoplastic B cells when investigating for residual disease. After CD19 CAR-T cell therapy, CD19 becomes unreliable in the detection of the tumor cells owing to development of CD19-negative subclones, observed in 10% to 20% of B-ALL following CAR-T therapy.[31] In 1 study, a novel combination of markers using the expression of CD22 or CD24 in conjunction with markers aberrantly expressed in B-ALL (CD10, CD20, CD34, CD38, and CD45) was effective in identifying CD19-positive and CD19-negative neoplastic blast populations.[32,33] For definite identification of the B-cell population, CD66b was used to exclude neutrophils that also express CD24. In another approach, Verbeek and colleagues[34] developed an alternative gating strategy for MRD evaluation in patients with B-ALL treated with CD19 targeting therapies. By their strategy, the evaluation is based first on identification of CD10-positive lymphoid cells or CD34-positive cells, with subsequent evaluation for abnormal expression patterns, such as aberrant positivity of CD66c/CD123 or CD73/CD304, or abnormal under/overexpression of CD38 or CD81. Possible leukemic lymphoblasts are back-gated on the forward scatter–side scatter and CD45 plots to ensure all cells form a uniform cluster.

Normal precursor cells must be distinguished from residual B-ALL lymphoblasts. There are normal progenitor cells with CD34 and CD22 expression but without CD24, which are present in small proportions in reactive or recovering bone marrows after chemotherapy. These populations may be observed following CD19 CAR-T treatment and need to be accurately identified to avoid false positive MRD diagnosis.[33]

CD22 CAR-T therapy has been used as an alternate treatment in patients who failed CD19 CAR-T therapy.[35] Similar to CD19 CAR-T treatment, antigen loss has been observed following CD22 CAR-T therapy. Thus, additional gating strategies to identify CD24-positive B-lineage cells, in addition to evaluation for CD19 and CD22, are necessary to detect leukemic B-lymphoblasts lacking CD22 expression. Some cases of B-ALL, especially those with *KMT2A* rearrangement, have decreased or absent expression of CD10, CD22, or CD24, and detection of residual disease in such cases is diagnostically challenging.[36] Alternate B-cell markers, including CD79a, as well as ancillary and molecular methods may prove useful in such scenarios.

Relapse of B-Lymphoblastic Leukemia/Lymphoma After Anti-CD19 Therapy

Relapsed B-ALL following anti-CD19 therapy (blinatumomab or CAR-T) may be CD19-negative yet have an otherwise similar or identical immunophenotype to the diagnostic disease (Fig. 2). Potential mechanisms leading to lack of CD19 expression include alternative splicing, which results in expression of CD19 isoforms with compromised target epitope, and reduced cell surface expression.[22,37] Braig and colleagues[38] and Shah and Fry[39] demonstrated that CD19 loss following treatment with blinatumomab may be mediated by disruption of CD19 membrane trafficking resulting in an interruption in the transport of CD19 from the Golgi apparatus to the cell surface.

Relapsed B-ALL uncommonly undergoes lineage switch and presents with a myeloid phenotype.[40] In 1 series, lineage switch from lymphoid to myeloid occurred in 12 of 163 cases (7.4%) of relapsed B-ALL following anti-CD19 CAR-T therapy.[41] Lineage transformation, both following anti-CD19 therapy and rarely after traditional chemotherapy, is associated with *KMT2A*-rearranged B-ALL. Lymphoid to myeloid lineage switch has been described for a patient with *TCF3::ZNF384* B-ALL following anti-CD19 CAR-T, and "monocytic switch" has been described in patients with *DUX4r*, *ZNF384r*, and *PAX5*-P80R–mutated B-ALL.[42–44] Mechanistically, the initial B-ALL and the acute myeloid leukemia at relapse may be derived from the same leukemia-initiating cell, which has the potential to differentiate into either myeloid or B-lymphoid lineage in response to specific intrinsic and extrinsic signals.[45] Treatment with CD19 CAR-T cells may trigger differentiation toward myeloid lineage. Cytokine release, including interleukin-6 (IL-6), has been well described in CAR-T treatment.[46] IL-6 has been shown to induce myeloid differentiation of a biphenotypic leukemia cell line[47] and can possibly explain the lineage switch.

ARTIFACT FROM THERAPEUTIC MONOCLONAL ANTIBODY THERAPY

Test interference from therapeutic mAb in flow cytometry has been rarely reported for both daratumumab[48] and alemtuzumab.[49] In a 2020 study, Jiang and colleagues[48] identified artifactual kappa light chain restriction on hematogones (normal B-lineage precursors) by flow cytometry in 7 patients on daratumumab therapy with appreciable hematogone populations; this finding was not seen in 5 control samples. In that study, the flow cytometry panels included either anti-kappa-allophycocyanin (APC) (clone C0222) or anti-kappa-fluorescein isothiocyanate (FITC) (clone F0434), and CD19-negative lymphocytes were used as the internal control population for surface light chain expression. It is hypothesized that the false kappa restriction represents cross-reaction of the fluorochrome-bound anti-kappa antibody with the daratumumab

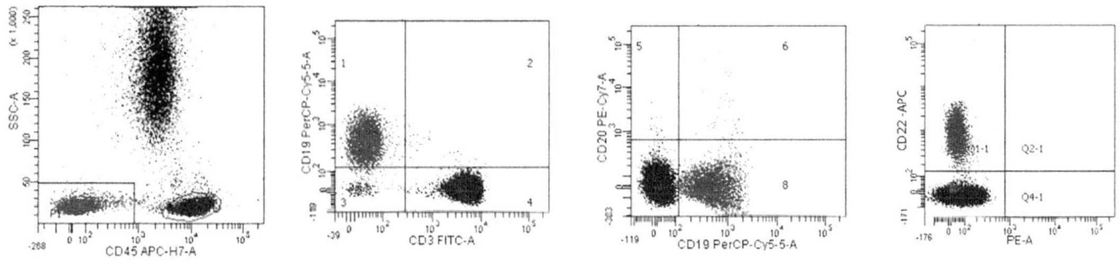

Fig. 2. Peripheral blood specimen from a patient with history of relapsed B-ALL currently 19 months status post CD19 CAR-T therapy with recovery of normal B cells at 6 months and treated with CAR-T boost at 9 months and 11 months after initial CAR-T therapy. A mature B-lymphocyte population is not identified by either CD19 or CD20 (mature lymphocytes are blue, corresponding to $CD3^+$ T cells); however, an abnormal $CD19^+$ B-cell population (*red*) is identified with the striking immunophenotypic abnormality of dim to negative CD45 expression. By additional evaluation, the abnormal population was determined to represent leukemic B-lymphoblasts positive for CD34, CD10, CD38, and TdT. The right-most plot shows surface expression of CD22. The patient subsequently received inotuzumab ozogamicin, an antibody-drug conjugate medication targeting surface CD22.

(immunoglobulin G1 [IgG1]-kappa) bound to CD38+ hematogones.

In an earlier 2019 study, Chen and colleagues[49] describe a case of artifactual surface kappa light chain restriction on a population of marrow hematogones in a patient treated with alemtuzumab (IgG1-kappa monoclonal antibody targeted against CD52) for T-prolymphocytic leukemia (T-PLL). They describe a second patient also treated with alemtuzumab for T-PLL with artifactual surface kappa light chain restriction on a population of residual neoplastic T-PLL cells. In both patients, background normal T cells also showed the pseudo-kappa restriction. By means of in vitro treatment of peripheral blood from healthy volunteer donor blood, the investigators provide supporting evidence for a direct mechanism of interference by the alemtuzumab. In that study, FITC-conjugated polyclonal rabbit F(ab')$_2$ fragment antibodies directed against kappa or lambda light chains were used to assess for light chain clonality. Isotype antibody-negative controls were used to determine fluorescent-positive from fluorescent-negative populations.

Although the authors have not formally studied this phenomenon in their flow cytometry laboratory, anecdotally they have also seen false kappa restriction on hematogones in selected clinical flow cytometry cases from patients on daratumumab (**Fig. 3**). In their laboratory, using FITC- or PE-conjugated polyclonal rabbit F(ab')$_2$ fragment antibodies directed against kappa or lambda light chains (Dako; Agilent Technologies, Santa Clara, CA, USA), the authors typically have background dim staining of monocytes and granulocytes by both kappa and lambda. In the setting of daratumumab, they have seen kappa, but not lambda, staining of hematogones at a similar level of intensity as the background (dimmer than that of mature B cells).

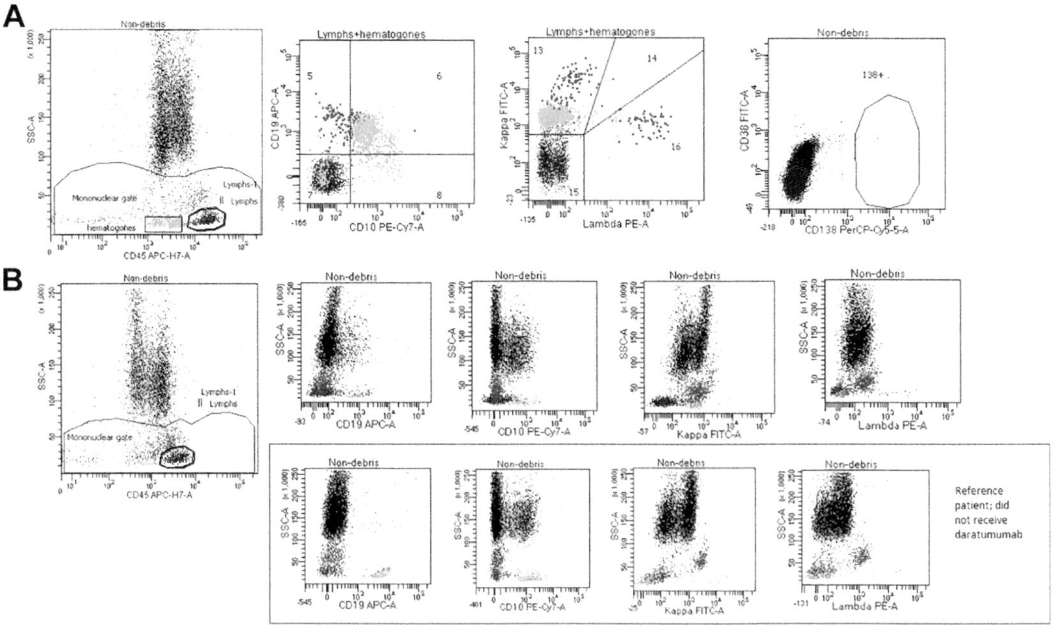

Fig. 3. (*A*) Bone marrow specimen from a patient 3 months status post autologous stem cell transplant for IgA lambda multiple myeloma; the patient received daratumumab as part of pretransplant therapy. No plasma cells were identified based on CD38 or CD138 expression (*right-most plot in panel*). Hematogones (normal B-lineage precursors; *light blue*) are identified based on their unique position on the side scatter versus CD45 plot (*left*) and coexpression of CD19 and CD10 (*second from left*), with differential intensity of staining. This population appears to show monotypic dim surface kappa light chain expression (*second from right*). Mature B cells are shown in red, whereas non–B-lineage lymphocytes are shown in dark blue. (*B*) Bone marrow specimen from a different patient 18 months status post autologous stem cell transplant for IgG lambda multiple myeloma on maintenance therapy with daratumumab and lenalidomide. Hematogones (*dark yellow*) are positive for CD19 and CD10 with dim CD45 expression and low side scatter. The hematogones show dim positivity for surface kappa, at a level similar to that of background monocytes and granulocytes (background staining). In the box (*lower panel*) are analogous plots from a patient who has not received daratumumab, showing the usual location for hematogones on the side scatter versus kappa plot (*second from right*). In the authors' laboratory, hematogones typically are negative for surface light chains, overlapping with background T lymphocytes.

EVALUATION FOR ANTIGEN EXPRESSION BY FLOW CYTOMETRY FOR THERAPEUTIC PURPOSES

Before starting a patient on therapy targeting a particular antigen, the treating clinician may need to assess for the presence of the marker on the population of interest. In the setting of hematolymphoid malignancies, flow cytometry can be a rapid and accurate method to assess cell surface marker expression on a particular cell population of interest. A challenge in this approach is the lack of standardization in flow cytometry across institutions. Nonstandardized flow cytometry panels and processing techniques can introduce variability in determination of antigen expression by flow cytometry. As an example, in a study comparing 5 different commercially available phycoerythrin-conjugated monoclonal antibodies against CD123, the investigators found significant differences in CD123 expression.[50] As another example, at the data interpretation step, there is variability in how flow cytometry laboratories define background populations (internal control populations vs isotype controls vs fluorescence-minus-one, FMO, controls) and decide on positive versus negative cutoff criteria (including percentage criteria vs mean fluorescence intensity). Such variation may alter patient selection and create difficulties in interpreting responses after exposure to targeted therapies.

FUTURE TRENDS

The rapidly and constantly changing landscape of targeted therapy makes it difficult for clinical flow cytometry laboratories to keep up with the increased demands imparted by monoclonal antibody therapy and CAR-T therapy. Identifying populations of interest will become particularly challenging if multiple population-defining markers are targeted. Ideally, evaluation for marker expression by flow cytometry to determine eligibility for targeted therapies will become more standardized, both within and outside of the clinical trial setting.

SUMMARY

The growing use of targeted therapy with therapeutic mAb or adoptive immunotherapy has important implications for diagnostic flow cytometry. Clinical flow cytometry laboratories need to be cognizant of the potential pitfalls and artifacts in flow cytometry interpretation introduced by patient use of these therapeutics.

CLINICS CARE POINTS

- Daratumumab therapy results in loss of CD38 expression by flow cytometry for up to several months. Alternative strategies to identify plasma cells beyond bright CD38 expression are needed in this setting. CD138 may not be the best alternative owing to downregulation in certain neoplasms and antigen loss with aging specimens. Alternative approaches to plasma cell identification in the setting of daratumumab therapy include VS38 and multiepitope CD38 antibodies.
- Minimal residual disease evaluation in patients with B-lymphoblastic leukemia/lymphoma treated with targeted therapies may be difficult. Using CD22 and CD24 expression to complement CD19 can help identify neoplastic B-cell populations, in addition to aberrant expression of markers, such as CD10, CD20, CD34, CD38, and CD45. Distinction from normal populations of cells, such as CD24-positive neutrophils or $CD34^+$, $CD22^+$ progenitor cells, is important.
- Relapsed B-lymphoblastic leukemia/lymphoma may be CD19-negative yet have an otherwise similar or identical immunophenotype to the diagnostic disease. Uncommonly, relapsed B-ALL undergoes lineage switch and presents with a myeloid phenotype, typically in the setting of anti-CD19 therapy.
- Artifactual kappa light chain restriction on hematogones has been reported in the setting of daratumumab (anti-CD38) and alemtuzumab (anti-CD52) therapy. Awareness of this artifact is important to prevent overinterpretation.

DISCLOSURE

The authors have nothing to disclose.

REFERENCES

1. Kaplon H, Reichert JM. Antibodies to watch in 2019. MAbs 2019;11(2):219–38.
2. Kaplon H, Chenoweth A, Crescioli S, et al. Antibodies to watch in 2022. MAbs 2022;14(1):2014296.
3. Castelli MS, McGonigle P, Hornby PJ. The pharmacology and therapeutic applications of monoclonal antibodies. Pharmacol Res Perspect 2019;7(6):e00535.
4. Leader B, Baca QJ, Golan DE. Protein therapeutics: a summary and pharmacological classification. Nat Rev Drug Discov 2008;7(1):21–39.

5. Golay J, Introna M. Mechanism of action of therapeutic monoclonal antibodies: promises and pitfalls of in vitro and in vivo assays. Arch Biochem Biophys 2012;526(2):146–53.
6. Salles G, Barrett M, Foa R, et al. Rituximab in B-Cell hematologic malignancies: a review of 20 years of clinical experience. Adv Ther 2017;34(10):2232–73.
7. Goebeler ME, Bargou R. Blinatumomab: a CD19/CD3 bispecific T cell engager (BiTE) with unique anti-tumor efficacy. Leuk Lymphoma 2016;57(5):1021–32.
8. Mocquot P., Mossazadeh Y., Lapierre L., et al., The pharmacology of blinatumomab: state of the art on pharmacodynamics, pharmacokinetics, adverse drug reactions and evaluation in clinical trials, *J Clin Pharm Ther*, 47 (9), 2022, 1337-1351.
9. Sadelain M, Brentjens R, Riviere I. The basic principles of chimeric antigen receptor design. Cancer Discov 2013;3(4):388–98.
10. Jacoby E, Nguyen SM, Fountaine TJ, et al. CD19 CAR immune pressure induces B-precursor acute lymphoblastic leukaemia lineage switch exposing inherent leukaemic plasticity. Nat Commun 2016;7:12320.
11. June CH, O'Connor RS, Kawalekar OU, et al. CAR T cell immunotherapy for human cancer. Science 2018;359(6382):1361–5.
12. Maude SL, Teachey DT, Porter DL, et al. CD19-targeted chimeric antigen receptor T-cell therapy for acute lymphoblastic leukemia. Blood 2015;125(26):4017–23.
13. Tasian SK, Gardner RA. CD19-redirected chimeric antigen receptor-modified T cells: a promising immunotherapy for children and adults with B-cell acute lymphoblastic leukemia (ALL). Ther Adv Hematol 2015;6(5):228–41.
14. Vitale C, Strati P. CAR T-cell therapy for B-cell non-Hodgkin lymphoma and chronic lymphocytic leukemia: clinical trials and real-world experiences. Front Oncol 2020;10:849.
15. Schuster SJ, Tam CS, Borchmann P, et al. Long-term clinical outcomes of tisagenlecleucel in patients with relapsed or refractory aggressive B-cell lymphomas (JULIET): a multicentre, open-label, single-arm, phase 2 study. Lancet Oncol 2021;22(10):1403–15.
16. Maude SL, Frey N, Shaw PA, et al. Chimeric antigen receptor T cells for sustained remissions in leukemia. N Engl J Med 2014;371(16):1507–17.
17. Kochenderfer JN, Dudley ME, Kassim SH, et al. Chemotherapy-refractory diffuse large B-cell lymphoma and indolent B-cell malignancies can be effectively treated with autologous T cells expressing an anti-CD19 chimeric antigen receptor. J Clin Oncol 2015;33(6):540–9.
18. Fry TJ, Shah NN, Orentas RJ, et al. CD22-targeted CAR T cells induce remission in B-ALL that is naive or resistant to CD19-targeted CAR immunotherapy. Nat Med 2018;24(1):20–8.
19. Ali SA, Shi V, Maric I, et al. T cells expressing an anti-B-cell maturation antigen chimeric antigen receptor cause remissions of multiple myeloma. Blood 2016;128(13):1688–700.
20. Lee DW, Kochenderfer JN, Stetler-Stevenson M, et al. T cells expressing CD19 chimeric antigen receptors for acute lymphoblastic leukaemia in children and young adults: a phase 1 dose-escalation trial. Lancet 2015;385(9967):517–28.
21. Gardner RA, Finney O, Annesley C, et al. Intent-to-treat leukemia remission by CD19 CAR T cells of defined formulation and dose in children and young adults. Blood 2017;129(25):3322–31.
22. Sotillo E, Barrett DM, Black KL, et al. Convergence of acquired mutations and alternative splicing of CD19 enables resistance to CART-19 immunotherapy. Cancer Discov 2015;5(12):1282–95.
23. Stroncek DF, Lee DW, Ren J, et al. Elutriated lymphocytes for manufacturing chimeric antigen receptor T cells. J Transl Med 2017;15(1):59.
24. Oberle A, Brandt A, Alawi M, et al. Long-term CD38 saturation by daratumumab interferes with diagnostic myeloma cell detection. Haematologica 2017;102(9):e368–70.
25. Courville EL, Yohe S, Shivers P, et al. VS38 identifies myeloma cells with dim CD38 expression and plasma cells following daratumumab therapy, which interferes with CD38 detection for 4 to 6 months. Am J Clin Pathol 2020;153(2):221–8.
26. Jourdan M, Ferlin M, Legouffe E, et al. The myeloma cell antigen syndecan-1 is lost by apoptotic myeloma cells. Br J Haematol 1998;100(4):637–46.
27. Flores-Montero J, Sanoja-Flores L, Paiva B, et al. Next Generation Flow for highly sensitive and standardized detection of minimal residual disease in multiple myeloma. Leukemia 2017;31(10):2094–103.
28. Mizuta S, Kawata T, Kawabata H, et al. VS38 as a promising CD38 substitute antibody for flow cytometric detection of plasma cells in the daratumumab era. Int J Hematol 2019;110(3):322–30.
29. Broijl A, de Jong ACM, van Duin M, et al. VS38c and CD38-multiepitope antibodies provide highly comparable minimal residual disease data in patients with multiple myeloma. Am J Clin Pathol 2022;157(4):494–7.
30. Muccio VE, Saraci E, Gilestro M, et al. Multiple myeloma: New surface antigens for the characterization of plasma cells in the era of novel agents. Cytometry B Clin Cytom 2016;90(1):81–90.
31. Park JH, Riviere I, Gonen M, et al. Long-term follow-up of CD19 CAR therapy in acute lymphoblastic leukemia. N Engl J Med 2018;378(5):449–59.
32. Cherian S, Miller V, McCullouch V, et al. A novel flow cytometric assay for detection of residual disease in patients with B-lymphoblastic leukemia/lymphoma

post anti-CD19 therapy. Cytometry B Clin Cytom 2018;94(1):112–20.
33. Cherian S, Stetler-Stevenson M. Flow Cytometric monitoring for residual disease in B lymphoblastic leukemia post T cell engaging targeted therapies. Curr Protoc Cytom 2018;86(1):e44.
34. Verbeek MWC, Buracchi C, Laqua A, et al. Flow cytometric minimal residual disease assessment in B-cell precursor acute lymphoblastic leukaemia patients treated with CD19-targeted therapies - a EuroFlow study. Br J Haematol 2022;197(1):76–81.
35. Pan J, Niu Q, Deng B, et al. CD22 CAR T-cell therapy in refractory or relapsed B acute lymphoblastic leukemia. Leukemia 2019;33(12):2854–66.
36. Hrusak O, Porwit-MacDonald A. Antigen expression patterns reflecting genotype of acute leukemias. Leukemia 2002;16(7):1233–58.
37. Fischer J, Paret C, El Malki K, et al. CD19 Isoforms Enabling Resistance to CART-19 Immunotherapy Are Expressed in B-ALL Patients at Initial Diagnosis. J Immunother 2017;40(5):187–95.
38. Braig F, Brandt A, Goebeler M, et al. Resistance to anti-CD19/CD3 BiTE in acute lymphoblastic leukemia may be mediated by disrupted CD19 membrane trafficking. Blood 2017;129(1):100–4.
39. Shah NN, Fry TJ. Mechanisms of resistance to CAR T cell therapy. Nat Rev Clin Oncol 2019;16(6): 372–85.
40. Kurzer J.H. and Weinberg O.K., To B- or not to B-: a review of lineage switched acute leukemia, *Int J Lab Hematol*, 44 Suppl 1, 2022, 64-70.
41. Lamble A., Myers R.M., Taraseviciute A., et al., Pre-infusion factors impacting relapse immunophenotype following CD19 CAR T cells, *Blood Adv*, 7 (4),2022, 575-585.
42. Novakova M, Zaliova M, Fiser K, et al. DUX4r, ZNF384r and PAX5-P80R mutated B-cell precursor acute lymphoblastic leukemia frequently undergo monocytic switch. Haematologica 2021;106(8): 2066–75.
43. Oberley MJ, Gaynon PS, Bhojwani D, et al. Myeloid lineage switch following chimeric antigen receptor T-cell therapy in a patient with TCF3-ZNF384 fusion-positive B-lymphoblastic leukemia. Pediatr Blood Cancer 2018;65(9):e27265.
44. Hirabayashi S, Butler ER, Ohki K, et al. Clinical characteristics and outcomes of B-ALL with ZNF384 rearrangements: a retrospective analysis by the Ponte di Legno Childhood ALL Working Group. Leukemia 2021;35(11):3272–7.
45. Zhou T, Wang HW. Antigen loss after targeted immunotherapy in hematological malignancies. Clin Lab Med 2021;41(3):341–57.
46. Murthy H, Iqbal M, Chavez JC, et al. Cytokine release syndrome: current perspectives. ImmunoTargets Ther 2019;8:43–52.
47. Cohen A, Petsche D, Grunberger T, et al. Interleukin 6 induces myeloid differentiation of a human biphenotypic leukemic cell line. Leuk Res 1992;16(8):751–60.
48. Jiang XY, Luider J, Shameli A. Artifactual kappa light chain restriction of marrow hematogones: a potential diagnostic pitfall in minimal residual disease assessment of plasma cell myeloma patients on daratumumab. Cytometry B Clin Cytom 2020;98(1):68–74.
49. Chen PP, Tormey CA, Eisenbarth SC, et al. False-positive light chain clonal restriction by flow cytometry in patients treated with alemtuzumab: potential pitfalls for the misdiagnosis of B-cell neoplasms. Am J Clin Pathol 2019;151(2):154–63.
50. Cruz NM, Sugita M, Ewing-Crystal N, et al. Selection and characterization of antibody clones are critical for accurate flow cytometry-based monitoring of CD123 in acute myeloid leukemia. Leuk Lymphoma 2018;59(4):978–82.

Diagnostic, Prognostic, and Predictive Role of Next-Generation Sequencing in Mature Lymphoid Neoplasms

Graham W. Slack, MD

KEYWORDS

• B-cell lymphoma • T-cell lymphoma • Next-generation sequencing • Gene mutation • Diagnosis • Prognosis • Therapy

Key points

- The mutational landscape of lymphoma has been revealed through next-generation sequencing (NGS).
- Gene mutations have diagnostic, prognostic, and therapeutic implications in various lymphoma subtypes and serve as useful genetic biomarkers.
- NGS is emerging as an important tool in the clinical laboratory that can be used to identify genetic biomarkers in lymphoma.

ABSTRACT

Lymphoma is a clinically and biologically heterogeneous disease. Next-generation sequencing (NGS) has expanded our understanding of this heterogeneity at the genetic level, refining disease classification, defining new entities, and providing additional information that can be used in diagnosis and management. This review highlights some of the NGS findings in lymphoma and how they can be used as genetic biomarkers to aid diagnosis and prognosis and guide therapy.

OVERVIEW

Lymphomas are a heterogeneous group of malignant neoplasms derived from lymphocytes. The fifth edition of the WHO Classification of Haematolymphoid Tumors recognizes more than 50 B-cell and 30 T-cell and NK-cell neoplasms, each defined by a constellation of clinical, morphologic, immunophenotypic, and genetic features.[1] Since 2006, high-throughput massively parallel sequencing technology, commonly referred to as next-generation sequencing (NGS), has been applied to lymphoid malignancies, expanding our understanding of these diseases at the genetic level, refining disease classification, defining new entities, and providing additional information that can aid in diagnosis, prognosis, and predicting response to different therapies.[2–4] Although this expanded understanding of lymphoid malignancy has come from the research setting, NGS technology is transitioning into the clinical laboratory, providing another tool for clinicians to use in the diagnosis and management of disease. The aim of this review is to describe a selection of lymphoid malignancies with a focus on our current understanding of their genetic alterations identifiable by NGS and how these can be used to aid in diagnosis and prognosis and predict therapy.

B-CELL LYMPHOMAS

A summary of the diagnostic, prognostic, and predictive genetic biomarkers in B-cell lymphomas, detectable by NGS, is presented in Table 1. For a more in-depth review of the genetics of mature

Department of Pathology & Laboratory Medicine, BC Cancer, 600 West 10th Avenue, Vancouver, BC, V5Z 4E6 Canada
E-mail address: gslack@bccancer.bc.ca

Surgical Pathology 16 (2023) 433–442
https://doi.org/10.1016/j.path.2023.01.010

Table 1
Diagnostic, prognostic, and predictive genetic biomarkers in B-cell lymphomas

Disease	Diagnostic	Prognostic	Predictive
LPL	*MYD88*	*MYD88, TP53*	*MYD88, CXCR4, BTK, PLCG2*
MZL	*KLF2, PTPRD*	*BIRC, NOTCH2*	
FL		*ARID1A, CARD11, CREBBP, EP300, EZH2, FOXO1, MEF2B*	*EZH2*
MCL		*TP53, (NOTCH1, NOTCH2, KMT2D)*	*CARD11, TRAF2, BIRC3, CCND1, BTK, PLCG2*
DLBCL-GCB		*FOXO1*	*EZH*
DLBCL-ABC	*MYD88*	*FOXO1*	*MYD88, BTK, CARD11, PLCG2*
BL	*ID3, TCF3*	*TP53*	

Abbreviations: ABC, activated B-cell type; BL, Burkitt lymphoma; DLBCL, diffuse large B-cell lymphoma; FL, follicular lymphoma; GCB, germinal center B-cell type; LPL, lymphoplasmacytic lymphoma; MCL, mantle cell lymphoma; MZL, marginal zone lymphoma.

B-cell lymphomas, the reader is referred elsewhere.[4]

LYMPHOPLASMACYTIC LYMPHOMA

Lymphoplasmacytic lymphoma (LPL) is a low-grade B-cell lymphoma characterized by the plasmacytic differentiation of the malignant lymphocytes. It occurs in older people and affects men with greater frequency. The bone marrow is the most common site of disease but lymph nodes and non-nodal sites such as the spleen, central nervous system, skin, and body cavities can also be involved. It is composed of small mature lymphocytes, plasmacytoid lymphocytes, and mature plasma cells and is most often associated with a serum M-protein: in 95% of cases an IgM M-protein is present, in the remaining 5% of cases an IgG or IgA M-protein is present or the disease may be nonsecretory with no detectable M-protein. Waldenström macroglobulinemia (WM) is defined as LPL associated with an IgM serum M-protein and disease involving the bone marrow.[1]

Next-Generation Sequencing Discoveries in Lymphoplasmacytic Lymphoma

Several NGS studies conducted during the past decade have evaluated LPL and WM. These studies have consistently identified gain-of-function mutations in *MYD88* as a driver mutation in this disease resulting in constitutive activation of the NF-κB pathway.[5] Greater than 90% of LPL/WM cases harbor a *MYD88* mutation, with a hotspot mutation at L265P found in more than 98% of the mutated cases; the remaining cases exhibiting mutations at alternate sites.[5–7] Approximately, 30% to 40% of LPL/WM cases harbor recurrent loss-of-function mutations in *CXCR4*, which are found almost exclusively in *MYD88*-mutated cases, and 17% of cases exhibit recurrent *ARID1A* mutations.[5,8] Non-IgM LPL is more frequently encountered in women and at extramedullary sites without marrow involvement. *MYD88* L265P and *CXCR4* mutations are seen in approximately 44% and 19% of these cases, respectively.[9] Wild-type *MYD88* cases of LPL are associated with lower serum M-protein, higher lymphocytosis, a higher lactate dehydrogenase level, an atypical CD27+ immunophenotype, and increased risk of transformation and death.[10,11] Studies have shown that these tumors exhibit a mutational profile that overlaps with diffuse large B-cell lymphoma, containing mutations that activate the NF-κB pathway downstream of MYD88 and Bruton tyrosine kinase (BTK), impart epigenomic dysregulation, and/or impair DNA damage repair, including *TP53* mutations.[12]

Genetic Biomarkers in Lymphoplasmacytic Lymphoma

Diagnosis

The detection of a *MYD88* L265P mutation is highly sensitive and specific for LPL/WM in the setting of low-grade B-cell lymphomas.[7,10]

Prognosis

MYD88 mutations are prognostic in LPL and WM with mutated cases showing a lower propensity to transform, whereas *TP53* mutations are associated with more aggressive disease.[9,11,13]

Predictive

The presence of a *MYD88* mutation predicts a positive therapeutic response to the BTK inhibitor, ibrutinib, whereas *CXCR4*, *BTK*, and *PLCG2* mutations are associated with a lack of response to ibrutinib, even when a *MYD88* mutation is present.[11,13,14]

Although the detection of a *MYD88* L265P mutation has proven diagnostic, prognostic, and predictive implications in LPL and WM, one study recently showed that a targeted NGS-based panel approach to testing yielded false-negative *MYD88* L265P results in approximately 30% of cases.[15] This highlights the need to standardize *MYD88* L265P mutation testing and emphasizes the importance of comprehensive validation when deploying NGS-based assays in the clinical laboratory.

FOLLICULAR LYMPHOMA

Follicular lymphoma (FL) is a B-cell lymphoma of germinal center type B cells. It is the most common indolent B-cell lymphoma in the Western world and typically affects older adults and men slightly more than women. Lymph nodes are usually involved with extranodal sites of disease frequently present, including bone marrow, spleen, gastrointestinal tract, soft tissue, ocular adnexa, and rarely testes. It is characterized by the proliferation of centrocytes and centroblasts in varying proportions with at least a partial follicular growth pattern in most instances. The genetic hallmark of FL, found in 80% to 95% of cases with classic features, is the t(14;18) (q32;q21)/ *IGH::BCL2*, which results in constitutive overexpression of the anti-apoptosis protein BCL2. Deletions of 1p36 (*TNFAIP3*) are frequent while translocations involving *BCL6* are present in 15% to 35% of cases and may be seen with or without concurrent *BCL2* translocations.[1]

Next-Generation Sequencing Discoveries in Follicular Lymphoma

Several studies have described the mutational landscape of FL. A central hallmark of the genetic landscape seen in FL is epigenetic dysregulation. Frequently reported recurrent mutations involve the epigenetic regulators *KMT2D*, *CREBBP*, *EZH2*, *EP300*, and *MEF2B*. Alterations are also seen in genes involved in other cellular processes including *ARID1A*, *BCL2*, *CARD11*, *CDKN2A*, *FOXO1*, *MYC*, *RRAGC*, *STAT6*, *TNFRSF14*, and *TP53*.[16-21]

Genetic Biomarkers in Follicular Lymphoma

Diagnosis

There are no gene mutations that are specific for FL; accurate pathologic diagnosis relies on careful evaluation and interpretation of morphologic, immunophenotypic, and cytogenetic features. The WHO classification does not recommend NGS in the routine workup of FL.[1]

Prognosis

The m7-FLIPI is a recently proposed prospective clinicogenetic risk model that incorporates the mutation status of 7 genes (*EZH2*, *ARID1A*, *MEF2B*, *EP300*, *FOXO1*, *CREBBP*, and *CARD11*) from diagnostic pretreatment biopsies, the follicular lymphoma International Prognostic Index score, and Eastern Cooperative Oncology group performance status.[22] This model dichotomizes patients into groups at low-risk and high risk for failing first-line immunochemotherapy and death. This model still requires evaluation and validation in prospective clinical trials.[23]

Predictive

Detection of *EZH2* mutation serves as a predictive biomarker in FL. *EZH2* encodes a histone methyltransferase, EZH2, that trimethylates Lys27 of histone H3 (H3k27). In 10% to 30% of FL, this gene exhibits recurrent gain-of-function mutations in its SET domain, which results in constitutive EZH2 activation. Tazemetostat is a first-in-class targeted inhibitor of EZH2 that has recently received U.S. Food and Drug Administration-approval for use in patients with relapsed or refractory FL with *EZH2* mutations.[24,25]

MANTLE CELL LYMPHOMA

Mantle cell lymphoma (MCL) is a B-cell lymphoma of CD5+ B cells derived from pregerminal center mantle zone B cells. It is a disease of older people and affects men more than women. Most patients present with disease involving lymph nodes and splenomegaly is common. Extranodal sites of involvement include bone marrow, gastrointestinal tract, and liver. Rarely, patients may present with leukemic non-nodal disease, which is associated with a favorable clinical course. MCL is characterized by a proliferation of small to medium-sized atypical lymphocytes in a mantle zone, nodal, or diffuse pattern. Aggressive variants can exhibit blastoid or pleomorphic cytology. The genetic hallmark of MCL, present in more than 95% of cases, is the t(11;14) (q13;q32)/*CCND1::IGH*, which results in constitutive overexpression of the cell cycle protein, cyclin D1. The rare cases lacking a *CCND1* rearrangement usually harbor rearrangements involving other cyclin genes, including *CCND2*, *CCND3*, and *CCNE*.[1]

Next-Generation Sequencing Discoveries in Mantle Lymphoma

Several NGS studies have evaluated the genetic landscape of MCL. The most commonly identified recurrently mutated genes are the DNA damage response genes, *ATM* and *TP53*, identified in upward of 60% and 30% of cases, respectively. Other recurrently mutated genes identified by NGS in MCL include *BIRC3*, *CARD11*, *CCND1*, *KMT2D*, *HNRNPH1*, *MEF2B*, *NOTCH1*, *NOTCH2*, *SMARCA4*, *TLR2*, *TRAF2*, *UBR5*, and *WHSC1*. Deletions of *CKDN2A* and *TP53* are also encountered in 10% to 40% of cases.[4,26–32]

Genetic Biomarkers in Mantle Cell Lymphoma

Diagnosis

There are no gene mutations that are specific for MCL; accurate pathologic diagnosis relies on careful evaluation and interpretation of morphologic, immunophenotypic, and cytogenetic features.[1]

Prognosis

Several studies have evaluated the prognostic significance of the known recurrent mutations in MCL. The most consistent predictor of a poor prognosis seems to be the presence of a mutation in *TP53*.[33] Mutations involving *NOTCH1*, *NOTCH2*, and *KMT2D* have also been reported to portend a worse prognosis but have not been upheld in some multivariate analyses and their significance remains uncertain.[27,32,34] Studies have also shown that patients harboring deletions of *TP53* have an unfavorable prognosis.[35]

Predictive

TRAF2, *BIRC3*, and *CCND1* mutations in MCL have been shown to confer resistance to ibrutinib therapy while *CARD11* mutations have been shown to confer resistance to ibrutinib and lenalidomide in vitro.[36–38] *BTK* and *PLCG2* mutations have also been linked to resistance to ibrutinib therapy.[14]

DIFFUSE LARGE B-CELL LYMPHOMA, NOT OTHERWISE SPECIFIED

Diffuse large B-cell lymphoma, not otherwise specified (DLBCL, NOS) is a clinically, morphologically, immunophenotypically, and genetically heterogeneous group of nodal and extranodal mature B-cell lymphomas that do not meet the diagnostic criteria for other defined B-cell neoplasms.[1] They are characterized by a proliferation of medium to large-sized lymphocytes with a diffuse growth pattern.

Gene expression profiling studies have shown that DLBCL can be divided into 2 groups of diseases based on their "cell of origin" and the differential expression of genes that recapitulate the expression of genes seen in normal germinal center B cells (DLBCL-GCB) and postgerminal center activated B cells (DLBCL-ABC). These 2 groups of DLBCL are prognostically significant, with DLBCL-GCB exhibiting a better response to front-line immunochemotherapy than DLBCL-ABC, and the current WHO classification states that it is desirable to assign a cell-of-origin when diagnosing DLBCL, which is usually performed with the assistance of immunohistochemical algorithms that act as surrogates for gene expression profiling in the clinical laboratory.[1,39,40]

Next-Generation Sequencing Discoveries in Diffuse Large B-cell Lymphoma

DLBCL is the most extensively studied lymphoid neoplasm using NGS. Several studies have revealed the mutational landscape of this heterogeneous disease and identified recurrently mutated genes that are enriched in either DLBCL-GCB or DLBCL-ABC or encountered in both entities. DLBCL-GCB is enriched with mutations in *EZH2*, *GNA13*, *SGK1*, *TET1*, *BCL2*, *BCL6*, and *MYC*, whereas DLBCL-ABC is enriched with mutations in *MYD88*, *CD79A*, *CD79B*, *CARD11*, *TNFAIP3*, and *PRDM1*. Both tumor types harbor mutations in *KMT2D*, *CREBBP*, *EP300*, *TP53*, *MEF2B, B2M*, *NOTCH2*, and *FOXO1*.[41–44]

Three independent studies have examined the genomics of DLBCL using a multiplatform approach, including NGS, leading to a refinement in our understanding of DLBCL beyond the cell-of-origin dichotomy, defining new molecular subtypes of DLBCL with distinct clinical and genotypic characteristics. These discoveries have the potential to open the door to the development of precision medicine approaches in this disease.[45–47] A probabilistic classification algorithm, LymphGen, has been developed that allows for the classification of DLBCL biopsies into 7 molecular subtypes in the clinical setting: MCD, characterized by *MYD88* and *CD79B* mutations; BN2, characterized by *NOTCH2* mutations and *BCL6* translocations; N1, characterized by *NOTCH1* mutations; EZB, characterized by *EZH2* mutations and *BCL2* translocations; ST2, characterized by *SGK1* and *TET2* mutations; A53, characterized by aneuploidy and *TP53* inactivation; "genetically composite," characterized by genetic alterations belonging to more than one molecular subtype; and "unclassifiable" tumors that could not be assigned to any of the defined molecular subtypes.[48,49]

Genetic Biomarkers in Diffuse Large B-cell Lymphoma

Diagnosis

Studies have consistently shown that *MYD88* mutations are exclusively seen in DLBCL-ABC, present in approximately 30% of cases, making it a genetic biomarker for the diagnosis of DLBCL-ABC when present in large B-cell neoplasms.[43,44,50,51] In addition, *MYD88* mutations are the hallmark genetic feature of the newly defined molecular subtypes of DLBLC (MCD).[46,48]

Prognosis

The presence of *FOXO1* mutations in DLBCL has been shown to be associated with decreased overall survival in patients treated with front-line immunochemotherapy, independent of cell-of-origin.[52]

The MCD and N1 molecular subtypes, characterized by *MYD88/CD79B* and *NOTCH1* mutations, respectively, exhibit inferior outcomes compared with the BN2 and EZB molecular subtypes, which are characterized by *NOTCH2* and *EZH2* mutations, respectively.[46]

Predictive

Studies have shown that DLBCL-GCB harbors recurrent mutations of the epigenetic regulatory gene, *EZH2*, the protein product of which can be targeted by drugs such as tazemetostat, and the use of which is currently being studied in clinical trials.[25,51]

DLBCL-ABC often exhibits chronic activation of the B-cell receptor/NF-κB signaling pathways, which includes a cascade of several proteins including CD79A, CD79B, MYD88, BTK, and CARD11. Ibrutinib targets BTK and may be useful in DLBCL-ABC that harbors activating mutations in genes upstream of *BTK*, including *MYD88* and *CD79B*; however, cases that harbor mutations in genes that encode proteins from BTK downward, including *BTK*, *CARD11*, and *PLCG2* are likely to exhibit resistance to ibrutinib therapy.[14,51,53]

Finally, the MCD and BN2 molecular subtypes of DLBCL are characterized by chronic active B-cell receptor signaling and may be amenable to therapy with agents that inhibit this pathway, including ibrutinib.[46]

T-CELL LYMPHOMAS

A summary of the diagnostic, prognostic, and predictive genetic biomarkers in peripheral T-cell lymphomas, detectable by NGS, is presented in Table 2. For a more in-depth review of the genetics of peripheral T-cell lymphomas, the reader is referred elsewhere.[3]

ANAPLASTIC LARGE CELL LYMPHOMA

Three types of anaplastic large cell lymphoma (ALCL) are recognized by the current WHO classification: ALK-positive ALCL, ALK-negative ALK, and breast implant-associated ALCL. These tumors share similar morphologic and immunophenotypic characteristics but are distinguished by their different clinical and genetic features.[1] Common to all of these tumors is the malignant hallmark cell, a large pleomorphic cell with lobulated or horseshoe-shaped nuclei, vesicular chromatin, and prominent nucleoli. Hallmark cells uniformly express CD30 by immunohistochemistry and are usually CD4+ cells that often express cytotoxic markers such as TIA-1, granzyme B, or perforin. Loss of other T-cell antigens is common.

ALK-positive ALCL is more common in children and young adults and characteristically harbors a gene rearrangement involving *ALK*, which can be detected by immunohistochemical staining for ALK, and shows superior response to therapy

Table 2
Diagnostic, prognostic, and predictive genetic biomarkers in T-cell lymphomas

Disease	Diagnostic	Prognostic	Predictive
EATL	*SETD2*		*JAK1*
MEITL	*SETD2, STAT5B*		
HSTCL	*SETD2, STAT3, STAT5B*		*STAT3, STAT5B*
ALCL, ALK+		*TP53*	*ALK, NOTCH1*
ALCL, ALK−	*MSC*	*JAK1, STAT3, TP53*	*JAK1, STAT3*
AITL	*TET2, DNMT3A, RHOA, IDH2, CD28*		*TET2, DNMT3A, RHOA, IDH2*
PTCL, TFH	*TET2, DNMT3A, RHOA*		*TET2, DNMT3A, RHOA*
PTCL, NOS		*TP53, FAT1*	
ENKTCL		*DDX3X, TP53*	*JAK3, STAT3, BCOR*

Abbreviations: AITL, angioimmunoblastic T-cell lymphoma; ALCL, ALK−, ALK-negative anaplastic large cell lymphoma, ALCL, ALK+, ALK-positive anaplastic large cell lymphoma; EATL, enteropathy-associated T-cell lymphoma; ENKTCL, extranodal NK/T-cell lymphoma; HSTCL, hepatosplenic T-cell lymphoma; MEITL, monomorphic epitheliotropic T-cell lymphoma; PTCL, NOS peripheral T-cell lymphoma, not otherwise specified; PTCL, TFH, nodal T-follicular helper cell lymphoma (not AITL).

than ALK-negative ALCL. ALK-negative ALCL is a disease of adults that lacks *ALK* rearrangements and has a worse prognosis than ALK-positive ALCL but better than peripheral T-cell lymphoma, NOS. *DUSP22* and *TP63* rearrangements are detected in 30% and 5% of ALK-negative ALCL cases, respectively. Breast implant-associated ALCL arises in the peri-implant capsule or serous cavity in association with a macrotextured breast implant. It does not exhibit rearrangements of *ALK*, *DUSP22*, or *TP63* and has a favorable prognosis if detected at an early stage when cells are confined to the capsule or serous fluid.[1]

Next-Generation Sequencing Discoveries in Anaplastic Large Cell Lymphoma

NGS studies examining the mutational landscape of ALCL are limited but have identified recurrent gene mutations in ALCL. Found in both ALK-positive and ALK-negative ALCL are mutations involving *TP53*, *LRP1B*, *KMT2D*, *EPHA5*, *TET2*, *PRDM1*, *ATR*, *NOTCH1*, *NOTCH2*, *EPHA3*, *KDR*, *SOCS1*, *ARID1A*, and *MSH6*. *KMT2C* and *EP300* mutations seem restricted to ALK-positive ALCL, whereas recurrent mutations of *MSC*, *JAK1*, and *STAT3* seem restricted to ALK-negative ALCL.[54,55]

Genetic Biomarkers in Anaplastic Large Cell Lymphoma

Diagnosis

MSC mutation has been reported in ~15% of ALK-negative ALCL but has not been identified in ALK-positive ALCL or other T-cell lymphoma types making *MSC* a specific genetic biomarker for the diagnosis of ALK-negative ALCL.[56]

Prognosis

STAT3 mutation in ALK-negative ALCL has been shown to predict a worse overall survival in response to therapy while *TP53* mutation in either ALK-positive or ALK-negative ALCL predicts a worse progression-free survival.[55]

Predictive

ALK kinase domain mutations may be present at diagnosis or emerge in response to therapy in patients with ALK-positive ALCL, which can lead to resistance to the ALK inhibitor crizotinib.[57] Conversely, in ALK-positive ALCL, recurrent *NOTCH1* mutations, T349P and T331P, may confer sensitivity to targeted therapy with gamma-secretase inhibitors, which may work with additive/synergistic effect with crizotinib.[58] *JAK1* and *STAT3* mutations are recurrent in ALK-negative ALCL and have been shown to be suitable targets to inhibition in both in vitro and in vivo studies making them a potential predictive genetic biomarker for this disease.[54]

NODAL T-FOLLICULAR HELPER CELL LYMPHOMA

The current WHO classification recognizes 3 types of nodal T-follicular helper (TFH) cell lymphoma: angioimmunoblastic-type, follicular-type, and NOS.[1] These tumors are grouped together because they share phenotypic and genetic features with effector TFH cells that are located in germinal centers. The malignant T-cells in these lymphomas usually express 2 or more TFH cell-associated proteins including PD1, ICOS, CXCL13, BCL6, and CD10.

Angioimmunoblastic-type is the most common and extensively studied of the 3 with well-defined clinical and pathologic features. It typically presents in middle-aged to older adults with systemic disease and diffuse lymphadenopathy. Involved lymph nodes contain a polymorphous lymphoid infiltrate in a vaguely nodular to diffuse pattern within a background of high endothelial venules surrounded by networks of follicular dendritic cells. Follicular-type also presents in older adults with advanced stage disease. Involved lymph nodes show partial or complete effacement of architecture by a lymphoid infiltrate in a follicular pattern; high endothelial venules and extrafollicular follicular dendritic cells typical of the angioimmunoblastic-type are not present. Nodal T-follicular cell lymphoma, NOS, is a diagnosis of exclusion. It is a nodal T-cell neoplasm that expresses CD4 and at least 2 TFH cell-associated proteins but does not exhibit the pathologic features of either the angioimmunoblastic or follicular-types.[1]

Next-Generation Sequencing Discoveries in Nodal T-Follicular Helper-Cell Lymphoma

NGS studies have examined the mutational landscape of nodular TFH cell lymphomas and have consistently shown these tumors exhibit recurrent mutations in a few genes with high frequency, including *TET2* (48%–75%), *DNMT3A* (10%–30%), *RHOA* G17V (60%), *PLCG1* (14%), *FYN*, and *VAV1*.[59,60] Recurrent mutations of *IHD2* R172 (33%–40%) and *CD28* have also been identified and seem to be restricted to the angioimmunoblastic-type.[60,61]

Genetic Biomarkers in Nodal T-Follicular Helper Cell Lymphoma

Diagnosis

NGS studies have shown that *TET2* mutations are enriched in nodal TFH cell lymphoma compared with peripheral T-cell lymphoma, NOS while *DNMT3A* and *RHOA* mutations are highly specific for these diseases.[60,62] Detection of these mutations may aid in the diagnosis of these tumors. In addition, within this group of tumors, *IDH2* and *CD28* mutations are restricted mostly to angioimmunoblastic-type disease, which can assist in making a definitive diagnosis in equivocal cases.[59,60]

Prognosis

There are no NGS studies that have identified genetic biomarkers that predict prognosis in nodal TFH cell lymphomas.

Predictive

Recent studies have shown that nodal TFH cell lymphomas, which contain recurrent mutations of the genes *TET2*, *DNMT3A*, *RHOA*, and *IDH2*, exhibit epigenomic dysregulation and a better response to histone deacetylase inhibitors (HDACi) compared with peripheral T-cell lymphoma, NOS, suggesting the detection of these mutations in T-cell lymphomas may predict the response to HDACi therapy.[63,64]

PERIPHERAL T-CELL LYMPHOMA, NOT OTHERWISE SPECIFIED

Peripheral T-cell lymphoma, not otherwise specified (PTCL, NOS) is a clinically, morphologically, immunophenotypically, and genetically heterogeneous group of nodal and extranodal mature T-cell lymphomas that do not meet the diagnostic criteria for other defined T-cell neoplasms.[1] PTCL, NOS occurs most frequently in adults, affecting men more than women. Many patients present with advanced stage and aggressive disease that responds poorly to current therapeutic regimens.

Gene expression profiling studies have identified 2 molecular subtypes of PTCL, NOS: tumors that show high expression of GATA3 and its target genes, and tumors that show high expression of TBX21 and its target genes.[65] GATA3-PTCL, NOS exhibits higher genomic complexity, is associated high *MYC* expression, a high proliferation signature, and inferior outcomes compared with TBX21-PTCL, NOS, which shows lower genomic complexity, NF-κB pathway enrichment, epigenetic dysregulation, and superior outcomes. These molecular subtypes can be predicted by a recently developed immunohistochemical algorithm.[66]

Next-Generation Sequencing Discoveries in Peripheral T-cell Lymphoma, Not Otherwise Specified

The mutational landscape of PTCL, NOS remains largely understudied because NGS studies are limited. Recurrently mutated genes that have been identified and variably reported include *TP53*, *TET2*, *CDKN2A*, *ATM*, *CD28*, HLA-B, *IKZF2*, *TRRAP*, *PRDM1*, *SOCS1*, *JAK3*, *ITPR3*, *ITPKB*, *PLCG1*, *PTPRC*, *FYN*, *VAV1*, *TET1*, *TET2*, *TET3*, *DNMT3A*, and *FAT1*. *TP53* mutations are enriched in GATA3-PTCL, NOS while *DNMT3A* mutations, although rare, are found in TBX21-PTCL, NOS.[62,67,68]

Genetic Biomarkers in Peripheral T-cell Lymphoma, Not Otherwise Specified

Diagnosis

There are no NGS studies that have identified genetic biomarkers that are sensitive and specific for the diagnosis of PTCL, NOS.

Prognosis

Two recent studies have identified genetic biomarkers of prognosis in PTCL, NOS: *TP53* mutations and *FAT1* mutations are both associated with an inferior prognosis compared with cases with wild-type genes.[67,68]

Predictive

There are no NGS studies that have identified genetic biomarkers that predict responses to alternative therapies in PTCL, NOS.

SUMMARY

NGS has advanced our knowledge of the mutational landscape in lymphoma and improved our understanding of the molecular pathways that lead to lymphomagenesis. NGS has also revealed genetic biomarkers that can aid in diagnosis and prognosis and assist in disease treatment. Because NGS technologies continue to make their way into the clinical laboratory we should expect that our understanding of the genetic changes that make up the different lymphoma types will evolve and more biomarkers will be discovered that can aid in the discovery and implementation of novel targeted therapies, moving us toward more precise medicine reducing morbidity and mortality in lymphoma.

DECLARATION OF INTERESTS

Dr G.W. Slack has received honoraria for participation in advisory boards sponsored by Seagen.

REFERENCES

1. Alaggio R, Amador C, Anagnostopoulos I, et al. The 5th edition of the World Health Organization

Classification of Haematolymphoid Tumours: Lymphoid Neoplasms. Leukemia 2022;36(7): 1720–48.
2. Slack GW, Gascoyne RD. Next-generation sequencing discoveries in lymphoma. Adv Anat Pathol 2013;20(2):110–6.
3. Vega F, Amador C, Chadburn A, et al. Genetic profiling and biomarkers in peripheral T-cell lymphomas: current role in the diagnostic work-up. Mod Pathol 2022;35(3):306–18.
4. Rosenquist R, Beà S, Du MQ, et al. Genetic landscape and deregulated pathways in B-cell lymphoid malignancies. J Intern Med 2017;282(5):371–94.
5. Treon SP, Xu L, Yang G, et al. MYD88 L265P somatic mutation in Waldenström's macroglobulinemia. N Engl J Med 2012;367(9):826–33.
6. Poulain S, Roumier C, Decambron A, et al. MYD88 L265P mutation in Waldenstrom macroglobulinemia. Blood 2013;121(22):4504–11.
7. Hamadeh F, MacNamara SP, Aguilera NS, et al. MYD88 L265P mutation analysis helps define nodal lymphoplasmacytic lymphoma. Mod Pathol 2015; 28(4):564–74.
8. Hunter ZR, Xu L, Yang G, et al. The genomic landscape of Waldenstrom macroglobulinemia is characterized by highly recurring MYD88 and WHIM-like CXCR4 mutations, and small somatic deletions associated with B-cell lymphomagenesis. Blood 2014;123(11):1637–46.
9. Varettoni M, Boveri E, Zibellini S, et al. Clinical and molecular characteristics of lymphoplasmacytic lymphoma not associated with an IgM monoclonal protein: A multicentric study of the Rete Ematologica Lombarda (REL) network. Am J Hematol 2019; 94(11):1193–9.
10. Jiménez C, Sebastián E, Chillón MC, et al. MYD88 L265P is a marker highly characteristic of, but not restricted to, Waldenström's macroglobulinemia. Leukemia 2013;27(8):1722–8.
11. Treon SP, Xu L, Guerrera ML, et al. Genomic Landscape of Waldenström Macroglobulinemia and Its Impact on Treatment Strategies. J Clin Oncol 2020; 38(11):1198–208.
12. Hunter ZR, Xu L, Tsakmaklis N, et al. Insights into the genomic landscape of MYD88 wild-type Waldenström macroglobulinemia. Blood Adv 2018;2(21): 2937–46.
13. Wang Y, Gali VL, Xu-Monette ZY, et al. Molecular and genetic biomarkers implemented from next-generation sequencing provide treatment insights in clinical practice for Waldenström macroglobulinemia. Neoplasia 2021;23(4):361–74.
14. Woyach JA, Furman RR, Liu TM, et al. Resistance mechanisms for the Bruton's tyrosine kinase inhibitor ibrutinib. N Engl J Med 2014;370(24):2286–94.
15. Kofides A, Hunter ZR, Xu L, et al. Diagnostic Next-generation Sequencing Frequently Fails to Detect MYD88(L265P) in Waldenström Macroglobulinemia. Hemasphere 2021;5(8):e624.
16. Okosun J, Bödör C, Wang J, et al. Integrated genomic analysis identifies recurrent mutations and evolution patterns driving the initiation and progression of follicular lymphoma. Nat Genet 2014; 46(2):176–81.
17. Morin RD, Johnson NA, Severson TM, et al. Somatic mutations altering EZH2 (Tyr641) in follicular and diffuse large B-cell lymphomas of germinal-center origin. Nat Genet 2010;42(2):181–5.
18. Pasqualucci L, Dominguez-Sola D, Chiarenza A, et al. Inactivating mutations of acetyltransferase genes in B-cell lymphoma. Nature 2011;471(7337): 189–95.
19. Bödör C, Grossmann V, Popov N, et al. EZH2 mutations are frequent and represent an early event in follicular lymphoma. Blood 2013;122(18):3165–8.
20. Li H, Kaminski MS, Li Y, et al. Mutations in linker histone genes HIST1H1 B, C, D, and E; OCT2 (POU2F2); IRF8; and ARID1A underlying the pathogenesis of follicular lymphoma. Blood 2014;123(10): 1487–98.
21. Huet S, Sujobert P, Salles G. From genetics to the clinic: a translational perspective on follicular lymphoma. Nat Rev Cancer 2018;18(4):224–39.
22. Pastore A, Jurinovic V, Kridel R, et al. Integration of gene mutations in risk prognostication for patients receiving first-line immunochemotherapy for follicular lymphoma: a retrospective analysis of a prospective clinical trial and validation in a population-based registry. Lancet Oncol 2015;16(9):1111–22.
23. Jurinovic V, Kridel R, Staiger AM, et al. Clinicogenetic risk models predict early progression of follicular lymphoma after first-line immunochemotherapy. Blood 2016;128(8):1112–20.
24. Morschhauser F, Tilly H, Chaidos A, et al. Tazemetostat for patients with relapsed or refractory follicular lymphoma: an open-label, single-arm, multicentre, phase 2 trial. Lancet Oncol 2020;21(11):1433–42.
25. Straining R, Eighmy W. Tazemetostat: EZH2 Inhibitor. J Adv Pract Oncol 2022;13(2):158–63.
26. Kridel R, Meissner B, Rogic S, et al. Whole transcriptome sequencing reveals recurrent NOTCH1 mutations in mantle cell lymphoma. Blood 2012;119(9): 1963–71.
27. Beà S, Valdés-Mas R, Navarro A, et al. Landscape of somatic mutations and clonal evolution in mantle cell lymphoma. Proc Natl Acad Sci U S A 2013;110(45): 18250–5.
28. Meissner B, Kridel R, Lim RS, et al. The E3 ubiquitin ligase UBR5 is recurrently mutated in mantle cell lymphoma. Blood 2013;121(16):3161–4.
29. Zhang J, Jima D, Moffitt AB, et al. The genomic landscape of mantle cell lymphoma is related to the epigenetically determined chromatin state of normal B cells. Blood May 8 2014;123(19):2988–96.

30. Sakhdari A, Ok CY, Patel KP, et al. TP53 mutations are common in mantle cell lymphoma, including the indolent leukemic non-nodal variant. Ann Diagn Pathol 2019;41:38–42.
31. Hill HA, Qi X, Jain P, et al. Genetic mutations and features of mantle cell lymphoma: a systematic review and meta-analysis. Blood Adv 2020;4(13): 2927–38.
32. Pararajalingam P, Coyle KM, Arthur SE, et al. Coding and noncoding drivers of mantle cell lymphoma identified through exome and genome sequencing. Blood 2020;136(5):572–84.
33. Eskelund CW, Dahl C, Hansen JW, et al. TP53 mutations identify younger mantle cell lymphoma patients who do not benefit from intensive chemoimmunotherapy. Blood 2017;130(17):1903–10.
34. Silkenstedt E, Linton K, Dreyling M. Mantle cell lymphoma - advances in molecular biology, prognostication and treatment approaches. Br J Haematol Oct 2021;195(2):162–73.
35. Delfau-Larue MH, Klapper W, Berger F, et al. High-dose cytarabine does not overcome the adverse prognostic value of CDKN2A and TP53 deletions in mantle cell lymphoma. Blood 2015;126(5):604–11.
36. Rahal R, Frick M, Romero R, et al. Pharmacological and genomic profiling identifies NF-κB-targeted treatment strategies for mantle cell lymphoma. Nat Med 2014;20(1):87–92.
37. Wu C, de Miranda NF, Chen L, et al. Genetic heterogeneity in primary and relapsed mantle cell lymphomas: Impact of recurrent CARD11 mutations. Oncotarget Jun 21 2016;7(25):38180–90.
38. Mohanty A, Sandoval N, Das M, et al. CCND1 mutations increase protein stability and promote ibrutinib resistance in mantle cell lymphoma. Oncotarget 2016;7(45):73558–72.
39. Rosenwald A, Wright G, Chan WC, et al. The use of molecular profiling to predict survival after chemotherapy for diffuse large-B-cell lymphoma. N Engl J Med 2002;346(25):1937–47
40. Hans CP, Weisenburger DD, Greiner TC, et al. Confirmation of the molecular classification of diffuse large B-cell lymphoma by immunohistochemistry using a tissue microarray. Blood 2004; 103(1):275–82.
41. Compagno M, Lim WK, Grunn A, et al. Mutations of multiple genes cause deregulation of NF-kappaB in diffuse large B-cell lymphoma. Nature Jun 4 2009; 459(7247):717–21.
42. Morin RD, Mendez-Lago M, Mungall AJ, et al. Frequent mutation of histone-modifying genes in non-Hodgkin lymphoma. Nature Jul 27 2011; 476(7360):298–303.
43. Pasqualucci L, Trifonov V, Fabbri G, et al. Analysis of the coding genome of diffuse large B-cell lymphoma. Nat Genet 2011;43(9):830–7.
44. Pasqualucci L, Dalla-Favera R. The genetic landscape of diffuse large B-cell lymphoma. Semin Hematol 2015;52(2):67–76.
45. Schmitz R, Wright GW, Huang DW, et al. Genetics and Pathogenesis of Diffuse Large B-Cell Lymphoma. N Engl J Med 2018;378(15):1396–407.
46. Chapuy B, Stewart C, Dunford AJ, et al. Molecular subtypes of diffuse large B cell lymphoma are associated with distinct pathogenic mechanisms and outcomes. Nat Med 2018;24(5):679–90.
47. Lacy SE, Barrans SL, Beer PA, et al. Targeted sequencing in DLBCL, molecular subtypes, and outcomes: a Haematological Malignancy Research Network report. Blood 2020;135(20):1759–71.
48. Wright GW, Huang DW, Phelan JD, et al. A Probabilistic Classification Tool for Genetic Subtypes of Diffuse Large B Cell Lymphoma with Therapeutic Implications. Cancer Cell 2020;37(4): 551–68.e14.
49. Morin RD, Arthur SE, Hodson DJ. Molecular profiling in diffuse large B-cell lymphoma: why so many types of subtypes? Br J Haematol 2022;196(4):814–29.
50. Ngo VN, Young RM, Schmitz R, et al. Oncogenically active MYD88 mutations in human lymphoma. Nature 2011;470(7332):115–9.
51. Bohers E, Mareschal S, Bouzelfen A, et al. Targetable activating mutations are very frequent in GCB and ABC diffuse large B-cell lymphoma. Genes Chromosomes Cancer 2014;53(2):144–53.
52. Trinh DL, Scott DW, Morin RD, et al. Analysis of FOXO1 mutations in diffuse large B-cell lymphoma. Blood 2013;121(18):3666–74.
53. Young RM, Staudt LM. Targeting pathological B cell receptor signalling in lymphoid malignancies. Nat Rev Drug Discov 2013;12(3):229–43.
54. Crescenzo R, Abate F, Lasorsa E, et al. Convergent mutations and kinase fusions lead to oncogenic STAT3 activation in anaplastic large cell lymphoma. Cancer Cell Apr 13 2015;27(4):516–32.
55. Lobello C, Tichy B, Bystry V, et al. STAT3 and TP53 mutations associate with poor prognosis in anaplastic large cell lymphoma. Leukemia 2021; 35(5):1500–5.
56. Luchtel RA, Zimmermann MT, Hu G, et al. Recurrent MSC (E116K) mutations in ALK-negative anaplastic large cell lymphoma. Blood 2019;133(26):2776–89.
57. Lovisa F, Cozza G, Cristiani A, et al. ALK kinase domain mutations in primary anaplastic large cell lymphoma: consequences on NPM-ALK activity and sensitivity to tyrosine kinase inhibitors. PLoS One 2015;10(4):e0121378.
58. Larose H, Prokoph N, Matthews JD, et al. Whole Exome Sequencing reveals NOTCH1 mutations in anaplastic large cell lymphoma and points to Notch both as a key pathway and a potential therapeutic target. Haematologica Jun 1 2021;106(6):1693–704.

59. Vallois D, Dobay MP, Morin RD, et al. Activating mutations in genes related to TCR signaling in angioimmunoblastic and other follicular helper T-cell-derived lymphomas. Blood 2016;128(11):1490–502.
60. Dobay MP, Lemonnier F, Missiaglia E, et al. Integrative clinicopathological and molecular analyses of angioimmunoblastic T-cell lymphoma and other nodal lymphomas of follicular helper T-cell origin. Haematologica 2017;102(4):e148–51.
61. Steinhilber J, Mederake M, Bonzheim I, et al. The pathological features of angioimmunoblastic T-cell lymphomas with IDH2(R172) mutations. Mod Pathol 2019;32(8):1123–34.
62. Heavican TB, Bouska A, Yu J, et al. Genetic drivers of oncogenic pathways in molecular subgroups of peripheral T-cell lymphoma. Blood 2019;133(15):1664–76.
63. Ma H, Davarifar A, Amengual JE. The Future of Combination Therapies for Peripheral T Cell Lymphoma (PTCL). Curr Hematol Malig Rep 2018;13(1):13–24.
64. Ghione P, Faruque P, Mehta-Shah N, et al. T follicular helper phenotype predicts response to histone deacetylase inhibitors in relapsed/refractory peripheral T-cell lymphoma. Blood Adv 2020;4(19):4640–7.
65. Iqbal J, Wright G, Wang C, et al. Gene expression signatures delineate biological and prognostic subgroups in peripheral T-cell lymphoma. Blood 2014;123(19):2915–23.
66. Amador C, Greiner TC, Heavican TB, et al. Reproducing the molecular subclassification of peripheral T-cell lymphoma-NOS by immunohistochemistry. Blood 2019;134(24):2159–70.
67. Watatani Y, Sato Y, Miyoshi H, et al. Molecular heterogeneity in peripheral T-cell lymphoma, not otherwise specified revealed by comprehensive genetic profiling. Leukemia 2019;33(12):2867–83.
68. Laginestra MA, Cascione L, Motta G, et al. Whole exome sequencing reveals mutations in FAT1 tumor suppressor gene clinically impacting on peripheral T-cell lymphoma not otherwise specified. Mod Pathol 2020;33(2):179–87.

Printed and bound by CPI Group (UK) Ltd, Croydon, CR0 4YY
03/10/2024
01040367-0002